Auditory Disorders in School Children

Fourth Edition

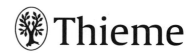

Auditory Disorders in School Children
The Law, Identification, Remediation

Fourth Edition

Ross J. Roeser, Ph.D.

Professor and Executive Director
UTD/Callier Center for Communication Disorders
School of Behavioral and Brain Sciences
University of Texas at Dallas
Dallas, Texas

Marion P. Downs, M.A., D.H.S.

Professor Emeritus
Department of Otolaryngology
Division of Audiology
Health Sciences Center
University of Colorado
Denver, Colorado

Thieme
New York · Stuttgart

Thieme New York
333 Seventh Avenue
New York, NY 10001

Editor: Melissa Von Rohr
Assistant Editor: Jennifer Berger
Director, Production and Manufacturing: Anne Vinnicombe
Production Editor: David R. Stewart
Marketing Director: Phyllis Gold
Director of Sales: Ross Lumpkin
Chief Financial Officer: Peter van Woerden
President: Brian D. Scanlan
Compositor: Compset, Inc.
Printer: Sheridan Books, Inc.

Library of Congress Cataloging in Publication Data is available from the publisher

Important note: Medical knowledge is ever-changing. As new research and clinical experience broaden our knowledge, changes in treatment and drug therapy may be required. The authors and editors of the material herein have consulted sources believed to be reliable in their efforts to provide information that is complete and in accord with the standards accepted at the time of publication. However, in view of the possibility of human error by the authors, editors, or publisher of the work herein, or changes in medical knowledge, neither the authors, editors, or publisher, nor any other party who has been involved in the preparation of this work, warrants that the information contained herein is in every respect accurate or complete, and they are not responsible for any errors or omissions or for the results obtained from use of such information. Readers are encouraged to confirm the information contained herein with other sources. For example, readers are advised to check the product information sheet included in the package of each drug they plan to administer to be certain that the information contained in this publication is accurate and that changes have not been made in the recommended dose or in the contraindications for administration. This recommendation is of particular importance in connection with new or infrequently used drugs.

Some of the product names, patents, and registered designs referred to in this book are in fact registered trademarks or proprietary names even though specific reference to this fact is not always made in the text. Therefore, the appearance of a name without designation as proprietary is not to be construed as a representation by the publisher that it is in the public domain.

Printed in the United States of America

5 4 3 2 1

TNY ISBN 1–58890–228–5
GTV ISBN 3–13–599804–5

Contents

SECTION III. REMEDIATION

Foreword

The Fourth Edition of *Auditory Disorders in School Children* by Ross J. Roeser and Marion P. Downs reflects the dramatic changes that have taken place in our field since the publication of their first edition in 1981. This newest edition, which is co-authored by the leading specialists in our field, thoughtfully covers the latest techniques for identifying and diagnosing hearing disorders in infants and children, the latest technologies and treatments for remediating hearing disorders, the latest protocols for managing children with hearing disorders, and the latest legal regulations governing educational programs for hard-of-hearing children. Each of these sections offers concrete information, along with subtle insights and shrewd practical guidance. The chapters are introduced with relevant "set-the-tone" quotations from philosophers (e.g., Emerson, Hippocrates, and Saint-Exupery) to audiologists (e.g., Carhart and Yoshinaga-Itano). Also included in the chapters are updated (1) glossaries of common terms, (2) appendices of resources for information or materials, (3) checklists, and (4) tables indexing state-of-the-art test materials and procedures. All of the chapters achieve impressive standards of excellence, bearing the editors' unmistakable stamp and style.

The overall goals of this newest edition remain similar to those of the original. In this edition, however, the authors emphasize ideas that were only "brewing" in the 20th century, but have become a reality in the 21st. We learn about auditory disorders in this new era, from legal, diagnostic, technological, remedial, educational, and social perspectives.

The latest edition begins by summarizing exciting new concepts that permeate the book, bringing previous dreams vividly to life. One new concept is "Hearing Deaf Children," children with hearing loss who receive early identification and intervention, and function successfully in "hearing" society due to advances in audiological, medical, and educational opportunities. Another is the "Audiology Home," a family-oriented service center coordinating and managing hard-of-hearing children's comprehensive array of multidisciplinary treatments and programs. This new era for the identification and treatment of children with auditory disorders, written in the strong voices of these authors, reads like one of the great success stories of our profession.

Clearly, this newest edition will continue to serve as the definitive resource for professional disciplines concerned with auditory disorders in school children.

Susan W. Jerger, Ph.D.
Ashbel Smith Professor and Director
Children's Speech Processing Laboratory
School of Behavioral and Brain Sciences
University of Texas at Dallas
Richardson, Texas

James F. Jerger, Ph.D.
Distinguished Scholar in Residence
School of Behavioral and Brain Sciences
University of Texas at Dallas
Richardson, Texas

Preface to the Fourth Edition

In 1979, when we first planned *Auditory Disorders in School Children*, never did we think we would be publishing a 4th edition more than 25 years later. At that time we were aware that a book like this was needed. Even though children with auditory disorders were being served in the schools there were many who were not, and the available technology and remediation strategies were not being utilized in all schools. The reasons were many and the issues were confounded by factors such as lack of funding and the need for teacher education. We believed that by providing a single source with updated material for students, school administrators, teachers, speech-language pathologists, and audiologists we would enhance the available screening, diagnostic, and educational services for school children with auditory disorders.

Our motive was simple and clear cut: to produce a textbook that was child-centered—focused on providing the very best programs for each child with an auditory disorder, whether it be a mild hearing loss, severe-to-profound hearing loss, or an auditory processing disorder. Providing the best possible programs for the individual child with an auditory disorder has remained the paramount focus for all editions of this textbook.

Today, our motive is the same. However, so many factors affecting children with auditory disorders have changed in the past quarter of a century that this edition of our book is quite different and unique. To name a few significant advances:

- New hearing screening tools with greater sensitivity are available and can be applied to younger and difficult-to-test populations
- Infants are now screened for hearing loss routinely within the first 48 hours of birth, before leaving the hospital
- Advanced technology has been applied to hearing aids to improve performance
- Cochlear implants have proven to be successful for use with children (and adults) with severe-to-profound deafness
- Assistive listening technology is available for use in the classroom
- New strategies for identifying and treating auditory processing disorders have been developed
- Remediation strategies have advanced and are more effective

While all of the above factors have had a major impact on school children with auditory disorders, without a doubt the most significant developments since publication of the first three editions of this book have been in neonatal hearing screening and cochlear implants. Neonates who have hearing loss are being identified before they leave the birthing hospital. Treatment strategies for infants found to have significant hearing loss are being implemented in the first weeks of life. Each child with hearing loss has the potential of receiving the critical services at an age early enough to allow for maximum benefit from intervention strategies.

Today, a little more than 10 years since they were approved by the FDA for use with children, cochlear implants have changed the way children with severe-to-profound deafness are educated. Before cochlear implants were available, children with severe-to-profound deafness were not expected to develop normal oral language skills. However, today, if provided with current technology and given the proper educational programming at an early enough age, these children can develop almost normal language and speech. Many children with cochlear implants are in classrooms with their normal hearing peers. The introduction of cochlear implants in the schools has challenged the traditional educational system. Today, we live in a new era for children with auditory disorders, much of it due to advances in cochlear implant technology.

The charge we gave to the contributors of the 4th edition of *Auditory Disorders in School Children* was to capture the recent innovations and advances in their chapters. We feel that not only did they meet our expectations, but have exceeded them in all areas. This book provides readers with child-centered materials that should enhance the well-being of school children having all types and degrees of auditory disorders.

Ross J. Roeser, Ph.D.
Marion P. Downs, M.A., D.H.S.

Acknowledgments

Major endeavors are seldom, if ever, carried out in isolation—they require the support of a team. This book is, by far, no exception to this rule. We are most appreciative of all those who worked very hard to produce yet another edition of *Auditory Disorders in School Children*. Most important are our contributors who, without exception, met our demanding publication schedule and accepted our editorial comments and suggestions in the spirit with which they were given. We selected some of the most enthusiastic and qualified authors that can be found anywhere to provide their thoughts and insights in each chapter of this book, and they proved us right in every respect. How fortunate we are to have such knowledgeable, capable, and cooperative contributors.

We also want to acknowledge the assistance of Dr. Jackie Clark, who served as an editorial consultant and proofreader. Her capable eye and excellent comments made our editing job significantly easier.

Ross J. Roeser, Ph.D.
Marion P. Downs, M.A., D.H.S.

Dedication

We dedicate the 4th Edition of *Auditory Disorders in School Children* to all those who have devoted their lives and efforts to help infants and children with auditory disorders.

Of particular note are the members of the Crystal Charity Ball, a Dallas-based philanthropic group of remarkable women who for over 50 years have worked tirelessly to help children in need in Dallas County. In 1993, and then again in 2003, the Crystal Charity Ball provided grants totaling over $1,200,000 for cochlear implant programs for children at the UTD/Callier Center for Communication Disorders. It is with financial support provided through caring efforts such as the Crystal Charity Ball that children with auditory disorders are able to benefit from the advances that are being made in technology and treatment strategies.

We also thank the Board of Trustees of the Foundation for the Callier Center for Communication Disorders who for over 40 years have supported programs serving children with auditory disorders, as well as other communication disorder programs for children and adults, at the UTD/Callier Center. Our board of respected community leaders continues to inspire us through the spirit of their active service, generous philanthropy, and loyal dedication.

As demonstrated by committed endeavors like the Crystal Charity Ball and the Foundation for the Callier Center, we salute individuals and organizations *everywhere* that are helping to prevent, diagnose, and treat auditory disorders in school children.

Ross J. Roeser, Ph.D.
Marion P. Downs, M.A., D.H.S.

Contributors

R. Ray Battin, Ph.D.
Clinical Neuropsychologist-Audiologist
The Battin Clinic
Houston, Texas

Paul Bauer, M.D.
Assistant Professor
Department of Otolaryngology–Head
 and Neck Surgery
Division of Pediatric Oncology
University of Texas Southwestern
 Medical Center
Dallas, Texas

Virginia Berry, M.S.
Assistant Professor
Speech and Hearing Sciences
University of Southern Mississippi
Hattiesburg, Mississippi

Jackie L. Clark, Ph.D.
Faculty Associate
UTD/Callier Center for
 Communication Disorders
University of Texas at Dallas
Dallas, Texas

Karen A. Clark, M.A.
Head, Educational Division
UTD/Callier Center for
 Communication Disorders
University of Texas at Dallas
Dallas, Texas

Carol G. Cokely, Ph.D.
Coordinator of Clinical Teaching in
 Audiology
UTD/Callier Center for
 Communication Disorders
University of Texas at Dallas
Dallas, Texas

Carl C. Crandell, Ph.D.
Associate Professor
Department of Communication Sciences
 and Disorders
University of Florida
Gainesville, Florida

Janet DesGeorges
President, Hands & Voices National;
Parent Consultant
Marion Downs National Center
University of Colorado
Boulder, Colorado

Marion P. Downs, M.A., D.H.S.
Professor Emeritus
Department of Otolaryngology
Division of Audiology
Health Sciences Center
University of Colorado
Denver, Colorado

Carol Flexer, Ph.D.
Professor, Audiology
School of Speech-Language Pathology
 and Audiology
The University of Akron
Akron, Ohio

Robert W. Keith, Ph.D.
Professor and Director
Division of Audiology and Vestibular
    Testing
University of Cincinnati Medical Center
Cincinnati, Ohio

Robert E. Kretschmer, Ph.D.
Associate Professor, Special Education
Teachers College
Columbia University
New York, New York

David M. Luterman, D.Ed.
Professor Emeritus
Department of Communication
    Disorders
Emerson College
Boston, Massachusetts

Helen McCaffrey Morrison, Ph.D.
Associate Professor
Department of Communication Sciences
    and Disorders
Texas Christian University
Fort Worth, Texas

Carolyn H. Musket, M.A.
Clinical Lecturer
Program in Communication Sciences
    and Disorders
UTD/Callier Center for
    Communication Disorders
University of Texas at Dallas
Dallas, Texas

Ross J. Roeser, Ph.D.
Professor and Executive Director
UTD/Callier Center for
    Communication Disorders
School of Behavioral and Brain Sciences
University of Texas at Dallas
Dallas, Texas

Peter S. Roland, M.D.
Professor and Chairman
Department of Otolaryngology–Head
    and Neck Surgery
University of Texas Southwestern
    Medical Center
Dallas, Texas

Susan P. Russell, M.A.
Division of Programs and Services
Montgomery County Public Schools
Montgomery, Maryland

Leeanne Seaver, M.A.
Executive Director
Hands & Voices National
Denver, Colorado

Angela G. Shoup, Ph.D.
Assistant Professor
Department of Otolaryngology–Head
    and Neck Surgery
University of Texas Southwestern
    Medical Center
Dallas, Texas

Joseph J. Smaldino, Ph.D.
Department Head and Professor
Communicative Disorders
University of Northern Iowa
Cedar Falls, Iowa

Diana L. Terry, M.S.
Educational Liaison
UTD/Callier Center for
    Communication Disorders
University of Texas at Dallas
Dallas, Texas

Phillip L. Wilson, Au.D.
Head of Clinical Audiology Programs
UTD/Callier Center for
    Communication Disorders
University of Texas at Dallas
Dallas, Texas

A New Era for the Identification and Treatment of Children with Auditory Disorders

ROSS J. ROESER AND MARION P. DOWNS

Nothing great was ever achieved without enthusiasm.
—Ralph Waldo Emerson

It is a new era for children with auditory disorders—those with mild and unilateral hearing loss; those with more severe hearing loss; those who are deaf; and those with auditory processing disorders who have hearing sensitivity within the normal range but who are unable to use sound for normal speech understanding. For professionals responsible for diagnosing and educating children with auditory disorders the challenges are no less than a revolution. Never before have technology and intensive habilitation combined to provide children having auditory disorders of all types with the opportunity to enter into a world of sound; to be able to develop their oral skills to a level that can equal those of their hearing peers. New understanding of how the brain processes sound and how treatments can improve performance are being uncovered each day. As we enter the new millennium, numerous changes bring joy to all who see the improved welfare of children with auditory disorders, but these same changes present a rigorous challenge for those in the educational system.

Many ideas brewing in the 20th century have come to fruition in the 21st. Today there is an influx of new technologies for children with loss of hearing; there is a cohort of children whose usual and unusual hearing losses were identified at birth and who were immediately enrolled in habilitation programs; there are medical and genetic breakthroughs that will sharply decrease the number of ear and hearing disorders (see Chapter 4); and there are improved surgical applications that can reach clear down to the first year of deafened lives. For children with auditory processing disorders each day brings new information on the plasticity of the central nervous system and how treatments can improve learning to hear and educational performance. This book was inspired by the new developments in identifying and managing children with auditory disorders; the material covers a wide variety of topics regarding the law, identification, and remediation.

As pointed out in Chapter 9, a regularly experienced phenomenon by all professionals serving children with special needs is that parents are better educated and are making greater and more informed demands—of physicians, audiologists, speech-language pathologists, teachers, and school administrators—to provide the very best programs for their children. This is a challenge, for sure, but also a boon for the child with hearing loss. Quintessential to this textbook is the well-established principle that *each child MUST be the focus of the programs provided by each and every professional serving that child.* It was this principle that authors were asked to focus on when preparing chapters for this text.

The chapters in this book cover the gamut of topics for professionals who work with all levels of auditory disorders. Each of the following sections provides an overview of the book.

The Child with Mild and Unilateral Hearing Loss

Until recent times the child with mild hearing loss was not considered at risk for educational delay. However, as pointed out in Chapter 10, studies have made it clear that children with hearing sensitivity once thought to be decreased by 15 to 20 dB, but "within normal limits," do, indeed, have potential delay. With the advent of screening programs outlined in Chapter 5, current technology makes it possible to identify children with minimal hearing loss and middle ear disorders, so that necessary measures can be provided for this at risk population. Newly acquired knowledge also makes it clear that children with unilateral hearing loss exhibit greater difficulty in understanding speech in the presence of competing background noise than do normal hearing children, which puts them at high risk for educational delay (see Chapter 10). Improving signal-to-noise levels in classrooms (see Chapter 12) and the use of classroom amplification (see Chapter 13) are important considerations for children with minimal/mild and unilateral hearing loss as well as for those with bilateral losses in the more severe ranges.

The Child with Moderate and Moderately Severe Hearing Loss

The child identified with moderate or moderately severe hearing loss has the added advantage of new technology in personal hearing aids that are more durable and reliable and have more sophisticated electroacoustic capabilities (see Chapter 11). There are also numerous resource materials to assist those who are educating children with hearing loss, as well as better classroom intervention strategies (see Chapter 18). As pointed out in Chapter 16, auditory training techniques and concepts have also become more sophisticated and effective.

The "Hearing Deaf" Child

Knocking at school doors are the families of children whose degree of hearing loss at birth would formerly have necessitated special oral classes, manual signing classrooms for children who were classified as Deaf, or even institutional placement. These are "New Era" children with hearing loss, and they make up what we will refer to as the "Hearing Deaf" population. If provided with the proper medical, audiological, and educational opportunities, Hearing Deaf children will gain admission into the classroom with their normal-hearing peers. It is now possible because the Hearing Deaf children will be speaking orally and intelligibly; their language level will be at or near their age level! If treated and educated properly these children will be able to function in society as hearing adults.

A fantasy? Hardly. Currently, universal newborn hearing screening (UNHS) is mandated by legislation in 32 states (see Chapter 5), and the success has spawned an increasing demand for new educational techniques for habilitation models. As UNHS programs successfully identify infants with significant unilateral or bilateral hearing loss, the demand for clinical and educational services is taking on new meaning. Laws are changing to accommodate these children (see Chapter 2). Most significantly, clinical and educational staff members are being required to provide services to children identified with hearing loss who are significantly younger, which is both desirable and challenging.

Prior to UNHS, the age of identification and intervention was consistently reported to exceed 2 years. Today, research has documented the desirable outcome for UNHS—

that identification and treatment are occurring significantly earlier (Harrison, Roush, & Wallace, 2003). Infants are being identified in birthing hospitals prior to discharge; it is not unusual in today's programs for parents to bring infants only weeks old to clinics for hearing aid fittings. The schools are being forced to step away from the tradition of grouping children with hearing loss into self-contained classes, and educators are being required to rethink the whole process of serving this New Era population with Hearing Deaf children.

Current technology and educational intervention now make it possible for each child with hearing loss, even those in the severe-to-profound range who are fitted with cochlear implants (see Chapter 15), to attain oral communication skills. Studies already document that Hearing Deaf children, if identified at birth and provided with appropriate habilitation, will show intelligible speech and are testing for language at levels near their hearing peers by school age. Among the leading investigators setting the pace for the New Era child are Christine Yoshinaga-Itano and her colleagues from the University of Colorado in Boulder and Mary Pat Moeller and her colleagues from The Boys Town Institute in Omaha.

Early Identification of Hearing Loss: A Critical Factor

Yoshinaga-Itano, Sedey, Coulter, and Mehl (1998) studied the language development of 150 children, 72 of whom had hearing loss identified prior to 6 months of age and were placed in intervention services at an average of 2 months after diagnosis. Another 78 children had hearing losses identified from 7 months to 30 months of age. All but four of the entire group had received immediate, appropriate intervention through public health or private agencies. All were given the Minnesota Child Development inventory, with both Receptive and Expressive Language Scales. The findings from this and similar studies are summarized in the following four sections.

The Importance of Early Identification

Children identified and habilitated before 6 months of age have receptive and expressive language quotients significantly higher than children whose hearing losses were identified after 6 months of age. The differences averaged 20 developmental quotient points. The impact of early identification was present and independent of gender, secondary disability, socioeconomic status, cognitive status, or type of habilitation services (viz., sign language, total communication, or auditory verbal training). From these data it is clear that infants and toddlers identified before 6 months of age had higher language quotients than those identified later. The importance of this finding stresses the need for universal neonatal hearing screening to improve the probabilities that normal language development will occur.

The Degree of Hearing Loss Has Little Relation to the Level of Language Skills

Those in the mild hearing loss group (26 to 40 dB) had an average language score only slightly better than the average language score than the more severe hearing loss groups, including the profound group (over 90 dB). The finding that degree of hearing loss has minimal effect on language development leads to a great deal of speculation. Is there a language center in the brain that requires a focused minimal amount of stimulation to develop maximally? Is there an effect from the lack of hearing during the 4 months that the normal fetus hears prenatally? One can only continue to speculate.

The Early Identification Advantage Persists into the School Years

Yoshinaga-Itano and Coulter (1998) followed 125 early-identified children until kindergarten and found that the advantage of early identification was still present as they entered school. Moeller (1998) provided longitudinal data on 150 deaf and hard-of-hearing children to the age of 7 years. Results from both studies clearly showed the early-identified group maintained their language advantage to the 7 years level. From this study it is clear that current technology and habilitative strategies are facilitating the means for normal language development, and it is logical to assume that the advantage will persist throughout the school years.

Intelligible Speech Shows an Advantage from Early Identification, but on Different Time Lines

Yoshinaga-Itano and Sedey (2000) evaluated speech intelligibility of 147 deaf or hard-of-hearing children from 14 months of age to 60 months using phonetic transcription. The strongest factor in predicting speech skills was the age of identification. By almost 5 years of age, even those with moderate-to-severe hearing loss had achieved significant intelligibility. The profound losses did not succeed in any recordable speech skills.

Findings from the preceding research have made it clear that the child with hearing loss born today has opportunities unlike any time before in history. Although these opportunities present themselves to every child living in a developed society where the technology and clinical and educational services are available, success is dependent on the coordination of technology with services—services that are provided in an effective way. Such services can be part of the Audiology Home described later.

Children with Auditory Processing Disorders

It has been recognized for many years that some children and adults have been classified as having "normal" hearing, but they are not able to "hear" and understand sounds, especially speech sounds, in the presence of noise. These individuals are unable to process sounds properly—thus they are classified as having an auditory processing disorder (APD). When evaluated with the standard audiological test battery (see Chapter 3) the majority of those with APD will have test results classified within normal limits.

The past 3 decades have brought significant changes in the diagnostic test battery and treatment strategies for children with APD. As detailed in Chapter 6, the level of sophistication in knowledge and understanding of APD has increased significantly. The diagnostic audiological test battery for APD has become more sensitive. Most notable is the report of the University of Texas at Dallas/Callier Center for Communication Disorders consensus conference on the diagnosis of APD in school children (Jerger & Musiek, 2002). The report suggests that screening for APD be considered; gives guidelines on how to screen for APD; provides assumptions, listener variables, and principles for differential diagnosis of APD; details a minimal test battery for APD in school children; and suggests areas for future research. The UTD/Callier Center APD consensus report represents a significant advancement for understanding and diagnosing APD.

Better diagnostic procedures for APD are accompanied by improved treatment techniques. Chapter 17 details a comprehensive array of classroom and therapy procedures for children with APD.

The Audiology Home

As treatments for children with auditory disorders have become more effective, they have also become more comprehensive, sophisticated, and complex. Oftentimes the necessary services for children with auditory disorders require a team of professionals, including medical specialists, audiologists, speech-language pathologists, teachers of hearing-impaired children, psychologists, and others. The Audiology Home (see Chapter 5) is a family-oriented service center where each child's treatment program can be centralized and coordinated (Jerger, Roeser, & Tobey, 2001). The Audiology Home should be the cornerstone for the successful management of infants and young children with auditory disorders. Given the nature of the disorder to be treated, the Audiology Home needs to be a multidisciplinary, family-oriented center providing all of the services necessary to attain maximal educational achievement.

Included in the array of services are audiological assessment and intervention, family counseling and support (see Chapter 19), community outreach and education, communication intervention, outcome assessments, and documentation of progress. To be most effective, the team should include, but not necessarily be limited to, physicians, audiologists, communication development specialists, counselors, and psychologists (see Chapters 7 and 8). A key ingredient for success is to have professionals in the Audiology Home meet regularly and interface with each other. Regular communications updating professionals with progress and setbacks will allow for program modifications. As the child ages, members of the Audiology Home should work in close collaboration with educational programs to ensure optimal intervention for maximal speech and language development.

Audiology Homes exist whenever and wherever multidisciplinary teams of professionals function to serve children with hearing loss. Audiology Homes can be found in community centers, hospitals, and schools. It is clear that in today's complex environment, to achieve the most desirable results, it takes a team to manage children with hearing loss effectively; it takes an Audiology Home. This text contains the essential information for professionals working in Audiology Homes to provide the very best services to each child served.

References

Harrison, M., Roush, J., & Wallace, J. (2003). Trends in age of identification and intervention in infants with hearing loss. *Ear Hear, 24*, 89–95.

Jerger, J., & Musiek, F. (2002). Report of the consensus conference on the diagnosis of auditory processing disorders in school-aged children. *Journal of the American Academy of Audiology, 11*, 467–474.

Jerger, S., Roeser, R.J., & Tobey, E. (2001). Management of hearing loss in infants: The UTD/Callier Center position statement. *Journal of the American Academy of Audiology, 12*, 329–336.

Moeller, M. (1998, June). *A diagnostic early intervention project: Strategies and outcomes.* Paper presented at the National Symposium on Infant Hearing, Denver, Colorado.

Yoshinaga-Itano, C., & Coulter, D. (1998, June). *Preliminary reports on the impact of early identification on language development of preschool-aged deaf and hard-of-hearing children in Colorado: Predictors of successful outcomes of deaf and hard-of-hearing children of hearing parents.* Paper presented at the National Symposium on Infant Hearing, Denver, Colorado.

Yoshinaga-Itano, C., & Sedey, A. (2000). Early speech development in children who are deaf or hard of hearing: Interrelationships with language and hearing. *The Volta Review, 100*, 181–212.

Yoshinaga-Itano, C., Sedey, A., Coulter, D., & Mehl L. (1998). Language development of early- and later-identified children with hearing loss. *Pediatrics, 102*, 1161–1171.

SECTION I

The Law

2

Special Education Law: A New IDEA for Students Who Are Deaf or Hard of Hearing

LEEANNE SEAVER AND JANET DESGEORGES

A deaf or hard of hearing child is, to some degree, without hearing. And yet the term "disabled" may be a misnomer. That same child is fully capable of developing language—spoken or manual—and becoming a complete person. A communication difference is not the same as a communication disability.
—Lawrence Siegel, J.D.

Deafness is a sensory difference. It only becomes a "disability" when the educational system fails the child and family.
—Christine Yoshinaga-Itano, Ph.D.

A child who is deaf or hard of hearing presents a paradoxical challenge to the American educational system. On the one hand, the child has a disability, clinically speaking. On the other hand, the child is completely *able* to accomplish the goals of education, while accessing communication differently than hearing students. In an environment of equal communication access, the concept of disability simply may not apply to students who are deaf and hard of hearing.

However, our American educational system is founded on *disability* as a qualifying condition. It is a deficits-based model programmed to react when the student digresses or fails in a way that can be tracked unquestionably to his or her "disabling" condition (U.S. Department of Education, 2002). Once this deficit has been established, the system goes about trying to accommodate for it through the mandate of special education. Statistically speaking, that system has failed to serve the unique needs of students who are deaf or hard of hearing. According to nationally standardized test (SAT) results, the deaf or hard of hearing student population graduates with an average grade-equivalent performance of 3.9 for reading comprehension, 5.0 for math problem solving, 4.5 for language, and 6.0 for spelling (Bloomquist Traxler, 2000).

Perpetuating Disability

Students who are able to overcome the negative impacts of their disability within a system that perpetuates failure may find themselves rewarded for their grade-appropriate academic outcomes by being booted off the special education caseload as no longer eligible. Ironically, these students may have to regress or fail to earn back the services that supported their achievement, and the cycle continues in its absurdity.

Nowhere is this dysfunction more apparent than in the case of babies whose deafness or hearing loss was identified at birth. With the advent of early identification and effective intervention, significant language delays and related problems associated with late identification of hearing loss have been virtually eliminated. The children who have

9

benefited from good early intervention arrive at the threshold of public education, usually at age 3, showing no deficits due to hearing loss. Their language and development is age-appropriate (Yoshinaga-Itano, Coulter, & Thomson, 2000). These are the very children who may be turned away from the doors of special education—and the supports that they need to maintain their accomplishment—because their early success disqualifies them from eligibility for services. Based on the special education eligibility criteria in many states, these children will need to regress before the educational system will consider them qualified for support.

Starting from the Beginning

The Individuals with Disabilities Education Act (IDEA) was passed in the mid-1970s (originally called the Educating All Handicapped Children Act) mandating programs of special education (i.e., specially designed instruction for students with disabilities) in public schools. According to IDEA, the purpose of special education was, and is, to "ensure that all children with disabilities have available to them a free and appropriate public education that emphasizes special education and related services designed to meet their unique needs and prepare them for employment and independent living." Students with special needs were eligible starting at age 3 through high school graduation under Part B of the law. (Part C of IDEA, which came into law in the late 1980s, covers special needs entitlements for the birth to age 3 population, also known as Early Intervention.)

Eligibility requirements as defined by IDEA essentially dictated that the student (1) had to have a disability, and (2) had to *need* specialized instruction. The need for specialized instruction was directly related to the student's deficits resulting from his or her disability. The determination of what that specialized instruction should look like was to be made by special education teachers, the student's parents or guardians, and others who would be working directly with the

student (e.g., speech-language pathologists, occupational therapists, parents, psychologists, interpreters, general educators, counselors, and other applicable representatives). This group would function as a team to create a document called the Individual Education Program (IEP), which sets forth the academic goals and objectives for students, based on their unique, individual needs.

Time for Change

Surely the earlier-mentioned success-equals-failure dynamic was never the intention of special education law. Although this short-sighted treatment (failure-perpetuation is only one of many examples) of deaf or hard of hearing students still operates at some level in all school districts across the nation, some important changes to IDEA have been incorporated into law. The act now requires IEP teams to address "special considerations" in order to meet the unique communication needs of students who are deaf or hard of hearing. Although we still have a long way to go, "special considerations" is a groundbreaking achievement for students who are deaf or hard of hearing. We have indeed come a long way already.

IDEA's Impact

IDEA enabled many students who were deaf or hard of hearing to attend the school in their own area, rather than board at the state's residence school for the deaf, which, prior to enactment of the law, had been a traditional placement for many deaf students. Beyond that, there was no obligation for public schools to accept students with disabilities who were considered to be "uneducable," or too difficult to educate. Their right to receive a "free and appropriate public education" (FAPE) was now an IDEA entitlement at whatever public school they would normally attend, based on where they lived. However, local education agencies (school districts) often found themselves unprepared for the special needs of this population. There was "not widespread understanding of the educational implications of deafness, even among special educators" (Deaf Students Education Services Policy Guidance Report, 1992). Further, given the low incidence of deafness, there wasn't always a critical mass of students to justify the existence of a program and staff with expertise in deafness or hearing loss. The solution for many school districts was to place deaf students in special education classrooms where other special needs (to use a term from those days, "retarded") children were taught. Academic expectations in many of these "self-contained" settings were homogenized and typically set so even the lowest achiever could accomplish them. Further complicated by a system that perpetuated failure, for deaf and hard-of-hearing students with normal cognitive abilities, this dynamic set in motion a trend of underachievement that has not been successfully reversed, statistically speaking, even today.

The Inclusion Movement

The spirit and the letter of the IDEA did not support the practice of segregating students with special needs exclusively into self-contained classrooms, but the practice was so common that many parents, advocacy groups, and even some philosophically aligned professionals protested vehemently. The call for "inclusion" of disabled students into general education classrooms was a powerful movement that swept the nation in the 1990s and was founded on the IDEA provision that "to the maximum extent appropriate, children with disabilities . . . are educated with children who are nondisabled . . . as close as possible to the child's home . . . in the school that he or she would attend if non-disabled" (IDEA Sec. 300.552 (b) (3) & (c)). This placement is considered the "least restrictive environment" (LRE) for students with special needs, but in fact, for many students who were deaf or hard of hearing, it created an environment of extreme isolation with no direct communication access to teachers or peers.

The Communication Conundrum

In 1992, the U.S. Department of Education's Office of Special Education Programs (OSEP) published the Deaf Students Education Services Policy Guidance Report in response to an earlier report by the now defunct Commission on Education of the Deaf. This program was concerned over the provision of FAPE for students who were deaf who had "significant obstacles to overcome in order to have access to FAPE, particularly with regard to communication access" (OSEP, 1992, p. 49274). The Deaf Students Policy Guidance Report intended to give direction to state and local education agencies on FAPE for students who were deaf or hard of hearing. It called for the consideration of certain factors in the development of an IEP for any student who was deaf, including:

1. Communication needs and the child's and family's preferred mode of communication
2. Linguistic needs
3. Severity of hearing loss and potential for using residual hearing
4. Academic level
5. Social, emotional, and cultural needs, including opportunities for peer interactions and communication

The Deaf Students Policy Guidance Report additionally recommended that children's needs be identified by professionals who are knowledgeable about the specific factors presented by the "nature and severity" of their deafness relative to the content and method of delivery of the curriculum. This reference pointed to the necessity of having educators who have expertise in deafness directly involved in the educational planning for students who are deaf or hard of hearing—a responsibility that was and is often left to professionals with no background in deafness or hearing loss.

A main thrust of the Deaf Students Policy Guidance report was that meeting the unique communication and related needs of a deaf student was fundamental to that individual's free and appropriate public education. It stated that:

> Any setting, including a regular classroom, that prevents a child who is deaf from receiving an appropriate education that meets his or her needs, including communication needs, is not the LRE for that child. Placement decisions must be based on the child's IEP. Thus the consideration of LRE as a part of the placement decision must always be in the context of LRE in which appropriate services can be provided. Any setting which does not meet the communication and related needs of a child who is deaf, and therefore does not allow for the provision of FAPE, cannot be considered the LRE for that child. The provision of FAPE is paramount, and the individual placement determination about LRE is to be considered within the context of FAPE. (p. 49274)

The report contended that some public agencies had "misapplied the LRE provision by presuming that placements in or closer to the regular classroom are required for children who are deaf" without considering the communication needs of the student. That said, the report also acknowledged that general education settings are appropriate and adaptable to meet the unique needs of particular deaf students, and that a continuum of placement options must be maintained, and that all placement decisions must be based on the IEP, with an emphasis on *individual* needs.

Incorporating New Policies

The 1992 Deaf Students Policy Guidance report evolved through the Deaf Education Initiative Project, composed of a task force of professionals from all arenas in deaf education, advocacy, and the deaf community. Under the direction of Dr. Robert Davila, former assistant secretary of education for the Office of Special Education and Rehabilitative Services, the Deaf and Hard of Hearing Students Educational Service Guidelines were published in 1994 for the National Association of State Directors of Education (NASDE) (Baker-Hawkins & Easterbrooks,

1994). Exhaustive, comprehensive, and communication-focused, this document became the definitive resource and reference on deaf education, from audiology to American Sign Language (ASL), to deaf cultural concepts to cued speech. It was distributed nationally, and remains a powerful source of still-practical, meaningful information specific to this population.

From Policies to Mandates

When IDEA was reauthorized in 1997, for the first time it included specific language that acknowledged the need for special considerations in the case of students who were deaf or hard of hearing (IDEA Sec. 300–346 (a) (2) (iv–v)). This was the result of active lobbying based on the Policy Guidelines (OSEP, 1992), and from that document came these new requirements. The 1997 reauthorization of the IDEA stated that:

> Sec.300.346 Development, review and revision of IEP.
> (a)(2) Consideration of special factors. The IEP team shall also . . .
> (iv) Consider the communication needs of the child, and in the case of the child who is deaf or hard of hearing, consider the child's language and communication needs, opportunities for direct communications with peers and professional personnel in the child's language and communication mode, academic level, and full range of needs, including opportunities for direct instruction in the child's language and communication mode; and
> (v) Consider whether the child requires assistive technology devices and services.

The challenge that this new language poses to parents, schools, and IEP teams is to apply its intention productively and practically to the day-to-day experience of deaf or hard of hearing students in school. How does the IEP team move past the theoretical consideration of these special factors and into a plan of action? This "consideration of special factors" can be broken into five main components:

1. Language and communication needs

2. Opportunities for direct communication with peers and professionals
3. Academic level
4. Full range of needs
5. Direct instruction in the student's communication mode or language

In addition to these five components, the use of assistive technology and services must also be addressed (IDEA Sec. 300.346 (a) (2) (v)).

1. Language and Communication Needs

Communication is at the heart of the matter when developing an individualized education program for a child who is deaf or hard of hearing. The team (including parents) must be fully aware of how the student is accessing communication in the environment and how that access may by necessity change. It may look different for the student with a cochlear implant than it does for the student using ASL. It may look different in a small classroom than during an assembly in the auditorium. It will look different when hearing aids or cochlear implants are removed to play certain sports. The point is that it does and will change or need adaptations, and the IEP team needs to consider that in the context of the student's communication mode or language. This is a different approach than the historical practice of placing a priority on the "method" of communication, rather than on the needs of children to fully access the communication in their world. The "child-centered" approach is essential to creating educational programming that is at the core driven by the right to access communication.

Possible issues considered based on the individual child include:

- Is there just one communication mode? More than one? Combinations of methods?
- How do the parents communicate with the child?
- How does the child communicate outside of school or with friends?
- How does the student access inferential learning?
- How have we objectively measured this student's ability to access information in his or her preferred mode of communication?
- How does this student access information in noise?
- How does this student access information in a room with poor acoustics?
- What type of technology does this student use? Hearing aid? FM system? cochlear implant? teletypewriter (TTY)? note-taking systems? real time captioning?
- What is the back-up plan when communication breaks down?
- Is the student's skill level in the chosen mode(s) of communication adequate for grade-level achievement?
- How can we assess his or her sign language or oral skill level?
- What kind of interpreter does this student need? Oral? ASL? Signed Exact English (SEE)? other?
- How can we assess functional hearing (beyond the audiogram)?
- How are tests administered in the classroom? Orally? In writing?
- Have we taken into consideration the "fatigue factor"?

Depending on the discussion, the IEP team may need to develop an action plan that addresses these special considerations based on the needs and modes of the individual student. It could include:

- Use of an educational sign language interpreter or teacher fluent with signing during instruction
- Parent training in sign language, auditory training, or both
- Acoustical adaptations to the environment
- Functional hearing test (link to www.handsandvoices.org/articles/education/ed/func_listening_eval.html)
- Classroom captioning
- Buddy system
- Use of FM system, personal or sound field system, hearing aids
- Adding sign or spoken language goals and objectives for the student
- Closed captioning on all television sets; captions for all movies to be shown

- Announcements given over the public address system also delivered or posted in writing
- Testing accommodations (e.g., extra time, no oral tests)
- Down time/break time

- Specialized seating arrangements
- Enhanced speech reading capabilities (no hands or projection equipment in front of the face, good lighting on the face, well-trimmed facial hair, no gum chewing)
- Other applicable ideas

Case Study 2–1: Unique Communication Needs   C.H. is 10 years old and has a mild/moderate hearing loss. She speaks well and is a good user of amplification. She is at her neighborhood school and is the only student with a hearing loss. People often remark that they would never know she has a hearing loss, her speech is "so good." But C.H. has had a hard time making friends and seems to be lagging behind in science. She was also reprimanded recently during PE for not following the rules. She sometimes fails to turn in homework assignments.

C.H. primarily uses her auditory ability to access information. However, she also lip-reads when she misses something. Unfortunately, her science teacher has a beard and tends to mumble. At lunchtime in the cafeteria, the acoustics are so poor that she misses out on a lot of the conversation that is going on around her at the table with her classmates. They wonder sometimes why she ignores them. Although she has an FM system that helps tremendously in noisy situations, the PE teacher has refused to wear it because she is afraid that it could be damaged in class, and besides, "PE is so physical and visual" she is sure that C.H. will just "catch on" to what's going on in class. The teacher announces the homework assignments at the end of the day but rarely writes the assignments down on the chalkboard.

IEP Action Plan: The IEP team must ensure that every teacher who comes in contact with Cheryl throughout the day uses and understands the need for the FM system. The "specials" teachers (PE, art, music, science labs, etc.) need to wear the FM system to reduce the impact of background noise. They need to understand that they must enunciate clearly, face the student, and use as many visuals, overheads, and supplemental written materials as possible to reinforce the "auditory input."

C.H. needs an opportunity to connect with other kids in a one-on-one environment. The kids should be shown how to get her attention before they talk to her (i.e., facing toward her, tapping on the shoulder). During class time when kids are in small group, they can pass the FM around so that the students get used to using the microphone. They can try the FM during lunchtime in the cafeteria. The teacher should write the homework assignment on the board every day and then check to make sure C.H. has written it down correctly.

---

2. Opportunities for Direct Communication with Peers and Professional Personnel

For many students who are deaf and hard of hearing, communication challenges can create isolation and loneliness—even in a room full of kids. The opportunity to communicate with and have meaningful relationships with other peers—be they hearing, deaf, or hard of hearing—must be considered in the development of the IEP. Morever, communicating directly with professional personnel, including teachers and interpreters, must be given special consideration.

For students who are placed at a center-based program or at the state school for the deaf, there may be natural opportunities for the student to directly connect with other students and professionals who use the same mode of communication. For students who are in a mainstream setting, there should be a discussion about how to effectively facilitate peer and professional interaction, regardless of the mode of communication used by the student (signed or spoken). Peers of like communication mode must be defined on a case-by-case basis. For example, a deaf child with a cochlear implant to develop speaking and listening skills may benefit from direct communication with typically oral communicating kids, either hearing or deaf. A native user of ASL must have opportunities to communicate with peers and professionals in that language. This is particularly important for young children who do not understand how to appropriately use an interpreter in the classroom and who may misunderstand the role of interpreter versus teacher.

Possible issues that should be considered based on the individual child include:

- Is the student in a mainstream or center-based/state school setting?
- Is the student in a rural or urban setting?
- Who are the student's current peers? (hearing kids? deaf or hard of hearing oral children? cueing children? deaf or hard of hearing signing children?)
- Does the student have access to peers in the same grade or age range?
- Do opportunities within the school district/region or state exist?
- Is there a deaf community in the student's geographical location?
- Does the student have access to the Internet to create friendships?
- Is there a deaf or hard of hearing adult role model program in the state?
- What are the parent's values about the child's participation in deaf or hard of hearing peer group activities?
- What are the student's values around being included with other deaf or hard of hearing students?
- If the student's peers include hearing kids, do those hearing peers know and understand sign language? or if oral, how to communicate effectively?

- How proficient is the professional(s) in the child's communication mode or language? Who is qualified to evaluate staff proficiency and/or qualifications?
- Are the qualifications of the staff serving the student linked to the child's individual needs (i.e., cochlear implant expertise, experience with student's age/grade level, etc.)?

Depending on the discussion, the IEP team may want to develop specific goals based on the consideration given to direct communication with peers and professionals and on the needs/modes of the individual student. These goals could be directly linked to academic achievement, or listed under "Related Services." Some examples include:

- Becoming an online (e-pen) pal with another student who's deaf or hard of hearing
- Developing special curricula that explore the contributions to society by individuals who are deaf or hard of hearing
- Identifying a section in the school library with resources on deaf issues, books written by deaf or hard of hearing authors, fiction that has deaf or hard of hearing heroines, and the like
- Offering sign language classes for the student body at the school
- Connecting to a state role model program, if available
- Networking mainstreamed students to center-based or state deaf residence schools for opportunities to gather socially
- Hooking up with local deaf community organizations (National Association of the Deaf, Self Help for Hard of Hearing)
- Adding information and projects about deafness (e.g., science fair projects that have to do with deafness, films about Helen Keller and others) to the general education curriculum
- Creating district/regional opportunities for deaf or hard of hearing kids to be together (e.g., track and field day, baseball camp, leadership trip to Washington, D.C., etc.)

Case Study 2–2: Direct Communication   J.S. is a sophomore in high school in a rural community. He is one of six students in his school district who is deaf or hard of hearing. However, he is the only one at the high school level. J.S. uses sign language primarily, and has an interpreter for his classes. His teacher doesn't call on him in class very often because she has trouble understanding his "deaf speech" and finds it distracting and disruptive to have an interpreter voice J.S.'s answers for him. J.S. doesn't raise his hand often because he's self-conscious about his speech intelligibility, and believes his teacher doesn't call on him because she doesn't like him or think he's smart enough to answer a question.

J.S. loves computers and baseball, but he's ambivalent about joining the baseball team. His interpreter leaves school promptly after the last class every day, so J.S. is worried that if he tries out for the baseball team, he won't be able to understand what the coach is saying. He hates his foreign language class and is having a hard time getting a C. He has two very close friends, both of whom are hearing. His parents are afraid if he hangs out with other deaf people, he might not learn to make it in the "hearing world." J.S. wishes he knew more deaf or hard of hearing kids with whom he could communicate less self-consciously.

J.S. lives in a rural community, but there is a small but active deaf community in the town 15 miles from where he lives. J.S.'s family has never had the opportunity to meet them. J.S. is a good lip-reader, but he really likes to just hang out with a couple of friends because when the group gets too big, the conversation moves too fast. His friends are very willing to learn sign language, but there aren't any classes available in their area.

IEP Action Plan: The IEP team, including J.S.'s parents, needs to include J.S. at the meeting and have a conversation about his peers. Does he want to meet other deaf or hard of hearing students? Are there really no other high school students within 50 miles of where J.S. lives who are deaf or hard of hearing? In fact, the state school for the deaf has an e-mail Listserv for all the students there. J.S. can access that on his computer at home to begin a relationship with other deaf or hard of hearing high school students. There is a leadership camp for high schoolers that are deaf or hard of hearing in the summer that Joe can attend. The school librarian can get a catalog from Gallaudet University with books that are available about contributions by deaf or hard of hearing adults. The team must understand that the law provides for access to school-sponsored activities, so J.S. can go out for the baseball team knowing that an interpreter must be provided. J.S. will have an opportunity to make new friends by being on the team. The local college has an ASL class that J.S. can take to fulfill his credit for a foreign language. His two close friends can take the class with him. Someone knows of a 22-year-old CODA (hearing child of deaf adult) who lives just 15 miles away and can introduce J.S. and his parents to some of the members of the deaf community in the area.

J.S.'s general education teacher needs some sensitivity training and awareness to be better prepared to communicate directly with him. The team writes goals into his IEP that include an increasing number of direct communications each week between her and J.S. They determine what subject must be discussed routinely (e.g., daily journal writing) and set specific times each week to meet one-on-one.

- Having a high school sports team from the state school for the deaf travel and do a presentation/exhibition for a mainstreamed students' high school
- Creating training goals and mentoring relationships for the mainstream staff to gain proficiency, if needed, in the student's communication mode or language
- Setting a goal for the student to communicate directly with the classroom teacher when asking or answering a question in class rather than defaulting to communicating through an interpreter

3. Academic Level

A deaf or hard of hearing student's academic level must be given special consideration, particularly if it is below expectations for standard grade-level achievement. Any discussion of the impact of the student's deafness or hearing loss on academic performance will demonstrate the interrelatedness of each "special consideration." In the case of the student who is below grade level academically, consider the following:

- Is it due to language delays resulting from late identification?
- How accessible is the classroom communication?
- Has communication inaccessibility created learning deficits that have been compounded year after year?
- Is the underachievement a reflection of the staff's lack of proficiency in the child's communication mode or language?
- What does it say about how the child's educational program is supported outside the classroom and at home?
- How effective are the parents in their role as "case managers" and advocates for their child?
- Does the student have peers to communicate with directly? Or is the student isolated and depressed, and, if so, is academic performance being affected?
- What is the student's emotional state? Stress level?

- Is the acoustical environment causing too much noise interference?
- Are there other learning differences or secondary conditions to consider?
- Is the student's communication mode effective in providing the best access to instructional information?
- Does the student need assistive technology to better access communication at school? At home?
- Is it appropriate to keep a seventh-grade deaf or hard of hearing student with a 2-year language delay in the fifth grade?
- Is the curriculum being taught to the deaf or hard of hearing student the same as it is taught to hearing students? (This is particularly problematic for students who are not mainstreamed.)

The IEP Action Plan: Consideration given to academic performance level is critical. It motivates the relationship between IEP goals and grade-level, standards-based benchmarks through the general curriculum. Those goals must be

- Measurable and objective; nonsubjective
- Not based solely on "teacher observation"
- Tied to the general curriculum of same-aged hearing peers
- Driven by communication access, based on the student's mode
- Formulated for appropriate grade-level achievement
- Designed to "place" the student in the optimal learning environment
- Remedial as necessary, without compromising the student's in-class, instructional time with pull-out time
- Reflective of collaboration strategies between the special education providers and the general education teachers
- Supported with best practice strategies like preteach, teach, and reteach methods

Academic level is also an important consideration relative to program placement of the student. Is the child best served at the state's residence school for the deaf? Is a center-based program in the school district the setting most appropriate for the child's needs? Or will the team decide that the student can be placed in the neighborhood school? What are the parent's goals for the child relative to placement? Placement of the student raises many challenging issues in the case of students who are deaf or hard of hearing, and the student's personality and natural inclinations must be a priority consideration. Placement is further discussed later in this chapter under Least Restrictive Environment versus Language Rich Environment.

4. Full Range of Needs

All students experience life at school both academically and socially. Many deaf or hard of hearing students communicate differently than hearing kids or teachers, and often those differences create communication barriers that stymie fluid, fluent exchange. We work diligently through IEPs to ensure communication access to academic information, but what about social information?

Often deaf or hard of hearing kids miss out on important news conveyed through inferential, or passive, learning—the things we pick up by simply overhearing a conversation, announcement, or exchange that may not have been intentionally directed at us. Whether that exchange was between Mom and Dad discussing a new job offer, a teacher scolding a student for disrespectful behavior, or classmates who are all planning to wear red and white to the football game on Friday, there's a lot to be learned by knowing what's being said around us. Passive learning is a normal and requisite process in which humans learn acceptable social behavior.

The deaf or hard of hearing child who doesn't hear his or her peers changing the rules to the game they're playing at recess is out of step and may be seen as misbehaving for not following the rules. Someone tells a teacher. The teacher notes that this is the fourth complaint this month, and this must be communicated to the principal. The child is not perceived as a team player, or may be seen as mentally impaired, especially if the speaking voice sounds different or if the

child uses a lot of hand gestures. All too often the result is avoidance by peers. The child's self-confidence and motivation to attend school plummet. Any sense or expression of injustice is misunderstood and dismissed by others, and the principal perceives the child as a behavior problem.

Most gaps in the social learning experience for many students who are deaf or hard of hearing can be directly traced to a lack of exposure to inferential knowledge and passive learning. To consider the deaf or hard of hearing student's *full range of needs* is to ensure that there are strategies to ensure opportunities for social learning and self-esteem building. Beyond a strictly academic agenda, the IEP team's considerations should include but are not limited to the following:

- Does the student have friends at school?
- Is the student involved in extracurricular activities?
- Is there good communication access at school-sponsored extracurricular activities?
- How can we make sure that the student knows not only what the teacher is saying but also what questions the other students are asking?
- Is the child benefiting adequately from the communication mode or language he or she is using?
- Is the child showing signs of emotional stress or depression?
- Is the home life healthy and supportive?
- Is the student experiencing the same rewards and consequences of his or her actions as everyone else?
- Can a class project be created that will highlight the student's abilities?
- Can the student council reserve a seat for a student who is deaf or hard of hearing?

Full range of needs encompasses academic and social needs, and all the things related to supporting them that sometimes are overlooked in the typical IEP meeting:

- Communication access in art, music, physical education class, athletics (sports teams), hallways, playground, cafeteria, school office

- Counseling and health services
- Special interest groups or after school clubs
- Telephone, TTY access at school
- School assemblies
- Field trips
- Transportation staff
- Janitorial, school cafeteria staff

Depending on the discussion, the IEP action plan could call for the following:

- Words of music written down for choir
- Use of visual supplements
- Interpreters for field trips
- Bus drivers who sign
- Captioning on all movies
- TTY
- Blinking light for alarms/bells
- Carpeting in hallways
- Buddy system for the playground
- FM system hooked up to sound systems during assemblies
- Outdoor education trip, interpreter? FM system?

- Video monitors with schoolwide news and announcements captioned or interpreted "on air" and/or posted announcements
- Pager systems
- Take home FM system to support the IEP agenda at home

5. Direct Instruction in the Student's Communication Mode or Language

The values inherent in IDEA's directives about a deaf or hard of hearing student's full range of needs are also represented in its requirement to consider opportunities for direct instruction in the child's language and communication mode. For the same reasons that we recognize the value of direct communication with peers and professionals (see no. 2 of this section), we must also acknowledge the value of direct instruction.

Direct instruction means that a deaf child using ASL, for example, is taught by his or her teacher directly in ASL. There is no intervention from an interpreter or paraprofessional. When a child receives or expresses

---

Case Study 2–3: Direct Instruction   J.M. is 4 years old and is in a center-based preschool program for children with special needs. She has a severe/ profound hearing loss and gets good benefit from wearing two hearing aids. There are three other children with different degrees of hearing loss, and several children in the class with other "special needs," including two children who have autism. The program philosophy is to offer the SEE signing system.

Consider the opportunities for direct instruction in J.M.'s language and communication mode. Her parents are deaf, and she is at age-level language skills in ASL. J.M. is able to have some auditory function as well. Her parents are concerned that she be given the opportunity to use her native language, maintaining her family's value of deaf culture and community. J.M. has begun to learn to read at a very young age.

IEP Action Plan: What can the IEP team do to create opportunities for J.M. for direct instruction in her primary mode of communication? Because the center program uses SEE sign language, but J.M.'s sign system is ASL, the team must accommodate her language. In a neighboring school district, a charter school offers teachers who use ASL in direct instruction to students. J.M.'s team believes that would be the best placement for her, given that they cannot accommodate ASL within their own program. J.M. will have an opportunity to be with other children who use ASL. With transportation provided by her home school district, J.M. begins attending the ASL charter school, and her parents become an important resource for the deaf culture and community program there.

communication directly with a teacher in his or her own communication mode or method, the relationship between them is more natural, personalized, and productive. Both teacher and student invest more of themselves in the teaching/learning dynamic and its outcome. Both benefit from a greater understanding of each other's style and expectations. And there is no chance that the teaching is compromised by the intervention of an interpreter who may substitute vocabulary, or lack knowledge of the subject and unintentionally misrepresent it to the student. Direct communication has the highest potential for mutual comprehension and fewer misunderstandings, so its importance in a teacher/student interaction cannot be underestimated.

Least Restrictive Environment versus Language Rich Environment

The considerations for both full range of needs and direction instruction in the child's mode or language are significantly impacted by the legal issue of LRE from literal and theoretical perspectives.

IDEA requirements for LRE placement start with the assumption that the student should attend the school that he or she would normally attend if nondisabled (IDEA Sec. 300.550–551), with the greatest degree of exposure to "typical" peers. But case law expands the understanding of LRE as a physical place to LRE as a concept. In this context, LRE is a setting in which students will experience the LRE based on their individual needs. This issue is critical to deaf or hard of hearing students.

When both sections of the law—LRE and special consideration of students who are deaf or hard of hearing—are taken into account, the IEP team needs to be very clear about which setting will provide the most conducive atmosphere to communication access. Depending on the political climate where you live, the push for a "full inclusion" model may be strong or weak. In other words, if one part of the law is given more weight than another (LRE over special con-

siderations for deaf or hard of hearing), the placement issue of the student may not be in his or her individual best interests. IDEA Sec. 300.552(a) states that the placement decision is made by a group of persons, including the parents and other persons knowledgeable about the child, along with evaluation data and the placement options. Possible issues considered based on the individual needs of the student could include:

- What sort of placement would be ideal?
- Does the school district have a center-based program for deaf or hard of hearing students? What modes of communication does the center-based program accommodate?
- Where is the state school for the deaf? What is the school's philosophy? Is it in writing?
- What kind of services would need to be implemented for the student to attend a "home/neighborhood" school? What kind of itinerant services are available?
- What kinds of programs are available in neighboring school districts?
- How much opportunity will there be for the student to communicate directly with peers and professionals in his or her communication mode or language?

Depending on the discussion, the IEP action plan based on the needs/modes of communication of the individual student could include:

- Student placement outside the school district into another program
- Revision or creation of a new program within the district
- Family relocation to another town (this happens!)
- Open enrollment
- Itinerant services in home/neighborhood school
- Center-based program that fits the communication needs of the student
- Continuum of alternative placements Sec. 300.551 (regular classes, special classes, special schools, home instruction, and instruction in hospitals and institutions)

Case Study 2–4: Least Restrictive Environment   L.R. is 7 years old and received a cochlear implant 3 years ago. She lives with her family in the suburbs of a fairly large city. She has been placed in her school district's center-based program that has a total communication (TC) model (personnel both sign and speak during the academic day). In the past, L.R.'s family used some sign language with her, but her oral skills have progressed to a point where she rarely uses sign language for expressive or receptive input. Her parents feel very strongly that L.R. needs strong spoken language models during her day. She has very strong auditory skills and is not fluent in sign language. The teachers at the TC program have not had experience with children who use cochlear implants, and they strongly believe all children should use sign language. L.R. loves math and science and learns best with a hands-on approach. She has made friends at her center-based program but doesn't have any friends in her own neighborhood.

L.R. was placed appropriately in the center-based program at the age of 4, but now at the age of 7 her needs have changed. The school district is not large enough to provide a distinct "oral" program option, so they have tried to meet the needs of all deaf or hard of hearing kids in one center-based program. There are very few kids out in the "mainstream" in that district. The speech therapist in the TC program has never worked with a child with a cochlear implant and has decided to "treat her like a child with a hearing aid." L.R.'s parents feel she's ready to be moved back to her neighborhood school and be fully mainstreamed with intinerant support from an educator who has training in deaf education and cochlear implant habilitation. The special education director recently learned that there is a program in the neighboring district that serves four children with cochlear implants and has a national grant to model support for students with cochlear implants.

IEP Action Plan: The team reviews L.R.'s IEP and agrees that their program may no longer be the best placement for her. Her parents believe that the center-based program is placing restrictions on her potential with the cochlear implant. L.R.'s mode of communication has changed over the last few years, and so her needs have changed too. The team agrees with the parents that L.R. should return to her neighborhood school for exposure to listening and speaking peers and staff. But the professionals working with L.R. need to have some skills, expertise, and experience working with kids who have cochlear implants. Because their school personnel have no expertise with cochlear implants, the special education director from L.R.'s school district contacts the neighboring district's cochlear implant staff. They begin to collaborate on a plan that creates ongoing mentor-training and in-service for the itinerant teacher who will be serving L.R. at her home school. Their collaboration includes work with L.R.'s new general classroom teacher who must understand and implement accommodations appropriate for this new student with a cochlear implant.

- State school for the deaf
- Information on other programs in the nation

Assistive Technology Devices and Services

In addition to the communication considerations for the student who is deaf or hard of hearing under the special considerations section of the law, there is an additional component regarding the student's need for assistive technology devices and services. As defined by law:

(1) the term "assistive technology device" means any item, piece of equipment, or product system, whether acquired commercially off the shelf, modified, or customized, that is used to

increase, maintain, or improve functional capabilities of a child with a disability. (2) the term "assistive technology service" means any service that directly assists a child with a disability in the selection, acquisition, or use of an assistive technology device. Such term includes; (A) the evaluation of the needs of such child, including a functional evaluation of the child in the child's customary environment; (B) purchasing, leasing, or otherwise providing the acquisition of assistive technology devises by such child; (C) selecting, designing, fitting, customizing, adapting, applying, maintaining, repairing, or replacing of assistive technology devises; (D) coordinating and using other therapies, interventions, or services with assistive technology devices, such as those associated with existing education and rehabilitation plans and programs; (E) training or technical assistance for such child, or, where appropriate, the family of such child; and (F) training or technical assistance for professionals (including individuals providing education and rehabilitation services), employers, or other individuals who provide services to, employ, or are otherwise substantially involved in the major life functions of such child. (20 U.S.C. 1401)

In today's world, now more than ever, technology allows people with disabilities to be more independent. As technology has advanced for all of society, so has the technology that specifically benefits students who are deaf and hard of hearing. For many students, the use of assistive technology devices and services is a vital element for achieving FAPE.

Assistive Technology Devices

Hearing aids, personal and classroom sound field FM systems, TTYs, closed-captioned TV sets, alerting devices (flashing alarms) and other assistive technology, and acoustical modifications must be considered by the IEP team. It should be noted that the audiologist along with the IEP team should determine which type of assistive listening device, if any, is most appropriate to meet the educational needs of the individual student. Parents can provide input into the decision

but cannot demand a specific brand or type of equipment. However, there's a principle in law which basically recognizes that there is diversity in what communication accommodation will work best for each individual. Therefore, when an individual (in this case the family) requests a particular assistive technology device or service, a public entity "must honor the choice, unless it can demonstrate that another equally effective means of communication is available, or that use of the means chosen would result in a fundamental alteration in the service, program . . . " (Americans with Disabilities Act, 28 CSR Sec. 35.160 (B) (2))

Case Study 2–5: Assistive Technology, Devices, and Services   V.S. is a student with mild/moderate hearing loss. Her school is next to a busy highway. The heating system is over 20 years old and makes a lot of noise. A functional listening evaluation has shown that the impact of background noise reduces V.S.'s speech perception by over 50% when she is wearing hearing aids only. When an FM system is added, speech perception is raised to 84%. The audiologist takes an audiometer reading in the classroom showing the reverberation and signal-to-noise ratio is at unacceptable levels. The IEP team determines that the use of acoustical accommodations will narrow the gap to an appropriate level in order for V.S. to be provided with FAPE. Carpet is added to the room, as well as acoustically treated ceiling tiles.

For the student who is deaf or hard of hearing, the use of technology devices and the services needed to provide FAPE are vital components in a student's IEP.

Assistive Technology Services

Beyond the "devices" themselves, services must be provided to ensure the usability and functionality of assistive technology devices. As stated above in the law, these services provide the framework for the student to receive meaningful benefit from such devices. Training and technical assistance to the student, school personnel, employers, and families is provided for under this section. In the provision of FAPE for a student the school district is required to ensure proper functioning of hearing aids. Section 300.303 states that "each public agency shall ensure that the hearing aids worn in school by children with hearing impairments, including deafness, are functioning properly" (Individuals with Disabilities Act of 1997, 20 U.S.C. 1412 (a)(2)).

Summary

The spirit and words of IDEA are based on values which ensure that all children with disabilities have available to them a free appropriate public education including special education and related services designed to meet their unique needs and prepare them for employment and independent living. Further, IDEA's directives serve to ensure that educators and parents have the necessary tools to improve educational results for children with disabilities by supporting systemic-change activities, coordinated research and personnel preparation, coordinated technical assistance, dissemination, and support (Individuals with Disabilities Education Act of 1997, 20 U.S.C – 1400(d) (1)(A)(3)).

There is no reasonable or acceptable solution to educating students who are deaf and hard of hearing, except to demand high expectations of a communication-based system of education. A communication-based system will improve the educational experience of many students with disabilities, but for a student who is deaf or heard of hearing, it is imperative. It is time for parents, educators, and deaf or hard of hearing consumers to stand together and raise the bar of educational opportunity for deaf or hard of hearing students in the educational system. We must ensure that these students have access to a quality education through appropriate access to communication, as supported by the law to the extent that it currently exists.

But laws alone will not turn the tides in the wake of deaf and hard-of-hearing student underachievement. Higher expectations for performance must be realized through better teacher and parent training, more general education support, greater access to standards-based curriculum, and universally consistent application of best practices. Across the nation, there are examples of greatness. Students from all walks of life, using any and all versions of signed or spoken communication, are achieving academic and social success by all standards. Whatever combination of factors contribute to that achievement, at a foundational level, full and effective access to communication must be given the credit. Understanding what constitutes quality communication is the charge of every parent and professional working with deaf or hard of hearing students. Creating academic and social environments where deaf or hard of hearing kids can experience full access to communication is our duty. The message we send to all children who are deaf or hard of hearing must be that they deserve the right to understand and be understood, and to know that their own contribution is greatly valued by school and family.

References

Americans with Disabilities Act (ADA)—Title II Technical Assistance Manual, II–7.1100.

Bloomquist Traxler, C. (2000). The Stanford Achievement Test, ninth edition: National norming and performance standards for deaf and hard of hearing students. *Journal of Deaf Studies and Deaf Education, 5,* 337–348.

Baker-Hawkins, S., & Easterbrooks, S. (Eds.). (1994). *Deaf and Hard of Hearing Students: Educational Service Guidelines.* Alexandria, VA: National Association of State Directors of Special Education.

Individuals with Disabilities Education Act of 1997 (IDEA), 20 U.S.C. 1400 (d) (1)); (IDEA Sec. 300.550 (b) (1); (IDEA Sec. 300–346 (a) (2) (iv–v), 20 U.S.C – 1400 (d)(1)(A)(3).

U.S. Department of Education, Commission on Excellence in Special Education. (2002). Report of the Commission. p. 3.

U.S. Department of Education, Office of Special Education Programs (OSEP). (1992, October). Deaf Students Education Services Policy Guidance Report. *Fed Register, 57*, 49274–49276.

U.S. Department of Education. (2001). Final regulations for the assistance to states for the Education of Children with Disabilities Program under part B on the Individuals with Disabilities Education Act. *Fed Register, 66*, 1474–1478.

Yoshinaga-Itano, C., Coulter, D., Thomson, V. (2000). The Colorado Newborn Hearing Screening Project: Effects on speech and language development for children with hearing loss. *Journal of Perinatalogy, 20*, S132–S137.

SECTION II

Identification

3

Behavioral and Physiological Measures of Hearing: Principles and Interpretation

ROSS J. ROESER AND JACKIE L. CLARK

There are in fact two things, science and opinion; the former begets knowledge, the latter ignorance.

—Hippocrates, 460–377 B.C.

The Physical Bases of Hearing

Sound

Most people are aware that the human ear responds to sound, but few are familiar with the technical aspects and physical characteristics of sound. An understanding of both is prerequisite to a working knowledge of and the possible difficulties that an individual has with hearing loss.

There are four elements required for sound production (Fig. 3–1). (1) An object, or vibrator, must be set into motion by a force causing molecular displacement or disruption of air particles, whereupon vibration or the movement of molecules in the air creates sound. (2) Vibration, the back-and-forth movement, or oscillation, of molecular particles gives rise to a sound wave. (3)Vibrations require an elastic medium, typically the air in our environment, to propagate. This implies that if a vibrator were set into motion in a vacuum, the sensation of hearing would not occur because no medium exists to transmit the vibrations. (4) The three elements of vibration, force, and medium can create sound. However, simply causing the physical conditions needed for sound may not be enough. Some also believe that to create sound, the presence of a hearing mecha-

nism (i.e., an ear) is required. Thus, if a force should set air particles into motion that were carried by a medium but no (hearing) person perceived the vibrations, sound did not occur.

Frequency and Intensity

Two parameters that define the basic characteristics of sound are frequency and intensity.

FREQUENCY

The physical measurement of what is psychologically perceived as pitch is frequency. Frequency specifies the number of back-and-forth oscillations, or cycles, produced by a vibrator in a given time as a sound is created. The term used to describe frequency is "hertz" (Hz), and this term specifies the number of cycles that occur in 1 second. For example, if a vibrator (tuning fork) were set into motion and completed 1000 back-and-forth cycles in 1 second, it would have a frequency of 1000 Hz. Frequency and pitch are related in that, as the frequency of a sound increases, the listener perceives a tone of an increasingly higher pitch.

A sound can be made up of only one frequency or, as in most instances, of many different frequencies. The simplest acoustic sig-

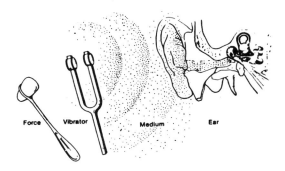

Figure 3–1. The four elements necessary for the production of sound.

nal is referred to as a pure tone and is created when only one frequency is present. In the example just given, the 1000 Hz vibrator was generating a pure tone because only one frequency occurred.

Pure tones do not exist in our everyday environment; they must be created electronically. However, pure tones are the basic acoustic signal used in auditory testing, primarily because they are the simplest form of sound to generate, the easiest to control, and, most important, they test the auditory system for frequency-specific problems.

Sounds we encounter in our everyday environment are complex and contain many different frequencies. The human ear responds to frequencies between 20 and 20,000 Hz. Frequencies that are below this range are infrasonic and those above this range, ultrasonic. For example, a sound with a frequency of 10 Hz is infrasonic and would not be perceived by the normal ear, and a sound with a frequency of 30,000 Hz is ultrasonic and would also not be perceived. Even though the ear responds to frequencies ranging from 20 to 20,000 Hz, frequencies primarily responsible for perceiving and understanding speech fall between 300 and 3000 Hz. This means that it would be possible for an individual to have essentially no hearing above 3000 Hz and have only marginal difficulty in speech understanding in a quiet environment. This observation is one reason why pure tones are important in assessing the auditory system.

In audiometric testing the standard frequencies evaluated range from 125 or 250 Hz through 8000 Hz. This frequency range is generally the most audible to the human ear and provides guidelines on how well the individual is able to perceive speech because the speech frequencies fall within this range. As part of a standard audiometric evaluation, pure tone thresholds are typically assessed at octave intervals and sometimes at half-octave intervals. Thus, the frequencies 250, 500, 1000, 2000, 4000, and 8000 Hz are routinely tested, and 750, 1500, 3000, and 6000 Hz are sometimes tested when additional information is warranted. However, it is becoming more customary to include 3000 and 6000 Hz in the standard audiometric evaluation, especially when hearing loss is present.

INTENSITY

The physical measurement of what is psychologically perceived as loudness is intensity. Intensity of a sound is determined by the amount of movement or displacement of air particles that occurs as a sound is created. As the amount of air particle displacement increases and becomes more intense, the sound becomes louder. Intensity is measured in units called decibels (dB), which literally means one tenth of a bell (named after Alexander Graham Bell). The decibel is technically defined as the logarithmic ratio between two magnitudes of pressure, or power.

As indicated by the technical definition, intensity is far more complicated than frequency, and to understand the decibel fully requires knowledge of advanced mathematical functions. The decibel is based on logarithmic function because the ear responds to a very large range of pressure changes, and logarithms allow these changes to be expressed by smaller numbers than would be required for a linear function. There are excellent references that the interested reader may consult for additional information on how to compute decibels using logarithms (Berlin, 1967).

Mathematical principles underlying the decibel are based on a logarithmic function and will not be covered in this chapter. However, a less difficult concept to understand is that the decibel is a relative unit of measurement. This means that simply saying, for example, 10 dB or 20 dB has no specific meaning without providing the reference for the measure. There are three decibel reference levels most often used in audiometric testing: sound pressure level (SPL), hearing level (HL), and sensation level (SL).

dB SPL. Perception of sound (hearing) occurs when pressure changes occur at the eardrum; the absolute pressure reference level for the decibel is dB SPL. The pressure reference used to determine dB SPL is 0.000204 dynes/cm², so 0 dB SPL is equal to a pressure force of 0.000204 dynes/cm², and 10 dB 20 dB SPL equals 10 or 20 dB above the 0.000204 dynes/cm² force. Because dB SPL is a physical measure, it is not affected by the frequencies present in sound. That is, 20 dB SPL is the same absolute pressure (20 dB SLP) irrespective of the frequency(ies) contained in the sound.

dB HL. The reference for the decibel used to express deviation from normal hearing sensitivity is dB HL. As will be pointed out later, the ear is not sensitive to all frequencies at the same intensity: hearing sensitivity changes as a function of the frequency of the sound (Fig. 3–2). Therefore, 0 dB HL represents an intensity equal to the threshold sensitivity of the normal ear at each frequency. Audiometers are calibrated in dB HL, so that any decibel value above 0 dB HL represents a deviation from normal hearing levels. For example, 25 dB HL is 25 decibels above the normal hearing threshold for that frequency.

In some instances, decibel hearing threshold level (HTL) will also be used. When dB HTL is used, it implies that the decibel value given was a measured threshold from a patient; that is, the value was an actual level obtained during threshold assessment.

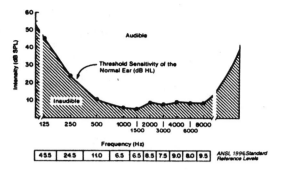

Figure 3–2. The threshold sensitivity of the normal ear as a function of frequency. The numbers at the bottom are the ANSI (1996) dB SPL values required to reach normal threshold sensitivity at each frequency.

dB SL. Individuals have their own threshold at each frequency, and dB SL uses the individual's threshold as a reference. For example, if a threshold of 20 dB HL is obtained at 1000 Hz, this value would represent 0 dB SL (threshold) for that individual. For this individual, an audiometric procedure using a presentation level of 30 dB SL means the audiometer intensity level would be 50 dB HL (20 dB HL = 0 dB SL + 30 dB SL = 50 dB HL). Despite variations in the threshold values between individuals or frequencies tested, dB SL allows for the presentation of stimuli at the same intensity above threshold.

Frequency and Intensity Function of the Human Ear

As described earlier, the ear responds to different absolute intensities, or different SPLs, as a function of frequency. Stated another way, it takes different intensities (SPLs) to reach the level at which the normal ear will perceive the sound (threshold level) at different frequencies. Figure 3–2 illustrates the threshold sensitivity function of the normal ear and gives the 1996 American National Standards Institute (ANSI) levels required to reach threshold at each frequency for normal ears (0 dB HL). As shown in Figure 3–2, the ear is most sensitive in frequencies around 1000 to 1500 Hz. Because audiometers are calibrated in dB HL, it is not necessary to know the absolute dB SPL/HL difference at each frequency. The audiometer automatically corrects for the dB SPL/HL difference as the frequency is changed; 0 dB HL represents the intensity in dB SPL at which the normal listener will perceive each frequency presented (threshold).

The Audiometer and Audiometry

The Audiometer

An audiometer is technically defined as an electronic device that generates signals used to assess hearing. There are various types of audiometers available from numerous manufacturers that vary from the simple screening to comprehensive diagnostic instruments. Signals in these audiometers can be generated from pure tones to more complex stimuli for comprehensive testing.

Basic Functions

Audiometers were first designed to generate the same frequencies as those produced by tuning forks; for example, 256, 512, and 1024 Hz. However, audiometer manufacturers have now standardized their instruments using a scale based on even thousands of Hertz. Therefore, audiometers today generate at least all of the following test frequencies: 250, 500, 750, 1000, 1500, 2000, 2500, 3000, 4000, 6000, and 8000 Hz.

Several models of audiometers with limited versatility have been recommended for screening. Concepts specific to screening audiometry are discussed in Chapter 5. Diagnostic audiometers provide, in addition to pure tones, a speech circuit and are designed to allow an audiologist to perform a variety of special diagnostic (site of lesion) auditory tests inside a commercially built, sound-treated room. Diagnostic audiometers are generally found in clinical or medical settings and are not usually available in the school setting.

Regardless of the make or model, all pure tone audiometers have certain basic controls and switches to perform the same basic functions. Despite the diversity found in commercially available audiometers, external controls and parts of the instruments are similar (Fig. 3–3). For school screening the child should be readily observable by the tester, but to prevent false responses the examiner should be out of the child's peripheral vision. Figure 3–3 (bottom) shows correct placement of the audiometer and how the examiner should be seated in relation to the child during screening.

Some functions of each of the basic components found on all audiometers include the power supply, power switch, hearing level dial, frequency selector dial, output selector switch, tone interrupter and tone reverse switch, masking dial, bone conduction oscillator, and earphones.

Power Supply. Power can be delivered to audiometers equipped with standard three-pronged plugs for 120 volt power, or with battery power in some portable screening audiometers. Battery-powered instruments are desirable because they can be used when power outlets are unavailable. However, the current drain may vary, resulting in great variability in the output of the test stimuli from battery-powered audiometers.

On-Off or Power Switch (1 in Fig. 3–3). After the audiometer has been plugged in, it should be turned on and allowed to warm up for approximately 10 minutes prior to testing. This procedure assures that the proper current has reached all parts of the instrument for optimal functioning. When testing is expected to continue for a number of hours, the audiometer should remain in the "on" position because turning it on and off several times during the day causes more wear on the electrical components..

Attenuator or Hearing Level Dial (2 in Fig. 3–3). This dial controls the intensity of the stimuli. The attenuator is actually a group of resistors built into the output circuit to control the intensity in small steps. Most attenuators are designed to operate in 5 dB steps, with a range of 0 to 110 dB HL for air conduction testing and 0 dB HL to as much as 70

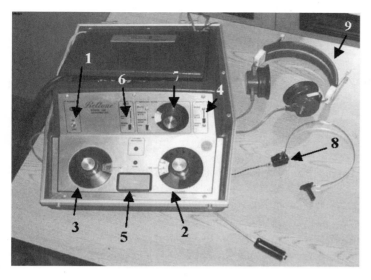

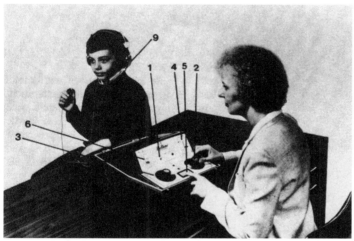

Figure 3–3. Components of two commercially available audiometers (see text for description). (Bottom, courtesy of Beltone Electronics.)

dB HL for bone conduction testing, depending on frequency. The maximum output for each frequency is specified on the frequency selector dial.

Frequency Selector Dial (3 in Fig. 3–3). The frequency selector allows stimuli to be varied in discrete steps from 125 to 8000 Hz in octave and half-octave intervals. As already mentioned, the frequency selector dial also shows, by use of smaller numerals on the dial, the maximum output (dB HL or dB HTL) that the audiometer is capable of producing at each test frequency.

Output Selector Switch (4 in Fig. 3–3). The output selector delivers test signals to the right earphone, left earphone, or bone conduction oscillator, or, in the case of diagnostic audiometers, through loudspeakers. The output selector switch determines which of these devices is activated.

Tone Interrupter (5 in Fig. 3–3) and Tone Reverse Switch (6 in Fig. 3–3). These can be either a button, bar, or lever used to present or interrupt the test stimuli, depending on the position of the tone reverse switch, and can allow the tone to be "normally on" or "normally off." In the normally on position, the tone is turned off by depressing the tone interrupter. In the normally off position, the tone is presented by depressing the tone interrupter. In audiometric testing the tone reverse switch should always be in the normally off position. Serious errors can result if the tone reverse switch is in the normally on position. The normally on position is used only during calibration and for special audiometric tests not performed as part of screening.

Masking Dial (7 in Fig. 3–3).   This can be used in instances when a masking sound must be applied to the nontest ear to ensure that crossover of the test signal is not occurring. The masking dial controls the level of the masking signal noise. Masking is an advanced skill used in diagnostic audiometry.

Bone Conduction Oscillator (8 in Fig. 3–3). The bone conduction oscillator is used to obtain threshold measures of bone conduction sensitivity. Bone conduction testing is a diagnostic procedure and should not be performed as part of routine screening unless specifically designed and supervised by an audiologist. The capability to perform bone conduction tests is not necessary in audiometers used in screening programs.

Earphones (9 in Fig. 3–3).   Earphones are secured in either a standard headband or foam plugs and transmit test tones to each ear individually according to a standardized color code: red for the right ear and blue for the left ear. Important points regarding earphones in general include: (1) earphones are calibrated to one specific audiometer and should always be considered an integral part of that particular instrument; (2) earphones should never be interchanged between audiometers unless the equipment is recalibrated; and (3) the tension of the headband, resiliency of the earphone cushions, and proper insertion of the foam plugs are important factors for reliable test results.

The standard audiometer earphone consists of a driver mounted in a supra-aural (MX-41/AR) noise excluding cushion (Fig. 3–4). Two other types of noise-excluding cushions, the circumaural cushion, and the combined (circumaural/supra-aural) cushion, attenuate ambient noise more effectively than the standard supra-aural cushions. Although supra-aural cushions are standard equipment on many audiometers, noise-excluding earphone cushions have been suggested for use in screening because they reduce (attenuate) ambient noise more effectively than the standard MX-41/AR cushion (Fig. 3–5). This feature implies that accurate tests may be performed in the presence of higher background noise levels. Research, however, has shown that there is no advantage for using the circumaural cushion in audiometry, due to the excessive volume created by incomplete coupling of the driver to the pinna (Roeser, Seidel, & Glorig, 1975). Due to size and complexity, noise-excluding earphones are also considered more difficult to use and have not been endorsed for general use in hearing screening in the schools.

Another type, insert earphones, which insert directly into the earcanals with a foam plug (Fig. 3–6), consist of two rectangular plastic cases containing the transducers that are coupled with plastic tubing to each foam plug. Insert earphones are especially helpful in performing threshold testing for children who fail the pure tone sweep-check screening. Those using this type of earphone must learn to insert the foam tip into the earcanal properly to achieve the maximum attenuation of background noise and reduce the false-positive identifications (Clark & Roeser, 1988). Some distinct advantages of insert-type earphones include: (1) better attenuation of external noise in the environment than with the standard earphones, which results in more accurate testing outside sound-treated rooms; (2) increased interaural attenuation leading to less of a problem of crossover to the nontest ear when unilateral hearing loss is present; (3) elimination of earcanal collapse created by the supra-aural cushions pressing down on the pinna; and (4) increased patient comfort.

A = Electro-Acoustic Driver
B = Supra-Aural Cushion (MX - 41/AR)
C = Resilient Cushion
D = Circumaural Done
E = Foam Filled Cavity
F = Enclosed Volume of Air

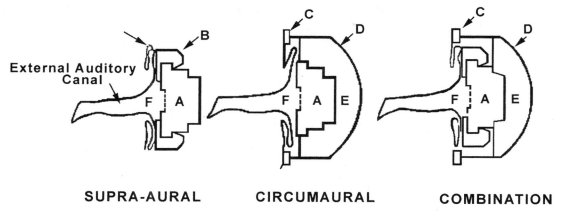

Figure 3–4. Schematic showing the components of a supra-aural earphone cushion, a circumaural cushion, and a combination-type (circumaural/supra-aural) cushion. (Reprinted with permission from Musket and Roeser, 1977).

Audiometer Calibration

Calibration is the process by which electronic equipment is checked and adjusted to ensure it meets minimum expected requirements set by established standards. Over the past 50+ years, five standards have been used to define operating characteristics for audiometers, including the absolute SPL levels (referred to as reference equivalent threshold sound pressure levels) at which the normal ear responds as a function of frequency: (1) the American Standards Association (ASA), adopted in 1951 (AMA, 1951); (2) the International Standards Organization (ISO), adopted in 1961 (ANSI, 1964); (3) the American National Standards Institute (ANSI), first adopted in 1969 (ANSI, 1970); and (4) revised in 1989 (ANSI, 1989) and (5) revised again in 1996 (ANSI, 1996). At present, all audiometers should conform to the 1996 ANSI standard. The ANSI S3.6–1996 can be obtained for a fee by writing to the American National Standards Institute at 25 W. 43rd Street, 4th Floor, New York, NY 10036, or the Acoustical Society of America at Suite 1N01, 2 Huntington Quadrangle, Melville, NY 11747–4502. Although not mandatory, it may prove to be helpful to those who test in the schools to have the standard if the school system has the basic equipment, such as a sound-level meter, necessary for electronic calibration.

Older studies have documented the unfortunate finding that audiometers used for school hearing screening often do not perform according to standards. For example, Walton and Wilson (1972) found that 82% of the 50 audiometers used in the schools had one or more calibration problems that could have interfered with test results. Problems with mechanical conditions, internal noise, intensity levels, attenuator linearity, and frequency accounted for the major errors. Audiometers today should be more durable and less variable in their performance because the electronic components incorporate integrated circuits and microchips. How-

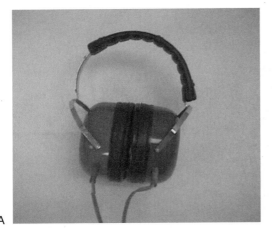

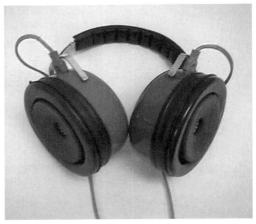

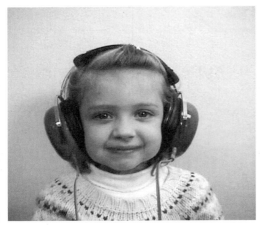

Figure 3–5. (A) A combination-type noise-excluding earphone system. Note in (B) that a standard cushion is contained within the plastic enclosure that surrounds the pinna. (C) Shows how they are placed on the child.

ever, recent data from field studies on more modern equipment are lacking.

Every user of an audiometer is responsible for checking the equipment regularly and ensuring that proper calibration is performed. There are four types of check/calibration schedules. These include a daily listening check, a monthly biological calibration check, a periodic electronic calibration (yearly), and an exhaustive electronic calibration (every 5 years).

Daily Listening Check

Prior to using the audiometer each day, and following an appropriate warm-up time (5 to 10 minutes), the tester should listen to the signal emitted from the audiometer at various intensities and at all frequencies for unwanted noise, transient clicks, or distortions in the signal. The tester should also determine that the signal is in the correct earphone. It is far better to discover a malfunction in the equipment at the beginning of testing than to face inappropriate referrals.

Biological Calibration Check

Each month that the audiometer is in use, a biological calibration check is required on at least one subject whose hearing threshold is known. The procedure involves obtaining baseline threshold measurements on three to

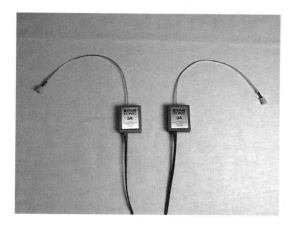

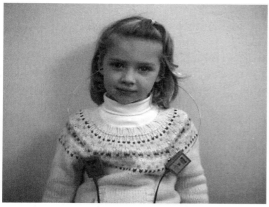

Figure 3–6. Etymotic, model ER3A, insert earphones. The top photograph shows the components of the system (see text for description), and the bottom photograph shows how they are placed on a child.

five individuals with normal hearing who will be available for comparison testing throughout the year. If on the monthly check, a threshold difference greater than 5 dB HL is found for one of the individuals for any test frequency between 500 and 6000 Hz, then the other subjects should be checked. If a shift greater than 5 dB in the same direction is confirmed by the additional biological checks, an electronic calibration of the audiometer is required. The results from each monthly biological calibration check should be recorded on a form that is kept in a calibration file maintained for each audiometer.

Periodic Electronic Calibration

At least once a year, every audiometer should have an electronic calibration to ensure that it meets the minimum standards defined by ANSI S3.6–1996. This service is provided by electronic or acoustic firms using specialized equipment. If it is necessary to ship the audiometer to another location for calibration, it should be packed carefully so that the instrument will be protected from damage in transit. As soon as the audiometer is returned from calibration or repair, the user should perform a biological check to reestablish new baseline threshold records on subjects, as just described.

Exhaustive Electronic Calibration

Every 5 years, each audiometer must have an exhaustive electronic calibration. This calibration is more comprehensive than the periodic electronic calibration and includes the testing of all settings on the frequency and intensity (HL/HTL) dials, as well as replacing switches, cords, and earphone drivers and cushions.

Basic Audiometric Tests

Pure tone and speech stimuli are used to perform routine audiometric testing, as well as diagnostic procedures as described below:

Pure Tone Audiometry

Pure tone stimuli are used to obtain air conduction and bone conduction thresholds and results are displayed on a pure tone audiogram. The term "threshold" is used to define the lowest or least intense level at which the individual being tested responds to the signal presented in a given number of trials; usually defined as two of four or three of six (50%). Standard psychophysical procedures have been developed for use in threshold assessment (Carhart & Jerger, 1959). Speech stimuli are used in obtaining speech reception/recognition thresholds (or spondee thresholds), and speech recognition scores. Results from speech testing are typically recorded in a table next to the pure tone audiogram.

Pure tone air conduction audiometry involves the measurement of auditory sensitivity using specific pure tones presented to the listener through standard or insert earphones, described earlier in this chapter. Pure tones are used for threshold testing and for screening (Chap. 5), and provide information regarding the differential effects of disorders in the inner ear.

Pure tone bone conduction audiometry is a diagnostic procedure in which thresholds are established in much the same manner as for air conduction thresholds. However, instead of using earphones, a single bone conduction oscillator, secured in a standard headband (see 8 in Fig. 3–3), is placed behind the ear on the mastoid bone or on the forehead. When the bone conduction oscillator is activated it sets the bones of the entire skull into motion, thus stimulating both inner ears (cochlea). Because both cochlea are stimulated simultaneously, the response obtained will reflect the auditory sensitivity of the cochlea with the lowest (best) thresholds, when one ear has better hearing. Thus, in bone conduction testing it is frequently necessary to mask the ear not being tested when a hearing loss is present. The addition of bone conduction thresholds allows the examiner to establish the type of hearing loss (conductive, sensorineural, or mixed) described in later sections.

Speech Audiometry

Many individuals first become aware that they have a hearing loss when their ability to detect and understand speech becomes impaired. Pure tone measurements only give limited information concerning communication difficulties. The purpose of speech audiometry is to quantify communication ability.

In standard speech audiometry, words can either be spoken into a microphone (monitored live voice presentation) or delivered using recorded presentation (tape or com-

pact disc) with the output signal regulated by the audiometer. While wearing earphones, the listener is instructed to repeat the test words, and one ear is tested at a time. Several standardized age-specific tests have also been developed using picture-pointing responses as well as written or spoken responses. Using these basic procedures, the threshold for speech and the ability to understand speech sounds is measured.

"Speech recognition threshold" (SRT) is currently the preferred term for measuring the threshold for speech, rather than "speech reception threshold," which was used for many years (ASHA, 1988). The SRT is a measure of auditory threshold sensitivity for speech routinely obtained using spondee words, which are compound or bisyllabic words, such as "railroad," "toothbrush," and "outside," presented with equal stress on both syllables. The purpose of the SRT is to validate pure tone thresholds, as well as set a reference level for speech recognition testing.

The SRT should be in agreement with thresholds that fall within the primary frequencies used for speech intelligibility (300 to 3000 Hz). Three octave frequencies tested within the 300 to 3000 Hz range, 500, 1000, and 2000 Hz, are used to calculate the pure tone average (PTA). For example, if thresholds are 60, 75, and 80 dB HL at 500, 1000, and 2000 Hz, the PTA would be 72 dB HL. One sign of patient reliability is seen with an agreement within 8 to 6 dB between the SRT and PTA (Hopkinson, 1978). In the preceding example, the SRT should be 64 to 78 dB HL, or within 5 dB of the 72 dB average, rounded to the nearest 5 dB increment (65 to 75 dB).

In some cases, when there is a large difference in one of the three frequencies, only two frequencies are used to calculate the PTA (Fletcher, 1950). If the PTA and SRT are not in close agreement, it suggests that the listener may not understand the task or may not be fully cooperating with the testing (pseudohypoacusis).

When hearing loss is in the severe to profound range, and speech recognition is very poor, a speech threshold to spondee words may not be obtainable. In such cases a speech detection threshold (SDT), sometimes referred to as a speech awareness threshold (SAT), is obtained. Rather than an SRT, the SDT simply quantifies the lowest level at which speech is detected. It would be expected that an agreement between SDT and the pure tone audiogram should be within 5 to 10 dB of the best (lowest) threshold on the audiogram. However, the SDT may also be influenced by the threshold at 125 Hz and, although this frequency is not routinely tested, it should be when the SDT does not agree with the pure tone audiogram.

The speech recognition score was originally referred to as a "speech discrimination test" until a suggestion was made to change the terminology to reflect the testing procedures more accurately, because in "discrimination" tasks individuals are asked to judge whether two stimuli are the same or different (Konkle & Rintelmann, 1983). Traditional tests use standardized, phonetically or phonemically balanced lists of single syllable (monosyllabic) words. "Phonetically/phonemically balanced" indicates that the distribution of phonetic elements in the lists approximates the distribution found in everyday conversation. Tests are increasingly being developed to use sentences, rather than words. To be more precise, many clinicians use the term "word recognition score" when words are used and "sentence recognition score" when sentences are used.

Speech recognition scores are calculated in percentage correct; a score of 100% means that all speech stimuli were recognized correctly. The following is a general guide for interpreting most standard speech discrimination test scores (Goetzinger, 1978):

90 to 100%—within the range of normal
75 to 90%—slight difficulty
60 to 75 %—moderate difficulty
50 to 60%—poor discrimination

An important procedural consideration is that, due to the high variability in data obtained when monitored live voice presentation is used for speech recognition testing,

standard clinical practice should use only recorded presentation. It is unfortunate that surveys of audiological practice have found that most audiologists continue to use monitored live voice presentation for speech recognition testing (Martin, Champlin, & Chambers, 1998). This practice needs to be changed!

The Audiogram

The audiogram is a graph or grid on which audiometric data are displayed. Many clinics use an audiogram to record their data, but some prefer to use a tabular form to record audiometric findings on a standard graphic audiogram and a tabular form (Fig. 3–7).

Clinics have used a wide variety of symbols and symbol systems to record results on audiograms; the diversity allows for confusion and misinterpretation, especially when records are exchanged between clinics (Martin & Kopra, 1970). Because of the possibility for misinterpretation, as illustrated in Figure 3–7, the American Speech and Hearing Association (ASHA) has developed a standard audiogram format and symbol system (Fig. 3–8) for audiograms (ASHA, 1990a). In constructing an audiogram, it is recommended that one octave on the frequency scale be equivalent in span to 20 dB on the HL scale. In addition, grid lines of equal darkness and thickness should appear at octave intervals on the frequency scale and at 10 dB intervals on the intensity scale. ASHA guidelines also recommend that, when "no response" is obtained at the maximum output of the audiometer, an arrow be attached to the lower outside corner of the appropriate symbol about 45 degrees outward from the frequency axis, pointing to the right for left ear symbols and to the left for right ear symbols.

Sound field tests are noted on the audiogram by placing the symbol "S" on the audiogram form. Sound field tests utilize one or two loudspeakers rather than earphones, and when unilateral hearing loss is present, thresholds represent sensitivity of the better ear only. When the presence of unilateral hearing loss is unknown, one must assume

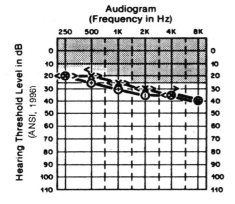

		RIGHT EAR				LEFT EAR				Sound Field
Freq.	AC	Mask	BC	Mask	AC	Mask	BC	Mask	
250	20		20		20		20		
500	25		15		20		20		
750									
1000	30		25		25		25		
1500									
2000	35		30		30		30		
3000									
4000	35		35		35		30		
6000									
8000	40				40				

Figure 3–7. Compares the same pure tone audiometric findings on a standard graphic audiogram form (left) and a grid-type form (right)

that the thresholds reflect only the sensitivity of the better ear, and thresholds under earphones must be obtained to complete the evaluation.

Because of potential confusion from using different symbol systems, audiograms should follow the ASHA guidelines. It is also important that the symbol system be used, and an explanation of any notations used should appear in a legend on the audiogram form.

Audiometric Interpretation

TYPES OF HEARING LOSS
AND AUDITORY DISORDERS

Three classical types of hearing loss can be identified with pure tone air and bone conduction tests: conductive, sensorineural, and mixed. Figure 3–9 illustrates the difference between these types of hearing loss based on the anatomic site involved. Classifications of auditory disorders require more advanced diagnostic procedures, and physiological measures include pseudohypoacusis (referred to as functional, nonorganic, or psychogenic hearing loss); auditory neuropathy (auditory dys-synchrony); and APDs.

Conductive Hearing Loss. This is by far the most common type of hearing loss found in school children and literally means that part or all of the mechanical conducting components of the auditory mechanism are

inefficient. These mechanical components of the auditory mechanism include the pinna, external earcanal, eardrum, middle ear ossicles and muscles, and middle ear cavity (Fig. 3–9). A purely conductive hearing impairment assumes no disorders of the inner ear (cochlea) or the auditory nerve.

Congenital anomalies of the outer ear may cause conductive hearing loss. However, most conductive loss acquired in childhood is the result of serous otitis media, an inflammation of the middle ear cavity accompanied by fluid (Northern & Downs, 2002). Impacted earwax (cerumen), perforated eardrum, and otosclerosis, a spongylike growth originating on the footplate of the stapes, are other common etiologies for conductive hearing loss.

Figure 3–10 presents the audiometric pattern for conductive loss, with thresholds for normal bone conduction and abnormal air conduction. In addition, with conductive hearing loss, immittance measures (described later) are most likely abnormal. Individuals with conductive hearing loss will demonstrate normal speech recognition ability when the signal is sufficiently loud. Moreover, speech production may be soft because individuals hear their own voices as louder than normal, due to an "occlusion effect" resulting from a "plugged" ear. Fortunately, with a conductive hearing loss, spontaneous recovery is frequent, or the loss can

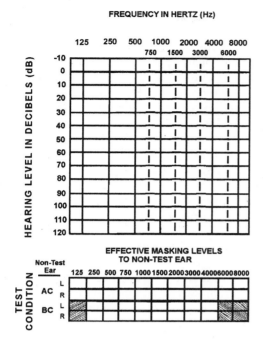

Response

MODALITY	EAR		
	LEFT	UNSPECIFIED	RIGHT
AIR CONDUCTION-EARPHONES			
UNMASKED	✗		○
MASKED	☐		△
BONE CONDUCTION-MASTOID			
UNMASKED	>	∧	<
MASKED	]		[
BONE CONDUCTION-FOREHEAD			
UNMASKED		∨	
MASKED	⌐		¬
AIR CONDUCTION-SOUND FIELD	✗	S	∅
ACOUSTIC-REFLEX THRESHOLD			
CONTRALATERAL		⋎	⊣
IPSILATERAL		⊤	⋏

Figure 3–8. Example audiogram form (top), showing approriate dimensions, and audiometric symbols (bottom) recommended by the American Speech and Hearing Association. Note that on the audiogram form 20 dB on the ordinate equals 1 octave on the abcissa.

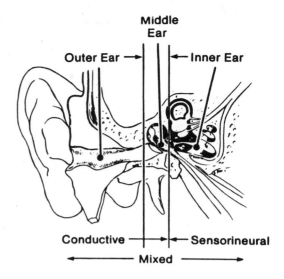

Figure 3–9. The three types of hearing loss classified according to anatomic site involved.

be reversed through either or both medical and surgical treatment.

Sensorineural Hearing Loss. Pathological changes in the inner ear or along the nerve pathway from the inner ear to the brainstem can cause sensorineural hearing lost. The inner ear contains the cochlea and sensory receptors or hair cells located on the basilar membrane, a structure within the cochlea.

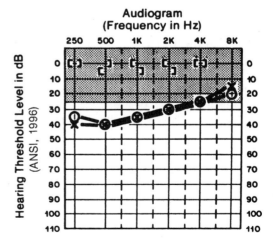

Figure 3–10. Pure tone air and bone conduction pattern for conductive hearing loss.

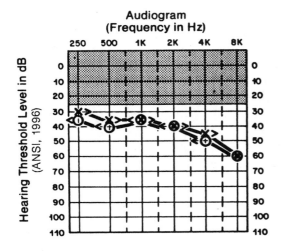

Figure 3–11. Pure tone air and bone conduction pattern for sensorineural hearing loss.

Hair cells transmit information to nerve fibers and the information is then fed to the temporal lobe of the brain via the eighth cranial nerve and auditory pathway. A pure sensorineural impairment exists when the sound conducting mechanism (outer and middle ear) is normal in every respect, but a disorder is present in the cochlea or auditory nerve, or both.

One example of a pure tone audiometric pattern for sensorineural hearing loss is shown in Figure 3–11. With sensorineural hearing loss, air and bone conduction thresholds are both elevated and within 10 dB of each other. Immittance measures of the tympanogram and static admittance (compliance), described later, are normal, and acoustic reflexes may be present, elevated, or absent, depending on the degree and etiology of the hearing loss.

Causes of sensorineural hearing impairment can be congenital (prior to or at birth) or acquired after birth. Congenital sensorineural hearing loss may result from hereditary factors, which cause underdevelopment or early degeneration of the auditory nerve, in utero viral infections, or birth trauma. Acquired sensorineural loss may be caused by factors such as noise exposure, acoustic tumor, head injury, or toxic effects of certain drugs. In virtually all cases, sensorineural hearing loss is not amenable to medical or surgical treatment.

Several symptoms characteristic of sensorineural hearing loss are shouting or talking in a loud voice, poor word recognition ability, and recruitment. Shouting or speaking in a loud voice may occur with sensorineural loss because the impaired person does not have normal hearing by bone conduction. Hence those with sensorineural hearing loss do not hear their own voice or other voices normally and may have difficulty regulating voice intensity level. Not all persons with sensorineural hearing loss speak loudly and not all with conductive loss speak softly; many learn to regulate their voice level appropriately.

Degradation in speech recognition is frequently associated with sensorineural hearing loss due to distortion of the speech signal caused by nerve fiber loss. A typical sensorineural hearing loss is characterized by better hearing in the low frequencies than in the high frequencies. Consonants contain high-frequency information, and vowels are predominantly low in frequency. Therefore, consonant sounds may be easily confused or not heard at all. Shouting at the individual with sensorineural loss may result only in agitation rather than improved comprehension because the person may be able to hear voices but not be able to understand the words.

The third symptom of sensorineural hearing impairment, recruitment, refers to a rapid growth in loudness once the threshold of hearing has been crossed. After the signal is intense enough to be perceived, any further increase in intensity may cause a disproportionate increase in the sensation of loudness. Because of recruitment and word recognition difficulty, individuals with sensorineural hearing loss experience difficulty in speech recognition in noisy surroundings. The presence of recruitment is a diagnostic finding that the site of the hearing loss is in the cochlea.

Mixed Hearing Loss. This type of hearing loss occurs when a significant conductive impairment is superimposed on a sensorineural hearing loss. Causes of mixed hear-

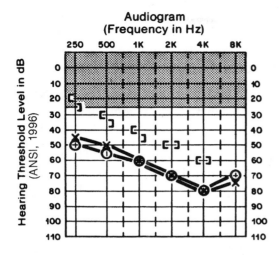

Figure 3–12. Pure tone air and bone conduction pattern for mixed hearing loss.

ing loss may be any combination of the causes described previously for conductive and sensorineural hearing loss. The conductive component of the mixed hearing loss may be amenable to medical treatment, but the sensorineural component is not reversible. Figure 3–12 shows audiometric data depicting a mixed hearing loss. With mixed hearing loss, air conduction and bone conduction thresholds are elevated, but bone conduction thresholds are better than air conduction thresholds by 10 dB or more.

Pseudohypoacusis. Also referred to as functional, nonorganic, or psychogenic hearing loss, "pseudohypoacusis" literally means false (pseudo), abnormally low (hypo) hearing (acusis). An audiological diagnosis of pseudohypoacusis is made when an individual claims to have a hearing loss, but discrepancies in audiometric test findings and behavior suggest that the loss does not exist or does not exist to the degree that is indicated by voluntary test results.

Several factors may explain causes for pseudohypoacusis. Some believe that emotional stress may lead an individual to unconsciously develop a "hearing loss" as a protective device or an escape from what seems to be an intolerable situation. Another motive for pseudohypoacusis may be pecu-

niary, and the individual may be well aware of the true status of auditory sensitivity. Whenever pseudohypoacusis is found in children, referral to a professional family counselor should be made to investigate the motives behind the need for feigning the loss of hearing.

Auditory Neuropathy. This is a recently discovered auditory disorder that involves an abnormal dysfunction of timing in the auditory system (Berlin, Hood, Hurley, & Wen, 1994; Starr, Picton, Sininger, Hood, & Berlin, 1996). Because the disorder involves a timing dysfunction, some believe the term "auditory dys-synchrony" better reflects the nature of the behavioral manifestations. It is believed that the underlying basis of auditory neuropathy is due to poor synaptic transmission between the inner hair cells of the cochlea and spiral ganglion within the auditory nerve to the brainstem. The result of such a problem is a lack of synchronous activity in the auditory nerve (Stein et al, 1996).

Symptoms of auditory neuropathy (dys-synchrony) include the following: the absence of auditory brainstem responses (ABRs) despite having adequate pure tone thresholds, indicating poor auditory neural function; the presence of otoacoustic emissions (OAEs), indicating the presence of normal outer hair cell function in the cochlea; and speech recognition abilities poorer than expected when compared with pure tone findings (Sininger & Oba, 2001). Pure tone thresholds can vary from normal hearing to mild to profound hearing loss. Parents and caregivers describe children with auditory neuropathy as having varying levels of difficulty with speech understanding, especially in noise—reports will vary from functionally deaf to relatively intact speech perception in quiet (Kraus, 2001).

Onset of auditory neuropathy can occur anytime from birth to adulthood, with the largest group showing symptoms prior to their second birthday. It appears that there is a fairly even gender distribution with slightly more males than females. There appears to be a genetic link for this disorder, but some patients (27%) have no apparent associated medical or family history (Sininger & Oba, 2001). Some of the neonatal risk factors, genetic predisposition, or syndromes associated with the disorder include hyperbilirubinemia toxemia; hereditary sensory-motor neuropathy (Charcot-Marie-Tooth, Type I or II); Freidreich's ataxia; Stevens-Johnson syndrome; Ehlers-Danlos syndrome, or Usher's syndrome.

Management of children with auditory neuropathy varies considerably, due to the heterogeneous and, at times uncertain, nature of the disorder. Foremost, referral of young children to educational programs emphasizing the visual communication modality is recommended. About half the children with auditory neuropathy and significant hearing loss appear to benefit from hearing aids. Those with severe-to-profound hearing loss who do not benefit from hearing aids appear to have success with cochlear implants.

Auditory Processing Disorder. APD occurs when children or adults are unable to utilize the auditory information they receive. An ASHA Task Force on "Central" Auditory Processing (1995) and a later UTD/Callier Center Consensus Conference (Jerger & Musiek, 2000) identified specific deficits that may occur individually or together in children having APD as sound localization and lateralization, auditory discrimination, auditory pattern recognition, temporal aspects of audition, auditory performance with competing acoustic signals, and auditory performance with degraded acoustic signals. Research provides evidence of neuromaturational and neuroplasticity differences between children and adults with normal and disordered auditory processing (Chermak & Musiek, 1997; Jirsa, 1994; Musiek, Baran, & Pinheiro, 1994). It is presumed that those who are diagnosed with APD have neurophysiological with concomitant behavioral manifestations affecting the auditory system. More males than females have auditory processing difficulties, possibly due to relatively more ge-

netic variability (Arcia & Connors, 1998). Generally, children with APD respond inconsistently to auditory stimuli, may listen attentively but have difficulty following simple or complex commands, frequently ask for information to be repeated, and have poor listening skills (Keith, 2000). Unfortunately, these behaviors are not unique to auditory processing behaviors; they can be exhibited by children having hearing loss, attention deficit disorder, allergies, or other problems. To determine the nature of such behaviors, there is a need for a complete diagnostic audiological evaluation, including auditory processing testing. The diagnosis and treatment of children with APDs are covered in Chapters 6 and 17.

DEGREE OF HEARING LOSS

Once a hearing loss has been identified, it becomes necessary to classify it according to the degree of difficulty experienced by the individual. The term "deaf," although sometimes used by nonprofessionals to refer to all persons who have a hearing impairment, is technically reserved for the individual with hearing loss whose auditory mechanism is so severely impaired that only a few or none of the prosodic and phonetic elements of speech can be recognized. Individuals who are deaf must rely mainly or entirely on speech reading or other forms of visual receptive communication for the perception of language (Boothroyd, 1988). Few individuals with hearing loss would be classified as being deaf under this definition.

On the other hand, the term "hard of hearing" refers to an individual with hearing loss who can identify enough of the distinguishing features of speech through hearing alone to permit at least partial recognition of spoken language. With the addition of the visual system, individuals with hearing loss may understand even more language, provided the vocabulary and syntax are within the linguistic code.

Although it is difficult to draw firm boundaries between individuals who are deaf and those who are hard of hearing on the basis of the loss demonstrated by pure tone findings alone, the following classification, based on the PTA (500, 1000, and 2000 Hz) is a general guide to the degree of hearing loss as it relates to children (Northern & Downs, 2002):

0 to15 dB HL—within normal limits
15 to 25 dB HL—slight
25 to 30 dB HL—mild
30 to 50 dB HL—moderate
51 to 70 dB HL—severe
70+ dB HL—profound

One classification used with adult populations is as follows (Goodman, 1965):

−10 to 25 dB HL—within normal limits
26 to 40 dB HL—mild
41 to 55 dB HL—moderate
56 to 70 dB HL—moderate to severe
71 to 90 dB HL—severe
91+ dB HL—profound

The relationship between the degree of hearing loss (PTA) and the degree of communication difficulty it presents is provided in Table 3–1.

In addition to the degree of loss, a complete description of an individual's hearing impairment should include whether one ear (unilateral) or both ears (bilateral) are involved and a statement regarding the type of loss. Besides the degree of loss through the speech frequencies, the overall effect of the hearing loss will depend on whether it involves one ear, both ears equally, or one ear to a lesser degree. For example, the child with significant hearing loss in one ear and normal hearing in the other will appear to hear normally, especially in a quiet listening environment. However, when noise is present, the child with unilateral hearing loss will have significant difficulty in discriminating speech.

Nonprofessionals calculating percent of hearing loss to designate a quantifiable amount of hearing loss is occasionally seen when there is a need to determine monetary award for hearing disability. Regardless of the need to use percent of hearing loss, it is not recognized as an accurate appraisal of an individual's communication function.

Table 3–2 lists common terms used to describe pure tone audiograms and provides the general contour for each (Roeser, 1986).

Table 3–1. Degree of Communication Difficulty as a Function of Hearing Loss

Communication Difficulty	Level of Hearing Loss (Pure Tone Average 500, 1000, 2000 Hz)	Degree of Hearing Loss
Demonstrates difficulty understanding soft-spoken speech; needs preferential seating and may benefit from speech reading training; good candidate for a hearing aid	25–40	Mild
Demonstrates an understanding of speech at 3 to 5 feet; requires amplification, preferential seating, speech reading training, and speech therapy	40–55	Moderate
Speech must be loud for auditory reception; difficulty in group and classroom discussion; may require special classes for hearing-impaired; plus all of the above needs	55–70	Moderate to Severe
Loud speech may be understood at 1 ft from ear; may distinguish vowels but not consonants; requires classroom for hearing-impaired and mainstreaming at a later date	70–90	Severe
Does not rely on audition as primary modality for communication; may work well with a total communication approach; may eventually be mainstreamed at higher grade levels	90	Profound

Adapted from Goodman (1965).

Table 3–2. Common Terms Used to Describe Pure Tone Audiograms

Term	Description	Audiometric Configuration
Flat	There is little or no change in thresholds (± 20 dB) across frequencies	
Sloping	As frequency increases; the degree of loss increases	
Rising	As frequency increases, the degree of loss decreases	
Precipitous	There is a very sharp increase in the loss between 1 and 2 octaves	
Scoop or trough shape	The greatest hearing loss is present in the mid frequencies, and hearing sensitivity is better in the low and high frequencies	
Inverted scoop or trough shape	The greatest hearing loss is in the low and high frequencies, and hearing sensitivity is better in the mid frequencies	
High frequency	The hearing loss is limited to the frequencies above the speech range (2000 to 3000 Hz)	
Fragmentary	Thresholds are recorded only for low frequencies, and they are in the severe to profound range	
4000 to 6000 Hz notch	Hearing is within normal limits through 3000 Hz and there is a sharp drop in the 4000 to 6000 Hz range, with improved thresholds at 8000 Hz	
Carhart's notch	There is a mixed hearing loss, and bone conduction thresholds have a characteristic configuration, with a maximum loss at 2000 Hz	

These terms will give those interpreting audiograms a general feeling for the configuration of the loss.

Audiometric Tests in Children

When standard audiological methods cannot be applied to young children successfully, or for children with special problems, procedures using behavioral methods are available. This section describes advanced tests used with these children. Though not used in school screening programs, they are presented to explain the types of tests that are available in the audiology clinic. Table 3–3 lists four procedures that are used by audiologists with young and difficult-to-test children: behavioral observation audiometry (BOA), conditioned orientation reflex (COR) audiometry/visual reinforcement audiometry (VRA), tangible reinforcement operant conditioning audiometry (TROCA), and play conditioning audiometry (PCA).

These specialized techniques require a calibrated sound field system, diagnostic audiometer, and sound-treated room. The procedure with BOA and COR/VRA involves placing the child in the sound-treated room, typically presenting stimuli in the sound field through calibrated speakers, and observing the child's behavior for expected reactions. Depending on the technique used, the child can be reinforced for responding to the sound. Although these are gross tests of hearing, valuable information can be obtained through BOA, COR, or VRA with children who are young and difficult to test. Because a child's attention and auditory function are being evaluated simultaneously, responses to signals are often referred to as minimal response levels rather than true thresholds.

Tests using speech stimuli are sometimes more successfully used with children who are young and difficult to test because speech is more meaningful than pure tones, and the child will respond more readily. In one common procedure, the audiologist presents the stimulus either through earphones or in the sound field and observes the child, or when possible, asks the child to respond by pointing to pictures. However, even if responses to speech are within normal limits, pure tone testing is required because speech stimuli do not test the high frequencies, and significant hearing loss could still be present.

Behavioral Observation Audiometry

BOA provides only minimal information about hearing sensitivity, but it is often the only successful behavioral test that can be applied to children 6 months to 2 years of age and those who are difficult to test. Testing usually takes place in the sound field, although if the child will accept earphones they are placed on the ears.

Tests using speech stimuli are sometimes more meaningful than pure tones and consequently more successfully used for the young child. Stimuli are presented to the child and behavioral responses are observed. Ideally, two evaluators should observe the child and a comparison of their observations made.

Testing must proceed quickly because the child may fatigue, lose interest, or become restless. Stimuli are initially presented at low to moderate intensities and if no response is noted an intense stimulus is presented to cause a startle response.

BOA has many limitations but is useful as a gross test of hearing sensitivity. Significant hearing loss can be ruled out, and conditioning levels for other behavioral test procedures can be determined. Results from BOA must be viewed cautiously because responses tend to be elevated and only represent sensitivity in the better ear when sound-field testing is used.

Conditioned Orientation Reflex/Visual Reinforcement Audiometry

COR/VRA relies on conditioning. That is, when a child (12 to 36 months) orients to a sound, reinforcement is provided by presentation of a visual reinforcer. This procedure is based on the visual orientation reflex; when a light stimulus is presented, a young child will turn reflexively toward the light source. By pairing an auditory stimulus with the light stimulus, the child can be condi-

Table 3–3. Summary of Audiological Evaluation Procedures for Infants and Children

Name of Test	Explanation of Technique	Indications for Use	Advantages/ Disadvantages
Behavioral observation audiometry (BOA)	*Conditioning:* None. A variety of test signals are presented through loudspeakers. Minimal intensity is determined where behavioral changes are observed (e.g., alerting, scanning, cessation or activity, or change in sucking during testing) *Reinforcement:* None	Infants under 6 months and older youngsters with severe developmental delays *Alternative:* Auditory evoked responses (particularly if test findings suggest a significant hearing loss)	*Advantages:* Can be used with unconditionable children *Disadvantages:* 1. Rapid habituation of unconditioned behavior 2. Unilateral losses may be missed 3. Can only rule out severe and profound losses because relatively high intensities are required to elicit unconditioned responses even in infants with normal hearing
Conditioned orientation reflex audiometry (COR)/visual reinforcement audiometry (VRA)	*Conditioning:* Establish bond between auditory signal and flashing lighted toy *Reinforcement:* Lighted toy as well as social praise during test phase	Toddlers from 6 to 24 months and many other children with developmental delays *Alternative:* Auditory evoked responses	*Advantages:* 1. Stimuli can be presented by earphones, bone conduction, or loudspeaker 2. Does not require voluntary response 3. Capitalizes on heightened visual alertness of children with hearing impairments *Disadvantages:* 1. Approximately 35% of infants under 12 months of age cannot be conditioned 2. Many toddlers will not accept earphones initially 3. If stimuli are presented in the sound field, a unilateral hearing loss may be missed

Table 3–3. Continued

Name of Test	Explanation of Technique	Indications for Use	Advantages/ Disadvantages
Tangible reinforcement operant conditioning audiometry (TROCA)	*Conditioning:* Connection is established between auditory stimuli and "button-pressing"	Preschoolers, especially those with short attention spans and those who work best with structure. Also many older mentally retarded children. *Alternative:* VRA (auditory evoked responses)	*Advantages:* 1. Stimuli can be presented by earphones, bone conduction, or loudspeakers 2. Can be used in conjunction with frequency-specific measures *Disadvantages:* 1. Time-consuming and requires repeated sessions to establish conditioning 2. Children will often insist upon eating the reinforcer between trials, thus increasing the length of the test session
Play conditioning audiometry (PCA)	*Conditioning:* Connection is established between auditory stimuli and play activity. *Reinforcement:* Play activity and social reinforcement during conditioning and testing. May also use visual reinforcement	Preschoolers, 30 months to 4 years, and older children with mild developmental delays. *Alternative:* TROCO or VRA (auditory evoked responses)	*Advantages:* Can be used in conjunction with any frequency-specific measures. *Disadvantages:* A variety of activities are needed to maintain interest in the activity; otherwise, response behavior habituates

tioned to orient to the light when the sound stimuli alone are perceived.

COR/VRA is a quick and efficient procedure. The main advantage is that the child need not perform a voluntary motor task, which makes it especially helpful when evaluating children younger than 3 years of age.

Tangible Reinforcement Operant Conditioning Audiometry

TROCA requires use of specially designed equipment that will dispense an object (tangible item) to reinforce a child's response to an auditory stimulus. The tangible reinforcer (e.g., candy, cereal; juice, soda; a small trinket or toy; or another object desired by the child) is paired with the auditory stimulus until a response activates a switch. Children who are difficult to test will require several conditioning trials and potentially a number of training sessions that last no longer than about 15 minutes to obtain reliable responses. Parents, teachers, or speech-language pathologists may include test training in their daily activities to expedite the testing.

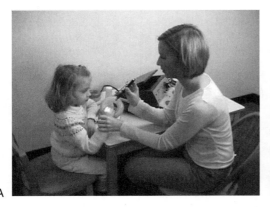

A

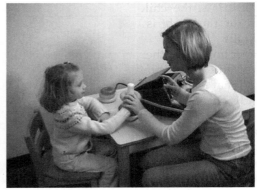

B

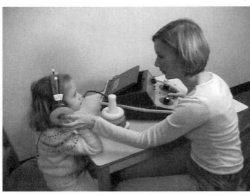

C

Figure 3–13. Play audiometry reinforcement using a flashlight (PARF). (A) Conditioning the child to respond to the light. (B) Teaching the correct response. (C) Transferring to the auditory-only stimulus.

Play Conditioning Audiometry

PCA is the most reliable testing method for children 2 to 5 years of age, by making the audiometric test a game. The child is trained to perform a simple motor task, such as dropping a block into a box, stacking rings, or snapping beads together, and is then given verbal praise as reinforcement.

PCA is first carried out by conditioning the child to presentation of suprathreshold stimuli and guiding the child through a response mode. This can be accomplished by laying the headphones on a table in front of the child and presenting the stimuli at high intensities (100 to 110 dB at 1000 Hz). When responses occur without the evaluator's urging or guidance, the headphones are placed on the child, the intensity is lowered to 50 to 60 dB, responses are reestablished, and the intensity is gradually lowered in 5 to 10 dB steps until

threshold is obtained. Thresholds obtained with PCA are considered very accurate.

A technique that is most helpful in PCA is play audiometry reinforcement using a flashlight (PARF). PARF is an effective procedure with very young children, as young as 2 to 2½ years of age, as well as older children who are difficult to test. PARF is used to initiate the test by teaching the child the correct task to be performed in response to light and then replacing the visual stimulus with the pure tone auditory stimulus.

The steps used in the ring stacking procedure, illustrated in Figure 3–13, are as follows. With the flashlight in the examiner's hand, the child holds a ring to the light (Fig. 3–13A). Once the light is flashed on and off briefly (1 to 2 seconds), the examiner takes the child's hand and moves it to the stack and helps the child to place the ring on the stack (Fig. 3–13B). Usually, after two or three trials, the child knows the response and the flashlight is placed completely out of sight.

Earphones are then placed on the child's ears, and the examiner takes the child's hand that has a ring in it and places it to the child's cheek (Fig. 3–13C). A 1000 Hz tone is presented at 50 dB HL, and the examiner guides the child's hand to the stack helping place the ring on the stack. If the child does not appear to respond at 50 dB HL, the tone intensity is increased in 10 dB steps until a response is obtained. Once the child learns the correct response, usually after three or four trials, the intensity is lowered in 20 dB steps until the stimuli are presented at 20 dB or higher if necessary. After 1000 Hz is tested, the procedure is continued at 2000 and 4000 Hz and then the other ear is screened.

Play conditioning can be used successfully with younger children. Generally, the procedure is limited when children are less than 30 months of age (Matkin, 1979).

Test training is used with PCA when children cannot be conditioned in one or two sessions with play techniques. This procedure involves teaching the child over a series of sessions to respond by block dropping, inserting pegs into a board, or performing some other overt behavior to the presentation of an auditory stimulus; essentially the same as those described for play conditioning, but the training occurs over several, sometimes numerous, sessions. The purpose of the training is to establish a behavior that can be used in screening or testing.

Sometimes only five to six sessions are required, and sometimes many more, to train a child; the number of sessions will vary with each child. It is important to keep sessions brief (10 to 15 minutes) and frequent (once or twice per school day).

Often the speech pathologist's schedule permits frequent, short contacts to provide the actual training. It is advisable to set up the test training program under the direction of the audiologist because children who are in this difficult-to-test category should

be tested by an audiologist after their behavior has been shaped.

PARF can also be used in test training. In fact, a rule to follow is that if a child will not condition to the visual stimulus with PARF it is highly unlikely that conditioning to an auditory stimulus will be possible. Auditory stimuli are more abstract than the visual stimuli used with PARF.

Physiological Measures

When behavioral audiometric tests cannot be used or are unreliable, valid information on hearing sensitivity and middle ear function can be obtained with physiological measures including: ABR audiometry, OAEs, and immittance measures. Physiological measures not only assess hearing sensitivity but also provide valuable data that can be used for diagnosis and treatment of hearing loss. An advantage of physiological measures is that they can be applied to those who cannot be assessed with behavioral measures because they do not require a volitional response such as raising the hand or repeating words.

ABR and OAE procedures are briefly described following here, and more comprehensive information on immittance measures is provided. It is unlikely that schools will have ABR equipment, and the role of OAE in school hearing conservation has yet to be determined. However, it is not uncommon for schools to have the capability of performing immittance tests.

Auditory Brainstem Response Audiometry

ABR, also termed brainstem-evoked response audiometry, is a highly reliable and successful procedure, especially with infants and young children. Infants are easily tested during sleep, but sedation may be necessary to maintain a nonactive state in young children. The procedure involves placing small electrodes on the patient's scalp. Clicks or tone bursts presented in rapid secession are delivered to the relaxed, preferably sleeping, patient. Minute, ongoing electroencephalographic (EEG) activity from the brain is picked up by the electrodes, digitized, and averaged by a computer. Three distinct peaks (out of seven) are analyzed by amplitude and time as a function of stimuli intensity. The resulting responses provide precise information regarding the function and integrity of the ear and auditory brainstem. An ABR threshold is considered the lowest intensity level in which a response is obtained and replicated.

One major limitation for the click-evoked ABR is that high frequencies (from 1000 to 4000 Hz range) are more reliably assessed. Thus only partial information is obtained regarding hearing sensitivity. Using tone bursts can facilitate frequency-specific ABR testing, but responses are more prone to artifact. Another limitation is that ABR evaluates only auditory sensitivity and not how an individual uses "hearing" or interprets sounds (i.e., cognitive interpretation of sound such as in speech audiometry). These two limitations make long-term monitoring of the child necessary until behavioral tests can be performed and more complete audiometric information obtained. Although these limitations do affect the predictive value of the ABR test, the technique has proven useful for those children who are impossible to test with behavioral methods. Hall (1992) provides a comprehensive overview of auditory evoked response procedures, including ABR.

OAEs are measured by coupling a small microphone to the external earcanal with a probe that is similar to the system used in immittance measures. By presenting clicks or tone pairs to the ear, averaging procedures similar to ABR testing are then used to detect the presence of energy reflected from the inner ear. Interpretation of OAE data is quite sophisticated. With heightened awareness of auditory neuropathy, OAEs are now used routinely in infant hearing screening programs (see Chapter 5) and are becoming an important part of the standard diagnostic auditory test battery for assessing cochlear function. When they are used appropriately by trained personnel, there is a high correlation with degree of hearing sensitivity.

There are two basic categories of OAEs: spontaneous OAEs (SOAEs) and evoked (or stimulated) OAEs (EOAEs). Implicit in the name, SOAEs occur in the absence of stimulation to the ear. SOAEs are low intensity sounds that usually are inaudible to the individual, and their presence is still not fully understood. EOAEs are recorded by introducing different types of stimuli to the ear. Stimulus type is the determinant for which of the three EOAEs will be recorded: transient evoked OAEs (TEOAEs), stimulus-frequency OAEs (SFOAEs), or distortion product OAEs (DPOAEs).

TEOAEs are produced after delivering a brief stimulus (click) to the ear. SFOAEs appear during the presentation of a tonal stimulus and occur at the frequency of the stimulus. DPOAEs are evoked by introducing two tonal stimuli simultaneously. DPOAEs occur at frequencies that are different from the stimulus frequencies and the observed response has a mathematical relationship to the frequencies of the primary stimuli.

The Immittance Instrument and Measures

Immittance Measures are based on the principle that, when a known quantity of sound (acoustic energy) is applied to the ear, a certain amount of measured energy is reflected; the amount of reflected energy will vary depending on the stiffness (immobility) or flaccidity (mobility) of the middle ear system. The stiffer or less flaccid or less compliant (mobile) the system, the greater the amount of energy that will be reflected (which means that less energy will be admitted). Conversely, the less stiff, more flaccid, or more compliant (mobile) the system, the smaller the amount of energy that will be reflected (which means that more energy will be admitted). Note that stiffness and admittance (compliance) are inversely related. As one increases, the other decreases.

Measuring middle ear function has become a standard of care that does not rely on behavioral responses. Although a semicooperative child can have middle ear function assessed in less than 1 minute per ear with little difficulty, the uncooperative child may require more testing time. Because little cooperation is required, immittance tests can be performed on younger children, as well as children who are difficult or impossible to test. However, the use of immittance measures does not eliminate the need for audiometric testing. A child can have perfectly normal findings on routine immittance tests and still manifest a significant bilateral sensorineural hearing loss. A more in-depth discussion regarding immittance principles and instrumentation follows.

Principles of Immittance Measurement

Terminology used for measures of middle ear function has changed over the past several years and can be confusing. The following definitions should help clarify this confusion.

Impedance: opposition to the flow of energy (in the outer and middle ear) expressed in ohms that is influenced by the mass, stiffness, and frictional resistance present in the system. The term "impedance measures" was first used to describe the clinical procedures involved in testing middle ear function.

Admittance: the ease with which acoustic energy is transmitted (in the outer and middle ear) expressed in mhos (mho is ohm spelled backward). The terms "admittance" and "compliance" are used synonymously.

Immittance: Because middle ear measures are electronically or electroacoustically based on the measurement of impedance or admittance, the term "admittance" was created to encompass both techniques (ASHA, 1979, 1990b).

Compliance: used synonymously with "admittance" is considered the inverse of stiffness as it relates to the ease of acoustic energy transmission (refer back to admittance). However, "admit-

tance" is the suggested terminology (ASHA, 1990b; Margolis & Heller, 1987). Compliance and admittance are measured in equivalent volumes of air using cubic centimeters or millimeters (1 cm^3 is the same volume as 1 mL; or 1.0 cm^3 = 1.0 mL). Because not all have adopted the use of the term "compliance," in this chapter "admittance" will be used.

Routine admittance measures do not assess hearing but provide objective information on the mechanical transfer function of sound in the outer and middle ear. That is, routine admittance measures assess the functional state of the conductive mechanism of the ear. Through such assessment, it is possible to detect and define disorders in the outer and middle ear system objectively.

Although the procedures used to administer admittance tests are relatively simple and can be learned in a matter of hours, the difficulty with the admittance testing lies in interpretation. To interpret the diagnostic value of the results from the admittance test battery, a thorough understanding of the auditory system and the principles of admittance are required. Such understanding includes a comprehensive knowledge of the acoustic and physiological principles underlying the admittance technique and auditory system, as well as the various pathological conditions that may affect the auditory system. This section presents the basics of the immittance technique as they apply to immittance screening and interpretation of results. Chapter 5 describes screening principles, pure tone, and immittance screening criteria and their application.

The Immittance Instrument

Various disorders in the outer and middle ear affect the stiffness of the system, which concomitantly affects mobility or admittance (compliance). When the reflected energy varies from a known normal range, many disorders affecting the outer and middle ear can be detected. This principle can be understood better by reviewing the mechanics of the immittance instrument itself.

Sometimes inappropriately called an immittance audiometer or an immittance bridge, the immittance instrument is composed of various complex components within this sophisticated system. An audiometer is a device used to assess hearing. Because immittance measures do not assess hearing, it is misleading to refer to an immittance instrument as an audiometer. The term "immittance bridge" was adopted because the instrument circuit contains an electronic component called a Wheatstone bridge, but the terminology is also not accurate.

The ANSI standard for immittance instruments is ANSI S3.39–1987 (1987). As with audiometers, the standard can be obtained for a fee by writing to American National Standards Institute as detailed previously. All current immittance equipment should meet the 1987 ANSI standards.

Initially, immittance instruments were operated manually, but with computer technology we now have microprocessor-based instruments that operate automatically. Figure 3–14 shows a microprocessor-based diagnostic immittance instrument. This instrument allows the user to perform simple screening testing as well as advanced diagnostic procedures (such as reflex decay and reflex latency) and can be used in an automatic mode or manually. The major components and functions of immittance instruments include the CRT screen, printout, manual control, pressure control, reflex-eliciting stimulus control, intensity control, probe, probe tips, and contralateral reflex-eliciting earphone

CRT Screen (1 in Fig. 3–14). The screen displays the data that are collected during immittance measurements.

Printout (2 in Fig. 3–14). The printout is a hard copy of the data shown on the CRT screen (see example in Fig. 3–18).

Manual Control (3 in Fig. 3–14). The manual control allows the user to run each applicable test procedure.

Pressure Control (4 in Fig. 3–14). The pressure control operates an air pump used to increase and decrease the air pressure in the external auditory canal during manual tympanometry. A manometer measures the pressure change as it occurs. The range of pressures available in most immittance instruments is from 200 to −400 or −600 daPa. Originally, immittance units measured pressure in millimeters of water pressure, and older equipment will express pressure in this terminology. Because decaPascals and millimeters of water are virtually the same in the pressure ranges used to perform immittance measures on the ear (97.8 daPa = 100 mm/H$_2$O), the two measures can be considered equivalent.

Reflex-Eliciting Stimulus Control (5 in Fig. 3–14). This control allows the examiner to choose either from pure tone stimuli at octave frequencies from 250 to 4000 Hz, or from broad band noise, low pass filtered noise, or high pass filtered noise.

Intensity Control (6 in Fig. 3–14). The intensity control allows the examiner to choose the intensity of the reflex eliciting stimuli from 35 to 110 dB HL for ipsilateral presentation and 35 to 120 dB HL for contralateral stimulation. Exposure to intensity

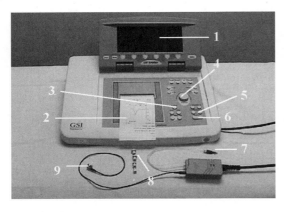

Figure 3–14. A diagnostic immittance instrument (see text for description).

levels above 110 dB HL can be harmful, and extreme care should be taken when presenting acoustic reflex stimuli at high intensities.

Probe (7 in Fig. 3–14). The probe is inserted into the external auditory canal; the ear into which the probe is inserted is the ear from which the immittance measures are being recorded.

Probe Tips (8 in Fig. 3–14). Probe tips of various sizes and constructed of plastic or rubber tips allow the probe to be inserted into the external auditory canal so that the necessary hermetic (airtight) seal can be obtained during immittance measures.

Contralateral Reflex-Eliciting Earphone (9 in Fig. 3–14). When using an insert-type earphone in combination with another insert type—or a standard supra-aural earphone, reflexes are elicited from the opposite ear (contralateral to) the probe ear. The reflex-eliciting earphone is used to present a signal to the ear opposite the probe ear to determine the presence or absence of acoustic reflexes.

Figure 3–15 shows how the probe is placed in the earcanal (top) and how the headset of the immittance instrument is placed for testing (bottom). With the headset in one position, immittance findings are obtained for one ear (the probe ear); the ipsilateral acoustic reflex stimulus is delivered to the probe ear, and the contralateral acoustic stimulus is delivered to the ear opposite the probe ear (contralateral reflex-eliciting ear). The headset is then reversed and the procedure is repeated.

In Figure 3–15, the immittance and ipsilateral reflex of the right ear are being measured. The contralateral acoustic reflex-eliciting signal is being delivered to the left ear; the acoustic reflex from the left ear stimulation is being recorded in the (contralateral) right ear. When describing immittance results, it is helpful to describe them in reference to the probe ear. In this way, no confusion will exist about the ear being described.

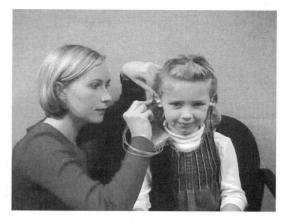

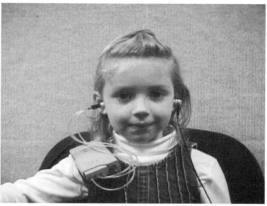

Figure 3–15. Placement of the probe into the external auditory canal (top). The bottom photograph shows how the instrument would be placed for obtaining the immittance values in the probe ear; the left earcanal has an insert earphone placed into it for stimulation of the contralateral acoustic reflex.

Figure 3–16 is a schematic representation of the principles used to determine the immittance in the probe ear. The diagram illustrates the closed cavity between the probe tip of the immittance instrument and the external earcanal: the area from the end of the probe tip to the tympanic membrane. As shown in Figure 3–16, the probe tip is connected to three components in the immittance instrument: a loudspeaker (2a), an air pump and manometer (4a), and a microphone (5a). The immittance probe apparatus measures the stiffness or admittance (com-

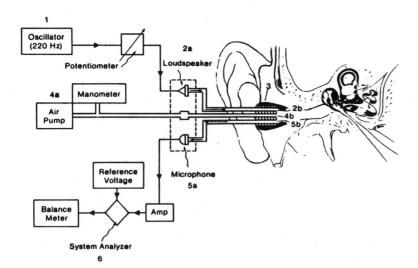

Figure 3–16. Principles of immittance measurement in the probe ear (see text for description).

pliance) of the middle ear system in the following way: a 220 Hz or 226 Hz (other probe frequencies are used when advanced tests are performed) probe tone emitted from the loudspeaker (2a) is introduced into the external earcanal through a port in the probe tip (2b). Depending on the state of the earcanal and middle ear, some energy is absorbed and transmitted to the inner ear and some energy is reflected. The reflected energy is picked up through a second port in the probe tip (5b) and delivered to the microphone (5a), and the system analyzer (6) compares the input signal to the reflected energy.

As already described, the immittance instrument acts like a small sound pressure measuring device in determining the state of the middle ear. The amount of reflected energy picked up by the microphone from the probe tone determines the functional state of the ear. A high amount of reflected energy means that the system is more stiff or less compliant than normal, and vice versa. Conditions such as otitis media and ossicular chain fixation result in high stiffness or low admittance (compliance); in such cases the reflected energy would be higher than normal. Conversely, low stiffness or high admittance (compliance) would be caused by conditions such as disarticulation of the ossicular chain or a scarred, flaccid tympanic membrane. Under these conditions, more

energy would pass through than normally, so the amount reflected would be less than normal.

The third port in the probe tip (4b) is connected to an air pump and manometer (4a). The air pump and manometer act together to increase, decrease, and measure the air pressure in the outer earcanal. This system is used in obtaining the tympanogram (described later).

Microprocessor (automatic) immittance units are being used more frequently in audiology clinics and in screening programs. This type of equipment is designed to be used in situations in which rapid assessment of middle ear function is required, such as in large-scale screening programs and with the pediatric population, where the child typically will not remain quiet for more than a few seconds. Figure 3–17 shows an automatic immittance unit in use during screening. The primary advantage of using this type of equipment is that obtaining an airtight seal requires only that it be held over the entrance of the earcanal, simplifying the procedure; and only about 5 to 10 seconds is required to perform tympanometry, static admittance, and ipsilateral acoustic reflex measures for each ear. Following the data collection, the information is displayed on a light-emitting diode screen, or a hard copy can be printed. An example is provided in Figure 3–18.

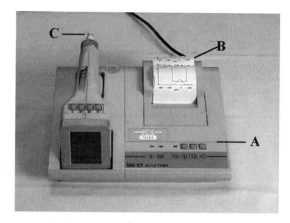

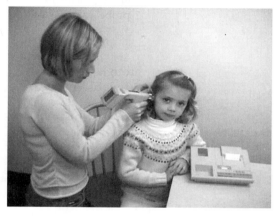

Figure 3–17. Example of a microprocessor-based screening immittance unit (top): A is the processor, B is the printer, and C is the probe tip. Data are obtained by holding the probe against the external auditory canal for about 5 seconds (bottom).

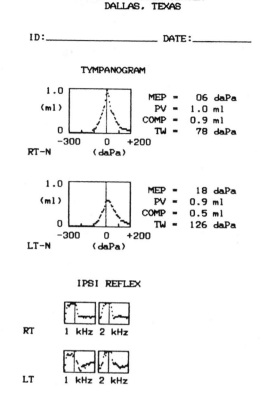

Figure 3–18. Example of printed findings obtained from a microprocessor-based screening immittance unit. Results shown would indicate normal middle ear function (see text for description).

Immittance Measures

Table 3–4 lists the four basic immittance procedures used to assess middle ear function: tympanogram, tympanogram height, physical volume, and acoustic reflex. In addition, a comparison is made between the classic (descriptive) immittance method and the absolute (microprocessor-based) method. As shown, the two procedures use essentially the same information but classify results differently for the tympanogram. The classic method describes the tympanogram shape (type A, B, and C) (Jerger, 1970). However, the absolute method pro-

vides objective measures of the tympanogram: Tympanometric peak pressure (TPP), tympanometric width/gradient (TW or GR), and tympanogram height (static admittance-peak Y) (ASHA, 1990b). Table 3–5 lists the mean norms for each of the basic immittance procedures and gives the 90% ranges for children and adults separately. Although each test provides significant information by itself, immittance tests are not performed or interpreted in isolation. Diagnostic capabilities are strengthened when

Table 3–4. Summary of Immittance Tests and Comparison of Classic and Absolute (Microprocessor-Based) Procedures

Procedure	Purpose	Classic Description	Units of Measurement	Absolute Description	Unit of Measurement
Tympanogram	Assess the pressure/compliance function of the eardrum	Static compliance	cm³/mL*	Tympanometric peak pressure (TPP)	daPa
				Tympanometric width (TW) gradient (GR)	daPa
Tympanogram height	Classification of tympanogram	Static compliance	cm³/mL*	Static admittance (peak Y)	mmho or cm³/mL*
Physical volume	Measures the equivalent volume of the space between the probe tip and the eardrum	Physical volume test	cm³/mL*	Equivalent earcanal volume (Vec)	cm³/mL*
Acoustic reflex (AR)	Indirect measure of stapedial muscle contraction to intense sound	AR	Relative change in eardrum admittance (compliance)	AR	Relative change in eardrum admittance (compliance)

*Cubic centimeters and milliliters are identical volumes (1 cm³ = 1 mL)

the results of all test procedures are interpreted together.

TYMPANOGRAM

The tympanogram measures eardrum admittance (compliance) or mobility as a function of mechanically varying the air pressure in a hermetically sealed external earcanal. Admittance (compliance) or mobility of the eardrum at an air pressure ranging from +200 to −400 daPa is recorded on a graph referred to as a tympanogram. The tympanogram is plotted by introducing the positive and negative air pressure into the probe ear and recording the admittance (compliance) of the ear, based on the amount of reflected energy.

To comprehend how varying air pressure in the external auditory canal affects the amount of reflected energy from the tympanic membrane, one must understand the pressure/admittance (compliance) principle. Figure 3–19 illustrates this principle in a normal ear. Recall that stiffness and admittance (compliance) are inversely related and that by measuring one of these characteristics, the other can be derived.

In Figure 3–19, the amount of reflected energy is at its lowest point when the pressure in the external auditory canal is at atmospheric pressure (0 daPa). Under this condition, in the normal ear: (1) there is equal pressure between the external and middle ear cavities; (2) the amount of energy absorbed by the tympanic membrane and middle ear structures from the probe tone is at the highest level; and (3) the amount of reflected energy from the probe tone is at its lowest level, which means that the admittance (compliance) is at its highest point. However, when either a positive or negative pressure is introduced into the external earcanal, the force exerted on the normal

Table 3–5. Mean Norms and 90% Ranges for Immittance Measures

Tympanometric Peak Pressure (TPP)	Tympanometric Width/Gradient (TW/GR)	Static Admittance/Compliance (Peak Y)	Earcanal Volume (Vec)
Borderline— 100 to −200 daPa	Children mean = 100 daPa 90% range +60 to −150 daPa	Children mean + 0.5 mmho/cm³/mL* 90% range+	Children mean = 0.7 cm³/mL* 90% range = 0.4 to 1.0 cm³/mL*
Abnormal more negative than −200 daPa	Adult mean = 80 daPa 90% range = 50 to 110 daPa	Adult mean = 0.8 mmho/cm³/mL* 90% range = 0.3 to 1.4, mmho/cm³/mL*	Adult mean = 1.1 cm³/mL* 90% range = 0.6 to 1.5 cm³/mL*

Adapted from the American Speech and Hearing Association Committee on Audiometric Evaluation (1979) and from Margolis and Heller (1987).
*Cubic centimeters (cm³) and milliliters (mL) are identical volumes (1 cm³ = 1 mL).

tympanic membrane stretches and stiffens it and other middle ear structures. As the system stiffens, a concomitant decrease in admittance (compliance) increases the amount of reflected energy. In Figure 3–19, the amount of reflected energy is greatest at 200 and −300 daPa, which indicates that admittance (compliance) is at its lowest point at these two pressures for this ear.

Modern, microprocessor-based immittance instruments are quick and efficient; the data are recorded automatically in just a few seconds by simply placing the probe into the earcanal. However, by using these automatic instruments, the examiner may not fully understand how the data are being collected. The procedure for manually plotting the data is more helpful in explaining the principles of immittance measurement.

Figure 3–20 shows a manually plotted tympanogram. Air pressure is introduced into the earcanal at 200 daPa. The 200 daPa pressure establishes a stiff system with low admittance (compliance), and the amount of reflected energy is greater than at atmospheric pressure. At this point, the first reading (1 in Fig. 3–20) is obtained; in the example in Figure 3–20 the reading is 1.4 mL. This reading also represents the equivalent physical volume of the system (see Physical/Earcanal Volume later).

In the normal ear, the admittance (compliance) obtained at +200 daPa will be low. The air pressure is then gradually reduced from +200 daPa until it reaches the point where the amount of reflected energy is the lowest, and the admittance (compliance) is the highest. This point is termed the point of maximum admittance (compliance) and indicates that the air pressure is equal between the external earcanal and the middle ear cavity. At this point, the second reading (2 in Fig. 3–20) is noted on the tympanogram. In the normal ear, the point of maximum admittance (compliance) is at or near atmospheric pressure (0 to −50 daPa). Finally, a third reading (3 in Fig. 3–20) is made at a more negative pressure, about −200 daPa less pressure than the

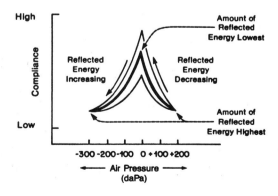

Figure 3–19. Schematic representation of how varying air pressure in the external earcanal affects the stiffness of the eardrum and the reflected energy of the probe tone (see text for description).

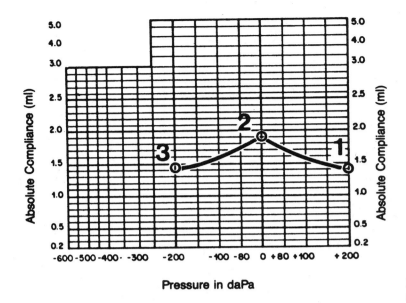

Pressure in daPa

O = Right Ear   X = Left Ear

Figure 3–20. Example of a manually plotted tympanogram (see text for description).

point of maximum admittance (compliance), to complete the tympanometric configuration. When the three points are connected, a pattern results that can be classified according to normal or various abnormal middle ear conditions.

Tympanograms can be plotted using a relative or absolute scale. Examples of the two methods are shown in Figures 3–18 and 3–20. Note that for relative measures the 200 daPa reading is always at 0 mL. With absolute measurements, the 200 daPa reading also provides specific information on earcanal volume (see Physical/Earcanal Volume later).

Classical (Descriptive) Method. Several systems have been proposed to classify tympanograms. Due to its simplicity, the classic (descriptive) method shown in Figure 3–21 has been the most popular. The three type A classifications represent normal middle ear pressure; the subclassifications of types A_d and A_s represent abnormally high and low admittance (compliance), respectively. The type B classification represents little or no admittance (compliance) in the conductive system, regardless of the air pressure in the

external ear. This is the most abnormal tympanogram that can be found. The type C classification represents abnormal negative pressure in the middle ear.

Absolute Method. Although the classic method for describing tympanograms is simple, it is subjective and not all tympanograms fall into the A, B, and C classifications. The absolute method quantifies tympanogram classification using TPP and TW or GR.

TPP is a direct measure of the air pressure in the middle ear at which the peak of the tympanogram occurs. Negative pressure occurs when the gas (air) is absorbed in the middle ear due to eustachian tube closure. Negative TPP is indicative of the early stages of otitis media; positive TPP is found in early stages of acute otitis media. Table 3–5 provides mean norms for TPP, as well as three other basic immittance measures. Normal middle ear pressure ranges between +50 and −100 daPa. As shown in Table 3–5, between −100 and −200 daPa middle ear function borderlines on abnormal, and beyond −200 daPa middle ear function is abnormal. Research has shown that large fluctuations

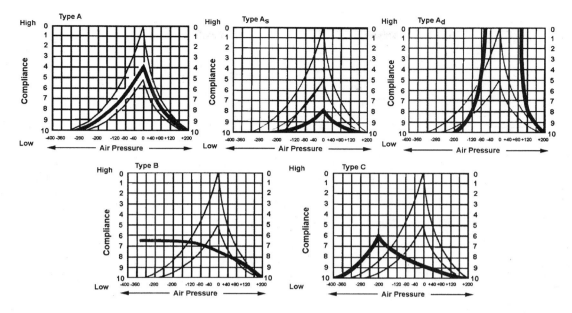

Figure 3–21. The classic (A, B, C) classification of tympanograms (Jerger, 1970).

can be found in TPP; abnormal TPP in the absence of other middle ear anomalies does not reflect significant changes in other middle ear function, and abnormal TPP cannot be observed reliably with an otoscope. It is important to note that some studies have shown that TPP is not a good predictor of middle ear effusion (Fiellau-Nikolajsen, 1983; Nozza, Bluestone, Kardatze, & Bachman, 1994). Due to these observations, TPP is not used as a unitary criterion for referral (see Chapter 5).

TW or GR describes the width and slope of the sides of the tympanogram surrounding the peak. TW/GR is calculated by measuring the pressure range corresponding to a percentage of reduction in static admittance from the maximum peak admittance. The procedure is as follows: (1) determine the peak (maximum) admittance (for example, 1.0 cm³/mL); (2) reduce the peak admittance by a percentage (e.g., 50%); (3) note the values on the positive and negative pressure tails of the tympanogram (at 0.5 cm³/mL); and (4) measure the distance between the positive tympanogram tail and negative tympanogram tail in decaPascal. The current

norms provided in Table 3–5 are based on a 50% criterion (ASHA, 1990b, 1997).

TW/GR measures appear to be sensitive to middle ear diseases that are not detected by other immittance measures or otoscopy (Fiellau-Nikolajsen, 1983; Nozza, et al, 1994). Normative data have been established with a number of studies involving 3- to 10-year-olds (Hunter, Margolis, Daly, & Giebink, 1992; Shanks, Stelmachowicz, Beauchaine, & Schulte, 1992). It should be noted that when tympanograms are flat (type B) the TW/GR cannot be measured properly.

TYMPANOGRAM HEIGHT: STATIC ADMITTANCE (COMPLIANCE)

In addition to peak pressure and width, proper interpretation of the tympanogram depends on specifying its height. Static admittance (compliance) provides objective information on tympanogram height by quantifying its peak relative to the tail value (obtained at 200 daPa).

Static admittance (compliance) measurement can be explained using the volume principle, which states that the absolute size

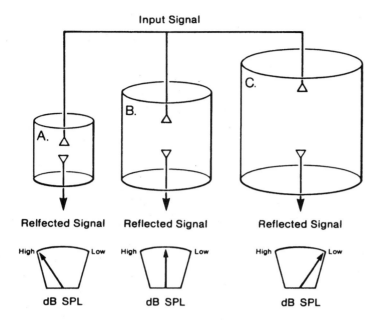

Figure 3–22. The effects of volume change on the input/output function of an acoustic signal for (A) a small cavity, (B) a medium cavity, and (C) a large cavity.

of a cavity of known physical characteristics (a hard-wall cavity) can be determined by knowing the amount of reflected energy from an input signal of known intensity. Figure 3–22 illustrates this concept. Figure 3–22A shows a fixed-volume cavity with an input acoustic signal and a reflected SPL value, which is high compared with Figure 3–22B and C. In Figure 3–22B, the same input acoustic signal is used, but the output SPL is reduced due to the increased volume in the larger cavity. With a larger cavity, there is more absorption, which causes less resistance, and, as a result, there is less reflection of energy. In Figure 3–22C, the same input acoustic signal is also used, but once again output SPL is reduced due to an even larger cavity. Based on this simple principle, the absolute volume of a cavity can be determined as long as the physical characteristics of the cavity are specified.

Static admittance is measured by introducing a positive pressure into the external auditory canal. In a normal ear the increased stiffness of the tympanic membrane sets up an artificial acoustical "wall." Under this condition, the volume of the cavity from the probe tip of the immittance instrument to the eardrum is measured in volume units

(cm^3 or mL) equivalent to a cavity of known physical characteristics. Note that the term "equivalent" is used because the physical characteristics of each earcanal will vary, and the reflected energy must be used in comparison to a standard cavity (a hard-wall cavity) of known physical characteristics. Once pressure is removed, the tympanic membrane returns to its natural resting place, and the artificial acoustical wall will no longer be present. Under this condition, the cavity from the probe tip, including the external canal and middle ear space, is measured in equivalent units.

The procedure used to obtain static admittance is to place the probe tip into the external earcanal, which directs the probe tone into the earcanal, and introduce a pressure of +200 daPa. The positive air pressure serves to stretch and stiffen the tympanic membrane, resulting in a large amount of reflected energy. An admittance (compliance) reading is obtained, which gives an equivalent volume (cm^3 or mL) at this positive air pressure setting. When the eardrum is intact, this reading is the equivalent volume of the external earcanal (sometimes referred to as the Cl reading). Air pressure is then adjusted from +200 daPa to the point of maximum admittance (compliance) (at or near 0 daPa in the normal ear) and a second reading is made (sometimes referred to as the C2 reading). This reading is the equivalent volume of the total outer and middle ear system. Static admittance (compliance) is calculated by subtracting the first reading (C1) from the second reading (C2). This derived value represents the equivalent volume of the middle ear system. In Figure 3–20 the static admittance (compliance) is 0.5 mL (1.9 mL minus 1.4 mL). With microprocessing immittance units, the user simply sees the resulting admittance value. In Figure 3–18 the static admittance (compliance) is 0.9 mL for the right ear (0.9 mL minus 0 mL) and 0.5 for the left (0.5 minus 0 mL).

Table 3–5 provides the mean normal values and 90% ranges for static admittance (compliance) for children and adults separately. As shown, for children the mean value is 0.5 mmho/cm³/mL with a range of 0.2 to 0.9 mmho/cm³/mL. For adults, the mean value is 0.8 mmho/cm³/mL, with a range of 0.3 to 1.4 mmho/cm³/mL.

PHYSICAL/EARCANAL VOLUME

In the presence of a flat tympanogram, static admittance (compliance) measures help to detect eardrum perforation and determine whether a pressure equalization (PE) tube (surgically placed in an eardrum) is patent (open). This additional information is available when the first reading (at +200 daPa; the C1 reading) is obtained. The measure is sometimes called the physical volume test (PVT) but the ANSI (1987) standard refers to this measure as "earcanal volume."

The PVT is accomplished by introducing positive air pressure into the external auditory canal and obtaining a reading at +200 daPa (a C1 reading). Mean earcanal volume norms and 90% ranges are provided in Table 3–5 for children and adults separately. For children, the mean is 0.7 cm³/mL with a 90% range of 0.4 to 1.0 cm³/mL. For adults, the mean is 1.1 cm³/mL with a 90% range of 0.6 to 1.5 cm³/mL. If a reading is unusually high, often exceeding 4.0 to 5.0 cm³/mL in

adults, and a flat (type B) tympanogram is obtained, a perforation is present, or if a PE tube was previously placed it is patent (open). In Figure 3–18 earcanal physical volume (PV) is given in digital form (1.0 mL for the right ear and 0.9 mL for the left). In Figure 3–20 the earcanal volume is provided on the tympanogram in absolute equivalent volume [1.4 mL, which is the admittance (compliance) reading at +200 daPa].

It should be recognized that the size and shape of the probe tip and its placement in the earcanal will influence the earcanal volume reading. This may result in some test/retest variability but should not change the interpretation of the test significantly.

When testing an ear with a perforation or open PE tube, the pressure may suddenly release when a positive pressure is introduced into the external earcanal. This finding would indicate that the eustachian tube is functioning. When a PE tube is present and earcanal volume is normal or below normal, the ventilating tube may be blocked.

ACOUSTIC REFLEXES

An acoustic reflex typically occurs in both ears (bilaterally) when a small muscle in the middle ear, the stapedius, contracts due to high intensity stimulation. The fact that the acoustic reflex is bilateral means that a signal directed to one ear can elicit a recordable reflex in the opposite (contralateral) ear.

When the stapedius muscle contracts in the normal ear, there is a resulting stiffening of the tympanic membrane. This stiffening of the tympanic membrane during contraction is detected by the immittance instrument as a change in the reflected energy from the probe tone. It is important to realize that the immittance procedure does not measure middle ear muscle contraction directly but measures the effect of middle ear muscle contraction on tympanic membrane stiffening. This has an important implication in interpreting the clinical value of acoustic reflex results because mechanical changes in the middle ear can obliterate recording the acoustic reflex when it occurs. That is, the presence of middle ear pathology will obliterate the effect of the middle ear contraction recorded with the immittance instrument.

Contralateral measurement of the acoustic reflex is achieved by presenting different acoustic signals through the reflex-eliciting earphone to one ear and measuring the change in stiffness that results due to the muscle contraction in the probe ear. This test should be performed with the middle ear system at the point of maximum admittance (compliance). If the reflex is not measured at the point of maximum admittance (compliance), it may be obliterated due to the pressure imbalance between the earcanal and the middle ear cavity.

Ipsilateral reflex measurement is achieved by stimulating and measuring the reflex in the same (probe) ear. The advantages of ipsilateral reflex measurement in diagnostic testing are reviewed by Jerger (1975).

Acoustic reflexes can be assessed by obtaining the threshold at which the reflex occurs, or screened by presenting the reflex-eliciting tone at a fixed intensity (100 or 105 dB HL). In the normal ear, acoustic reflexes are elicited between 85 and 95 dB HL. Once threshold is established at one frequency, the level is recorded and other frequencies can be tested. However, in immittance screening only one frequency is typically screened at a fixed intensity of about 100 dB (see Chapter 5).

Figure 3–23 provides graphic displays of acoustic reflex threshold measurement from two different ears; for both measures only ipsilateral reflexes were obtained. In Figure 3–23 (top) the test frequencies were 1000 and 2000 Hz, and the thresholds were 85 dB HL at 1000 Hz and 95 dB HL at 2000 Hz. In Figure 3–23 (bottom) the test frequencies also were 1000 and 2000 Hz; the thresholds were 85 dB HL for both frequencies. Note how the amplitude changes in the recordings by varying the intensity of the eliciting signal.

The presence of reflexes within normal limits at all frequencies is consistent with normal middle ear function; there is also a high probability that auditory sensitivity is within normal limits. However, acoustic reflexes may occur at expected intensities at all

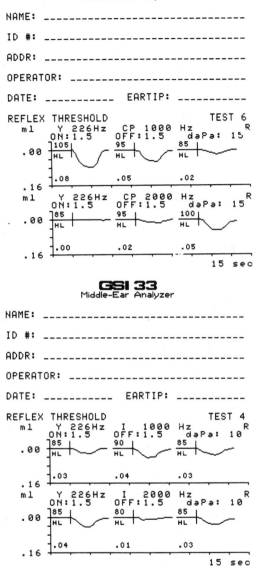

Figure 3–23. Two examples showing ipsilateral acoustic reflex recordings. The presence of a reflex is indicated by a downward deflection of the tracing (see text for additional description).

frequencies when mild or moderate to severe sensorineural hearing loss is present. For this reason, acoustic reflexes cannot be used to predict hearing threshold sensitivity with absolute assurance. Hearing threshold sensitivity must be assessed behaviorally if there are questions regarding hearing loss.

If reflexes are absent, some form of middle ear disease may be indicated. Absent reflexes may also indicate a moderate to severe sensorineural hearing loss without recruitment, or a paralysis of the seventh cranial nerve in the central auditory pathways. Absent reflexes have also occasionally been observed in individuals with normal or near-normal hearing, which may indicate middle ear disease or neurological involvement of the eighth or seventh nerve.

Partial or elevated reflexes may also be recorded. "Partial" means that a reflex is present at some frequencies tested and absent at others, and "elevated" refers to reflexes that are present at a hearing level exceeding 100 dB HL. Partial or elevated reflexes may indi-

cate the presence of a hearing loss at those frequencies in which they are absent.

Acoustic reflex measures provide a powerful diagnostic assessment of middle ear function and neurological functioning of the auditory system, as well as an index of auditory sensitivity. However, as pointed out in Chapter 5, because of their high level of sensitivity, acoustic reflexes are not used as a referral criterion for screening.

Application of Audiometric and Immittance Principles

The following four cases will be used to integrate and clarify the audiometric and immittance principles discussed in this chapter. Figure 3–24 shows findings for normal hearing and normal middle ear function bilater-

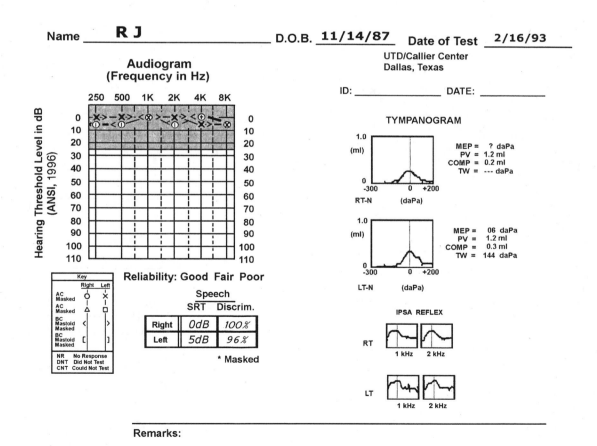

Figure 3–24. Audiometric and immittance findings within normal limits bilaterally.

ally. On the audiogram, thresholds are no poorer than 5 dB HL at any test frequency. As expected, speech audiometry reveals normal SRTs, agreeing with PTAs, and speech recognition scores within the normal range (90 to 100%). Tympanograms are type A bilaterally, with tympanometric peak pressure [Figs. 3–24 through 3–27 show tympanometric peak pressure as middle ear pressure (MEP)], static admittance/compliance (COMP), and TW within the normal range for the left ear; static COMP is at the lower range of normal for the right ear, which explains why MEP and TW were not recordable. Ipsilateral acoustic reflexes are present bilaterally at 1000 and 2000 Hz. Immittance results are consistent with normal middle ear function.

Figure 3–25 shows findings for a mild to severe bilateral sloping sensorineural hearing loss. Thresholds are within the range of normal limits at 250 and 500 Hz and drop into the moderate to severe range at higher frequencies. SRTs are within normal limits and agree with the two-frequency PTA (500 and 1000 Hz). In this case, because of the large difference between thresholds at 1000 and 2000 Hz, only 500 and 1000 Hz are used to calculate the PTA. Speech recognition scores are reduced bilaterally, with a poorer score in the left ear (70%) than in the right (82%).

Normal tympanograms (type A) with MEP, static COMP, and TW within normal limits are shown bilaterally. Note that acoustic reflexes are present bilaterally despite the

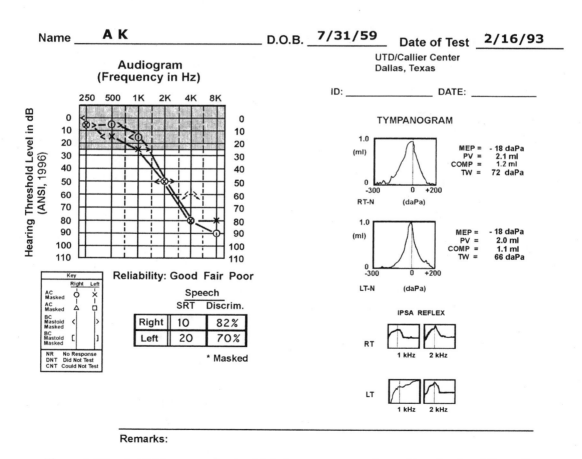

Figure 3–25. A mild to severe sloping high-frequency sensorineural hearing loss bilaterally.

presence of the high frequency hearing loss. Immittance results are consistent with normal middle ear function.

Individuals with audiometric findings like those shown in Figure 3–25 would be difficult to identify without pure tone audiometric tests. Such individuals will usually respond to speech within normal limits because of the normal thresholds in the 250 to 1000 Hz range. However, such individuals will have considerable difficulty in speech recognition, especially in the presence of background noise; and this difficulty may not be readily apparent to others. In addition, abnormal speech production may be present because high frequency fricative and sibilant sounds would be distorted. Only through audiometric screening/test-

ing would individuals with audiometric results like those shown in Figure 3–25 be detected.

Results in Figure 3–26 show normal hearing in the right ear with a mild rising conductive hearing loss in the left ear. SRTs are in agreement with the PTA for both ears and support the degree of hearing loss in the left ear. Speech recognition scores are within normal limits bilaterally.

Immittance findings support normal middle ear function for the right ear and the presence of a conductive hearing loss in the left ear. For the right ear, the tympanogram is normal (type A), with MEP, static COMP, and TW within the normal range. The left ear shows a flat (type B) tympanogram with immeasurable static COMP. Note that the

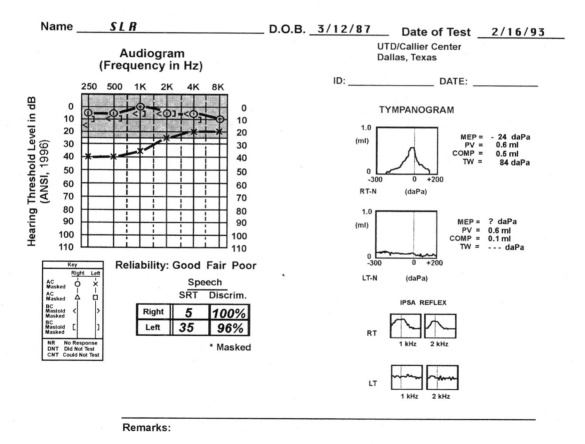

Figure 3–26. A mild left ear rising conductive hearing loss with normal hearing in the right ear.

PV for the left ear is within normal limits, suggesting that the eardrum is intact. Acoustic reflexes are present in the right ear and, due to the conductive pathological condition, absent in the left ear. Contralateral acoustic reflexes were not measured but would be absent bilaterally.

Figure 3–27 shows audiometric results for a hearing loss in the severe to profound range bilaterally. Thresholds between 250 and 500 Hz range from 65 dB HL; no responses were recorded at 110 dB HL above 1000 Hz. SRTs and speech recognition scores could not be obtained due to the severity of the loss. Note that, even though the SRTs could not be measured, SATs were obtained and agreed with thresholds in the 250 Hz region. Response by bone conduction was obtained at 250 Hz at

maximum limits of the audiometer (40 dB HL) for each ear, but no responses were obtained above this frequency. Because bone conduction threshold responses were present only at 250 Hz at equipment limits (40 dB HL), they are considered tactile stimulation rather than auditory; the child felt them rather than heard them.

The tympanogram was normal for the left ear, but abnormal (flat; type B) with low static COMP for the right ear. The physical volume was within the normal range for the right ear, indicating that the eardrum was intact. As expected, due to the degree of hearing loss present, acoustic reflexes were absent bilaterally.

The data in Figure 3–27 point out the value of immittance measures when severe to profound hearing loss is present. Due to

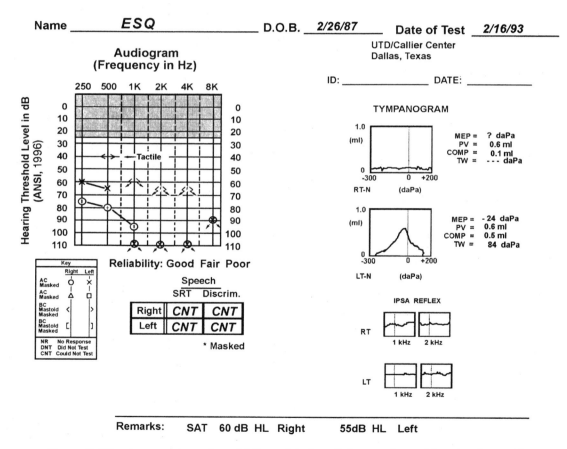

Figure 3–27. A severe to profound bilateral (primarily) sensorineural hearing loss with abnormal immittance findings for the right ear.

the output limitations of bone conduction testing, it is impossible to detect conductive hearing loss when air conduction thresholds exceed 70 dB HL. Therefore, the only means available to detect conductive disorders with a loss this severe is through the use of immittance testing. The results in Figure 3–27 suggest the presence of a significant conductive disorder and the child should be referred for medical examination.

What Families Want to Know about Diagnosis

Families will respond in unique and different ways to the life-changing diagnosis of their child's hearing loss. For example, one family may react with an expressive emotional outbreak, while another family will have a very quiet and stoic demeanor. Yet, both forms of reactions are indicative of an underlying concern for the well-being of the family's child. It is the clinician's skills and experience that will determine success in building rapport to address each family's emotional and informational needs. Rapport will develop once family needs are established.

Surveys have shown that families expect professionals to provide very specific information about hearing loss. Primarily families suggest that information should include how the loss will affect the child's cognitive and emotional development, and describe the expected ramifications upon the family (Martin, George, O'Neal, & Daley, 1987; Roush, 2000; Williams & Darbyshire, 1982). Roush and Harrison (2002) mailed two questionnaires to 600 families having children 3 months to 5 years and 10 months with newly identified hearing loss; two thirds of the parents reported that they had children with a severe-to-profound hearing loss. The first questionnaire was completed at initial diagnosis and the second a few months following the initial diagnosis. Parents were asked to rate priorities as high, medium, or low for a number of topics dealing with the initial diagnosis of their child's hearing loss. Those

topics prioritized at diagnosis, beginning with the highest priority, were:

> Causes of hearing loss
> Coping with the emotional aspects of hearing loss
> Understanding the audiogram
> Learning to listen and speak
> Understanding the ear and hearing

Interestingly, the priorities changed on the questionnaire completed following initial diagnosis. Beginning with the highest priority parents were more concerned with:

> Learning to listen and speak
> Realistic time lines for learning to listen and speak
> Cochlear implants
> Communication options
> Responsibilities of early intervention agencies
> Legal rights of children with hearing loss

It is clear from these data that families want to make informed decisions about their child's hearing health care by acquiring as much information as possible. Professionals must be prepared to provide as much information to parents as possible, as well as direct parents to sources of information when requested.

Genetic Counseling

Congenital hearing loss occurs in 1 out of 1000 births and 50% of the losses are genetically based. Available technology and knowledge make it possible to determine the genetic makeup of hearing loss in many families and also to calculate probabilities for hearing loss in additional children. It is imperative that families with infants and children having newly identified hearing loss undergo genetic studies and counseling. There are a number of centers focusing on the genetics of hearing loss across the United States that provide educational information for professionals and families. A few of the major facilities include:

American Society of Human Genetics, 9650 Rockville Pike, Bethesda, MD 20814 (www.society@ashg.org)

U.S. Department of Energy Office of Science, Human Genome Project (www.ornl.gov/TechResources/Human_Genome)

Numerous organizations and societies dealing with genetics (www.faseb.org/genetics)

Summary

This chapter reviews the principles and procedures used for behavioral and physiological audiological assessment of infants and children and provides examples of how they are applied. Sophisticated audiological procedures now available facilitate the identification of infants and children with hearing loss at an increasingly earlier age. Professionals in the schools need an understanding of the procedures available to provide the most effective educational programs.

References

American Medical Association (AMA). (1951). Specification of the council on physical medicine and rehabilitation of the American Medical Association. *JAMA, 146,* 255–257.

American National Standards Institute (ANSI). (1964). Standard reference zero for calibration of pure-tone audiometers: ISD recommendation R389. New York: American National Standards Institute.

American National Standards Institute (ANSI). (1970). Specifications for audiometers (ANSI S3.6–1969). New York: American National Standards Institute.

American National Standards Institute (ANSI). (1987). American National Standard specifications for instruments to measure aural acoustic impedance and admittance (ANSI S3.39–1987). New York: American National Standards Institute.

American National Standards Institute (ANSI). (1989). Specifications for audiometers (ANSI S3.6–1989). New York: American National Standards Institute.

American National Standards Institute (ANSI). (1996). Specifications for audiometers (ANSI S3.6–1996). New York: American National Standards Institute.

Arcia, E., & Connors C. (1998). Gender differences in ADHD. *J Dev Behav Pediatr, 19,* 77–83.

American Speech and Hearing Association (ASHA). (1979). Committee on Audiometric Evaluation: Guidelines for acoustic immittance screening of middle ear function. *ASHA, 21,* 283–288.

American Speech and Hearing Association (ASHA). (1988). Guidelines for determining threshold level for speech. *ASHA, 30,* 85–88.

American Speech and Hearing Association (ASHA). (1990a). Guidelines for screening hearing impairment and middle ear disorders. *ASHA, 32* (Suppl. 2), 17–24.

American Speech and Hearing Association (ASHA). (1990b). Guidelines for audiometric symbols. *ASHA, 32* (Suppl. 2), 25–30.

American Speech and Hearing Association (ASHA). (1995). Task force on central auditory processing consensus development. Washington, DC: American Speech Hearing Association.

American Speech and Hearing Association (ASHA). (1997). Guidelines for audiological screening. Rockville, MD: American Speech-Language-Hearing Association.

Berlin, C.I. (1967). Programmed instruction in the decibel. In: J.L. Northern (Ed.), *Hearing Disorders* (pp. 279–296). Boston: Little, Brown.

Berlin, C.I., Hood, L., Hurley, A., & Wen, H. (1994). Contralateral suppression of otoacoustic emissions: An index of the function of the medial olivocochlear system. *Otolaryngol Head Neck Surg, 110,* 3–21.

Boothroyd, A. (Ed.). (1988). *Hearing Impairment in Young Children.* Washington, DC: Alexander Graham Bell Association for the Deaf.

Carhart, R., & Jerger, J. (1959). Preferred method for clinical determination of pure tone thresholds. *J Speech Hear Disord, 24,* 330–345.

Chermak, G., & Musiek, F. (1997). *Central Auditory Processing Disorders: New Perspectives.* San Diego: Singular.

Clark, J., & Roeser, R. (1988). Three studies comparing performance of the ER-3A tubephone with TDH-50P earphone. *Ear Hear, 9,* 268–274.

Fiellau-Nikolajsen, M. (1983). Tympanometry and secretory otitis media: Observations on diagnosis, epidemiology, treatment, and prevention in prospective cohort studies of three-year-old children. *Acta Otolaryngol,* (Suppl. 394), 1–73.

Fletcher, H. (1950). A method of calculating hearing loss for speech from an audiogram. *J Acoust Soc Am, 22,* 1–5.

Goetzinger, C. (1978). Word discrimination testing. In: J. Katz (Ed.), *Handbook of Clinical Audiology* (pp. 149–158). Baltimore: Williams & Wilkins.

Goodman, A. (1965). Reference zero levels for pure tone audiometers. *ASHA, 7,* 262–263.

Hall, J. (1992). *Handbook of Auditory Evoked Responses.* Boston: Allyn & Bacon.

Hopkinson, N. (1978). Speech reception threshold. In: J. Katz (Ed.), *Handbook of Clinical Audiology* (pp. 141–158). Baltimore: Williams & Wilkins.

Hunter, L., Margolis, R., Daly, K., & Giebink, G. (1992, February). *Relationship of tympanometric estimates of middle ear volume to middle ear status at surgery.* Paper presented at the Midwinter Research Meeting of the Association for Research in Otolaryngology, St. Petersburg Beach, Florida.

Jerger, J. (1970). Clinical experience with impedance audiometry. *Arch Otolaryngol, 92,* 311–324.

Jerger, J., & Musiek, F. (2000). Report of the consensus conference on the diagnosis of auditory processing disorders in school-aged children. *J Am Acad Audiol, 11,* 467–474.

Jerger, S. (1975). Diagnostic use of impedance measures. In: J. Jerger (Ed.), *Handbook of Clinical Impedance Audiometry* (pp. 128–140). Acton, MA: American Electromedics Co.

Jirsa, R. (1994). The clinical utility of the P3 AERP in children with auditory processing disorders. *J Speech Hear Disord, 35,* 903–912.

Keith, R. (2000). Diagnosing central auditory processing disorders in children. In: R. Roeser, M. Valente, H. Hosford-Dunn, (Eds.), *Audiology Diagnosis* (pp. 337–353). New York: Thieme.

Konkle, D., & Rintelmann, W. (1983). Introduction to speech audiometry. In: W. Rintelmann (Ed.), *Principles of Speech Audiometry* (pp. 1–10). Baltimore: University Park Press.

Kraus, N. (2001). Auditory neuropathy: An historical and current perspective. In: A. Starr (Ed.), *Auditory Neuropathy: A New Perspective on Hearing Disorders* (pp. 1–14). San Diego: Singular.

Margolis, R., & Heller, J. (1987). Screening tympanometry: Criteria for medical referral. *Audiology, 26,* 197–208.

Martin, F., Champlin, C., & Chambers, J. (1998). Seventh survey of audiometric practices in the United States. *J Am Acad Audiol, 9,* 311–313.

Martin, F., George, K., O'Neal, J., & Daley, J. (1987). Audiologists' and parents' attitudes regarding counseling of families of hearing-impaired children. *ASHA, 29,* 27–33.

Martin, F., & Kopra, L. (1970). Symbols in pure tone audiometry. *ASHA, 12,* 182–185.

Matkin, N. (1979). The audiologic examination of young children at risk. *Ear Nose Throat J, 58,* 297–302.

Musiek, F., Baran, J. & Pinheiro, M. (1994). *Neuraudiology: Case Studies* (pp. 7–28). San Diego: Singular.

Musket, C., & Roeser, R. (1977). Using circumaural enclosures with children. *J Speech Hear Res, 20,* 325–333.

Northern, J.L., & Downs, M. (2002). *Hearing in Children.* Baltimore: Lippincott Williams & Wilkins.

Nozza, R., Bluestone, C., Kardatze, D., & Bachman, R. (1994). Identification of middle ear effusion by aural acoustic admittance and otoscopy. *Ear Hear, 15,* 310–323.

Roeser, R. (1986). *Diagnostic Audiology.* Austin: Pro-Ed.

Roeser, R., Seidel, J., & Glorig, A. (1975). Performance of earphone enclosures for threshold audiometry. *Sound Vibration, 10,* 22–25.

Roush, J. (2000). Implementing parent-infant services: Advice from families. In: R. Seewald (Ed.), *A Sound Foundation Through Early Amplification: Proceedings of an International Conference, Stafa, Switzerland* (pp. 159–165). Chicago, IL: Phonak.

Roush, J., & Harrison, M. (2002). What parents want to know at diagnosis and during the first year. *The Hearing Journal, 55,* 52–54.

Shanks, J., Stelmachowicz, P., Beauchaine, K., & Schulte, L. (1992). Equivalent earcanal volumes in children pre- and posttympanostomy tube insertion. *J Speech Hear Res, 35,* 936–941.

Sininger, Y., & Oba, S. (2001). Patients with auditory neuropathy: Who are they and what can they hear? In: A. Starr (Ed.), *Auditory Neuropathy: A New Perspective on Hearing Disorders* (pp. 15–36). San Diego: Singular.

Starr, A., Picton, T.W., Sininger, Y., Hood, L., & Berlin, C.I. (1996). Auditory neuropathy. *Brain, 119,* 741–753.

Stein, L., Tremblay, K., Pasterak, J., Benerjee, S., Lindermann, K., & Kraus, N. (1996). Brainstem abnormalities in neonates with normal otoacoustic emissions. *Semin Hear, 17,* 197–213.

Walton, W., & Wilson, W. (1972). Stability of routinely serviced portable audiometers. *Lang Speech Hear Serv Sch, 3,* 36–43.

Williams, D., & Darbyshire, J. (1982). Diagnosis of deafness: A study of family responses and needs. *Volta Review, 84,* 24–30.

4

Medical Aspects of Disorders of the Auditory System

PETER S. ROLAND AND ANGELA G. SHOUP

The desire to take medicine is perhaps the greatest feature which distinguishes man from animals.

—Sir William Osler, 1849–1919

For school-age children, the initial referral to obtain services from either or both the otolaryngologist and the audiologist often comes from the school nurse, speech-language pathologist, teachers, or parents. In evaluation and management of infants and children, school personnel may encounter various indicators associated with medically treatable conditions requiring appropriate referral. The otolaryngologist and audiologist often work closely in the treatment of children with auditory and vestibular disorders. Referrals for evaluation and treatment are reciprocal. In some cases, a physician will refer a child to an audiologist in order to obtain additional information about the auditory or vestibular system or for appropriate nonmedical treatment of auditory impairment. The audiologist identifies medically relevant indicators for referral of patients to the otolaryngologist for evaluation and treatment.

In cases of initial identification of hearing impairment at any age, the audiologist strives to quantify the disorder and obtain appropriate intervention services. The physician evaluates the need for medical treatment and attempts to determine etiology in order to recommend appropriate medical intervention and provide prognostic information. This chapter focuses on selected auditory and vestibular conditions encountered in the pediatric population.

History

As with any evaluation, the initial step when a patient presents with auditory or vestibular difficulties is a problem-focused case history. In the evaluation of children, developing rapport with the parents is as important as relating well to the child. Even older children may have difficulty explaining their experiences to strangers. Parents are the experts on their children, and their observations should be encouraged.

Children present to the otolaryngologist with a limited number of complaints. Some of the more commonly reported symptoms that will be discussed are tinnitus (internally generated sound in the ear), hearing loss, otalgia (ear pain), otorrhea (drainage from the ear), and vertigo (a form of dizziness). Adequate evaluation requires complete elucidation of difficulties. In addition to a general birth and medical history, the following information should be gathered for each presenting symptom:

1. When the symptom was first noted
2. Whether the symptom is constantly present or intermittent

3. If the symptom is intermittent, how often it occurs and how long it lasts with each occurrence
4. Severity of the symptom
5. Whether, in general, the symptom is improving or worsening
6. Whether the symptom is bilateral or unilateral. If bilateral and intermittent, does it occur in each ear simultaneously or independently? If bilateral, did it begin simultaneously in both ears?
7. If more than one symptom is troubling the patient, one must establish if the symptoms occur independently or are clustered to form a symptom complex (syndrome).

Tinnitus

Millions of persons experience varying degrees of tinnitus; indeed, at some time or another almost everyone experiences brief episodes of tinnitus, usually in quiet environments. Most individuals are not bothered by such brief episodes, but when tinnitus remains sustained they may experience considerable discomfort. Some persons find the symptom annoying. Others are kept awake at night and may have difficulty concentrating during the day. A few individuals find the tinnitus disabling and are prevented from pursuing their usual daily activities. An occasional individual may find the experience so torturous that suicide is contemplated.

Children may have much greater difficulty in expressing and describing their subjective sensations. On the whole, tinnitus seems to be a less bothersome symptom in the pediatric age group than it is among adults. Nonetheless, some children have their hearing loss first identified as part of an evaluation for tinnitus. Although the etiology of tinnitus is often unknown, tinnitus can be associated with otologic disease that may benefit from treatment. Children who report tinnitus may also experience hearing loss or dizziness. For these reasons, children should be referred for medical evaluation if they report hissing or ringing sounds in their ears.

Hearing Loss

Although formal audiometric testing is the most critical component in assessing hearing loss, it is often useful to gain some understanding of how much difficulty the child experiences due to hypoacusis, and in what circumstances. This can be somewhat difficult, especially in younger children. Consultation with family and teachers is critical. Parents are usually acute observers of their own child's hearing acuity and may be aware of fairly subtle changes. Although parents can be (and often are) manipulated by children who exhibit nonorganic hearing loss, a parent's report of suspected auditory dysfunction should be sufficient to warrant additional testing.

Various congenital disorders or diseases may be associated with hearing loss (Fig. 4–1). Some of these are genetic, and presence of a family history of hearing loss can provide prognostic and diagnostic information in evaluation of the hearing-impaired child. If other family members have hearing loss, the nature of such losses should be explored and audiograms obtained. The time at which children first noted hearing loss, how they noted it, and its rate of progression should always be determined if possible. Individuals should be specifically evaluated to see if their hearing fluctuates and, if so, under what circumstances, how frequently, and with what severity. Any association of the hearing loss with vertigo or tinnitus, otalgia, otorrhea, upper respiratory infection, nasal stuffiness, headache, dysarthria (speech disorder involving motor control of the articulators), dysphagia (swallowing disorder), visual changes, numbness or tingling in the extremities, or focal motor weakness should all be established.

The time course of the hearing change is the most useful piece of historical information. Losses that have occurred many years prior to the current evaluation and are stable are not likely to require medical intervention. In making such determinations the availability of previous audiograms is extremely helpful. Inquiries should be made into the circumstances of longstanding

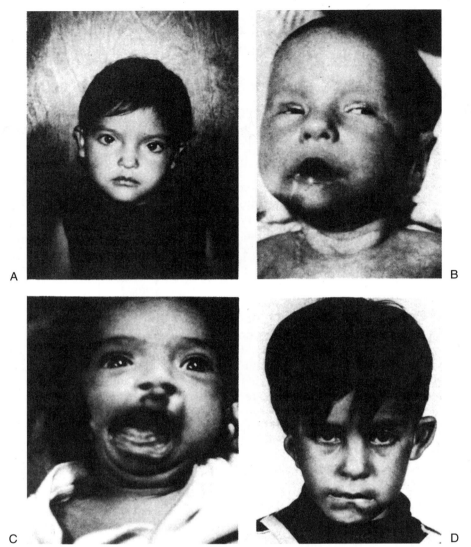

Figure 4–1. Examples of genetic birth defect syndromes with associated hearing loss. (A) Waardenburg's syndrome. This patient does not have a white forelock; she has the increased medial intercanthal distance, severe hearing loss, and brilliant blue eyes. (B) Rubella syndrome. This infant had microcephaly, microphthalmia, carp-shaped mouth, large abnormal ears, a bulbous nasal tip, and a fixed stapes. (Reprinted with permission from Hemenway, Sardo, & McChesney, 1969). (C) Treacher Collins syndrome with severe facial malformations including a very small mandible, which caused the tongue to obstruct the airway and led to his death. Temporal bone pathological findings showed a malformed monopod stapes, and the facial nerve exited directly from the side of the skull. (Reprinted with permission from Sando, Hemenway, & Morgan, 1968). (D) Microtia-atresia. Both the malformed right ear and the normal-appearing left ear had conductive losses. The left ear hearing loss was due to stapes fixation. (Reprinted with permission from Bergstrom, 1976).

losses, and any association with febrile illness, antibiotic therapy, noise exposure, trauma, or surgery must be noted.

Otalgia

Otalgia (ear pain) precipitates many physician visits and has a myriad of causes. In a high percentage of adults, otalgia is not otogenic. It is estimated that in the primary care setting, only 50% of cases of ear pain in adults are caused by ear disease. Although nonotogenic otalgia is less common in children, they may also experience pain as occurring within the structures of the ear when it is, in fact, referred from other related structures. Pain of otologic origin is usually dull, aching, and relatively constant. Pain that comes and goes frequently during the day is rarely otogenic. Referred otalgia is commonly due to disorders affecting the larynx, pharynx, and tonsils. Tonsillitis and pharyngitis are two common causes of referred otalgia in children. Disorders of the muscles of mastication and the temporomandibular joint are also often perceived as ear pain.

Many important otologic conditions such as cholesteatoma, other forms of chronic otitis media, Meniere's disease, and acoustic tumor may not be associated with pain. Otogenic ear pain may be due to cerumen impaction, infection, and, quite rarely, neoplasms. The most common cause of otogenic ear pain is infection. Both external otitis and acute otitis media may cause excruciating pain that precipitates a physician visit, usually on an emergent basis. Because most such cases are treated in the primary care setting, the incidence of ear pain due to otologic disease is actually lower in a referral otolaryngology practice than it is in a general practice.

Otorrhea

With the rare exception of cases in which spinal fluid drains through the ear, otorrhea (drainage from the ear) is related to infection. When otorrhea is present, the child's history and associated symptoms are especially important. Painless drainage is usually the result of chronic otitis media or its complications. These may be cholesteatoma, chronic mastoiditis due to irreversible mucosal disease, and tympanic membrane perforation or chronic reflux through the eustachian tube. Otorrhea may occur sporadically as the result of an otherwise asymptomatic tympanic membrane perforation, especially if water has inadvertently entered the middle ear space. Children with a history of painless drainage going back for months or years are highly suspect of harboring a temporal bone cholesteatoma. This is especially true if the drainage fails to resolve after vigorous treatment with systemic and topical antibiotics. Drainage associated with pain is more likely to be caused by an acute infectious process. Otitis media that results in rupture of the tympanic membrane may be preceded by very severe ear pain. Acute external otitis is frequently manifested by the simultaneous occurrence of aural drainage and acute ear pain.

Vertigo

Vertigo (dizziness) has myriad causes, many of which are entirely unrelated to the temporal bone and ear. A detailed history is the single most important piece of information in establishing a diagnosis. The following points should be clearly elucidated in every patient history:

1. What exactly does the child mean by "dizziness"? What does he or she experience?
2. When did the symptom first occur, how often does it occur, and how long does it last when it does occur?
3. What is the shortest and longest time the dizziness has lasted?
4. Is the dizziness associated with nausea, vomiting, or sweating?
5. Is the child aware of any change in hearing before, during, or after the dizzy spell?
6. Do any activities reliably bring on the dizzy spell?

7. Is the dizzy spell associated with any difficulty in swallowing or speaking or any change in vision?

8. Is consciousness ever completely lost during a dizzy spell?

9. Is there associated tinnitus or feeling of aural fullness?

10. Can the child tell when a dizzy episode is about to occur?

11. Does the child have headaches before, during, or after each episode of vertigo or disequilibrium?

12. Is there is a familial history of migraine?

Careful evaluation of the history in light of basic audiometry will usually establish whether the vertigo is likely to be otogenic in etiology and will probably suggest a diagnosis. Descriptions of vertigo vary dramatically. Vertigo arising from the vestibular system generally has as its principal component "the illusion of motion." This may be a sense of rotation or the sense of falling to one side or the other. When the child uses such terms as "light-headed," "giddy," "confused," or "faint" the sensation is not likely to be labyrinthine in origin. Finding out about possible headaches is also of importance. Migraine is a much more common cause of episodic vertigo in childhood than in adulthood and accounts for a substantial number of children with intermittent dizzy spells. Once additional information has been obtained through careful questioning and review of the patient's history, further diagnostic tests can be ordered to confirm or deny the initial conclusions.

Physical Examination of the Ear

Once historical information has been obtained and clarified, examination of the ear begins with the auricle. The size and shape of the auricle and its position should be carefully noted. Some children will have no auricle (anotia) due to congenital aural atresia, some will have one that is abnormally small (microtia) or poorly formed (Fig. 4–1D), and other children may have an auricle placed either unusually low with respect to the remainder of the facial skeleton or unusually high (melotia). The area around the auricle should also be assessed. Presence of auricular pits, fistulas, accessory tags, and cysts may be indicative of abnormalities in other parts of the auditory system. Postauricular scars should be noted because their presence suggests previous surgeries. The mastoid should be inspected for any evidence of tenderness or swelling.

The size and adequacy of the external auditory canal should be ascertained. Children with very narrow, or stenotic, earcanals may be more at risk for cerumen impaction. Extremely narrow earcanals also may be associated with other developmental anomalies within the auditory system. Some children have collapsing external auditory canals with a slitlike opening. This should be noted prior to audiometry so that insert earphones can be used to evaluate the tympanic membrane and middle ear conduction mechanism.

To assess the likelihood of collapse and the adequacy of the size of the external auditory canal, the auricle should be drawn backward and upward. This opens the lateral portion of the cartilaginous canal and permits assessment of the bony canal. The presence of flaking skin, which suggests chronic seborrheic dermatitis, should be noted at this time. An otoscope may then be used to examine the external auditory canal and tympanic membrane. Preliminary examination of the size of the canal will allow the appropriate-sized speculum to be selected. The largest speculum that can be comfortably inserted into the patient's external auditory canal should be chosen. Specula for use in the external auditory canal are designed in such a way that they rarely protrude further into the ear than the cartilaginous portion of the external auditory canal. This portion can be stretched and manipulated with minimal or no discomfort. Should the speculum reach the inner third of the earcanal, even the slightest pressure will be extraordinarily painful. For optimum visualization, the patient's head should be tilted toward the opposite shoulder to account for the normal upward direction of the earcanal.

It will often be necessary to remove cerumen from the external auditory canal to examine the tympanic membrane. This may be accomplished by a trained health care professional using an ear syringe or Waterpik for the instillation of water to "flush" the cerumen out of the external auditory canal. Water irrigation should not be used in patients who have tympanostomy tubes [pressure equalization (p.e.) tubes] or perforations of the tympanic membrane. Alternatively, cerumen may be removed using small curettes or a cerumen spoon with or without the adjunctive use of an operating microscope. Cerumen that has been impacted into the external auditory canal by the repeated use of Q-tips may be difficult to remove. Such children should be referred to an otolaryngologist who can remove the cerumen using the operating microscope if irrigation techniques have failed. Occasionally, a general anesthetic will be required for cerumen removal.

Inspection of the earcanal may also reveal foreign bodies. These may include insects, beads, beans, grains, rocks, etc. Sometimes the foreign body may cause irritation and inflammation of the canal. The foreign body must be removed by physical extraction or suction. Irrigation should be used with caution because some foreign bodies may expand when wet (e.g., beans, grains). In addition, living insects may need to be immobilized prior to removal.

Once the earcanal is clear, every attempt should be made to visualize the entire tympanic membrane. Otoscopic or microscopic examination of the ear cannot be considered complete until the entire tympanic membrane, including the pars flaccida, has been visualized. Figure 4–2 shows the landmarks on the tympanic membrane. The annulus tympanicus should be followed anteriorly and posteriorly until it meets the anterior and posterior malleolar folds. The pars flaccida lies between these two folds. Perforation or deep retraction of the pars flaccida is virtually always diagnostic of a choleste-

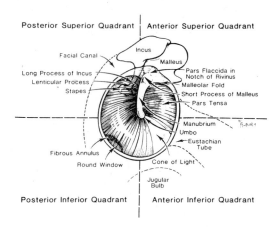

Figure 4–2. Diagram of the lateral surface of the tympanic membrane. Special note should be made of the pars flaccida. Failure to examine the pars flaccida is a common cause of missed cholesteatoma. The head of the malleus and incus are not normally seen. When the heads of these ossicles can be seen, this reliably indicates the presence of bony erosion almost always due to cholesteatoma. (Reprinted with permission from Meyerhoff & Carter, 1984).

atoma. Both the long and short process of the malleus can be seen through the normal tympanic membrane, and their presence should be noted. The long process of the incus and chorda tympani can frequently, although not invariably, be seen as well (Fig. 4–3). However, if the head of the malleus or body of the incus is seen, there has been erosion of the superior external auditory canal and lateral wall of the middle ear space. This is seen almost exclusively in cholesteatoma.

Occasionally, a retracted tympanic membrane lies directly on the incudostapedial joint, forming a "myringostapediopexy." In such circumstances, long-term retraction, probably due to eustachian tube insufficiency, can be assumed. Surprisingly, hearing can often be near normal in such situations. The examiner should also be wary of the "dimeric tympanic membrane," which results when perforations of the tympanic membrane heal without the middle fibrous layer regenerating in normal fashion. The dimeric tympanic membrane is an extremely thin "secondary" membrane that is always

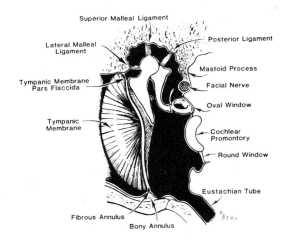

Figure 4–3. Diagram of the middle ear space seen in coronal cross section. The funnel shape of the tympanic membrane can be clearly seen. One can appreciate that the heads of the ossicles should not normally be visible. A very close relationship between the facial nerve and the footplate of the stapes is readily apparent in the diagram. The inferior position of the round window should also be noted. (Reprinted with permission from Meyerhoff & Carter, 1984.)

translucent and often transparent. Such secondary membranes may be indistinguishable from perforations without the use of the operating microscope.

Masses behind the tympanic membrane may be caused by a variety of pathological processes. Color is important and may be a clue to etiology. White masses suggest cholesteatoma, tympanosclerosis, or, very rarely, middle ear osteoma. Dark blue masses suggest venous vascular structures, such as a high jugular bulb. Dark red masses suggest highly vascular tumors such as glomus tympanicum tumors or granulation tissue. The presence of pulsations within a mass strongly suggests that it is arterialized and vascular in etiology. This can sometimes be confirmed by applying positive pressure to the tympanic membrane using the pneumatic otoscope. Positive pressure reduces blood flow within the mass and causes blanching of the drum overlying the middle ear mass. Such blanching is referred to as a positive Brown's sign and strongly suggests

a vascular neoplasm. Occasionally, a red blotch will be seen in the area of the oval window. This may not be a mass but may represent the hypervascular bone characteristic of an active focus of otosclerosis.

Visual evaluation of tympanic membrane function can be accomplished with a pneumatic otoscope. The pneumatic otoscope is used to create positive or negative pressure on the tympanic membrane. Such pressure changes normally cause visible movement; thus, using the pneumatic otoscope, the examiner can assess the degree of mobility of the tympanic membrane. Chronic middle ear effusion, for example, usually promotes a sluggish or immobile tympanic membrane. In addition, brisk tympanic movements virtually exclude the possibility of tympanic membrane perforation. Pneumatic otoscopy using the handheld otoscope may occasionally induce movement in healed secondary (dimeric) membranes, which makes it apparent that the drum is indeed intact although quite thin. Tympanometry (Chapter 3) is an objective measure of tympanic membrane function used by audiologists.

No otologic examination is complete without examination of the facial nerve. Patients should be asked to frown, smile, wrinkle their nose, whistle, show their teeth, and shut their eyes. Any asymmetry between sides or the inability to perform any of these motions should be clearly noted. The earliest and most subtle sign of facial weakness is lagophthalmos. The eyelid closes a bit more slowly on the affected side than on the normal, contralateral side. This is clearly evident when the patient blinks spontaneously: the blink on the affected side appears to lag behind its normal contralateral partner.

Diseases of the External Auditory Canal

A variety of conditions, most of which occur in children, affect the external auditory canal. Of special importance are the congenital aural atresias that are generally diagnosed in childhood and require staged management of both the auditory and cosmetic components.

Congenital Aural Atresias

Malformations of the external and middle ears occur approximately once in every 10,000 to 20,000 births. Congenital aural atresias can involve the pinna, external auditory canal, middle ear space, ossicles, and/or the inner ear. Such anomalies may occur alone or in association with other regional or distant defects. Fortunately, the atresia occurs unilaterally four times more frequently than it does bilaterally.

A variety of syndromes associated with malformations of the ear have been identified (Table 4–1). It appears that a significant percentage of cases of atresia are not due to genetic causes. The etiology in unilateral cases often remains obscure, but many may be acquired as the result of vascular injury to the branchial arches, which can occur in utero. Because embryological development of the ear is finished by week 28 of gestation, injuries that occur in late pregnancy will not affect development of the ear. Portions of the external auditory canal and middle ear develop from the same underlying embryological structures, so middle ear malformations are frequently associated with malformations of the external auditory canal. Fortu-

Table 4–1. Syndromes Associated with Congenital Aural Atresia or Malformations of the Ear

Apert's syndrome
Crouzon's disease
Franceschetti syndrome
Marfan syndrome
Treacher Collins syndrome
Pierre Robin syndrome
Goldenhar's syndrome
Nager's acrofacial dysostosis
Wildervanck's syndrome
Juvenile Paget disease
Möbius' syndrome
Levy-Hollister's syndrome (LADD)
CHARGE syndrome
Fraser's syndrome
Noonan's syndrome

nately, however, the cochlea, semicircular canals, and eighth cranial nerve are rarely affected. Thus, the hearing loss encountered with aural atresia is usually conductive. The anatomical course of the facial nerve is frequently altered in malformations of the ear and temporal bone, which makes surgical correction somewhat more hazardous, but facial nerve function is rarely affected by the malformation. The tympanic membrane is frequently replaced by a bony plate, and there are a large variety of identified malformations and deformities of the ossicles.

When there is gross malformation of the auricle, atresia is usually identified promptly, often on the day of birth. When the pinna is normal, identification of the stenotic or atretic external auditory canal may be delayed for a number of years if universal newborn hearing screening is not implemented at the birthing facility. In such cases, identification may await the child's failure to meet developmental guidelines or failure of screening audiometric tests in school.

Management of the child with congenital aural atresia should begin with a complete evaluation to detect any associated abnormalities. If there is an external auditory canal present, it should be carefully inspected to determine whether it becomes stenotic or atretic medially. Careful inspection of the external auditory canal is often difficult in the small child and occasionally requires radiographic imaging, especially if the earcanal is extremely narrow (stenotic). Radiographic imaging can also be used to verify the status of the middle ear structures and the bony cochlea as well as the position of the temporomandibular joint in candidates for surgery.

More important than radiographic assessment is accurate determination of hearing thresholds. Differentiation of conductive from sensorineural components is important but often difficult in the young child, and ear specific sensory sensitivity may be impossible to ascertain in patients with bilateral atresia. The use of both air and bone conduction auditory brainstem response (ABR) for threshold assessment may be pivotal in assessing patients who cannot reliably complete behavioral audiometric testing.

In patients with unilateral atresia, if hearing is normal in the nonatretic ear, parents should be counseled about the difficulties encountered by a child with unilateral hearing loss. An FM system may be recommended for use in the classroom. Because hearing rehabilitation must occur long before children with bilateral atresia are surgical candidates, amplification needs to be considered even in those individuals who may later benefit from reconstructive operations. The need for hearing restoration is immediate and should not be delayed even a few weeks beyond birth. Educational and social development can be retarded by hearing loss and the restoration of hearing after the critical developmental period may not compensate for the handicapping effects of early hearing loss. The available options include the use of conventional amplification, externally applied bone conduction hearing aids, and implantable bone conduction hearing aids. As a general rule, when conventional amplification can be used, it is the treatment of choice. The BAHA, an implanted bone conduction system, is preferred, when appropriate, in patients with unilateral or bilateral maximal conductive hearing losses and normal bone levels if they cannot be successfully fitted with conventional hearing aids. The implanted BAHA system is FDA cleared to treat children age 5 years and older. However, the BAHA Softband can be used in children under 5 years of age. Using an adjustable elastic band to connect to the sound processor and hold it comfortably against the skin, the BAHA Softband allows young children to experience the benefits of the BAHA until they are old enough to receive the complete system (Fig. 4–4).

Repair of the external auditory canal, tympanic membrane, and middle ear space can be accomplished by a variety of surgical techniques. Favorable outcomes are more likely in individuals with the least severe abnormalities. Whether surgical repair should be undertaken depends entirely on the patient and parents. It is often useful to wait until the child is old enough to participate in the decision for surgical repair of congenital atresia. Surgical intervention is not without risks and complications. Frequently, the air–bone gap can be closed to 30 dB or less but failure to close the air–bone gap is the most common problem associated with reconstructive surgery. It is also relatively common for the external auditory canal to gradually narrow again after surgery. Finally, although the rate remains low, facial nerve injury occurs significantly more commonly after repair of congenital lesions than after repair of acquired lesions. In patients with only conductive hearing losses, even if maximal, the continued use of amplification may provide perfectly adequate hearing restoration, thus negating the need for surgery.

Dermatitis

Two types of dermatitis affect the external auditory ear with some frequency. These are seborrheic and atopic dermatitis. Seborrheic dermatitis, the most common, is usually manifested by chronic itching of the external auditory canals and frequently associated with dry, flaky skin over the conchal bowl and medial portions of the external auditory canal. Careful physical examination often reveals the complete or near absence of cerumen. The condition is important not only because itching is subjectively distressing, but chronic irritation of the skin of the external auditory canal reduces its effectiveness as a barrier to infection. Thus, children with chronic seborrheic dermatitis are much more susceptible to chronic bacterial external otitis (swimmer's ear) than are the unaffected, normal population. Indeed, after careful questioning, many children who have recurrent episodes of external otitis will be discovered to have chronic dry, flaking, and itchy external auditory canals. In some children the same condition waxes and wanes on an irregular and unpredictable basis. Many children will have little or no difficulty for years, with sporadic "flareups" lasting weeks or months. Seborrheic dermatitis of the external auditory canal responds favorably to the use of very low dose

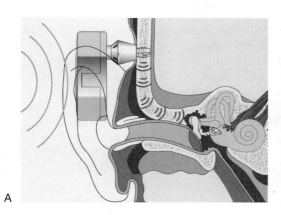

A

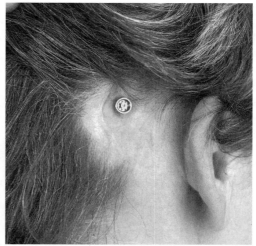

B

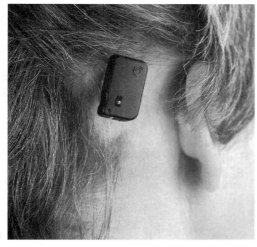

C

Figure 4–4. Bone-Anchored Hearing Aid (BAHA; Entific Medical Systems, reprinted with permission): (A) Diagram of the BAHA system producing sound movement through direct bone conduction. (B) External abutment as seen in position on the mastoid of an individual. (C) The BAHA sound processor attached to the abutment.

steroid preparations at infrequent intervals. The use of 2% hydrocortisone cream applied to the conchal bowl and medial external auditory canal two or three times a week is frequently sufficient. In more difficult cases, the use of a steroid-containing antibiotic drop that is placed into the external auditory canal may also be required. Some cases respond to the simple application of mineral oil or other emollient without the use of medication.

The other dermatitis that is seen with some frequency is allergic or atopic dermatitis. The majority of these cases occur in response to exogenous materials placed in or around the external auditory canal. Many allergic reactions are seen in response to topi-cal antibiotic drops. Neomycin is especially likely to produce topical sensitization and result in allergic reaction. Allergic reactions to neomycin (and other topical antibiotics) occur in two somewhat distinct forms. A fulminant form (sudden, severe) is occasionally encountered that results in massive swelling of the external auditory canal and a dramatic drug eruption involving the conchal bowl, lobule, and, frequently, the skin of the neck. The eruption is associated with cutaneous weeping of serosanguinous fluid and is accompanied by intense pain and tenderness. Such reactions, of course, require the immediate discontinuance of the offending agent and often the use of both topical and systemic steroid medications. A more indolent form (gradual, mild) of hypersensitivity is manifested simply by the failure of a typical external otitis to resolve in response to what appears to be appropriate antibiotic therapy. Long-term drainage, edema of the external auditory canal, pain, and tenderness persist in the presence of the use of both topical drops and mechanical cleansing. Discontinuing the offending agent and treating the external otitis with a nonantibiotic drop containing an antiseptic with or without a topical steroid can adequately treat such reactions.

Also possible are atopic reactions to the materials from which both ear molds and earplugs are made. Again, the reaction may be fulminant with obvious swelling, pain, and tenderness or may be more indolent with only minimal swelling and moderate tenderness. The mainstay of treatment is replacement of the offending agent with a more hypoallergenic material.

Bacterial External Otitis

The most common cause of bacterial infections of the external auditory canal is bacterial external otitis or "swimmer's ear." Bacterial external otitis is characterized by edema and erythemia of the earcanal. The patient may report a sensation of heat or "fever" in the canal, or pain and itching. If swelling is severe, collection of debris in the earcanal may lead to some conductive hearing loss. Otoscopic inspection may reveal shedding of the epithelium and either a serous or mucopurulent exudate. The disorder is of relatively sudden onset and is characterized by severe pain localized to the affected external auditory canal. An important diagnostic feature is extreme sensitivity to any movement of the auricle or tissues surrounding the external auditory canal. This is helpful in distinguishing external otitis from middle ear problems, in that even fairly vigorous auricular movement does not cause pain in patients with middle ear infections. In many cases of external otitis it is not possible to examine the tympanic membrane fully because of the exquisite tenderness of the canal and a marked amount of canal

swelling. The disorder is rarely, if ever, associated with fever, malaise, or other signs of systemic infection.

In more than 60% of cases, the offending organism in bacterial external otitis is *Pseudomonas aeruginosa*. This organism is relatively ubiquitous in the environment and in the appropriate circumstances may be pathogenic. It is, however, extremely sensitive to the local acidity (pH) of its environment. *Pseudomonas* is incapable of growing or reproducing in acid media. One of the functions of cerumen appears to be maintenance of a slightly acidic environment, which prevents the growth of *Pseudomonas*. Introduction of water into the external auditory canal by swimming (or other means) washes out the normal acidity of the canal and may substitute a nonacid environment. In such circumstances, the commonly occurring *Pseudomonas* may produce a purulent bacterial infection. The incidence of acute bacterial external otitis is significantly higher in June, July, and August because most swimming occurs during these months. In addition, the incidence is greater in people under the age of 18. As already mentioned, the presence of an impaired skin barrier, as can occur with seborrheic dermatitis, may significantly increase the chances of the development of bacterial external otitis.

Treatment follows logically from the known etiology of the infection. Reacidification of the external auditory canal is almost always sufficient to cure the disorder, unless the external auditory canal is so swollen as to prevent the acidifying fluids from entering or there is so much accumulated mucopurulent debris that the drops do not come in contact with the infected tissues. An external canal that is swollen closed can be dealt with effectively by placing a small wick into the external auditory canal. The wick is made of an expandable material and draws the acidifying solution into the canal. When a large amount of mucopurulent debris has accumulated, mechanical removal using the operating microscope and suction is essential and often crucial to successful management. In severe cases, such cleansing may need to be done two or three times every other day.

Antibiotic drops should be continued at least a week beyond remission of pain.

Although antibiotic drops directed against *Pseudomonas* are effective in eliminating infection, they are generally unnecessary and should only be used in severe cases as described above. The use of antibiotic drops carries with it the risk of producing a topical allergic reaction and the promotion of fungal external otitis.

Fungal External Otitis

The normal earcanal houses many types of fungi. Most fungal growth that occurs within the external auditory canal is saprophytic. The "dead" debris these fungi grow on includes desquamated epithelium, cerumen, or the mucopurulent debris from a previous bacterial infection. True fungal external otitis with tissue invasion of fungal elements is uncommon and almost completely limited to individuals who are significantly immunocompromised. Individuals taking high-dose steroids, using immunosuppressive agents, or with immunodeficiency disorders are candidates for such infections. An exception to this general rule may be healthy individuals who have had long-term treatment with systemic antimicrobials or topical antibiotics. In such individuals, fungi are frequently cultured from a chronic draining external auditory canal, and they may be etiologically important.

Patients with fungal external otitis, sometimes referred to as otomycosis, may report tinnitus and itching, but rarely experience pain. Otoscopic inspection may reveal hairlike cilia in the earcanal. An aural discharge may be present that is usually gray or black because the primary organism is often *Aspergillus niger*. A white, furry discharge may be present if *Candida albicans* is the offending organism. Fungal external otitis is best treated by withdrawal of the antibiotic therapy, if appropriate, and the use of topical antiseptics like Mercurochrome or gentian violet. Antiseptics have the advantage of being fairly universal in their toxicity. Thus they are much less likely to select out resistant organisms, which can then grow unrestrained by their usual bacterial competitors. Acidifying agents are also useful in the treatment of fungal external otitis because many of the fungi are sensitive to ambient pH. Occasionally, especially in immunocompromised individuals, the use of topical or even systemic antifungal agents may become necessary.

Disorders of the Tympanic Membrane, Middle Ear, and Mastoid

Tympanic Membrane Perforations

Tympanic membrane perforations can arise as a consequence of either infection or trauma. Acute otitis media frequently results in perforation of the tympanic membrane. Generally speaking, such perforations heal spontaneously, but occasionally the perforation fails to heal and is left as a permanent feature of the tympanic membrane. Chronic infection with an unusual organism, such as *Mycobacterium tuberculosis*, produces a much higher rate of permanent tympanic membrane perforation than occurs in the epidemic otitis media of school children.

Various types of trauma can produce tympanic membrane perforation. Penetrating objects, such as Q-tips or sticks, are occasionally involved. Blast trauma, however, is much more common. An example of blast trauma occurs from a slap to the side of the head in which the external auditory canal is completely occluded, thus forcing a column of air onto the tympanic membrane and rupturing it. Another type of blast injury is most frequently responsible for the tympanic membrane perforations associated with water skiing.

Perforations of the tympanic membrane diagnosed on physical examination should be first categorized as to their location. They may occur in either the pars tensa or the pars flaccida. Perforations of the pars flaccida may be assumed to be cholesteatomas and should be managed as such. Perforations in the pars tensa can be divided into those that are central and those that are marginal. A central perforation has a small rim of intact tympanic membrane around it. Marginal perforations extend all the way to the bony annulus of the external auditory canal. It is often difficult and sometimes impossible to determine whether an anterior perforation is marginal because the anterior canal wall makes it difficult to see the most anterior portion of the tympanic membrane. The distinction between central and marginal perforations is important because marginal perforations have the potential to develop into cholesteatomas and, therefore, should be considered dangerous. Central perforations, on the other hand, are unlikely to develop into cholesteatomas and are sometimes referred to as "safe" perforations. The size of the tympanic membrane perforation should also be determined. Size can be recorded in terms of either an estimate of diameter in millimeters or an estimate of the percentage of tympanic membrane involved in the perforation.

Both location and size are important factors in determining the amount of conductive hearing loss associated with the particular type of perforation. Small pinpoint perforations may have no associated hearing loss, and larger perforations may produce losses up to 50 dB. Perforations directly over the round window niche may produce significant hearing loss because of phase cancellation effects. Conductive hearing losses > 40 to 50 dB suggest associated ossicular discontinuity or fixation.

Most tympanic membrane perforations heal spontaneously and without significant or meaningful residual complications. However, when infection is present with an acute tympanic membrane perforation, the probability of spontaneous healing is significantly reduced. Injuries involving water or traumatic tympanic membrane perforations contaminated with water shortly after their occurrence are less likely to heal, leaving a chronic tympanic membrane perforation. Three sorts of difficulties arise from chronic perforations of the tympanic membrane: (1) formation of cholesteatoma, (2) significant conductive hearing loss, and (3) recurrent infection.

By permitting the ingress of bacteria from the external auditory canal into the middle ear space, perforations may lead to recurrent infections of the middle ear and mastoid. If water is allowed to enter the external auditory canal, it may carry bacteria into the middle ear space and further increase the likelihood of infection. For this reason, some physicians recommend protection of the middle ear space from waterborne bacterial contamination through the use of ear protection for swimming or bathing when a patient has patent tympanostomy tubes or a chronic perforation of the tympanic membrane.

The treatment of tympanic membrane perforations is surgical repair. In individuals with marginal perforations, the propensity of these perforations to form cholesteatomas is sufficient to warrant surgical repair in most cases. Repair of central perforations, however, is entirely elective.

Middle Ear Infections

The general term used for infections of the middle ear is "otitis media." If the infection is characterized by fluid in the middle ear space, the term "otitis media with effusion" may be used. Otitis media with effusion is the most common cause of conductive hearing loss in children. For this reason, chronic or recurrent cases of otitis media in early childhood may also lead to delays in speech and language development. In addition, development of central auditory pathways may be affected by fluctuating hearing loss; thus the child may experience difficulties with speech perception in noise and paying attention in class when distractions are present (see Chapter 17).

EUSTACHIAN TUBE DYSFUNCTION

Eustachian tube dysfunction is often responsible for the advent of otitis media. Figure 4–3 shows the middle ear space and the eustachian tube. The eustachian tube plays an important role in ventilating the middle ear space, equalizing pressure between the middle ear and atmospheric pressure, and clearing the space of foreign agents. The normally functioning eustachian tube remains closed at rest but should open episodically to equalize middle ear pressure with ambient barometric pressure. The eustachian tubes are opened by active muscular contraction of small palatal muscles during swallowing or yawning. If the eustachian tube is always open (patulous), then bacteria-laden secretions from the nasopharynx may enter the middle ear and produce infection. In fact, such secretions may be forced into the middle ear if the eustachian tube is open during active sneezing or nose blowing. If the tube remains chronically shut, negative pressure will develop in the middle ear. Negative middle ear pressure may result in the development of a retracted tympanic membrane and middle ear effusion. Over time, such fluid may thicken and become mucoid ("glue" ear). If bacteria find their way into such an effusion, acute purulent bacterial otitis media will rapidly develop. By producing swelling of the mucous membranes of the eustachian tube and inhibiting normal ciliary function, middle ear effusions (either infected or uninfected) may themselves produce dysfunction of the eustachian tube and perpetuate their own condition.

Otitis media is more prevalent in infants and young children, with the incidence usually decreasing as children approach school age. This is partially due to structural differences in the adult and pediatric eustachian tubes, which lead to poorer eustachian tube function in children. The eustachian tubes in infants and children are more horizontal, shorter, and wider than those of adults. Palatal muscle function, as with muscle function generally, is less efficient in infants and small children than it is in adults; therefore, the active tubal opening is less reliable and vigorous.

Blockage of the eustachian tube can occur due to intrinsic and extrinsic factors. Inflammation of the nasal end of the eustachian tube can produce sufficient swelling to obstruct it mechanically. Such inflammation may result from viral (a cold) or bacterial infection, chemical irritation (tobacco smoke, chlorinated pool water), or inhalant allergy. Extrinsically, lymphoid and adenoid tissues may block the eustachian tube. The consequences of long-term eustachian tube dysfunction include not only persistent or recurrent middle ear effusions with or without infection, but also pathological alterations of the tympanic membrane and complications associated with the inner ear, mastoid, or central nervous system.

OTITIS MEDIA

There are a variety of types of otitis media. Essentially, otitis media can be classified based on either or both the time course of the disease and the type of fluid. Temporal classification includes acute, subacute, chronic, and recurrent. Acute otitis media lasts from 0 to 3 weeks, subacute from 3 to 8 weeks, and chronic for longer than 8 weeks. Types of fluid evident in otitis media may be serous (thin, watery), mucoid (thick, tenacious), purulent (containing pus), or mixed. Mixed fluid is most common and generally consists of purulent and mucoid fluids. A sample must be taken and analyzed to determine the type of fluid.

Acute otitis media is one of the most common diseases of early childhood and affects at least 70% of children prior to the age of 6 years. It is the most frequent reason for the administration of antibiotics to children. Prior to the use of antibiotic medications, acute otitis media was the cause of significant mortality in infancy and childhood. Fortunately, current antimicrobials have significantly reduced (but not completely eliminated) the incidence of life-threatening complications. The peak incidence of otitis media is between 6 and 24 months of age. It occurs more frequently during the winter months. Exposure to secondhand cigarette smoke and placement in day-care centers seem to increase the incidence of acute otitis media significantly. Males are diagnosed with otitis media more frequently than females, as are certain ethnic groups (American Indians, Eskimos, and Hispanics). The disease appears to have a genetic component and also seems to be associated with allergies. Furthermore, the disease is more prevalent in urban centers and in patients from lower socioeconomic groups.

In general, otitis media begins with edema, hyperemia, and hemorrhage in the subepithelial space of the middle ear mucosa. This is then followed by the local infiltration of white blood cells and the accumulation of pus within the middle ear space. Typically, acute otitis media is of relatively sudden onset. Because it represents the accumulation of pus within a closed body cavity, it is associated with significant systemic signs of infection, such as elevated temperature, malaise, and elevated white blood cell count. The ear is exquisitely painful, although there is no tenderness in the area of the auricle or periauricular tissues as is seen with external otitis. In untreated cases, the condition often resolves with spontaneous rupture of the tympanic membrane. The opening in the tympanic membrane allows the pus to drain into the external auditory canal. Rupture of the tympanic membrane is associated with very rapid relief of pain. In more than 90% of cases, the tympanic membrane heals spontaneously and there is no residual damage.

Otitis media is caused by infection with a number of relatively common bacteria. If spontaneous recovery does not occur, otitis media generally responds to the institution of prompt antibiotic therapy. A single episode of otitis media treated with appropriate antibiotics will generally produce an effusion that clears within 1 month. In 90% of cases, an effusion due to an initial episode of acute otitis media clears within 3 months.

When the middle ear space continues to harbor fluid for more than 2 months after an episode of otitis media, the condition has become chronic otitis media with chronic middle ear effusion. Although culture of fluid reveals a small number of viable bacteria, the condition is not an infection in the usual sense of the word. There is no associated pain, fever, or development of pus. Indeed, the condition is frequently asymptomatic and 50% of cases are "silent." Such cases can be diagnosed only on routine "well-baby" evaluations. The persistence of fluid behind the tympanic membrane presents difficulties if and only if it either produces significant conductive hearing loss or promotes frequently recurrent acute otitis media. The presence of this fluid in and of itself is medically of no great consequence. Therefore, an estimate of hearing threshold is crucial in the intelligent management of chronic middle ear effusion. A child with normal hearing thresholds who has relatively few middle ear infections need not be treated aggressively for the mere presence of middle ear fluid.

When persistent middle ear fluid causes significant conductive hearing loss (> 15 dB in a child) or is associated with more than four to six episodes of otitis media per year, treatment should be implemented. The use of prophylactic antibiotics has been advocated for many years. However, the rapid development of antimicrobial resistance in the organisms commonly responsible for acute otitis media now makes such protracted antibiotic treatment controversial. Concern has recently developed that antibiotic resistance may increase the prevalence to the point where serious life-threatening complications are again common. Because many of these conditions are caused by chronic eustachian tube dysfunction, the use of antihistamines or decongestants would seem to make sense. However, several good clinical studies have shown that antihistamines and decongestants are of essentially no use whatsoever in the treatment of persistent middle ear fluid in children. The use of steroids remains controversial but can be effective. If effusions persist for > 12 weeks and are associated with significant hearing loss, consideration should be given to the insertion of tympanostomy tubes. However, the mere presence of fluid will not be a compelling reason for surgical intervention. This is especially true if the effusion is unilateral. In children with bilateral effusion who have conductive hearing losses > 15 or 20 dBs, justification for tympanostomy tube insertion is considerably reinforced. One must remember that the conductive hearing loss associated with middle ear effusions is variable, and audiometric evaluation may occur when a child is hearing relatively well. The observations of parents or teachers should be given great credence. When there is a documented or even suspected problem with the acquisition of speech and language skills, or difficulty in school, then insertion of tympanostomy tubes should be considered to eliminate the possibility of mild conductive hearing loss as an etiologic or confounding variable (Case Study 4–1).

Some children have special predisposing factors for otitis media with effusion. Children with cleft palate or Down syndrome and patients with craniofacial syndromes such as Treacher Collins syndrome or Crouzon's disease are especially predisposed to otitis. These patients should be evaluated individually, bearing in mind their congenital anomalies. Almost all will benefit from tympanostomy tubes. In children with concurrent sensorineural hearing loss the use of tympanostomy tubes may be more urgent. If the sensorineural component is severe or profound, elimination of the conductive component may make the difference in successful remediation with amplification. Children with other medical problems that produce febrile conditions or with drug allergies may benefit from the early insertion of tympanostomy tubes to eliminate acute otitis media as a confounding variable. Children readily subject to febrile seizures may have little tolerance for the acute episodes of otitis media that most children deal with easily.

The insertion of tympanostomy tubes is a relatively simple procedure. In many chil-

---

Case Study 4–1   J.M. is a 4-year-old child who had a 1- to 2-year history of multiple recurrent episodes of otitis media. He had been on antibiotics for almost 12 out of the last 18 months. This included one 3-month period during which he received prophylactic antibiotics in an attempt to eliminate middle ear infections. However, even during this period of time he developed one episode of acute otitis media. He was referred for an evaluation for speech and language delay and attention deficit disorder. He was deemed to be approximately 3 to 6 months behind in the acquisition of both expressive and receptive language skills. He had difficulty concentrating, could not attend well to tasks, and fell asleep easily and frequently during the day. He had chronic nasal congestion and was a chronic mouth breather, according to his parents. He snored loudly at night and gagged on his food during meals.

Examination showed that he had bilateral middle ear effusions with no evidence of infection. He had mucus coming from both nostrils and was breathing loudly and heavily through his mouth. Intraoral examination showed very large hypertrophic tonsils that met at the midline ("kissing").

Audiometric evaluation showed that he had bilateral, flat, 40 dB conductive hearing loss, tympanograms were flat bilaterally (Audiogram 4–1). Soft tissue lateral x-ray of his neck showed that in addition to his large, obstructive tonsils he had large pads of adenoid tissue that completely prevented movement of air through his nose.

He underwent bilateral adenotonsillectomy with insertion of tympanostomy tubes. His snoring resolved immediately and many of the symptoms of his attention deficit disorder disappeared. He no longer fell asleep during the day and was able to concentrate much better because he was getting a good night's sleep. Approximately 6 months after the operative intervention he had "caught up" and had age-appropriate speech and language skills.

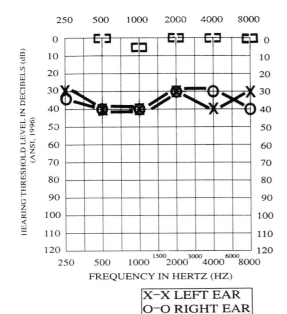

X–X LEFT EAR
O–O RIGHT EAR

Audiogram 4–1. Audiometric configuration showing binaural flat conductive hearing loss. (See Case Study 4–1.)

dren over the age of 7 or 8 years it can be performed as an outpatient office procedure, as is generally done with adults. However, in younger children, a short general anesthetic is necessary. The tympanostomy tubes act as prosthetic eustachian tubes. At the time of tympanostomy tube insertion, the fluid is mechanically aspirated from the middle ear space. The tympanostomy tube then permits effective pressure regulation, equalizing the ambient pressure between the earcanal and the middle ear space and draining middle ear fluid through the tube into the earcanal. In patients over the age of 4 years, a number of studies have now shown that hypertrophied adenoid tissue plays a significant etiologic role in the persistence of middle ear effusion. In children more than 4 years old with persistent fluid, consideration should be given to simultaneous adenoidectomy at the time of tympanostomy tube insertion.

Tympanostomy tubes are spontaneously extruded from the tympanic membrane after about 1 year. Although the tympanic membrane heals completely after extrusion of tympanostomy tubes in 97 to 98% of cases, in 2 to 3% the tympanic membrane fails to heal after extrusion of the tube. This is more common with larger tubes and is more likely to occur when the tube is extruded in the presence of active infection. In the vast majority of such cases, the infection can be effectively eliminated with a 5- to 7-day course of topical antibiotic drops placed into the external auditory canal. Even though the rate of permanent perforation related to tympanostomy tube placement is low, tympanostomy tube insertion has become sufficiently frequent so that this now accounts for a significant number of permanent tympanic membrane perforations in young children. Persistent tympanic membrane perforation occurs in about 3% of patients and may require operative repair after tube extrusion.

Complications related to the insertion of tympanostomy tubes are relatively infrequent. Ten to 25% of patients will develop drainage from the middle ear through the tympanostomy tube into the earcanal at some time. Tympanosclerosis of the tympanic membrane can occur but is generally of no consequence. Such complications need to be compared with the rather serious complications of persistent otitis media and the developmental and educational consequences of persistent conductive hearing loss.

Complications Associated with Otitis Media. There are a variety of conditions that can result from otitis media. Recurrent infection can deposit hyalin (a calcium-like substance) in the middle ear. These hyalin deposits, termed "tympanosclerosis," may be limited to the tympanic membrane or may involve the heads of the ossicles within the middle ear space. Tympanosclerotic plaques limited to the tympanic membrane are easily noticed but, although they may present a dramatic appearance, rarely produce hearing loss or other alteration of middle ear function. On the other hand, tympanosclerotic deposition around the heads of the ossicles will produce fixation and maximum conductive hearing loss. The processes of the development of tympanosclerosis of the tympanic membrane and middle ear space appear to be independent. Although there is good evidence that development of tympanosclerosis of the tympanic membrane is associated with injury to the drum (tympanic membrane perforation), the apparent etiology of middle ear tympanosclerosis is entirely unknown. Fortunately, middle ear tympanosclerosis is uncommon.

Chronic or repeated retraction of the tympanic membrane will produce stretching and thinning. A chronically retracted tympanic membrane may rest on the long process of the incus and incudostapedial joint and produce ossicular erosion, ossicular discontinuity, and moderate to severe conductive hearing loss. Further atrophy will leave the tympanic membrane draped over the medial wall of the middle ear. This will produce functional elimination of the middle ear space. When the eardrum is left in this configuration for an extended period of time, fibrosis and scarring will occur, and the process will become irreversible (adhesive otitis media). If thinning and retraction of the tympanic membrane occur in the posterior quadrant, and portions of the drum are sucked into the mastoid cavity, a cholesteatoma may develop.

In the absence of antibiotic therapy, most cases of acute otitis media will resolve after spontaneous perforation. However, a significant minority will not resolve. A variety of complications can occur due to unresolved otitis media. As previously noted, conductive hearing loss can occur that can have a deleterious effect on development. Chronic tympanic membrane perforation may result, eventually leading to cholesteatoma in some cases. The affected child may also develop chronic mastoiditis, sigmoid sinus thrombosis, facial nerve paralysis, labyrinthitis with complete sensorineural hearing loss, meningitis, or brain abscess. Some of these complications can be fatal.

Cholesteatoma

As previously mentioned, marginal perforations of the tympanic membrane, especially in the pars flaccida, may develop into cholesteatomas. Cholesteatomas are also a complication observed with otitis media. Less frequently, cholesteatomas may be congenital or caused by previous surgeries of the ear.

The lateral surface of the tympanic membrane consists of skin and, like skin in other portions of the body, it sheds epithelial cells (desquamates). The normally functioning external auditory canal removes these shed components as they are produced. If a sufficient portion of the tympanic membrane is retracted far enough into the mastoid, these shed epithelial cells can no longer escape from the external auditory canal; they accumulate as a mass of dead skin within the temporal bone and erode the bone slowly through a combination of pressure necrosis and enzymatic activity. Such a collection of dead skin trapped within the middle ear space or temporal bone and increasing slowly in size is termed a "cholesteatoma." The condition may also be referred to as a "keratinoma" or an "epidermoid inclusion cyst" or, in the older otologic literature, as a "pearly tumor." The dead skin components at the center of these skin-filled cysts are an excellent medium for bacterial growth, and eventually infection will develop. Infection accelerates the process of bony destruction. Infections in such cysts are difficult to eradicate because bloodborne antibiotics are not delivered to these nonvascular areas and topical drops cannot penetrate to the core of the mass of dead skin.

As cholesteatomas expand, they do so only at the expense of surrounding normal structures. Thus cholesteatomas may result in any one of the following complications:

1. Destruction of one or all of the ossicles, producing conductive hearing loss
2. Erosion of the bone of the labyrinthine capsule with penetration of the membranous labyrinth, causing a severe or

Case Study 4–2   B.Q. is an 8-year-old who had been treated for right-sided "external otitis" for the last year. He had virtually continuous, foul-smelling, mucopurulent drainage from the right ear. It was not associated with pain. He had multiple episodes of otitis media and middle ear effusion as a younger child and had two sets of tympanostomy tubes. Audiograms performed between the ages of 3 and 5 years showed mild conductive hearing loss that fluctuated 10 to 15 dB. However, after extrusion of his second set of tympanostomy tubes at the age of 5 years, he had two entirely normal audiograms.

Examination showed a normal left tympanic membrane except for the presence of some tympanosclerosis. The pars tensa of the right tympanic membrane also had some tympanosclerosis. However, in the area of the pars flaccida a perforation could be seen. A large amount of mucopus could be seen issuing from this perforation. After extensive cleansing and careful evaluation with the Zeiss operating microscope, a small amount of squamous epithelium could be removed from the perforation. It was apparent that the perforation represented the open neck of a large cholesteatoma. Audiometric evaluation was normal, including tympanometry.

The nature of cholesteatoma was carefully explained to the parents and the necessity for surgical removal emphasized. The child's father, however, had recently taken a new position and wished to wait 9 months until the child's cholesteatoma would be covered by their insurance policy.

Six months after his initial presentation, the child's parents called because B.Q. had woken up acutely dizzy. He was seen immediately that day and audiometric evaluation showed a significant neurosensory hearing loss. He was, therefore, taken to the operating room immediately. A large cholesteatoma found filling the mastoid had eroded into the horizontal semicircular canal. The cholesteatoma was carefully removed and a piece of tissue placed over the open semicircular canal. The vertigo remitted promptly, but he was left with a significant neurosensory hearing loss (Audiogram 4–2).

profound sensorineural hearing loss and overwhelming vertigo (labyrinthine fistula; Case Study 4–2)

3. Bacterial infection of the labyrinthine fluids producing bacterial labyrinthitis. Because the fluids within the labyrinth are in direct communication with the cerebrospinal fluid, bacterial meningitis frequently develops as a consequence of bacterial labyrinthitis. Untreated bacterial meningitis may be fatal within a matter of only a few hours.

4. Erosion into the cranial cavity producing either meningitis or brain abscess

5. Thrombosis or infection of veins in the brain, producing brain swelling, stroke, coma, and death

6. Thrombosis and infection of the major venous outflow tract (sigmoid sinus); may produce metastatic infection, brain abscess, and death

7. Erosion into and paralysis of the facial nerve

Patients with cholesteatomas may present with vertigo, tinnitus, headaches, pain, and fever. Otoscopic inspection may reveal a marginal perforation, often in the pars flaccida, and purulent fetid otorrhea. Audiometric evaluation may reveal a variety of findings, including hearing within normal limits, conductive hearing loss, or mixed hearing loss.

Surgical removal is the only reliable treatment and requires mastoidectomy in virtually all cases. Because the complications of cholesteatoma may be fatal, surgical therapy has as its goal complete removal of the

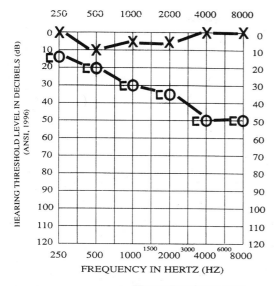

X–X LEFT EAR
O–O RIGHT EAR

Audiogram 4–2. Audiometric evaluation showing significant neurosensory hearing loss in the right ear. (See Case Study 4–2.)

cholesteatoma and creation of a "safe" ear not subject to recurrent disease. Reconstruction of the disrupted middle ear transformer mechanism is of secondary importance. Even so, every effort is made to restore hearing when this is consistent with elimination of serious disease. In most cases, the surgeon will recommend a second procedure approximately 6 months after the first in order to verify that the cholesteatoma was completely excised and regeneration has not occurred. At this time, ossicular reconstruction may be performed to improve hearing.

Otosclerosis

In the active phase, otosclerosis is more properly termed "otospongiosis." However, the term "otosclerosis" is so ensconced in the literature that its continued widespread use is irresistible. During the otospongiosis phase, vascular spongy bone growth occurs to replace the normal hard bone of the labyrinthine capsule. When this "new" bone

growth hardens, the term "otosclerosis" is appropriate. This new growth occurs most frequently in the area of the oval window. In about 10% of affected individuals the otosclerotic process extends to involve the footplate and annular ligament. When this occurs, mobility of the footplate will be progressively reduced and a conductive hearing loss will slowly develop. There is evidence to support the notion that release of toxic enzymes into the perilymphatic spaces of the inner ear may cause progressive sensorineural hearing impairment and that this can be arrested by treatment with sodium fluoride. However, the diagnosis is difficult, especially in patients without concurrent stapes fixation, and the frequency with which "cochlear" otosclerosis occurs is not known.

The disease is hereditary in many (but certainly not all) cases and occurs more frequently in Caucasians. Three quarters of all patients will develop disease in both ears. Females exhibit otosclerosis more frequently than males, and the disease is usually identified when they are between 30 and 40 years of age. Although otosclerosis is rare in childhood, it can be evident in the mid-teenage years.

Definitive diagnosis depends on middle ear exploration with visualization of the otosclerotic focus and mechanical verification of stapes fixation. Presurgical diagnosis is based on the presence of slowly progressive conductive hearing loss in the absence of concurrent or preceding chronic ear disease. Presurgical diagnosis is accurate in about 90% of cases. The cardinal audiometric finding in otosclerosis is a progressively increasing conductive hearing loss. Early in the course of the disease, when only the anterior portion of the stapes is fixed, a marked, low frequency loss is seen. As footplate fixation becomes complete, high frequencies become involved and the loss becomes a flat, conductive hearing loss. A sensorineural component may be seen in some individuals but not all. Depression of bone conduction scores isolated to the 2000 Hz range is characteristic of otosclerosis and referred to as Carhart's notch.

When surgical correction is desired, the fixed stapes is completely or partially removed and replaced with a prosthesis. The operation takes about 45 minutes and may be performed under local anesthesia as a day surgical procedure that does not require hospitalization. A wide variety of prostheses and techniques have been used and most have produced excellent results. Indeed 95% of patients undergoing surgery for otosclerosis will experience a closure of the air–bone gap to within 10 dB. Three to 5% of patients will experience no improvement and will therefore continue to be good candidates for amplification. The biggest risk associated with stapedectomy is the 1 to 2% chance of complete and profound sensorineural hearing loss associated with the operative procedure. The reason for such catastrophic loss has never been completely clarified, but it does not seem to be necessarily related to technical intraoperative difficulties.

Ossicular Discontinuity

In some cases, conductive hearing loss may be due to discontinuity of the ossicular chain. Disruption of the integrity of the bones in the middle ear can occur as a complication from many of the outer and middle ear disorders discussed. For example, in children ossicular discontinuity occurs most frequently due to recurrent or persistent middle ear infection or effusion. Ongoing disease in the middle ear can lead to necrosis of the long process of the incus. In most such cases, the ossicular discontinuity is not complete, but rather the necrotic distal segment of the long process of the incus is replaced by a thin band of fibrous tissue. The connection between the long process of the incus and the capitulum of the stapes thus becomes fibrous rather than bony. Transmission of sound becomes inefficient and a significant conductive hearing loss is apparent. However, it is uncommon for the conductive hearing loss to be maximal in nature. A considerable percentage of these children have a rather interesting audiometric finding in that the conductive hearing loss is greater in the higher frequencies than in the lower.

Ossicular discontinuity can also be due to previous surgical procedures. Oftentimes, surgery for cholesteatoma requires removal of part or all of one or more of the ossicles. Most frequently, the incus needs to be removed because of irremediable involvement with cholesteatoma. The head of the malleus may have to be removed and, frequently, the capitulum of the stapes. In many cases, bony destruction of the ossicles by the cholesteatomatous process has occurred prior to surgical intervention.

Trauma can produce ossicular dislocation. In general, trauma produces inferior dislocation of the incus. The long process loses contact with the capitulum of the stapes. The incudomalleolar joint can be disrupted at the same time. Less frequently, the trauma involves the inner ear as well if it produces subluxation of the stapes into the oval window. When this occurs, there may be associated dizziness and sensorineural hearing loss as well as a conductive hearing loss. If such a situation is suspected, then immediate surgical intervention should be recommended to limit the amount of sensorineural hearing loss and to close the opening between the inner and middle ear space (perilymph fistula).

Treatment of ossicular discontinuity or dislocation is called ossiculoplasty. Repair of the ossicular chain is possible in most cases. Unfortunately, results are not as good with repair of defects involving the malleus and incus as stapes replacement is for repair of otosclerosis. Closure of the air–bone gap to 10 dB probably occurs in less than three quarters of all patients but depends somewhat on the nature of the hearing deficit. When the malleus, incus, and stapes superstructure are gone and a total ossicular replacement prosthesis must be used, closure of the air–bone gap to within 30 dB is considered a good result. On the other hand, when the conductive hearing loss is caused by necrosis of the long process of the incus, complete closure can frequently be obtained.

Inner Ear and Internal Auditory Canal

Sensorineural Hearing Loss

"Sensorineural hearing loss" refers to hearing loss that is due to pathology of the inner ear or auditory nervous system pathways. Such hearing losses usually cannot be corrected medically, but require amplification, aural habilitation/rehabilitation, and/or other services (i.e., sign language). There are a variety of causes for both congenital and acquired sensorineural hearing loss, including genetic and nongenetic etiologies. In many cases the cause of sensorineural hearing loss may not be known.

CONGENITAL SENSORINEURAL
HEARING LOSS

Approximately 50% of moderate to profound childhood sensorineural hearing loss is due to genetic factors. Congenital sensorineural hearing loss may occur in isolation or as part of a pattern of associated symptoms (syndrome). There is a large variety of known genetic inner ear hearing loss syndromes. Fortunately, the majority of congenital genetic sensorineural hearing losses occur in isolation.

A variety of nongenetic sensorineural hearing losses that are congenital in nature have also been described. Prenatal infections are probably the most common. For example, prior to the 1970s, maternal rubella syndrome was responsible for causing deafness associated with congenital cataracts and heart disease in many infants (Fig. 4–1B). The availability of vaccines to prevent this disease has significantly reduced the incidence of hearing loss attributable to rubella. Currently, cytomegalovirus (CMV) is a more prevalent cause of either or both congenital and progressive hearing loss. This virus can also cause other serious complications, including cerebral palsy, kidney disease, jaundice, and microcephaly. Although there is no known cure, early treatment with gancyclovir may reduce the symptoms. Toxoplasmosis and syphilis are other infections that can involve the developing embryo and produce congenital as well as progressive sensorineural hearing loss.

Other difficulties at birth can lead to sensorineural hearing loss. Infants who have jaundice, or hyperbilirubinemia, with serum bilirubin levels > 20 mg/100 mL of plasma serum may develop a neurological disorder known as kernicterus. Kernicterus has been associated with sensorineural hearing loss as well as other symptoms. Maternal/infant Rh incompatability can lead to sensorineural hearing loss, cerebral palsy, brain damage, and kernicterus. Ototoxic drugs given to the mother during pregnancy may produce congenital hearing loss. Hypoxia during intrauterine development may produce significant injury to the auditory system. Injury to the vascular system of the branchial arches can produce either unilateral or bilateral hypoplasia of the membranous labyrinth. Perinatal hypoxia due to birth trauma may also result in sensorineural hearing loss, as may intracranial hemorrhage complicating delivery.

ACQUIRED SENSORINEURAL
HEARING LOSS

Acquired sensorineural hearing loss can also be divided into genetic and nongenetic forms. There are a large variety of genetic causes for delayed sensorineural hearing loss. Cochlear otosclerosis has already been mentioned as one such manifestation. Progressive sensorineural hearing loss can be attributed to a large variety of syndromes displaying musculoskeletal features. Among them are Alport's syndrome and all of the mucopolysaccharidoses, such as Hunter's syndrome and Hurler's syndrome. Other well-documented syndromes are associated with visual as well as hearing problems, such as Alström syndrome, Refsum's syndrome, and Cockayne's syndrome. However, the largest variety of delayed, genetically mediated sensorineural hearing losses occur sporadically as a consequence of a recessive inheritance pattern and are fortunately not associated with specific syndromes.

The nongenetic etiologies are well known and probably consist most frequently of those losses due to infection, neoplasm, the administration of ototoxic agents, or trauma. Noise-induced hearing loss falls into this category.

PROGRESSIVE SENSORINEURAL
HEARING LOSS

Some children with hearing impairment develop progressive sensorineural hearing loss. Many of these children have well identified syndromes such as Alport's, renal tubular acidosis, branchio-oto-renal syndrome, Refsum's syndrome, Norrie's disease, osteopetrosis, or mucopolysaccharide storage diseases. Some will have familial tumors. Others will have an infection/virus associated with progressive hearing loss, such as CMV, toxoplasmosis, or syphilis.

In many cases the etiology of progressive sensorineural hearing loss may be unknown. Some children may develop hearing loss due to exposure to loud noise (Brookhouser, Worthington, & Kelly, 1991, 1992) or trauma (perilymph fistula). For these reasons, it is important to monitor the hearing of children with identified hearing loss and rescreen or evaluate hearing in children who begin to exhibit difficulties attending in the classroom.

Perilymph Fistula

Perilymph fistula should be suspected if sensorineural hearing loss develops or progresses during or after a bout of otitis media. Perilymph fistula should also be suspected if hearing loss develops after head trauma or barometric trauma. Vertigo or disequilibrium may accompany the hearing loss. Reilly and Kenna (1989) documented that up to 6% of all children with sensorineural hearing loss had perilymph fistula. Perilymph fistula can be difficult to diagnosis without surgical exploration. Operative repair may prevent further deterioration and, although infrequently, in some patients may improve hearing (Case Study 4–3) .

Meniere's Disease

Meniere's disease or syndrome is a disorder with four principal clinical features: (1) episodes of whirling vertigo lasting several minutes to several hours; (2) low-pitched roaring tinnitus occurring or worsening during a vertiginous attack; (3) fluctuating, low frequency sensorineural hearing loss; and (4) a sense of fullness or pressure in the affected ear that can be very severe. Meniere's disease can occur in childhood, albeit rarely. Only about 3 to 4% of patients with Meniere's disease present in the pediatric age group. When endolymphatic hydrops or Meniere's disease is suspected, comprehensive evaluation is required for diagnosis. Electrocochleography and electronystagmography can be useful in documenting unilateral labyrinthine dysfunction and confirming the diagnosis of Meniere's disease.

Most children are entirely asymptomatic between episodes, although some experience a chronic, mild disequilibrium, tinnitus, or aural fullness. The disease is usually progressive. Early in the course of the disease, hearing often returns completely to normal between attacks, but over months or years a permanent hearing loss usually develops. The hearing loss may follow any pattern, but low frequency losses are more common in the early course of the disease. Children with long-standing disease, on the other hand, are more likely to have flat losses.

It is not possible to predict the course of the disease in individual patients. Some children will experience a relatively indolent variety with attacks separated by years, others will lose all hearing and balance function over a period of several months. Most children follow a middle course, with attacks coming in clusters lasting several weeks and separated by months or even years of symptom-free periods. The development of anacusis is uncommon. The disease is bilateral in 15 to 20% of patients. Older children with Meniere's disease frequently complain of dysacusis and diplacusis, which are relatively unusual symptoms. Word recognition scores are variably affected but often well

Case Study 4–3   C.F. is an 8-year-old child who first presented to the otolaryngology department because of a cerebrospinal fluid leak in her left ear. She had two previous episodes of meningitis due to cerebrospinal fluid leak. The leak was identified using special radiographic techniques. Audiometric evaluation at the time of the first visit showed that she had no hearing in her left ear and a 60 dB hearing loss in her right ear (Audiogram 4–3A). However, her speech and language development was much better than one would expect with such a hearing loss, and it was assumed she had had better hearing when younger and that it had progressively deteriorated. At that time, she was taken to the operating room where the left inner ear was completely filled with muscle and the ear closed off to prevent further spinal fluid leakage and meningitis. She did well for 2½ years, after which she had an additional episode of meningitis. She was, therefore, seen again in the otolaryngology department. Review of her computed tomography scans confirmed that she had bilateral Mondini's deformity. It was apparent that she now had developed cerebrospinal fluid leakage from her other ear. Audiometric evaluation at this time showed approximately a 90 dB "corner" audiogram (Audiogram 4–3B). To prevent recurrent meningitis, it would be necessary to "pack" completely the cochlea with muscle or fat. This would eliminate C.F.'s residual hearing. It was, therefore, elected to place the electrode array of a Nucleus cochlear implant into the cochlea at the time of surgery. At operation, she was found to have multiple congenital defects of her stapes footplate. Insertion of the implant was accomplished even though she had only a single "common" cavity. Because the electrode array was "coiled" within the common cavity, only the middle electrodes were stimulated. Postoperatively, she did well. She had no recurrent meningitis and her hearing was functionally better than preoperatively. She is doing well in a regular classroom situation.

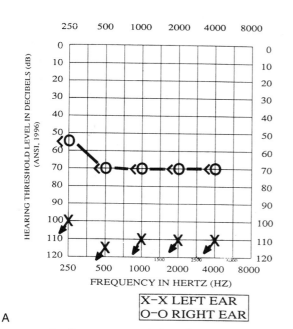

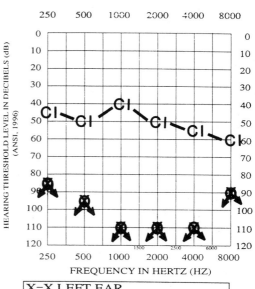

A

B

Audiogram 4–3.   (A) Audiometric evaluation showing no hearing in the left ear and hearing loss in the right ear. (B) Audiometric evaluation showing a 90 dB "corner" audiogram. (See Case Study 4–3.)

preserved. Definitive diagnosis is difficult and depends on the documentation of a fluctuating, low-tone sensorineural hearing loss associated with abnormal vestibular function. Abnormal electrocochleography strongly reinforces the diagnosis.

Primary therapy consists of vigorous salt restriction and the use of diuretics. When such therapy fails, consideration can be given to endolymphatic sac decompressive surgery. Endolymphatic sac decompressive surgery is helpful in 75% of patients in terms of relieving vertiginous symptoms. However, the evidence for hearing improvement is equivocal.

Tumors of the Internal Auditory Canal and Cerebellopontine Angle

Children may develop tumors of the temporal bone or cerebellopontine angle that can produce unilateral hearing loss and vestibular dysfunction (Fig. 4–5). Acoustic neuroma or meningioma accounts for the large majority of tumors that affect hearing in children. Children with acoustic neuromas frequently have neurofibromatosis type II (von Recklinghausen's disease) and in such individuals there may be a positive family history because the disease exhibits autosomal dominant inheritance. Other varieties of benign and malignant tumors occur sporadically in the pediatric population.

All children with unilateral otologic symptoms should be evaluated for tumors. Symptoms of mass lesions involving the

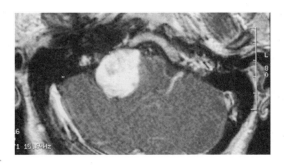

Figure 4–5.   MRI showing an acoustic neuroma in the cerebellopontine angle.

temporal bone or cerebellopontine angle may be subtle and slow to develop. Classically, the child experiences progressive, high frequency sensorineural hearing loss over several months or years. Older children may complain of associated tinnitus. As the tumor enlarges, nerves in the surrounding area may become sufficiently distorted and stretched so as to produce numbness of the external auditory canal or face, or weakness of facial muscles and facial paralysis. Continued growth results in compression of the brainstem with obstruction of the normal flow of cerebrospinal fluid, consequent hydrocephalus, and death.

Because some tumors are malignant, early diagnosis is critical and may permit lifesaving intervention. Even when the tumor is benign, early diagnosis permits the tumor to be removed much more easily and safely with lower surgical morbidity and mortality. The ability of the surgeon to preserve normal function of the facial nerve while achieving total tumor removal correlates directly with tumor size at the time of the diagnosis in benign tumors. The larger the tumor the more likely permanent facial weakness becomes. Diagnosis depends on a high incidence of suspicion and the frequent use of ABR examinations in children with unilateral complaints. At a minimum, the evaluation should include assessment of word recognition and interpeak latencies on the ABR. More than 90% of children with cerebellopontine angle or temporal bone tumors affecting hearing will have abnormal ABRs. Stapedius reflex testing frequently shows stapedius reflex decay when there is compression of the eighth cranial nerve. In many cases, radiographic imaging should be obtained.

Summary

Identification and treatment of the child with either or both auditory and vestibular disorders requires a team of professionals. The teachers and other school personnel must be alert to indications that the child needs evaluation or services from another professional. The focus of this chapter was to provide guidance on indications for medical and audiological referral. In addition, some insight was offered into diagnostic processes and treatment options for disorders of the outer, middle, and inner ear. Once these issues have been resolved, difficulties with auditory perception possibly due to nervous system dysfunction, such as central auditory processing disorders or auditory neuropathy, can be assessed, if indicated (see Chapter 17).

References

Bergstrom, L. (1976). Congenital deafness. In: G.M. English (Ed.), Otolaryngology Loose Leaf Series, Vol. 1. Philadelphia: Harper and Row.

Brookhouser, P.E., Worthington, D.W., & Kelly, W.J. (1991). Unilateral hearing loss in children. *Laryngoscope, 101,* 1264–1272.

Brookhouser, P.E., Worthington, D.W., & Kelly, W.J. (1992). Noise-induced hearing loss in children. *Laryngoscope, 102,* 645–655.

Hemenway, W.G., Sando, I., & McChesney, D. (1969). Temporal bone pathology following material rubella. *Arch Exp Ohren Nasen Kehlkopflceilkd, 195,* 287–300.

Meyerhoff, W.L., & Carter, J.B. (1984). Scope of the problem and fundamentals. In: W.L. Meyerhoff (Ed.), *Diagnosis and Management of Hearing Loss.* Philadelphia: WB Saunders.

Reilly, J.S., & Kenna, M.A. (1989). Congenital perilymphatic fistula: An overlooked diagnosis? *Am J Otol, 10,* 496–498.

Sando, I., Hemenway, W.G., & Morgan, R.W. (1968): Histopathology of the temporal bones in mandibulofacial depostosis. *Trans Am Acad Opthalmol Otolaryngol, 72,* 913–924.

5

Screening for Auditory Disorders

Ross J. Roeser and Jackie L. Clark

A few honest men are better than numbers.

—Oliver Cromwell, 1599–1658

Screening is the general process by which groups of people are separated into those who manifest some defined disorder and those who do not. In this sense, it is a binary process—either passing the individual who is considered a likely candidate *not* to have the disorder, or *not* passing the individual who is considered a likely candidate to have the disorder. When screening for hearing loss is performed in hospitals or schools, the goal is to identify as early as possible those who have loss of hearing that will affect their development. However, identifying those having hearing loss through effective screening programs is only one component of a comprehensive program of "hearing conservation." Hearing conservation involves effectively screening populations for possible hearing loss, ensuring referral for diagnostic evaluation of those who are unable to meet the screening criteria, and providing comprehensive treatment programs for those confirmed to have significant hearing loss. Treatment programs can range from treating a transient medical condition to involving educational intervention with appropriately fit hearing aids or even cochlear implants. Effective treatment programs also often involve providing services to the family, as well as the child, because family dynamics often play an important role in the success of the child.

Experience suggests that the vast majority of hearing conservation programs are effective in screening infants and children with hearing impairment, but oftentimes are ineffective in follow-up and providing comprehensive services to those who are identified. Once an infant or child is identified as having significant hearing impairment, it is imperative that provisions be made for proper audiological diagnosis, as well as medical and educational follow-up. For example, amplification may be indicated. In all cases, special educational intervention should be considered. Without provisions for these comprehensive follow-up services, infants and children with significant hearing loss will continue to be sensorially deprived and will not attain their maximum educational potential.

Traditionally, hearing screening programs have used air conduction hearing tests to identify children with peripheral hearing impairments. Such tests have proven to be effective in identifying significant hearing loss, but it is now well established that there are serious limitations in identifying middle ear pathological conditions with air conduction tests. A number of studies have pointed out that audiometric screening alone will fail to detect about one half of the children with confirmed middle ear disease (Brooks, 1980; Cooper, Gates, Owen, & Dickson, 1975; Eagles, Wishik, & Doerfler, 1967; Melnick, Eagles, & Levine, 1964).

This chapter reviews basic principles underlying screening. Guidelines are presented for auditory screening of neonates, infants, toddlers, and school-aged children. Topics covered include neonatal hearing screening, screening for hearing loss in preschool and school-aged children, screening for middle ear disorders, and screening for auditory processing disorders. Readers who are not completely familiar with audiometric and immittance principles should review Chapter 3.

Screening Principles

The Concept of "Pass," "Fail," and "Refer"

Hearing screenings aid in identifying individuals with a defined disorder as early as possible, who would otherwise not have been identified, and to administer treatment at a time when it will either remediate the disorder or retard its rate of development. Although screening is an either/or process, disorders may exist on a continuum from "not present at all" to "present in the most severe form." Based on this principle, it is incorrect to think that those individuals who pass the screening are completely free from the disorder for which the screening is being conducted. Instead, one should view those who pass the screening as individuals who do not manifest the disorder for which the screening is being conducted in a form severe enough to warrant consideration for additional testing.

This viewpoint is especially relevant for the screening of auditory disorders in infants and children because of the constraints that typically are put on such screening programs. As will be pointed out in later sections of this chapter, the procedures used for identifying auditory disorders in children are limited, due to the nature of the tests themselves and the environment in which they are performed. Therefore, if a child successfully passes an auditory screening test, it is not appropriate to think that the child's auditory system is completely normal, because the child may, in fact, have some auditory impairment. However, if the criteria are appropriate and the child passes the school screening, one can say that the child's audi-

tory system is not impaired to the extent that it will interfere with educational achievement, and if hearing loss does exist, it is not significant enough to warrant additional audiological testing.

To illustrate, a child's hearing is screened in the schools at 500, 1000, 2000, and 4000 Hz at 25 dB HL, and the pass/fail criterion is failure to respond to two frequencies in the same ear. Although it has been estimated by the school's screening criteria that the child's hearing loss will not cause significant educational problems, the child still does have hearing loss; hearing is not "normal." This concept of "pass" and "fail" must be maintained throughout the development and implementation of all hearing conservation programs, especially those in the schools.

Reliability and Validity

Four related terms are used to describe the general effectiveness of any type of screening test: "reliability" and "validity," and "sensitivity" and "specificity." Reliability deals with the consistency of the test. That is, if the test is administered and then repeated by a different or the same tester at another time, will the test results be the same (i.e., test–retest or within- or intraexaminer reliability)? Without a high degree of reliability, the screening tool is ineffective because the results of the test will vary from test session to test session and from tester to tester.

It is not difficult to envision how poor reliability will have serious consequences on screening tests; the reliability of a test must be high for the test to be effective. However, even if a screening test is reliable, it may not be an effective test if it fails to identify the problem for which the screening is being conducted. To illustrate, one could use the color of children's hair as a screening test for deafness, and in all probability this measure would have a high degree of test–retest and intraexaminer reliability. However, hair color is a very poor index of deafness because it is not a valid test for deafness. Another more realistic example would be the use of pure tone screening tests to identify middle ear disorders. As has already been stressed, pure tone testing fails to identify about one half of the children with middle ear disorders. Therefore, pure tone testing is not a valid measure to assess the state of the middle ear and should not be used for identifying middle ear problems.

The validity of a screening test, then, is the degree to which results are consistent with the actual presence or absence of the disorder. In other words, validity determines whether the test is actually measuring the trait for which the screening is being conducted. It is important to realize that newly developed screening procedures must be validated in some way before they are put into widespread use. Such assessment would involve calculating the percentage of false-positive and false-negative identification, and the sensitivity and specificity of the test.

False-Positive and False-Negative Identifications

It would be ideal if a screening test was 100% accurate in its classification, and if all those with and without the disorder were correctly identified. However, this situation is rarely if ever the case, and there are always an expected number of false-positive and false-negative identifications. These two conditions are illustrated in the tetrachordic table in Figure 5–1. As shown in Figure 5–1, screening test results are represented on the

vertical axis whereas diagnostic test results that confirm the presence or absence of a disorder are shown on the horizontal axis.

As an example, the diagnostic procedure for hearing loss would be pure tone threshold tests performed in a sound-treated room. Results from the screening test, shown on the ordinate in Figure 5–1, can either be positive, indicating the presence of the disorder, or negative, indicating the absence of the disorder. These cells represent all possible outcomes once the results of both the screening and the diagnostic tests are known. There are three possible outcomes from the analysis: correct identification of the abnormal and normal subjects (cells A and D), false-positive identifications (cell B), and false-negative (cell C) identifications. As illustrated, a false-positive identification occurs when an individual fails the screening test but actually does not have the disorder. A false-negative identification occurs when an individual passes the screening test but has the disorder. The formulas in Figure 5–1 show how the percentage of false-positive and false-negative identifications can be calculated. Examples of how the formulas are used are presented later.

Neither false-positive nor false-negative identifications are desirable in screening programs, and they represent a liability or "cost" to the screening process. The cost can be the actual dollars that are spent as a result

DIAGNOSTIC TEST RESULTS

	Disorder Present	Disorder not Present
POSITIVE (Fail)	A — Correct Identification of Abnormal Subjects	B — False Positive
NEGATIVE (Pass)	C — False Negative	D — Correct Identification of Normal Subjects

SCREENING TEST RESULTS

Percent of False Positive = $\dfrac{B}{B + D} \times 100$

Percent of False Negative = $\dfrac{C}{A + C} \times 100$

Figure 5–1. Tetrachordic table classifying results into correct identifications (cells A and D), false-positive identifications (cell B), and false-negative identifications (cell C).

of the screening, or the needless expenditure of time, effort, or any other resource. Frankenberg (1971) lists the following as costs of false-positive identifications: (1) the cost associated with retrieving the child for further evaluations, (2) the cost of additional screening or diagnostic tests that will fail to confirm the disorder, (3) the mental anguish of the parents and the child, and (4) the cost and danger of unnecessary treatment if the absence of the disease is not detected by diagnostic tests.

False-positive results are most likely to interfere with the overall acceptance of the screening program in the community it serves. This is especially true for hearing screening because the cost of false-positive identifications may be high. An office visit to an otolaryngologist or audiologist can be expensive, and it is quite disconcerting for parents to be charged a fee to be told that their child is "normal." Only a few parents voicing their dissatisfaction over this unnecessary visit would be needed before false-positive identifications would ultimately jeopardize acceptance of the program. Thus,

from the perspective of the administrator of the screening program, false-positive identifications must be avoided.

Costs of false-negative identifications are: (1) the loss of the benefits associated with early identifications and diagnosis, and (2) false reassurance, which will delay correct identification of the child's problem, even when symptoms persist. In the case of hearing impairment, time lost in providing the necessary educational and possibly medical intervention is detrimental to the child; if this delay is too great, the child may be deprived of full educational potential.

Sensitivity and Specificity

Sensitivity and specificity are used to measure the validity of a screening test. Sensitivity of a test is the accuracy in correctly identifying the disordered subjects. Specificity is the test's accuracy in correctly identifying the subjects without the disorder. Figure 5–2 is an extension of Figure 5–1, and illustrates how these two terms are applied. Cell A represents those subjects who failed the screen-

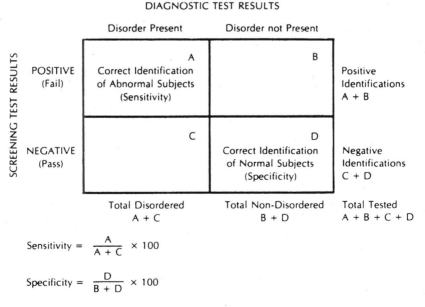

DIAGNOSTIC TEST RESULTS

	Disorder Present	Disorder not Present	
SCREENING TEST RESULTS — POSITIVE (Fail)	A — Correct Identification of Abnormal Subjects (Sensitivity)	B	Positive Identifications A + B
NEGATIVE (Pass)	C	D — Correct Identification of Normal Subjects (Specificity)	Negative Identifications C + D
	Total Disordered A + C	Total Non-Disordered B + D	Total Tested A + B + C + D

$$\text{Sensitivity} = \frac{A}{A + C} \times 100$$

$$\text{Specificity} = \frac{D}{B + D} \times 100$$

Figure 5–2. Correct identification of abnormal subjects-sensitivity (cell A) and normal subjects-specificity (cell D) for a screening test.

ing test and actually had the disorder. Data from cell A are used to calculate the sensitivity of the screening test. Cell D represents subjects who passed the screening and did not have the disorder. Data from this cell are used to calculate the specificity of the screening test. The sensitivity and specificity of a given test are computed using the formulas provided at the bottom of Figure 5–2.

Figure 5–3 presents data showing how the false-positive, false-negative, sensitivity, and specificity values of a screening test can be calculated using hypothetical data from a hearing screening test on 1000 children. Of these 1000 children, diagnostic test results showed that 92 actually had hearing loss (cells A + C), and 908 actually were free from hearing loss (cells B + D). The screening test identified 96 children with hearing loss (cells A + B), and 904 children without hearing

loss (cells C + D). Based on the data presented in Figure 5–3, the sensitivity of this test is calculated to be 95.7% and the specificity 99.1%. Stated differently, the screening test correctly identified 95.7% of those subjects who actually had hearing loss and 99.1% of the subjects who were free from hearing loss. The false-negative and false-positive rates were calculated to be 4.3% and 0.9%, respectively.

Hypothetical data provided in Figure 5–3 would strongly support the validity of screening tests being used to detect hearing loss because both the sensitivity and specificity are high, and the false-positive and false-negative rates low. This is a desired result that one attempts to achieve in any screening program.

In designing a screening test, sensitivity and specificity must be considered together

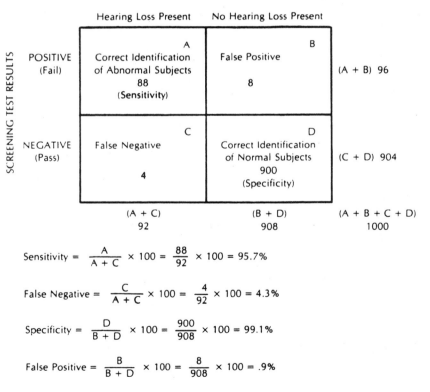

DIAGNOSTIC TEST RESULTS

		Hearing Loss Present	No Hearing Loss Present	
SCREENING TEST RESULTS	POSITIVE (Fail)	A Correct Identification of Abnormal Subjects 88 (Sensitivity)	B False Positive 8	(A + B) 96
	NEGATIVE (Pass)	C False Negative 4	D Correct Identification of Normal Subjects 900 (Specificity)	(C + D) 904
		(A + C) 92	(B + D) 908	(A + B + C + D) 1000

$$\text{Sensitivity} = \frac{A}{A + C} \times 100 = \frac{88}{92} \times 100 = 95.7\%$$

$$\text{False Negative} = \frac{C}{A + C} \times 100 = \frac{4}{92} \times 100 = 4.3\%$$

$$\text{Specificity} = \frac{D}{B + D} \times 100 = \frac{900}{908} \times 100 = 99.1\%$$

$$\text{False Positive} = \frac{B}{B + D} \times 100 = \frac{8}{908} \times 100 = .9\%$$

Figure 5–3.   Calculating the sensitivity, false-negative rate, specificity, and false-positive rate for a hypothetical screening test administered to 1000 subjects.

because they are related and directly influence the false-positive and false-negative rates. The overall goal is to maintain a balance between the factors that determine validity of the test so that the sensitivity and specificity, as well as the related false-positive and false-negative rates, are within a predetermined acceptable range for the screening that is being conducted. An extreme example is the case in which the screening test pass/fail criteria would be set at an extremely low intensity, such as 10 dB HL, and virtually all of those tested would fail (cells A or B). Such a test will produce 100% sensitivity. However, the false-positive rate would also be 100%, and the specificity and false-negative rates each 0%, making the test worthless. Conversely, redesigning the same test so that the pass/fail criteria would be set at an extremely high level, such as 50 dB HL, a great many would pass the test, resulting in 100% specificity. However, in this case the false-negative rate would be very high, maybe even 100%, and the sensitivity and false-positive rates 0%, also providing a worthless test.

Co-positivity and Co-negativity

It is possible to compare two different types of screening tests that are screening for the same disorder and to evaluate the performance of a given tester by comparing the test results with those obtained by an expert. In either case, for the results obtained, the co-positivity and co-negativity can be determined. The co-positivity is the extent to which the two tests agree in identifying those with the disorder (the positive results), and the co-negativity is the agreement in identifying those without the disorder (the negative results). An example of two different audiometric tests would be the comparison of results from a test using speech signals to those using pure tones presented at a fixed intensity. To compare tester performance, results that are obtained by the tester would be compared directly to those obtained from the same subjects by a certified audiologist.

The co-positivity and co-negativity of a test are calculated using the same formulas for calculating sensitivity and specificity, respectively. However, unlike sensitivity and specificity, measures of co-positivity and co-negativity, while providing valuable information on the reliability of a screening test, do not measure the test's validity.

Program Evaluation

Program evaluation should be an integral part of any screening process and can occur at a number of levels, from evaluation of the equipment to evaluation of the procedures and personnel used in the program. Of course, routine calibration checks of the equipment are mandatory (see Chapter 3). With the information previously given, it is possible to conduct a methodological evaluation of the screening procedures and personnel, provided one of two steps is added to the screening process—either the reliability of the procedures can be evaluated by comparing test results from those individuals who perform routine screening with those obtained by an audiologist (co-positive and co-negativity), or the validity of the procedures can be evaluated by comparing screening results with diagnostic findings (sensitivity and specificity).

EVALUATING CO-POSITIVITY
AND CO-NEGATIVITY

An example of evaluating the reliability of the program by calculating its co-positivity and co-negativity follows: Two audiometric support personnel separately screen 868 children and the school's audiologist immediately rescreens the children. Figure 5–4 shows the data after they have been categorized into a tetrachordic table. The co-positivity and co-negativity for Support Person 1 were 76% and 94%, respectively, with commensurate false-negative and false-positive rates of 24% and 6%, respectively. However, for Support Person 2 the respective values were 97% and 99.3% for co-positivity and

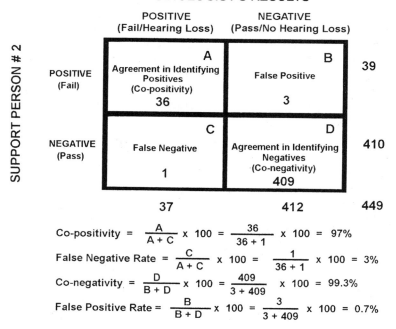

Figure 5–4. Calculating co-positivity and co-negativity of a screening test for two support personnel.

co-negativity and 3% and 0.7% for the false-negativity and false-positive rates.

The data in Figure 5–4 would indicate that for some reason the results of the screenings performed by Support Person 1 are inferior to those obtained by Support Person 2, when compared with the audiologist's results. In fact, these hypothetical data would be alarming if they were actually obtained through program evaluation because of the high false-negative rates found for Support Person 1. To check Support Person 1, the equipment being used would be examined to ensure that it is in proper calibration and there are no malfunctions, and the actual test procedures used in the screening would be evaluated carefully. If findings similar to those in Figure 5–4 were revealed through program evaluation, careful scrutiny of the performance of Support Person 1 should be made until it is within limits similar to those for Support Person 2.

EVALUATING SENSITIVITY AND SPECIFICITY

Whenever results from a screening test can be compared to results from a diagnostic test, the sensitivity and specificity of the screening test can be calculated to determine the validity of the results. Such an evaluation can be performed retrospectively, after the results have been obtained and reported, or a theoretical model can been created based on prevalence figures to judge sensitivity and specificity of specific procedures.

It is unfortunate that most hearing conservation programs do not routinely evaluate the sensitivity and specificity of their programs. Program evaluation does require extra time on the part of the personnel in the program, which ultimately translates into added dollars. However, without appropriate evaluation, the basic issue of the program's effectiveness will always be subject to questions. With the advent of the two-step otoacoustic emission/auditory brainstem response (OAE/ABR) neonatal screening approach, sensitivity and specificity can be measured when procedures are compared if all babies screened are screened with both techniques.

Practical Considerations for Auditory Screening

Considerations relevant to both infant and school-aged screenings include screening expectations, equipment upkeep and maintenance, test environment, visual inspection of the earcanals; and awareness of normal auditory developmental milestones. When addressed, each of these practical considerations can either facilitate or create a stumbling block for any screening program.

Screening Expectations

Discrepancies found between screening programs such as the type of tests used, the instrument(s) used to perform the tests, the training of the testers, environmental noise present during hearing screening, and the pass/fail criteria influence the overall effectiveness of the program. However, even when these factors are controlled as closely as possible, variability still exists. For example, Table 5–1 presents results from audiometric screening of 54,370 children in the Dallas Public Schools using a pure tone sweep check test at 500, 1000, 2000, and 4000 Hz at a level of 25 dB HL. Six different testers performed the screening, but the procedures, equipment, and pass/fail criteria were identical, and all testers had the same training. Despite this uniformity in the program, the percentage of failures between testers ranged from 0.9 to 3.4%; and all of the values were lower than the nominal 5% value for prevalence of hearing loss suggested by many studies. What, then, can account for interexaminer differences? This question can be answered on the basis of data gathered from epidemiological studies of auditory disorders in children.

Epidemiology is technically defined as the study of frequencies and distributions of disorders and the relationship between the various factors that contribute to their occurrence (Newman, 1975). When an epidemiological study is conducted, all of the factors that relate to a particular disease process are considered, including age, sex, social and cultural characteristics, climate, and so on.

Table 5–1. Screening Data from the Dallas Independent School District

Tester	No. Children Screened	Percent Failing Test
1	10,129	1.0
2	8,525	3.4
3	9,680	1.4
4	7,997	2.1
5	9,351	1.2
6	8,688	0.9
Total	**54,370**	**Average 1.7**

Once an epidemiological study is completed, it is possible to assess how the factors studied affect the incidence of the disorder and its severity.

We are now able to make the following generalizations about auditory disorders: hearing loss and ear disease are more prevalent in young children and in certain populations, such as American Indians (Weit, 1979) and Eskimos (Kaplan, Fleshman, Bender, Baum, & Clark, 1973); low socioeconomic status may increase the incidence of hearing loss and ear disease (Fay, Hochberg, & Smith, 1972); the incidence of hearing loss and ear disease changes with climate and specific seasons of the year (McEldowney & Kessner, 1972); and high-frequency sensorineural hearing loss is more prevalent in older males in grades 9 through 12 (Hull, Mielke, & Timmons, 1971; Weber, McGovern, & Fink, 1967). A summary of literature dealing with screening in special populations has been published by Northern (1978). These factors make it impossible to estimate the expected incidence of hearing loss or ear disease in a population of school-age children on an a priori basis, regardless of screening techniques used.

Equipment Upkeep and Maintenance

Specific descriptions of the necessary equipment most appropriate for each type of screening program are described later in this chapter and in even more detail in Chapter

3. However, an important criterion that should be used in selecting equipment for use in the screening program is the quality and availability of maintenance and calibration service. All audiometric equipment must be serviced on a regular basis, and the location and efficiency of the service center should be considered before making a purchase. It would not be advisable to purchase an instrument from the dispenser 1000 miles away, when a local dealer who provides direct service is available.

Test Environment

Testing environments should have low ambient noise levels, be well lit and well ventilated, and be of adequate size to accommodate the tester and equipment. A most critical requirement of the test environment is the ambient noise level because false-positive identifications will occur in hearing screening if the background noise levels are too high. The most desirable space for hearing screening is located as far away as possible from heating units, air conditioners or other mechanical equipment, and high traffic areas such as the cafeteria, shop areas, and restrooms. The exact location depends entirely on the facility itself and the daily schedule of activities.

Testing in settings with high environmental ambient noise levels may potentially result in the test stimulus itself being masked and inaudible. High ambient noise levels have a limiting effect on the frequencies and intensity at which hearing screening can be performed and are the reason for imposing many of the recommended guidelines for hearing screening. Most noise found in a typical school environment will have its main energy concentrated in the frequencies below 1000 Hz. This is the primary reason why screening guidelines recommend testing at 1000 Hz and above, even though some important data can be obtained at 500 and 250 Hz. Moreover, screening tests performed at intensities of 10 to 15 dB HL can be severely affected by noise, even though these intensities are more sensitive to marginal hearing loss.

It has been reasoned by some that if background noise level is too high, simply increasing the intensity level of the test stimuli will solve the problem. However, this solution is not acceptable because test sensitivity would be reduced for those children who actually have hearing loss, resulting in more children fallaciously passing the hearing screening. In no case should the levels of the test stimuli be increased above those specified by the screening program, and an alternate test site should be selected.

Some solutions to resolve the problem of ambient noise would include use of sound-isolated rooms, mobile test vans or trailers, or small portable hearing test booths. These would all ensure that acceptable background noise levels would be present all of the time. However, with the constant demands and limitations on hospital or school finances, such equipment may be beyond the scope of most budgets.

A final solution for eliminating unwanted background noise is the use of noise-excluding earphone enclosures and insert-type earphones (described in Chapter 3). Certain types of these enclosures are generally more effective in reducing background noise than the standard headsets (see Chapter 3) (Roeser & Glorig, 1975; Roeser & Musket, 1976; Roeser, Seidel, & Glorig, 1975). Furthermore, laboratory and field studies in the pediatric population have proven their overall effectiveness (Musket & Roeser, 1977; Stark & Borton, 1975). Despite the studies supporting their use, noise-excluding headsets do present inherent problems, such as earphone placement. Thus they should be

utilized only by highly experienced examiners who are aware of the difficulties that may occur with their use. Noise-excluding earphones should not be used routinely in hearing conservation programs. Insert-type earphones not only attenuate background noise but also reduce earcanal collapse and have higher interaural attenuation.

A simple biological check should always be made prior to screening to assess the appropriateness of the test environment before any testing is performed. A biological check can be performed by screening normal-hearing volunteers (e.g., the tester and one other person) as they listen to the screening stimuli. Obviously, if these individuals fail to perceive the test stimuli within the test environment, it is most likely an unsatisfactory environment, provided that proper equipment calibration has been verified. For those who may have access to a sound-level meter, Table 5–2 provides allowable decibel sound pressure levels (SPLs) for conducting screening according to ANSI (1999) standards.

Visual Inspection of the Ear

Visual inspection of the ear includes gross examination of the pinnae and external earcanal with an otoscope. Medical referral should be made for any gross defects of the pinnae and earcanal because structural defects may suggest the presence of other otologic abnormalities needing attention. Examples are abnormal position or structure of the external ear, ranging from complete absence of the pinnae and atresia (underdevelopment) of the earcanal to more subtle ab-

Table 5–2. Allowable Octave-Band Ambient Noise Levels (SPL; 20 µPa) for Threshold Measurements at 0 dB HL (ANSI, 1999) and for Screening at the ASHA (2002) Recommended Levels

Test Frequency	500	1000	2000	4000
Octave-band cutoff Frequencies	300 600	600 1200	1200 2400	2400 4800
Octave-band levels: Ear covered (MX-41/AR cushion)	19.5	26.5	28.0	34.5
Plus ASHA screening level	20	20	20	20
Resulting maximum allowable noise level for ASHA screening	39.5	46.5	48.0	54.5

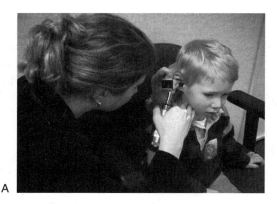

A

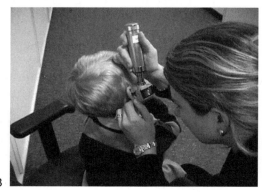

B

Figure 5–5. Otoscopic inspection of the earcanal can be accomplished using two different methods: (A) with the handle of the otoscope held in the palm of the examiner's hand and extended below the child's head, and (B) with the handle of the otoscope held between the examiner's thumb and forefinger and above the child's head. In each case the examiner's hand holding the otoscope must be in contact with the child's head to prevent the possibility of forcing the instrument into the ear in the event of sudden movement, such as coughing.

normalities, such as malpositioned pinnae or preauricular pits and tags. Discharge from the earcanal may be seen as dry crusty material and needs immediate referral.

Otoscopy is the process by which the earcanal and tympanic membrane are inspected by an examiner, with an otoscope (Fig. 5–5). Otoscopic inspection aims to assess the condition of the outer ear and tympanic membrane and is highly dependent on the training and skill of the examiner. Accordingly, the procedure should be adminis-

tered by individuals with supervised training and experience in visual examination of the ear. Notations should be made by the examiner regarding any blockage due to a foreign object or cerumen in the earcanal and the following eardrum conditions: abnormal color (red, yellow, or dull gray), bulging eardrum, fluid line or bubbles behind the eardrum, perforation, and retraction pockets.

Until recently, the use of otoscopes by audiologists has been somewhat equivocal; many audiologists have routinely used otoscopes for years and others have not. However, in 1991 the American Speech-Language-Hearing Association (ASHA) legislative council passed a resolution that specifically states that both otoscopy and cerumen management are within the scope of practice of audiology (ASHA, 1991). It is now clear that audiologists not only should, but must, perform routine otoscopic examination on their patients. In addition, cerumen management is within the scope of practice for audiologists and, depending on state licensure, they are able to clean earcanals when otoscopic inspection reveals excessive or impacted cerumen.

Musket and Dowraczyk (1980) described an otoscope that is disguised as a puppet in order to reduce the level of fear a child, especially preschoolers, might encounter during otoscopic inspection. Since this early description of otoscope modifications, there have been a variety of otoscope accessories produced for commercial use. Some of the child-friendly products include modified otoscopes or creative accessories mounted on the otoscope speculum. Commercially available products range from an otoscope modified with a small plastic bear sitting atop the viewing piece (EarBear® Company) or a small plastic elephant (Elly the Elephant®); or whimsical and colorful cartoon faces that attach to large or small otoscope speculae (EARnimals®) in a variety of characters including a lightning bug, elephant, frog, bear, whale, and hummingbird (Fig. 5–6). As Musket and Dowraczyk (1980) suggest, with a little creativity it is possible to

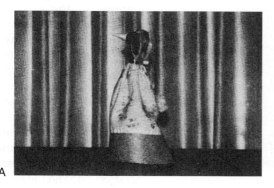

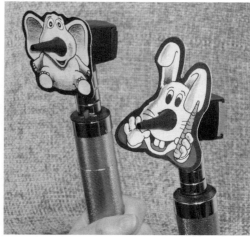

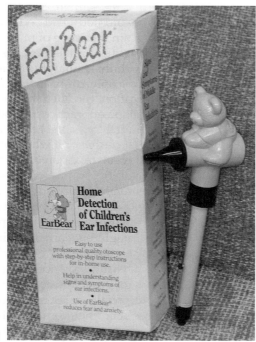

Figure 5–6. Modifications of an otoscope. (A) Otoscope disguised as a puppet (Musket & Dowraczyk, 1980). (B) Commercially available EarBear® otoscope. (C) Commercially available EARnimals® cartoon faces that attach to otoscope speculae.

make otoscopic inspections less frightening for the very young child.

Awareness of Normal Auditory Behaviors

Many behaviors have been associated with auditory impairment in children, and consequently it is important that professionals and parents become familiar with behavioral signs or physical symptoms of hearing loss that might give them clues as to a child's need for audiological examination. Behaviors and physical symptoms that may indicate auditory impairment in a child are listed in Table 5–3. Although these signs may also be associated with other types of learning problems, any child exhibiting one or more should be referred for audiometric screening, and diagnostic evaluation when indicated.

Table 5–3. Behaviors and Physical Symptoms in Children That May Indicate Hearing Loss

Behaviors

a. Frequently asks to have this repeated
b. Turns one side of head toward speaker
c. Talks too loudly or too slowly
d. Shows strain in trying to hear
e. Watches and concentrates on teacher's lips
f. Is inattentive in classroom discussion
g. Makes frequent mistakes in following directions
h. Makes unusual mistakes in taking directions
i. Tends to isolate self
j. Tends to be passive
k. Is tense
l. Tires easily
m. Has a speech problem
n. Is not working up to apparent capacity
o. Has academic failure following severe illness

Physical Symptoms

a. Mouth breathing
b. Draining ears
c. Earaches
d. Dizziness
e. Reports of ringing, buzzing, or roaring in ears (tinnitus)

Newborn and Infant Hearing Screening

Profound hearing loss occurs in 1 in 1000 births worldwide. Based on the results from several neonatal hearing screening program estimates there are between 8000 and 16,000 newborns a year identified with hearing loss in the United States (O'Neal, Finitzo, & Littman, 2000), making hearing loss the most prevalent birth defect in the United States. These statistics clearly document the need for infant hearing screening. However, current research has shown an urgent need to begin habilitative programs with infants identified with significant hearing loss by 6 months of age so that developmental milestones may occur closer to age expectations (Yoshinaga-Itano, Sedey, Coulter, & Mehl, 1998). Several governmental and professional organizations, including the National Institute on Deafness and Other Communication Disorders (1993); the U.S. Public

Health and Human Services (1990, 2000); and the Joint Committee on Infant Hearing (JCIH) (2000), have strongly supported implementing hearing screening programs nationwide for all neonates using objective, physiological measures within hours of birth, and immediately remediating any hearing disorders uncovered during the screening process. Currently 37 states and the District of Columbia have mandated, through legislative procedures, hospital-based newborn hearing screening programs for the purposes of identifying hearing loss and initiating necessary intervention before 6 months of age. There are untold numbers of hospitals in the remaining states that have opted to voluntarily implement their own programs without mandated infant hearing screening programs within their state.

To ensure that every hospital provides a comprehensive, timely, coordinated, and accessible early hearing detection and intervention (EHDI) program, the JCIH Position Statement (2000) proposed eight principles on which to build EHDI foundations: (1) all infants have access to hearing screening using physiological measures; (2) all infants who do not pass the birth admission screen and any subsequent rescreening begin appropriate audiological and medical evaluations before 3 months of age; (3) all infants with confirmed hearing loss receive interdisciplinary program services before 6 months of age; (4) all infants who pass screening but have risk indicators for other auditory disorders receive ongoing audiological and medical monitoring; (5) infant and family rights are guaranteed through informed choice; (6) infant hearing screening and evaluation results are afforded privacy and confidentiality without compromising the ability of health and education to provide care; (7) information systems are used to measure and report the effectiveness of EHDI services; (8) EHDI programs provide data to monitor quality, compliance, and cost effectiveness.

While keeping all eight principles in mind, there are a number of development and maintenance EHDI program issues within each hospital to be resolved. Program costs for most facilities are challenging. After conducting a survey, the National Campaign for Hearing Health (2000) reported that costs for newborn hearing screening within multiple hospitals ranged between $20 and $60. Importantly, screening for hearing loss costs less than one tenth of the cost for screening for phenylketonuria (PKU), hypothyroidism, or sickle cell anemia, which are less prevalent than hearing loss and are screened in nearly every state (Johnson, Mauk, & Takekawa, 1993). Clearly, the resulting developmental delays and life-threatening consequences in extreme cases that can result from the above endocrine anomalies allow hospitals to justify screening charges for these conditions as of medical necessity for all infants. However, the ramifications brought by hearing loss can arguably be considered a long-term (lifelong) strain to most families and communities, ranging from educational to emotional to financial.

In establishing a new program an important consideration is that each hospital have clearly defined procedures, protocols, and structural features in which the staff operate. When developing screening procedures the routine daily activities of the hospital need to be considered, including procedures for chart documentation, the schedule for collecting and recording infant vital signs, "rooming-in" times, specific times when the hospital is quieter or noisier, times and location of routine nursery procedures (e.g., circumcisions, etc.), and proximity of procedure rooms (which can be noisy). A survey of the hospital's daily routine is needed before decisions regarding personnel, protocol, equipment, and diagnostic follow-up support services are made for the program. Newborn hearing screening programs are built on the premise that initial screening will take place within 24 to 48 hours after birth and prior to discharge. Cost effectiveness and patient confidentiality must be strictly maintained.

Personnel

A team comprising audiologists, physicians, nursing personnel, speech-language pathologists, and trained technical staff plays an instrumental role in an EHDI program. Two particular team members who shoulder much of the responsibily for implementing and carrying out the program are the program manager and the screener(s). Fiscal constraints often dictate who within the institutional professional staff should act as program manager. Due to third-party reimbursement limitations, very few hospitals are able to rationalize the necessary costs for hiring an audiologist to oversee the program. As a result, it is not unusual to find speech-language pathologists or nurses designated as the EHDI program manager to oversee the general operations, training, and monitoring of technical personnel; the education of the immediate medical community and families; and the follow-up procedures for those infants who do not pass the screening, as well as to act as program advocate, benchmark the program, and maintain and report screening results to the necessary state agencies. Methods to ensure confidential communications to the parents as well as reports to physicians are chosen by the program manager. Ultimately, the program manager determines the appropriate protocol and equipment utilized in the facility's universal screening program. In short, the program manager is responsible for merging the hospital infrastructure with the development and implementation of the EHDI protocols and for assessing the effectiveness of the protocols.

Day-to-day responsibilities of conducting screenings in the nursery are oftentimes assigned to a technical support staff. Although screeners are responsible for conducting the physical assessment with accuracy and in a quiet environment, they must also document results in the hospital chart, advise hospital staff of a completed screening, alert the program manager of equipment malfunctions or failures, and advise all necessary team members of any infants who are to be referred for further testing. Depending on the number of neonates to screen and the time restrictions within the hospital environment, there may be multiple times for screenings to occur daily.

Protocol: Otoacoustic Emission versus Auditory Brainstem Response

Despite the broad variety of screening protocols being used, hospital neonatal hearing screening programs have been successful in identifying those with hearing loss (Arehart, Yoshinaga-Itano, Thomson, Gabbard, & Stredler Brown, 1998; Finitzo, Albright, & O'Neal, 1998; Gravel et al, 2000). Objective physiological measures called for by JCIH (2000) can include either OAE or ABR tests (see Chapter 3). Those using OAEs can choose either distortion product otoacoustic emissions (DPOAE) or transient evoked otoacoustic emissions (TEOAE). As more states engage in legislatively mandated newborn hearing screening programs, the demand for simpler, smaller, and automated equipment has increased dramatically. A program manager can choose any number of commercial devices that are readily available, with reportedly exceptionally high hearing screening sensitivity (Finitzo et al, 1998).

Otoacoustic emission screening devices are noninvasive and can be housed in either a portable handheld or computer-driven unit (Fig. 5–7). Screenings conducted with OAEs only assess the integrity of the outer hair cells within the cochlea. A subsequent assumption is made about general hearing status depending upon testing results (Gorga et al, 1993; Prieve et al, 1993). Some OAE devices can measure frequency-specific responses via distortion product (DPOAE) whereas others measure the overall spectral responses via transient evoked (TEOAE). All OAE devices will have a requisite microphone coupler with a removable probe tip. Both stimuli delivery and recording are carried out in one microphone coupler system. Probe tips covering the microphone coupler can be of varying sizes and shapes best fitting an infant's earcanal. Neonates are more prone to having debris or vernix caseosa within the earcanal, and placement of a probe tip into the earcanal can further impact any debris already present. Once debris impaction occurs there is an increased possibility, especially for very newborn babies, not to pass the initial screening. Clearly, any

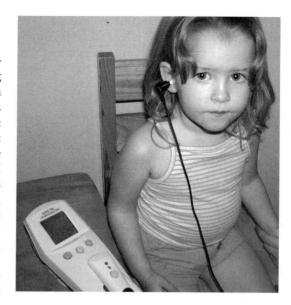

Figure 5–7. Portable otoacoustic emission screening system requires a probe to be placed in the earcanal.

debris in the earcanal will create a conductive hearing loss and render an inaccurate finding even if the condition is of a temporary nature.

With heightened awareness of auditory neuropathy, some hospitals are opting to conduct screenings with ABR rather than or in addition to OAE devices (Chapters 6 and 17). Discovered 3 decades ago, the ABR is still considered the gold standard for nonbehavioral threshold prediction and is often used with the difficult-to-test population. Results are based on the assumption that normal brainstem and auditory system integrity is predictive of normal hearing (Gorga et al, 1993). ABR, like OAE screening, is a noninvasive test using computer-based devices that can be housed in either a portable handheld or laptop unit (Fig. 5–8). More peripheral attachments are required for operating the ABR than the OAE, but overall costs between disposable accessories can be similar between the two technologies. The ABR stimuli delivery and recording systems are carried out differently than the OAE. In addition to a requisite microphone coupler with removable probe tips,

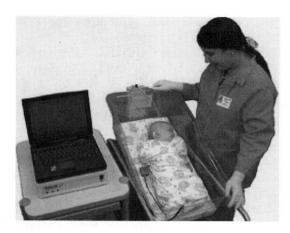

Figure 5–8. Auditory brainstem response screening system requires electrodes to be placed on the head of the infant and a probe be placed in the earcanal.

there are also three or four electrode leads that must be affixed to the infant's scalp with tape.

Three forms of stimuli are currently used in the ABR screening: click, tone-burst, and steady-state. A click stimulus is not frequency specific, but instead provides a broad range of higher frequencies. Though considered more frequency specific, the tone-burst stimulus can be difficult to record and observed at near-threshold levels. A newer ABR, the auditory steady-state response (ASSR), is believed to provide a simultaneous presentation of frequency-specific stimuli at threshold intensity levels (Cone-Wesson, Parker, Swiderski, & Rickards, 2002; Dimitrijevic, John, & Van Roon, 2002). However, for the time being, the ASSR does not have its own current procedural terminology code for third-party payment considerations and is not a clinically feasible method of screening neonates.

As mentioned earlier, some programs opt to perform a two-tiered screening that utilizes OAE for an initial screening and a second tier with ABR screening for those infants who do not initially pass. Current literature indicates that either device, when used appropriately by trained personnel, can provide the necessary information for a successful screening program and both are

highly correlated with the degree of peripheral hearing sensitivity (Finitzo et al, 1998; Mason & Hermann, 1998; Vohr, Carty, Moore, & Letourneau, 1998). Once a hospital determines the specific type of screening protocol (i.e., OAE or ABR) best suited to their nursery environment, a decision about types of equipment to use easily follows.

Pass/Refer Criteria

Rather than "pass/fail," current screening terminology categorizes results as either "pass" or "refer." That is, if an infant does not pass the initial screen, the results are designated as "refer," avoiding the implication that the infant "failed" the test. This choice of terminology is believed to reduce parental or family emotional anguish or alarm over the screening results. There could still be a need to continue monitoring some infants' hearing status if a progressive condition that could lead to hearing loss is suspected or discovered.

Each hospital is responsible for determining follow-up protocol for each refer finding. As mentioned earlier, a second screening using an OAE or ABR may be conducted prior to discharge. This second screening just prior to discharge is a viable means of reducing the number of false-positives during the screening process. Oftentimes, when the second screening is conducted, extraneous factors that might have resulted in the refer finding, such as debris (vernix caseosa) in the earcanal or high noise levels, have had time to be resolved.

Communicating screening results through the routine nursery channels, from the infant's nurse and primary physician to the parents, is accomplished through a variety of means chosen by the program manager. Standardized medical record forms specific to each hospital found in the infant's chart are adequate to alert the medical staff and document screening results as well as recommend follow-up procedures. Handouts detailing screening results and brochures relevant to the findings are provided for the infant's parents. Of course, materials provided to parents must be printed using terminology and language that the parents are most comfortable reading and understanding.

Benchmarks

Benchmarks are considered quality control indicators or efficiency standards of specific programs within a facility, such as the effectiveness of personnel performing certain tasks, or the number of individuals being positively affected by services, and so forth. Each hospital is given the extra responsibility of managing and maintaining all screening results. Defined as the quantifiable goals or targets by which an EHDI program may be monitored and evaluated, benchmarks can be used to evaluate progress and point toward the necessary steps for program quality assurance (O'Donnell & Galinsky, 1998). While utilizing benchmarking data for program quality, it is still necessary to maintain patient and family confidentiality as defined by state regulations. Recommended benchmark and quality indicators for birth admission screenings include the following: screen a minimum of 95% of infants during their birth admission or before 1 month of age; maintain a referral rate for medical or audiological management of 4% or less; and, ideally, achieve a return for follow-up of 70% or more of infants (JCIH, 2000).

Effective information management systems should be capable of compiling infant data and the EHDI follow-up service providers. By using the information management system to track infants and families it is possible to quantify the number of infants requiring and receiving services and those services provided, and to identify infants lost to follow-up at any stage of the process. It has been argued that a mandatory centralized, statewide tracking system will reduce the inherent problems associated with the transition of infants and families from screening to confirmation of and intervention for hearing loss (Diefendorf & Finitzo, 1997). Currently, the Maternal and Child Health Bureau (MCHB) requires that each state report the number of live births and the number of newborns screened for hearing

loss during the birth admission. The Pilot National Data Set proposed in 1999 by the Centers for Disease Control and Prevention (CDC) in conjunction with the Directors of Speech and Hearing Programs in State Health and Welfare Agencies (DSHPSHWA) outlined multiple components necessary to create a national database that would supercede the state requirements. JCIH has endorsed a national database that will document aggregate state data providing demographics, including prevalence and etiology, as well as provide national benchmark and quality indicators across the United States. Some elements required of each state in the Pilot National Data Set include number of live births; number of newborns screened before discharge from the hospital; number of infants referred for audiological evaluation before 1 month of age; number of audiological evaluations before 3 months of age; number of infants with permanent congenital hearing loss; mean, median, and minimum age of diagnosis of hearing loss for infants identified in newborn hearing screening programs; and number of infants with permanent hearing loss receiving intervention by 6 months (JCIH, 2000).

Hearing Screening for Preschool and School-Aged Children

Despite the success of many newborn hearing screening programs, there is still an ever-present need to detect hearing loss in school-aged children. Because some states do not have mandated newborn hearing screening programs, the possibility of false-negative results exists, and some children will have acquired hearing loss. Consequently, toddlers, youngsters, and school-aged children need to be screened routinely for undetected hearing loss.

Northern and Downs (1991) indicate that there were 42,000 children with severe hearing impairment attending special schools or classes for the hearing-impaired in the United States in 1991. Bess, Dodd-Murphy, and Parker (1998) evaluated 1218 school-aged children and found the prevalence of mild sensorineural hearing loss to be 5.4% (1 in 20 children). When all degrees and type of hearing loss are included, based on a screening level of 25 dB or more through the speech frequencies, more recent prevalence estimates for school-aged children are between 11.3 and 14.9% (Bess et al, 1998). ASHA (2002) suggest that prevalence rates would result in an average of 131 for every 1000 school-aged children with some degree of hearing loss.

The inclusion of minimal sensorineural hearing loss is considered crucial because of the recognized life altering effects (Bess et al, 1998). Research has demonstrated that a significant number of children with minimal sensorineural hearing loss fail at least one grade; exhibit some dysfunctional traits in behavior, energy levels, stress levels, social and self-esteem; and have greater difficulty in communicating in general (Bess et al, 1998; Blair, Peterson, & Viehweg, 1985; Quigley & Thomason, 1968).

These most recent prevalence rates are, indeed, higher than those reported in early identification studies (Anderson, 1978; Berg, 1970) and are cause for concern. The apparent increase in prevalence could potentially be explained by a number of factors, such as the definition of the level at which "hearing loss" is detected. Other factors contributing to increased prevalence of hearing loss in children are believed to include greater exposure to high noise levels during leisure activities at earlier ages (Montgomery & Fujikawa, 1992); markedly increased episodes of middle ear disease (Hunter et al, 1996); and improved survival rate of premature at-risk infants being treated in the neonatal intensive care units (Salamy, Eldredge, & Tooley, 1989).

Personnel

Two levels of personnel may be utilized in school hearing conservation programs, one supervisory and one technical (ASHA, 1975; Darley, 1961). Ideally, the supervisor of the program should be an audiologist. As the supervisor of the program, the audiologist is responsible for the higher administrative functions of the program, such as selecting the screening procedures to be used, training and monitoring the technical staff, ensuring proper equipment calibration, performing or referring those who do not pass the screening for diagnostic audiological testing, and discussing test results with medical personnel.

In smaller school systems, resources may not be available to have a full-time audiologist to supervise the hearing conservation program. In such cases it is possible in most areas of the country to have a part-time audiologist consultant who will monitor the activities just listed. The consultant's primary role is to set up the program and train the technical staff as thoroughly as possible. Only when special problems arise is the consultant required to be available in the school system itself.

The technical or support personnel perform the screening tests and carry out the day-to-day activities of the program, such as performing daily calibration checks and filling out statistical reports. Many school systems use nurses or speech-language pathologists in this role. Because of their training, such professionals are effective but still require in-service training to familiarize them with the general area of hearing, hearing disorders, and audiometric testing. Such sessions should be held for no less than 1 full day before the individual begins to function in the program. A very helpful way to avoid any confusion in the program, and to keep it uniform, is to develop a written manual describing the screening program and procedures used.

When paraprofessionals or professionals with no training in auditory disorders and screening are used for technical support, additional training is mandatory. The National Conference on Identification Audiometry recommended that for such persons the training course be conducted over a 2- to 6-week period, with at least half of the time devoted to supervised practice in testing (Darley, 1961). Because the success of the entire hearing conservation program rests on the support personnel, the need for adequate training cannot be overemphasized. The absolute minimum training period for

Table 5–4. Topics to Be Included in Paraprofessional Training Programs for Auditory Screening in the Schools

1. Basic physical principles of sound
2. Anatomy and physiology of the auditory system
3. Disorders of the ear and types of hearing loss
4. Use, care, maintenance, and calibration of audiometers
5. Screening procedures
6. Threshold measurement and referral procedures
7. Record keeping

the paraprofessionals should be 5 days, with half of the time in supervised practicum. As a guide, topics that should be included in the training program are listed in Table 5–4.

Protocol: Pure Tone Sweep Check Test

The individual pure tone sweep check screening test, originally described by New-hart (1938) and recommended by the ASHA Committee on Audiometric Evaluation, is the preferred screening test for school-aged children (ASHA, 1975, 1985). The pure tone sweep check test involves presenting stimuli at predetermined frequencies and fixed intensity levels, and the child is instructed to respond by raising a hand, raising a finger, or responding in some other manner. Earphones are placed over both ears of the child and a practice tone is presented at a level above the test tone (i.e., 40 dB HL) to acquaint the child with the type of signal to be heard. All of the test stimuli are first presented to one ear and then the other, and a record is made as to the presence or absence of a response at each frequency; no attempt is made to alter the attenuator dial to determine the threshold level when the child fails to respond. The sweep check procedure can be successfully administered to both school-age and preschool children in about 2 minutes per child (Hood & Lamb, 1974).

FREQUENCY

Differences exist concerning the frequencies and intensities to test in the individual pure tone sweep check test. In general, the frequencies recommended have been in the 500 to 6000 Hz range. Tones at and below 500 Hz are not recommended because they are more easily masked by room noise and do not provide significant information to the testing procedure; most recent guidelines do not recommend using frequencies at and below 500 Hz (ASHA, 1975, 1985). The use of 6000 Hz in screening has also been questioned due to its variability (House & Glorig, 1957).

Although data are available to support limited frequency screening, (Ventry & Newby, 1959) conclusive data suggest that limited frequency screening procedures are not as effective as the pure tone sweep check test. Siegenthaler and Sommer (1959) evaluated the audiometric test results of more than 19,500 children and estimated that 35% of those failing the sweep check test did not demonstrate losses at 4000 Hz. Stevens and Davidson (1959) report similar observations on 1784 audiograms. These findings suggest that limiting the screening to a single frequency, or even to two frequencies, significantly reduces the sensitivity of hearing screening, at least in school children. In light of these data, it is apparent that screening should be performed at three or four frequencies.

INTENSITY

The recommended intensity or intensities at which screening should occur have generally varied between 20 and 30 dB HL (ANSI, 1996). In selecting the screening level, two factors should be considered. First is the effect of the background noise and second is the sensitivity of the test in detecting even slight hearing loss. Background noise was discussed previously in this chapter. However, as the screening level decreases, the ambient noise will have a greater effect on the test signal. This one factor has prevented schools from screening at or below 15 to 20 dB HL.

By decreasing the level at which the test is performed, the sensitivity of the test can be increased and children with even slight hearing loss can be identified. Because audiologists believe that even slight hearing loss affects the development of speech and language, the goal of many programs is to reduce the intensity at which the screening is performed to identify children with minimal hearing loss. However, we are forced into accepting screening levels of 20 to 25 dB HL because of the conditions under which most screening is performed. It is unfortunate, but reduction of the screening level to 10 or 15 dB HL would significantly increase the number of overreferrals because of false-positive identification due to background noise.

PASS/FAIL CRITERIA

The specific pass/fail criteria used in the program will depend entirely on the frequencies and intensities at which the screening is performed. However, results from several studies make it quite clear that referral should be based on failure of two screening tests given several hours apart on the same day or several days apart. In this procedure only children who fail the second screening test are referred for follow-up. A second test is recommended due to various temporary factors, such as inattentiveness, noise in the test environment, nervousness, and transient conductive hearing loss. Once these variables are allowed to abate, the number of overreferrals can be reduced. Melnick et al (1964) found that the inclusion of a second screening reduced the number of overreferrals by 23%. Wilson and Walton (1974) rescreened 411 children in grades K through 5 who failed an initial screening test and found that slightly more than 50% passed the rescreening. Results from these two studies certainly support the need for rescreening before referral.

Table 5–5 summarizes six pure tone sweep check procedures developed over a number of decades. Although these protocols in no way exhaust the possible screening guidelines that have been proposed, they represent the wide range of screening procedures used in the schools. In 2002, ASHA published *Guidelines for Audiology Service Provision in and for Schools*. As shown in Table 5–6, these guidelines are summarized by procedure, frequency, pass/fail intensity criteria, and follow-up recommendations for four groups of children. Those four groups of children defined by age include birth through 6 months; infants and toddlers (7 months to 2 years); preschool children (3 to 5 years); and school-aged children (5 to 18 years). Infants up to 6 months of age cannot participate in the same conditioned audiological protocol as older children; instead they require more objective tests of physiological function such as ABRs or OAEs. With the exception of the birth through 6 month and 7 months through 2 years of age population, the recommended frequencies are 1000, 2000, and 4000 at 20 dB. These same frequencies are also suggested for those 7 months through 2 years old, however the pass/fail intensity criterion of 30 dB is dependent upon the Visual Reinforcement Audiometry, and 20 dB is dependent upon Conditioned Play Audiometry.

Not responding to any frequency in either ear is considered a failure that requires rescreening within 1 to 3 months after initial screening. One exception, again, is found with newborns to 6-month-olds, who must be immediately rescreened when a fail occurs, then rescreen within 1 to 3 months if the second rescreen is failed. The ASHA procedures are intended to detect those children with educationally significant hearing loss. However, unless the loss is in the severe range and also affects 3000 Hz, those who fail at 4000 Hz only should not experience significant auditory problems in the classroom; 4000 Hz falls outside of the standard speech range (Chapter 3). Detecting high-frequency hearing loss is important because there are medical and audiological conditions that need to be identified. As an example, noise-induced hearing loss first manifests itself in the 4000 to 6000 Hz range. Children failing only at 4000 Hz need to be referred for a complete audiological follow-up with appropriate treatment and counseling.

A limiting factor of the ASHA guidelines is that they do not detect minimal or mild hearing loss (Chapter 10); however, the relatively high noise levels in the schools prevents screening at lower intensity levels. A possible method for identifying a child with

Table 5–5. Comparison of Recommended Test Frequencies, Intensity Levels, and Pass/Fail Criteria for School Hearing Screening

Source	Test Frequencies	Intensity Level	Pass/Fail Criteria
ASHA, 1985	1000, 2000, and 4000 Hz	20 dB	Fail to respond to one tone in either ear
Anderson, 1978	1000, 2000, and 4000 Hz	20 dB	Fail to respond to any one signal in any ear
Downs et al, 1965	1000, 2000, 4000, and 6000 or 8000 Hz	15 dB	Fail to respond to either 1000 or 2000 Hz or to both 4000 and 6000 to 8000 Hz in either ear
National Conference on Identification Audiometry	1000, 2000, 4000 and, 6000 Hz	20 dB at 1000, 2000, and 6000 Hz 30 dB at 4000 Hz	Fail to hear any signals at these levels in either ear
Northern & Downs, 1991	1000, 2000, 3000, and/ or 4000 and 6000 Hz	25 dB	Fail to respond to one tone at 1000 or 2000 Hz; or Fail to respond to two of three tones at 3000, 4000, and 6000 Hz
State of Illinois Department of Public Health	500, 1000, 2000, and 4000 Hz	25 or 35 dB	Fail to respond to one tone at 35 dB in either or respond to any two tones at 25 dB in the same ear

ASHA, American Speech-Language-Hearing Association.

an abnormal auditory system is to perform immittance screening in conjunction with hearing screening. Often minimal hearing loss is typically associated with conductive pathology that is associated with abnormal middle ear functions and associated middle ear disease. However, as pointed out following here, routine screening of middle ear disorders is not a standard practice in school hearing conservation programs for a number of reasons.

The availability of OAEs for audiological testing has raised the question of their effectiveness as a single alternative for identification of hearing loss in school children. Several studies have been conducted on this topic using both TEOAEs and DPOAEs (see Chapter 3) (Kruger & Ladonna, 2002; McPherson & Smith, 1997; Nozza & Sabo, 1992; Sabo, Winston, & Machias, 2000). Because the recording of an OAE is dependent on having normal middle ear function, one of the advantages of using emissions is that they might be sensitive to both hearing loss

and middle ear disorder. However, current data do not support using OAEs as an alternate for school hearing screening. It appears that current technology renders the OAE procedure less sensitive than the pure tone sweep check test (Sabo et al, 2000). Perhaps technological advances might improve to the level that OAEs are appropriate for school hearing screening. At present, for students capable of performing behavioral tasks, pure tone testing with middle ear measures is the preferred method of school hearing screening. OAEs can provide an additional option for children with developmental disabilities who are untestable with pure tone audiometry.

Periodicity of School-Based Testing

Few would argue that the ideal screening program would test every child every year from birth through high school graduation. However, screening all children annually is not practical most of the time, and many

Table 5–6. ASHA (2002) Guidelines for Audiological Screenings: Infants through 18 Years

Population	Procedure	Frequency	Intensity Pass/ Fail Criteria	Follow-up
Birth through 6 months	Automated ABR DPOAE TEOAE	Click 2000, 3000, 4000 Hz 2000, 3000, 4000 Hz	Min. 35 dB nHL 55/65 dB (F1/F2) 80 dB	Immediate rescreen, then 1 to 3 months after initial screen
Infants and toddlers (7 months to 2 years)	VRA CPA	1000, 2000, 4000 Hz 1000, 2000, 4000 Hz (use inserts receivers only if possible)	30 dB HL 20 dB HL	Rescreen 1 to 3 months after initial screen
Preschool children 3 to 5 years)	CPA	1000, 2000, 4000 Hz (use inserts receivers only if possible)	20 dB HL	Rescreen 1 to 3 months after initial screen
School-age children 5 to 18 years)	CPA Conventional	1000, 2000, 4000 Hz	20 dB HL	Rescreen 1 to 3 months after initial screen

ABR, auditory brainstem response; CPA, conditioned play audiometry; DPOAE, distortion product otoacoustic emissions; TEOAE, transient evoked otoacoustic emissions; VRA, visual reinforcement audiometry.

compromises have been suggested. Virtually all published guidelines support two general principles with regard to periodicity of testing (Bess, 1980; Grifing, Simonton, & Hedgecock, 1967).

1. There is a greater need for screening younger children.
2. There are populations of children with a higher incidence of hearing loss and ear disorders who warrant testing outside of the routine schedule.

Rationales for the focus of screenings on younger children are based on two observations. First, during the early years there is a higher prevalence of transient hearing loss due to middle ear disease; second, mild and frequency-specific hearing losses are often undetected. Based on these principles, annual screening of all infants, preschool children, and children in grades K through 3 is highly recommended.

Controversy exists on the cost–benefit ratio of screening after grade 3. After analyzing the data from 14,800 tenth graders, Downs, Doster, and Weaver (1965) concluded that audiometric screening programs should be relaxed in the upper grades. This conclusion is based on the low yield of previously undetected hearing impairment in the upper grades.

Although there is a general reduction in the incidence of hearing loss in the upper grades, studies have shown that the incidence of high frequency loss significantly increases in the 4000 to 6000 Hz region beyond grade 8, especially in males. Weber et al (1967) reviewed the audiometric configurations from 1000 students failing the screening procedures performed by the Colorado Department of Health. Thirty percent of the losses identified were in the 4000 Hz region, with 24.9% in males and 5.1% in females. As age increased to 16 years or older, there was a significant increase in the losses at 4000 Hz. Hull et al (1971) report data from 38,568 children in grades 1 through 12. In comparing all grade levels across frequencies, the highest incidence of hearing loss exceeding 25 dB HL (ANSI, 1996) was at 4000 Hz in the male population in grades 11 and 12.

Woodford and O'Farrell (1983) documented the high noise levels in school band rooms and vocational education areas, and found that students involved in high-sound-level activities are more likely to have high-frequency hearing loss. In addition, they, unfortunately, found that few industrial arts programs furnish hearing protection or are aware of the need for such protection. A survey by Allonen-Allie and Florentine (1990) found similar results in 27 schools, but also revealed that teachers desired training in hearing conservation.

Because hearing loss is more prevalent in males who engage in noisy activities, implementing a hearing conservation program for the students exposed to high noise levels in the schools (e.g., industrial arts programs) is important because these students most likely are those who will be exposed to high noise levels in later life. In addition to identifying existing hearing loss, through education these students will become aware of the effects of noise on their hearing, which may prevent occupational hearing loss from noise exposure in later years (Roeser, 1980).

With respect to special populations and high-risk children, the following guidelines should be applied. Annual hearing conservation should be performed on students who:

1. Are new to the school or to the school district
2. Repeat a grade
3. Have delayed or impaired speech and language before they are enrolled in therapy
4. Are returning to school after a serious illness
5. Appear to be delayed
6. Are having emotional or behavior problems
7. Were absent during a previously scheduled screening examination
8. Are involved in course work that places them at risk for noise exposure (band, woodworking, and auto mechanics)

Regardless of grade level, annual testing should also be performed on pupils discovered by previous tests to have hearing impairment and on pupils enrolled in adjustment or remedial classes.

Pitfalls to Avoid in Hearing Screening

The following factors are often found in hearing screening programs and can have a detrimental effect on the results of the screening; steps must be taken to avoid them.

1. Child observing the equipment. This should be avoided at all times because children will respond to the visual cues. The child should be seated at an oblique angle so the tester and audiometer are out of the child's peripheral vision, or a blockade should be placed between the examiner and the child.
2. Examiner giving visual cues (such as facial expression, eye or head movements)
3. Incorrect adjustment of the headband and earphone placement. Care must be taken to place the earphones carefully over the ears so that the protective screen mesh of the earphone diaphragm is directly over the entrance of the external auditory canal. Misplacement of the earphone by only 1 inch can cause a threshold shift as great as 30 to 35 dB.
4. Vague instructions about the child's listening task or mode of response
5. Noise in the test area. False-positive identifications will result from excessive noise in the test environment. If there is a question about the noise levels present, the examiner should perform tests on individuals with known normal hearing (the examiner's hearing, if it is normal). If they do not pass the test, the noise levels are too high.
6. Prolonged or extended test sessions. The screening should require only 3 to 5 minutes. If a child requires significantly more time than this, the routine screening should be discontinued and a short rest taken. If the child continues to be difficult to test, play conditioning should be used.
7. Test tone presentation too long or too short. The test stimulus should be presented for 1 to 2 seconds. If the stimulus is presented for a shorter or longer time than this, inaccurate responses may be obtained.

Case Management

In many traditional hearing conservation programs, all children who do not pass the screening are immediately referred for audiological, medical, and educational follow-up. Such referrals are important to identify significant auditory and medical problems. Screening tests must be considered only as a preliminary indication of the presence of hearing loss. Before the exact nature and extent of the loss can be determined, comprehensive audiological testing must be undertaken under acceptable testing conditions to confirm the existence of hearing loss.

The Medical Home and the Audiology Home

It would be ideal if all children were referred to a clinic with both medical and audiological facilities. In such facilities, the physician and audiologist can work together to assess the nature and extent of the problem and provide appropriate treatment and follow-up. This setting would be the "Medical Home." The American Academy of Pediatrics (1992) proposed the concept of Medical Home that would identify and access services needed for children's health, identify the etiology of hearing loss, provide habilitative care for children identified with hearing loss, recommend medical treatment, and refer to other sources. In a Medical Home the pediatrician or other primary care provider (PCP) acts in partnership with the parents. Traditional medical ethics require that children failing screening be referred to the family physician, who is typically a general practitioner or pediatrician. The general medical practitioner plays a very important role in the overall management of the family's medical needs but often does not have the expertise required for the diagnosis and management of otologic problems. For this reason, those children failing the screening program will be best served if they are referred directly to an ear specialist (otologist). Feedback from the physician should be requested and records kept on all medical referrals. Anderson (1978) and Barrett (1985) provide examples of forms that can be used for follow-up purposes. With the advent of health maintenance organizations (HMO) and preferred care providers into the health care delivery system, decisions regarding referral sources for those failing the screening are becoming predetermined administrative decisions.

An audiology home will provide case management of infants and children with hearing loss based on the principle of a one-stop, family-oriented resource that provides clinical services related to audiological assessment and intervention strategies (Jerger, Roeser, & Tobey, 2001). As a multifaceted service center the audiology home team includes professionals with expertise in audiology, communication development, counseling, education, and technology. These professionals are dedicated to facilitating the needs of families with hearing-impaired children.

Upon arriving at the audiology home, many parents may have preconceived ideas and outdated information regarding communication options and current technologies available. As the expert in hearing loss the audiologist becomes the resource facilitator to help the family make good, informed decisions for a child's habilitation. Regular interactions and updates implemented by the audiology home team with the medical caregiver and educational personnel as the child ages will ensure that intervention strategies are optimized. Five principles suggested to ensure the implementation of any screening program include (1) identification and specifications of degree, type, configuration, and asymmetry of hearing loss; (2) family and parental counseling that provides information regarding hearing loss with modes of communication and educational strategies available; (3) introduction of the available sensory aid technology; (4) promotion of optimal social–emotional, auditory, and cognitive development; and (5) ongoing multidimensional documentation of all aspects of communication development (Jerger et al, 2001).

Early Childhood Intervention Services and Educational Follow-Up

In many cases, the hearing loss will be transient and the extent and duration of the impairment will depend on the nature of the abnormal condition. However, even for these children, special provisions will need to be made in the home or classroom. Early childhood intervention (ECI) services and schools must be notified when hearing loss is found so that special provisions can be made to accommodate the child's needs in the home or school. ECI professionals are trained in a variety of academic disciplines, such as speech-language pathology, education of hard of hearing and deaf children, or early childhood special education.

Frequently cited principles of effective intervention include age at which services began, duration of services provided, contact hours and intensity of intervention at home or in school, center-based and home-based learning experiences, spectrum of services provided (i.e., breadth and flexibility), recognition and adaptation to individual differences, family involvement and other support mechanisms (JCIH, 2000; Meadow-Orleans, Mertens, Sass-Lehrer, & Scott-Olson, 1997). An education professional is able to monitor the timeliness of services and provide information regarding program options, funding sources, communication options, and emotional support.

Screening for Middle Ear Disorders

Prior to 1970, there were no practical tools for routine screening of middle ear disorders, especially in school children. The only valid procedure was to examine the ear with an otoscope, and this procedure requires a trained observer and is not sensitive to many types of middle ear disease. However, with the emergence of immittance measures of the ear (described in Chapter 3), a feasible method of identifying middle ear disorders in school children is available. From a theoretical point of view, few audiologists and other health professionals would argue that immittance is a valuable part of school hearing conservation and belongs in every program. Such a statement is based on the validity and reliability of immittance tests and the relative ease with which immittance measurements are performed.

Historical and current literature is replete with studies showing the advantages and disadvantages of screening for middle ear disorders in school children using immittance tests. Support for immittance screening is most notable with unanimous documentation that pure tone screening tests alone are not sensitive to middle ear disorders. The advantage of immittance screening is an increase in overall accuracy of the screening program, a reduction in the number of children needing retests prior to referral, and an increased probability in identifying children with otologic problems. In addition to these factors, there is compelling evidence that significant delays in speech and language development and educational retardation may be related to chronic ear disease in children, especially during the early years.

National guidelines do not recommend universal mass screening with immittance on a routine basis for the detection of middle ear disorders (Bess, 1980). However, it should be emphasized that regular screening using immittance is not discouraged for special populations of children. Because of the effects of middle ear disease on speech and language development and the high incidence of middle ear disorders in special populations, immittance screening should be performed routinely on these children. Included are Native Americans and individuals with sensorineural hearing loss, developmental delay, mental impairment, and craniofacial anomalies, including cleft palate and Down syndrome (Bluestone, Fria, & Arjona, 1986).

Personnel involved in hearing screening programs may be those used in the immittance screening program, but with more extensive training. Technical personnel must be thoroughly familiar with the mechanics of the instrumentation used in the program, the proper use of the instrumentation, and problems that can be encountered with the instrument and how to troubleshoot such problems. They must also be familiar with interpretation of test results and thoroughly knowledgeable about disorders of the ear. Because the addition of immittance screening requires more technical expertise, there is a far greater need for a certified audiologist to be available to the program.

Screening for Auditory Processing Disorders

Only recently has the possibility of screening to identify children with auditory processing disorders (APD) been considered. Although there are currently no stardardized screening protocols for APD in children, Jerger and Musiek (2000), as part of the Callier Center Consensus Conference on Auditory Processing Disorders, recommended three possible procedures: questionnaire, psychometric testing, or a combination of the two. Ultimately, those initially failing an APD screening would be referred to an audiologist for diagnostic evaluation.

Screening questionnaires become a necessity for children under 5 years of age due to the lack of age-appropriate psychometric screening tests available for younger children. Elements of the screening via questionnaire should reflect identifiable observation of suspect behaviors. Some of those questionable behaviors would include difficulty hearing/understanding in the presence of reverberation or background noise, difficulty understanding degraded speech, difficulty following spoken instructions in the classroom, difficulty discriminating and identifying speech sounds, and inconsistent responses to auditory stimuli or inconsistent auditory attention (Jerger & Musiek, 2000).

Psychometric screening instruments should be chosen with minimal cognitive, attentional, and linguistic demands on the child. Ideally, the procedures are kept to no more than 15 minutes in length. Direct screening tests should contain an open set dichotic digit test and a gap detection test with short

silent gap in the presence of broadband noise (Jerger & Musiek, 2000). Both elements minimize the linguistic challenge placed upon the child.

Clearly, whether questionnaire, psychometric screening instruments, or both forms are chosen, specific pass/fail criteria are needed. The screening procedure will be age dependent and will be influenced by available resources (type of equipment and screening environment). It is critical to design an APD screening protocol that minimizes the influence of nonauditory factors (e.g., language or memory).

Summary

This chapter covers the topic of screening for auditory disorders in infants and school children. Technical advances made in the past decade have made it possible to screen effectively for hearing loss in infants, which has allowed for early identification and referral. School children can be effectively screened using the age-old pure tone sweep check test. Screening for middle ear disorders is not a standard practice but can be used for selected students. The more recent concept of screening for auditory disorders in school children has been introduced recently and awaits the development of a standardized screening test.

References

Allonen-Allie, N., & Florentine, M. (1990). Hearing conservation programs in Massachusetts' vocational/technical schools. *Ear Hear, 1,* 119–120.

American Academy of Pediatrics. (1992). Ad hoc task force on definition of the medical home team. *Pediatrics, 90,* 5 (RE9262).

American National Standards Institute (ANSI). (1996). Specification for audiometers (ANSI S3.6–1996). New York: American National Standards Institute.

American National Standards Institute (ANSI). (1999). Maximum permissible ambient noise for audiometric testing (ANSI S3.1–1999). New York: American National Standards Institute.

American Speech-Language-Hearing Association (ASHA). (1975). *Guidelines for Identification Audiometry.* ASHA Committee on Audiometric Evaluation. Rockville Pike, MD: ASHA.

American Speech-Language-Hearing Association (ASHA). (1985). Guidelines for identification audiometry. *ASHA, 27,* 49–52.

American Speech-Language-Hearing Association (ASHA). (1991). External auditory canal examination and cerumen management. *ASHA, 35*, 64–66.

American Speech-Language-Hearing Association (ASHA). (2002). *Guidelines for Audiology Service Provision in and for Schools*. Rockville Pike, MD: ASHA.

Anderson, C. (1978). Conservation of hearing. In: J. Katz (Ed.), *Handbook of Clinical Audiology* (2nd ed.) (pp. 48–60). Baltimore: Williams & Wilkins.

Arehart, K.H., Yoshinaga-Itano, C., Thomson, V., Gabbard, S.A., & Stredler Brown, A. (1998). State of the states: The status of universal newborn screening, assessment, and intervention systems in 16 states. *Am J Audiol, 7*, 101–114.

Barrett, K. (1985). Hearing and immittance screening of school-age children. In: J. Katz (Ed.), *Handbook of Clinical Audiology* (4th ed.) (pp. 621–641). Baltimore: Williams & Wilkins.

Berg, F. (1970). Definition and incidence. In: F. Berg, & S. Fletcher (Eds.), *The Hard of Hearing Child* (pp. 121–142). New York: Grune & Stratton.

Bess, F. (1980). Impedance screening for children: A need for more research. *Ann Otol Rhinol Laryngol, 89* (Suppl. 68), 228–232.

Bess, F., Dodd-Murphy, J., & Parker, R. (1998). Children with minimal sensorineural hearing loss: Prevalence, educational performance, and functional status. *Ear Hear, 19*, 339–354.

Blair, J., Peterson, M., & Viehweg, S. (1985). The effects of mild sensorineural hearing loss on academic performance of young school-age children. *Volta Review, 87*, 87–93.

Bluestone, D., Fria, T., & Arjona, S. (1986). Controversies in screening of middle ear disease and hearing loss in children. *Pediatrics, 77*, 57–70.

Brooks, D. (1980). Impedance in screening. In: J. Jerger, & J. Northern (Eds.), *Clinical Impedance Audiometry* (pp. 164-182). Acton, MA: American Electronics Corp.

Cone-Wesson, B., Parker, J., Swiderski, N., & Rickards, F. (2002). The auditory steady-state response: Full-term and premature neonates. *J Am Acad Audiol, 13*, 260–269.

Cooper, J., Gates, G., Owen, J., & Dickson, M. (1975). An abbreviated impedance bridge technique for school screening. *J Speech Hear Disord, 40*, 260–269.

Darley, F. (1961). Identification audiometry for school-age children: Basic procedures. *J Speech Hear Disord (Monogr)*, (Suppl. 9), 26–34.

Diefendorf, A.O., & Finitzo, T. (1997). The state of the information. *Am J Audiol, 6*, 91.

Dimitrijevic, A., John, M., & Van Roon, P. (2002). Estimating the audiogram using multiple auditory steady-state responses. *J Am Acad Audiol, 13*, 227–235.

Downs, M., Doster, M., & Weaver, M. (1965). Dilemmas in identification audiometry. *J Speech Hear Disord, 30*, 360–364.

Eagles, E., Wishik, S., & Doerfler, L. (1967). Hearing sensitivity and ear disease in children: A prospective study. *Laryngoscope (Monogr)*, (Suppl.), 1–274.

Fay, T., Hochberg, I., & Smith, C. (1972). Audiologic and otologic screening of disadvantaged children. In: A. Glorig, & K. Gerwin (Eds.), *Otitis Media* (pp. 141–156). Springfield, IL: Charles C Thomas.

Finitzo, T., Albright, K., & O'Neal, J. (1998). The newborn with hearing loss: Detection in the nursery. *Pediatrics, 102*, 1452–1460.

Frankenberg, W. (1971). Selection of diseases and tests in pediatric screening. *Pediatrics, 54*, 41–56.

Gorga, M., Neely, S., Bergman, B., Beauchaine, K., Kaminiski, J., Peters, J., & Jesteadt, K. (1993). Otoacoustic emissions from normal-hearing and hearing-impaired responses. *J Acoust Soc Am, 93*, 2050–2060.

Gravel, J., Berg, A., Bradley, M., Cacace, A., Campbell, D., Dalzell, L., DeCristofaro, J., Greenberg, E., Gross, S., Orlando, M., Pinheiro, J., Regain, J., Spivak, L., Stevens, F., & Prieve, B. (2000). The New York State universal newborn hearing screening protocol on inpatient outcome measures. *Ear Hear, 21*, 131–140.

Grifing, T., Simonton, K., & Hedgecock, L. (1967). Verbal auditory-screening for pre-school children. *Trans Am Acad Ophthalmol Otolaryngol, 71*, 104–111.

Hood, B., & Lamb, L. (1974). Identification audiometry. In: K. Gerwin, & A. Glorig, (Eds.), *Detection of Hearing Loss and Ear Disease in Children* (pp. 68–79). Springfield, IL: Charles C Thomas.

House, H., & Glorig, A. (1957). A new concept in auditory screening. *Laryngoscope, 67*, 661–668.

Hull, F., Mielke, P.J., & Timmons, R. (1971). The national speech and hearing survey: Preliminary results. *ASHA, 13*, 501–509.

Hunter, L., Margolis, R., Rykken, J., Le, C., Daly, K., & Giebink, G. (1996). High frequency hearing loss associated with otitis media. *Ear Hear, 17*, 1–11.

Jerger, J., & Musiek, F. (2000). Consensus Conference on APDs in children. *J Am Acad Audiol, 11*, 467–475.

Jerger, J., Roeser, R., & Tobey, E.A. (2001). Management of hearing loss in infants: The UTD/Callier Center position statement. *J Am Acad Audiol, 12*, 329–336.

Johnson, J., Mauk, G., & Takekawa, K. (1993). Implementing a statewide system of services for infants and toddlers with hearing disabilities. *Semin Hear, 14*, 105–119.

Joint Committee on Infant Hearing (JCIH). (2000). Year 2000 Position Statement: Principles and guidelines for early hearing detection and intervention programs. *Am J Audiol, 9*, 9–29.

Kaplan, G., Fleshman, J., Bender, T., Baum, R., & Clark, W. (1973). Long-term effects of otitis media: A ten-year cohort study of Alaskan Eskimo children. *Pediatrics, 52*, 577–585.

Kruger, W.O., & Ladonna, F. (2002). A comparison of screening methods in school-aged children. *Otolaryngol Head Neck Surg, 127*, 516–519.

Mason, J., & Hermann, K.R. (1998). Universal infant hearing screening by automated auditory brainstem response measurement. *Pediatrics, 101*, 221–228.

McEldowney, D., & Kessner, P. (1972). Review of the literature: Epidemiology of otitis media. In: A. Glorig, & K. Gerwin, (Eds.), *Otitis Media* (pp. 24–39). Springfield, IL: Charles C Thomas.

McPherson, B., & Smith, V. (1997). Hearing screening for school children with otitis media using otoacoustic emission measures. *Asia Pac J Speech Lang Hear, 2*, 69–82.

Meadow-Orleans, K.P., Mertens, D.M., Sass-Lehrer, M., & Scott-Olson, K. (1997). Support services for parents and their children who are deaf or hard of hearing. *Am Ann Deaf, 142*, 278–288.

Melnick, W., Eagles, E., & Levine, H. (1964). Evaluation of a recommended program of identification audiometry with school-age children. *J Speech Hear Disord, 29*, 3–13.

Montgomery, J., & Fujikawa, S. (1992). Hearing thresholds of students in second, eighth, and twelfth grades. *Lang Speech Hear Serv Sch, 23,* 61–62.

Musket, C., & Dowraczyk, R. (1980). Using an otoscope with preschoolers in acoustic immittance screening programs. *Lang Speech Hear Serv Sch, 11,* 109–111.

Musket, C., & Roeser, R. (1977). Using circumaural enclosures with children. *J Speech Hear Disord, 20,* 325–333.

National Campaign for Hearing Health. (2000). Infant screening background information: What newborn screening costs. Available online: www.infanthearinghealth.net/pages/factstats/index.html (accessed July 2002).

National Institute on Deafness and Other Communication Disorders. (1993). *National Institutes of Health Consensus Statement: Early Identification of Hearing Impairment in Infants and Young Children.* Bethesda, MD: NIDCD.

Newhart, H. (1938). A pure tone audiometer for school use. *Arch Otolaryngol, 28,* 777–779.

Newman, M. (1975). Hearing loss. In: M. Strom, (Ed.), *Differential Diagnosis in Pediatric Otolaryngology* (pp. 138–152). Boston: Little, Brown.

Northern, J. (1978). Impedance screening in special populations: State-of-the-art. In: E. Harford, F. Bess, & D. Bluestone (Eds.), *Impedance Screening for Middle Ear Disease in Children* (pp. 229–248). New York: Grune & Stratton.

Northern, J., & Downs, M. (1991). *Hearing in Children* (4th ed.). Baltimore: Williams & Wilkins.

Nozza, R.J., & Sabo, D.I. (1992). Transiently evoked OAE for screening school-age children. *The Hearing Journal, 45,* 29–31.

O' Neal, J., Finitzo, T., & Littman, T.A. (2000). Neonatal hearing screening follow-up and diagnosis. In: R. Roeser, M. Valente, & M. Hosford-Dunn (Eds.), *Audiology Diagnosis* (pp. 527–544). New York: Thieme.

O'Donnell, N.S., & Galinsky, E. (1998). Measuring progress and results in early childhood system development. New York: Families and Work Institute. Available online: www.familiesandwork.org (accessed November 2003).

Prieve, B., Gorga, M., Schmidt, A., Neely, S., Peters, J., Schulte, L., & Jesteadt, K. (1993). Analysis of transient evoked otoacoustic emissions in normal-hearing and hearing-impaired ears. *J Acoust Soc Am, 93,* 3308–3319.

Quigley, S., & Thomason, F. (1968). *Some Effects of Hearing Impairment upon School Performance.* Springfield: Illinois Office of Education.

Roeser, R. (1980). Industrial hearing conservation programs in the high schools. *Ear Hear, 1,* 119–120.

Roeser, R., & Glorig, A. (1975). Pure tone audiometry in noise with auraldomes. *Audiology, 14,* 144–151.

Roeser, R., & Musket, C. (1976). *Noise Attenuating Earphone Systems.* Series 15, Report 4. Minneapolis: Maico Aud Library.

Roeser, R., Seidel, J., & Glorig, A. (1975). Performance of earphone enclosures for threshold audiometry. *Sound & Vibration, 10,* 22–25.

Sabo, P.S., Winston, R., & Machias, H.D. (2000). Comparison of pure tone and transient otoacoustic emissions screening in a grade school population. *Am J Otol, 21,* 88–91.

Salamy, A., Eldredge, L., & Tooley, W. (1989). Neonatal status and hearing loss in high risk infants. *J Pediatr, 114,* 847–852.

Siegenthaler, B., & Sommer, R. (1959). Abbreviated sweep check procedures for school hearing testing. *J Speech Hear Disord, 24,* 249–257.

Stark, E., & Borton, T. (1975). Noise excluding earphone enclosures for audiometry. *Audiology, 14,* 232–237.

Stevens, D., & Davidson, G. (1959). Screening tests of hearing. *J Speech Hear Disord, 24,* 258–261.

U.S. Department of Health and Human Services. (1990). *Healthy people 2000.* Paper presented at the National Promotion and Disease Prevention Objectives for the Nation, Washington, DC.

U.S. Department of Health and Human Services. (2000, January). *Healthy people 2010.* Conference Edition. Washington, DC.

Ventry, I., & Newby, H. (1959). Validity of the one-frequency screening principle for public school children. *J Speech Hear Disord, 2,* 147–151.

Vohr, B.R., Carty, L., Moore, P., & Letourneau, K. (1998). The Rhode Island Hearing Assessment Program: Experience with statewide hearing screening (1993–1996). *J Pediatr, 133,* 353–357.

Weber, H., McGovern, F., & Fink, D. (1967). An evaluation of 1000 children with hearing loss. *J Speech Hear Disord, 32,* 343–354.

Weit, P. (1979). Patterns of ear disease in the Southwestern American Indian. *Arch Otolaryngol, 105,* 381–385.

Wilson, W., & Walton, W. (1974). Identification audiometry accuracy: Evaluation of a recommended program for school-age children. *Lang Speech Hear Serv Sch, 5,* 132–142.

Woodford, C., & O'Farrell, M. (1983). High-frequency loss of hearing in secondary school students: An investigation of possible etiological factors. *Lang Speech Hear Serv Sch, 14,* 22–28.

Yoshinaga-Itano, C., Sedey, A., Coulter, D.K., & Mehl, A.L. (1998). Language of early and later identified children with hearing loss. *Pediatrics, 102,* 1161–1171.

6

Auditory Processing Disorders

ROBERT W. KEITH

My own primary interest is in assessing communication efficiency rather than concentrating on applications to medical diagnosis.

—Raymond Carhart, 1970

Definition of Auditory Processing Disorders

This chapter discusses approaches to the assessment of auditory processing and the identification of children with auditory processing disorders (APDs). The term "auditory processing disorders" has evolved over the years and has been variously described as a central auditory processing disorder (CAPD), auditory perceptual disorder, auditory language-learning disorder, and auditory processing disorder. The term "APD," which will probably be universally adopted (and will be used in this chapter), was adopted by the University of Texas at Dallas (UTD)/Callier Center Consensus Conference on the diagnosis of auditory processing disorders in school-aged children (Jerger & Musiek, 2000). In spite of lingering controversy about the treatment of children with this problem, there is little doubt about the reality of auditory processing disorders in children.

An American Speech-Language-Hearing Association (ASHA, 1996) ad hoc committee defined CAPDs as deficits in information processing of audible signals not attributed to impaired hearing sensitivity or intellectual impairment. Specifically, the committee stated that "APD" refers to limitations in the ongoing transmission, analysis, organization, transformation, elaboration, storage, retrieval, and use of information contained in audible signals. More simply stated, the auditory system is responsible for:

- Sound localization and lateralization
- Auditory discrimination
- Auditory pattern recognition
- Temporal aspects of audition including resolution, masking, and ordering
- Performance with competing signals
- Performance with degraded signals

Subsequently the UTD/Callier Center Consensus Conference on the diagnosis of APD in school-aged children suggested, "An APD may be broadly defined as a deficit in the processing of information that is specific to the auditory modality" (Jerger & Musiek, 2000). The panel concluded that the problem may be exacerbated in unfavorable acoustic environments. It may be associated with difficulties in listening, speech understanding, language development, and learning. "In its pure form, however, it is conceptualized as a deficit in the processing of auditory input." What is suggested in both of these definitions is the construct that APD contributes to developmental language disorders and interferes with academic achievement in the classroom.

Table 6–1. Auditory Processing Skills Important to the Learning Process

Discrimination	To differentiate sounds of different frequency, duration, or intens
Localization	To localize the source of sound
Auditory attention	To direct attention to relevant acoustic signals and sustain that attention for an appropriate amount of time
Auditory figure ground separation	To identify a primary speaker from a background of noise
Auditory discrimination	To discriminate among phonemic elements of speech that are acoustically similar
Auditory closure	To understand the whole word or message when part is missing
Auditory synthesis	To merge or blend isolated phonemes into words
Auditory analysis	To identify phonemes or morphemes embedded in words
Auditory association	To attach meaning to words
Auditory memory	To store and recall stimuli in the appropriate order or sequence

In an effort to be systematic, various authors have attempted to identify and define those auditory processing skills that may be important to a child's learning through hearing. Some abilities commonly listed by authors are shown in Table 6–1, although other auditory processing abilities can be identified. A direct cause-and-effect relationship between the abilities listed in Table 6–1 and achievement in language acquisition, reading, or academics has not been established. Many children who fail to achieve in these areas have auditory processing problems, but some children who achieve normally also have poor auditory processing skills, and some poor readers and students with low achievement have normal auditory processing abilities.

As with learning disabilities that are multidimensional, APD can exist in combination with or as a result of other disorders. For example, auditory perceptual problems may stem from neurological problems or brain injury resulting from head trauma, meningitis or other viral infections, seizure disorders, congenital anomalies such as agenesis of the corpus callosum, or other factors. Maternal drug and alcohol abuse may also result in APD in offspring. Additionally, there are undoubtedly genetic factors involved because many family members have similar educational histories of auditory learning problems. Some children with attention deficit hyperactive disorders (ADHD) have comorbidity with APD, and a diagnostic assessment is sometimes necessary to identify the primary problem.

Prevalence of Auditory Language-Learning Deficits

The prevalence of learning disabilities in the school-age population between 6 and 17 years is estimated to be 4 to 5% (Macmillan, 1993; Roush, 1995), although that percetage increases if children with ADHD are included. Many of these children have APD. For example Chermak and Musiek (1997) estimate that the prevalence of APD is 2 to 3% of children, with a 2:1 ratio between boys and girls. One difficulty in establishing the prevalence of children with APD is that the definition of the condition is problematic. Thus estimates of prevalence will vary, depending on definitions used in different localities and from author to author. Another problem with prevalence studies is that mild cases of auditory processing disorders are inconspicuous or easily compensated for when educational demands are at a minimum. With increased pressure for academic achievement, however, mild disorders can become educationally significant. In truth, until consensus is reached on a definition of APD, prevalence estimates are just that, informed guesses.

Behaviors of Children with Auditory Processing Disorders

When asked what behaviors were typical of children with APD, a teacher described tham as seeming to be "in a fog" and saying "Huh?" frequently. The teacher explained that such children often do not do their schoolwork, do not follow directions, and do not respond to auditory stimuli. She remarked, "When I talk to children with that kind of problem, they just look at me."

The following observations appear to be characteristic of children with auditory processing problems:

1. Most are male.
2. They have normal pure tone hearing thresholds.
3. They generally respond inconsistently to auditory stimuli. They often respond appropriately, but at other times they seem unable to follow auditory instructions.
4. They have a short attention span and fatigue easily when confronted with long or complex auditory learning activities.
5. They are distracted by auditory stimuli. Brutten, Richardson, and Mangel (1973) describe these children as being at the mercy of their environment. They are unable to block out irrelevant stimuli and must respond immediately and totally to everything they see, feel, or hear, no matter how trivial.
6. They may have difficulty with auditory localization skills. This may include an inability to tell how close or far away the source of the sound is and an inability to differentiate soft and loud sounds. There have been frequent reports that these children become frightened and upset when they are exposed to loud noise, and often hold their hands over their ears to stop the sound.
7. They may listen attentively but have difficulty following long or complicated verbal commands or instructions.
8. They frequently request that information be repeated.
9. They are often unable to remember information presented verbally for both short-term and long-term memory. They may have difficulty counting, reciting the alphabet, or remembering the days of the week and months of the year or addresses and telephone numbers.
10. They may be slow to respond to auditory information, as if it takes longer to think through and process what was heard.

Cohen (1980) points out that, in addition, many of these children have significant reading problems, are poor spellers, and have poor handwriting. They may have articulation or language disorders. In the classroom they may act out frustrations that result from their perceptual deficits, or they may be shy and withdrawn because of the poor self-concept that results from multiple failures. These examples are only a few of the behaviors that are associated with APD. Not every child with an auditory processing problem will exhibit all of the behaviors mentioned. The number of problems experienced by a given child will be an expression of the severity of the auditory learning disability.

The reader will recognize that the behaviors just listed are not unique to children with APD. They are common to children with peripheral hearing loss, attention deficit disorders, allergies, and other problems. It should not concern professionals to find similar behaviors among children with various language-learning disorders. Children may have very different underlying causes for similar behaviors, but they do not represent a homogeneous group. It is the clinician's task to determine the underlying deficit or deficits among children with similar behaviors and to recommend the appropriate remediation approach for each child.

Identification and Assessment of Auditory Processing Disorders

Peripheral Hearing Loss

Before any attempt is made to diagnose a child as having APD, it is necessary to rule out the presence of peripheral hearing loss of a conductive or sensorineural type. A conductive hearing loss results from damage or disorders to the sound-conducting mechanism, including the external earcanal, eardrum, middle ear space, or bones of the middle ear. Examples of a conductive loss include foreign body or wax (cerumen) occluding the earcanal, a perforated eardrum, or fluid in the middle ear from a cold or allergy. A hearing loss in the cochlea (inner ear) is called a sensorineural hearing loss (SNHL). SNHL is caused by genetic factors, viral and bacterial infections, head trauma, and other acquired, syndromatic, or congenital factors. When an SNHL is severe, it is relatively easy to identify because the child will not respond to sound, and speech-language will be delayed. When an SNHL is mild the diagnosis may be more difficult. See Chapters 3 and 4 for an expanded discussion of hearing loss in children.

Peripheral hearing losses, whether mild and flat or sloping high frequency, are likely to result in inconsistent auditory responses, poor auditory attention, and other behaviors that indicate difficulty in learning through the auditory channel. Therefore, any child who exhibits these behaviors, or any child with speech or language delays, must be tested to rule out a peripheral hearing loss. It is vitally important to recognize that pure tone hearing screening tests done in the schools are not sensitive to the presence of fluid in the middle ear or limited damage to the cochlea, and fail to identify mild conductive hearing loss or SNHL. Tympanometry gives additional information about middle ear function and is a necessary component of school hearing screening programs. Oto-acoustic emissions are also a valuable addition to the screening protocol. See Chapter 5 for an in-depth discussion of screening for hearing loss and middle ear disorders.

It is also important to keep in mind that a single hearing test performed on a child may not be adequate. Fluctuating hearing loss associated with allergies or colds, or the possibility that an SNHL is progressive, makes it unwise to plan a child's long-term educational experience on the basis of a single hearing test.

A final word about conductive hearing loss; until recently, little information was available on the long-term effects of early and prolonged otitis media with static or fluctuating hearing loss on auditory processing abilities. There is evidence that otitis media can cause auditory learning problems and is not the innocuous disease that it was once considered to be (Menyuk, 1992). The residual effects can be auditory processing problems that may cause language and learning delays long after the middle ear disease has been resolved. Therefore, children with histories of frequent colds or chronic middle ear disease should be carefully watched for signs of auditory language-learning problems.

For peripheral assessment a minimal test battery should include pure tone thresholds at octave frequencies between 250 and 8000 Hz, tympanometry and otoacoustic emissions (OAEs). In order to be valid pure tone testing needs to be conducted in a quiet room that meets standards for allowable background noise. Screening for hearing loss at 25 dB HL or testing outside of a controlled area raises the specter of false-negative findings; that is, failure to identify a mild but educationally significant hearing loss.

Assessment Procedures

When a peripheral hearing loss has been ruled out in a child and when behaviors indicate the possibility that an APD is present, a thorough evaluation of auditory processing abilities should be performed. According to the ASHA Consensus Conference, the diagnosis of APD is accomplished using a variety of indicators:

- Case History
- Systematic observations of auditory behavior
- Audiological tests
  Temporal processing—ordering, discrimination, resolution (e.g., gap detection), and integration
  Localization and lateralization
  Low-redundancy monaural speech (time compressed, filtered, interrupted, competing, etc.)
  Dichotic stimuli including nonsense syllables, digits, words, and sentences
  Binaural interaction (e.g., masking level difference [MLD])
  Electrophysiological procedures may also be useful
- Speech-language pathology measures

Case History

When possible, an in-depth history from the child's caregiver should be taken. Rosenberg (1978) called the case history "the first test" because of the value of the information obtained. This reference, although old, is as true today as when it was first written. Rosenberg pointed out that a carefully taken history can be extremely useful in differentiating among various problems, supplements results from auditory tests, and helps in making decisions about the child's educational management.

The case history should be taken systematically to avoid missing important information. When taking the history an opportunity should be provided for the caregiver to state any concerns about the child, describe the child's behaviors, and express any other related concerns. Specific information that should be requested includes information about (1) the family; (2) the mother's pregnancy; (3) conditions at birth and the child's growth and development, health, and illnesses; (4) general behavior and social–emotional development; (5) speech and language development; (6) hearing and auditory

behavior; (7) nonauditory behavior; and (8) educational progress. The specific questions asked of parents will depend on the setting in which the testing is being done and the purpose of the examination. Areas to be investigated in the history when an APD is suspected are given in Table 6–2.

Checklists of Auditory Processing Disorders

Several checklists exist to assist school personnel in identifying children who may benefit from assessment of auditory processing abilities. The Fisher's Auditory Problems Checklist (Fisher, 1976) is a 25-item checklist of a broad base of listening and attention problems. Benson (1995) classified each item on Fisher's checklist but our center has found the results to have poor specificity. We find that the checklist has poor norms and has never been subjected to validation studies.

One useful tool that can be used to systematically collect and quantify the observed listening behaviors of children's auditory behavior is the Children's Auditory Performance Scale (CHAPS) (Smoski, Brunt, & Tannahill, 1992). CHAPS is a scaled questionnaire consisting of 25 items used to rate listening behavior in a variety of conditions. Responses from parents and teachers can be quantified and the child's listening behaviors profiled. According to the authors, the clinical applications of this scale include identifying children who should be referred for an evaluation of auditory processing abilities and to prescribe and measure the effects of intervention.

Two other questionnaires include the Evaluation of Classroom Listening Behaviors (ECLB) (VanDyke, 1985) and the Screening Instrument for Targeting Educational Risk (S.I.F.T.E.R.) (Anderson, 1989). The ECLB is useful in educational settings as a pre- and postobservation instruction instrument for students using personal and classroom assistive listening devices in order to determine if there is an improvement in listening skills. Similarly, the S.I.F.T.E.R. utilizes 15 questions to compare the student's functional ability performance to the stu-

Table 6–2. Information Model for Taking a Case History

Area	Information Needed
Family history	History of any family member's difficulty in school achievement The primary language spoken in the home
Pregnancy and birth	Unusual problems during pregnancy or delivery Abnormalities present at the child's birth
Health and illness	Childhood illnesses, neurological problems, psychological disorders, head trauma or injury, middle ear disease, allergies Drugs or medications prescribed by a physician
General behavior and social–emotional development	Age-appropriate play behavior Social isolation or withdrawal Impulsiveness Aggression, tact, and sensitivity to others Self-discipline
Speech and language development	Evidence of articulation, voice, or fluency problems Ability to communicate ideas verbally Ability to formulate sentences correctly Appropriateness of verbal expression to subject or situation
Hearing and auditory behavior	Ability to identify the source of sound and listen selectively in the presence of noise Reaction to sudden, unexpected sound Ability to ignore environmental sounds Consistency of response to sound Need to have spoken information repeated Ability to follow verbal instructions Ability to listen for appropriate length of time Ability to remember things heard Ability to pay attention to what is said Ability to comprehend words and their meaning, to understand multiple meanings of words, and to understand abstract ideas Discrepancies between auditory and visual behavior

dent's peers, and to track a child's performance over time. It has also been used to evaluate a child's performance before and after introducing a classroom amplification system.

Assessment of Auditory Processing Abilities

The assessment should begin with careful observation of the child, with particular attention to the auditory behavior patterns described previously in this chapter. Care should be taken to identify strengths as well as weaknesses and to note performance in other modalities, including vision, motor coordination, tactile response, speech, and language. According to UTD/Callier Center Consensus Conference panel (Jerger & Mu-

siek, 2000) auditory processing and methods of assessing auditory processing can be influenced by other disorders that can impact auditory function, including:

- ADHD
- Language impairment
- Reading disability
- Learning disability
- Autistic spectrum disorder
- Reduced intellectual functioning

There are at least two different approaches to the assessment of auditory processing abilities. Each depends on the examiners' understanding of APD and their viewpoint based on professional training. The speech-language pathologist's (SLP) approach is from the cognitive perspective, which stresses information processing strategies. This approach is a top-down model of auditory processing. The SLP approach is very different from the audiologist's assessment approach, which is targeted at understanding deficiencies that are *specific* to the auditory system. To accomplish this task, the audiologist's assessment battery attempts to evaluate the individual's ability to process auditory signals along the entire auditory pathway from the cochlea to the auditory cortex and association areas; this represents a bottom-up approach.

The Speech-Language Evaluation

The ASHA (1996) consensus panel recommended "nonstandardized but systematic observation of auditory behavior." Lasky and Cox (1983) describe a systematic approach to observation of the child's auditory behavior in their assessment and remediation model. They recommend observational evaluation of the child under different conditions of signal and its *presentation*, and *environment*, while evaluating the child's *responses*, and *strategies* (SPERS). The SPERS evaluation utilizes increasingly difficult signals, presentation, listening environments, and response requirements to analyze the strategies a child employs in listening and processing auditory information. Levels of difficulty that disrupt or enhance performance are noted and incorporated into remediation plans.

Some of the auditory abilities that are assessed during formal testing include auditory attention, discrimination, closure, analysis, blending, and memory, as well as language assessment.

Auditory Attention

The ability to sustain attention over time can be assessed by observing children in comparison with their peers. A child should have the ability to direct attention toward a relevant acoustic signal, whether speech or music, and to sustain that attention for an appropriate length of time. When a child is not tuned in to listen, the child cannot learn auditorily. Observation of a child's behavior

in various listening situations may be supplemented by tests of auditory vigilance when describing a child's auditory attention. For example, the Auditory Continuous Performance Test (ACPT) (Keith, 1994a) contains a list of 100 monosyllabic words presented at the rate of 1/s. Within each word list are embedded 20 random presentations of a target word, "dog." The list is repeated six times without interruption, resulting in a test of approximately 10 minutes. Measurement of performance decrements in identifying the target word over the duration of the test is a way of objectively determining a child's auditory vigilance.

Auditory Discrimination

Auditory discrimination is the skill necessary to discriminate among words and sounds that are acoustically similar. Auditory discrimination can be assessed at many levels. For example, repeating a monosyllabic word correctly, the child has demonstrated an ability to discriminate speech sounds at the imitative level. When syllables or word pairs are presented orally and the child is asked to report whether they were exactly the same or different another level of processing is introduced. In that case, the child must understand the concept of the same and different, and a cognitive aspect to auditory discrimination is introduced. When children can repeat words correctly but cannot tell whether the sounds are the same or different, the problem is cognitive and not auditory discrimination because the decision-making process is a higher order.

Some tests of auditory discrimination require the child to point to a picture in response to stimulus words. The conceptual difficulty with any picture-pointing test is that it is cross-modality, requiring visual recognition of all of the pictures and an auditory–visual association between word and picture. In today's parlance it would be said that these tests are not "auditory specific." Because these tests rely on visual perception and auditory–visual integration it is difficult to attribute any breakdown to auditory discrimination in the narrow sense. Nevertheless, because they are common behaviors asked of a child, an inability to respond appropriately to a picture-pointing task indicates a possible delay in the child's development.

The Lindamood Auditory Conceptualization Test is another level of auditory discrimination (Lindamood & Lindamood, 1971). In this test, the child is asked to associate sounds with colored blocks and manipulate them to demonstrate their ability to discriminate one speech sound from another; and their ability to perceive the number, order, and sameness or difference of speech sounds in different sequences. This highly cognitive task is on the opposite end of the continuum of auditory discrimination abilities that range from imitation to cognition. In the assessment of auditory discrimination abilities, the examiner should determine the level at which the child's auditory discrimination abilities break down.

Auditory Closure

Auditory closure is the ability to understand the whole word or message when the part is missing or missed. In noisy environments this skill is used to comprehend messages when parts of words are unintelligible because they are masked. As a linguistically based cognitive ability, auditory closure can be assessed using tasks that require the child to fill in missing parts of a word. A different approach to testing auditory closure is to eliminate certain frequency components of spoken words by electronic low-pass filtering. Eliminating the high frequencies of speech results in a signal that sounds muffled. Research has shown that low-pass filtered speech effectively separates children with learning problems from those who are normally achieving (Keith & Farrer, 1981). Filtered words testing is one subtest of the SCAN-C auditory test battery (Keith, 2000b).

Auditory Analysis

The ability to identify phonemes, syllables, or morphemes embedded in words requires both auditory and linguistic processing abilities. Some diagnostic reading tests contain subtests of auditory analysis abilities. The Auditory Analysis Test (Rosner & Simon, 1971) requires the child to form a new word when a phoneme or syllable is removed from a larger word. For example, the examiner will ask the child to say "gate" and then repeat it again without "g" as "ate." Similarly, in the initial and final positions, "trail" without "t" is "rail" and "please" without "z" is "plea." The inability to perform this task may indicate that the child is unable to isolate individual sounds within words, which has implications for reading and spelling.

Auditory Blending

Sometimes called auditory synthesis or phonemic synthesis, auditory blending is the ability to merge isolated phonemes into words. This auditory ability is considered by many to be a fundamental requisite to learning to read by a phonic method. The child must combine those sounds to tell what the word is. Examples of stimuli are: f-oot (foot), t-oa-st (toast), and k-e-tch-u-p (ketchup). Katz has supported phonemic synthesis training for years (Katz & Harmon, 1981; Katz, Stecker, & Henderson, 1992) and recently introduced a Phonemic Synthesis Test for use with younger children with norms between ages 4 and 7 years.

Auditory Memory

As is the case with auditory discrimination, memory exists at many levels, including perceptual or echoic memory, short-term memory, long-term memory, and episodic memory. Many parents do not recognize these several levels, and it is difficult for them to reconcile the fact that a child can remember an incident from the distant past but cannot remember a spelling lesson between the previous evening's practice and the next day's test. Therefore, innumerable tests have been designed to assess verbal working memory using all kinds of speech stimuli, including phonemes, sentences, paragraphs, and short stories. Two aspects of memory that are typically assessed are memory span and sequential memory (e.g., as administered in the Test of Auditory-Perceptual Skills–Revised) (Gardner, 1996). Ac-cording to Chelfont-Evans (Chelfonte Evans, 2001) a number of investigators suggest that deficits in verbal working memory are pre-dicted to have widespread negative effects on language learning, including the produc-tion of utterances with increased length and/or syntactic complexity. Because of this relationship between verbal working mem-ory and linguistic performance (i.e., recep-tive and expressive language) it is important to assess verbal working memory.

Language Assessment

In the continuum from auditory awareness to use of language the evaluation of recep-tive and expressive language resides at the top of the hierarchy. There is a break in the continuum between auditory processing skills and language, described years ago by Katherine Butler as "half way up the down staircase." In a model proposed by English (English, 2001), although a gray area exists between auditory processing and receptive language, "when two or more words are combined, the listener uses receptive lan-guage skills, which must be assessed with instruments designed for that purpose." An example of such an instrument is the Clini-cal Evaluation of Language Fundamentals-Third Edition (CELF®-3) Screening Test (Semel, Wiig, & Secord, 1995). The CELF-3 Screening Test is a measure designed to screen students for language disorders, whereas the CELF-3 is used to assist in the diagnosis of the language disorder and to identify areas of relative strength and weak-ness. For example, the receptive language subtests (depending on age of the subject) include word structure, formulated sen-tences, recalling sentences, and sentence as-sembly. In particular, those interested in au-ditory processing disorders are concerned about marked discrepancies between recep-tive and expressive language CELF-3 scores.

Comment

In the previous paragraphs, many different auditory skills have been discussed as if they each occurred in isolation. It may be possible to describe the components of audi-tory perception, but it is virtually impossible to actually test auditory abilities independ-ent of each other. A number of specialists have noted that each of these skills overlap and are inseparable. Nevertheless, attempts to describe auditory processing subskills in a child who is having problems with lan-guage and learning can be important for de-veloping an effective remediation program.

Uncertainty exists whether the specific au-ditory skills, as they have been defined, form the basis of learning language, or whether these skills are acquired as a result of having learned language. Some experts state that auditory perception is fundamen-tal to learning language and that auditory processing deficits cause disorders in areas of language, reading, and learning. These experts further state that auditory percep-tion can be readily broken down into spe-cific deficits that are amendable to training, that a hierarchy of auditory perceptual skills exists with processes moving from simple to complex, and that remediation should fol-low the same order. Others believe that poor performance on auditory skills may result from a language disorder because these chil-dren do not have sufficient linguistic, se-mantic, and cognitive skills to enable them to develop strategies for dealing with the au-ditory tasks.

These different positions are discussed here because the selection of remedial tech-niques will depend directly on which philos-ophy is adopted. If one holds that specific auditory deficits, such as auditory closure, auditory blending, and so forth, are respon-sible for the language deficit, then remedia-tion would proceed via training of those specific skills on a hierarchical basis. If, on the other hand, one takes the position that auditory processing problems result from a language disorder, then remediation would proceed on a language basis, in which the therapist would use intervention strategies such as those described in Chapter 16.

A further point is that many of the tests purported to measure specific auditory skills are actually measures of language.

That is, to perform on these tests, the child must have developed relatively sophisticated language skills, and the more advanced the child's language, the better the child will perform. To assess auditory abilities, therefore, it is critical to evaluate each test for prelinguistic and linguistic or precognitive and cognitive language content. A prelinguistic task is one in which a stimulus sound is simply imitated, without the need to understand, define, or associate a visual object with it. For example, to repeat the nonsense syllables "ba" and "da" is the simplest form of imitation and is a prelinguistic skill, but to know whether these two sounds are the same or different requires higher linguistic competence. Repetition of syllables or words heard in the presence of a background noise at a favorable signal-to-noise (S/N) ratio is a low-level cognitive imitative speech task. When the intensity of the noise is equal to or exceeds the intensity of the speech, direct masking occurs, and the task becomes a higher-level cognitive task of auditory closure. Repeating pairs of words that are minimally acoustically different is a simple imitative task, but once the child is asked to state whether the words sound the same or different and where the difference occurs, the task becomes one of language.

The purpose of this discussion is simply to raise the issue of differences between low linguistic auditory perceptual and cognitive-based tests of auditory processing. They are important concepts when considering whether a child's problem is one of auditory perception (auditory specific) or receptive language.

The Audiological Evaluation

A second and different approach to assess auditory processing disorders is used by audiologists. This approach evaluates the child's ability to respond under different conditions of signal distortion or competition, and, increasingly, to examine the auditory system using electrophysiological measures. Most of these tests require an imitative speech response that is not cognitively based. The principle of this test approach assumes that a person who has a normal auditory system can tolerate distortions of speech and still understand it. A listener with an auditory processing deficit will encounter difficulty with the distorted speech due to "internal distortion" (Teatini, 1970). Results of distorted speech tests (sometimes called sensitized speech tests) can be used to infer the development status of the child's central auditory nervous system and to help determine whether APD may form a basis for language or reading problems. Although the cause-and-effect relationship between auditory perception and language is not clearly understood, there is reason to believe that growth of language is related to progressive maturation of the auditory nervous system including the corpus callosum and the cerebral cortex. When it is shown that prelinguistic auditory processing abilities are poorly developed, the child may not have the neurological potential necessary to organize and develop a linguistic system, or development may be slower than normal. The greater the severity of the auditory processing abnormalities the greater the presumed effect on the acquisition of language. When auditory abnormalities occur in combination with problems of other sensory systems (for example, a visual perceptual disorder), or when associations among auditory, visual, tactile, vestibular sensory systems are not established, the effect is more devastating, and the child will have marked difficulty in overall learning.

Screening for Auditory Processing Disorders

The increasing burden of referrals for auditory processing evaluation made to educational audiologists and those in the private sector demands improved methods for determining who are possible candidates for a full diagnostic battery. The UTD/Callier Center Consensus Conference on diagnosing APD in children (Jerger & Musiek, 2000) specifies three approaches to screening: (1) screening questionnaire, (2) testing, or (3) a combination of questionnaire and testing. Questionnaires were discussed in the preceding paragraphs. The conference recommended that screening by test "should include the following elements: a dichotic digit test consisting of two digits in each ear and a free-recall response mode, a gap-detection test in which a short silent gap is inserted in a burst of broadband noise." In a statement of concern a group of audiologists (Katz et al, 2002) suggest that the screening tests mentioned in the consensus document "do not meet acceptable psychometric standards."

There are actually few well-standardized screening tests available to identify children with auditory processing disorders. One test marketed as screening test for APD is the Selective Auditory Attention Test (SAAT) (Cherry, 1980). The SAAT obtains speech recognition scores in quiet and in the presence of a semantic distractor in the same ear at 0 dB signal-to-noise ratio. Children point to pictures using the Word Intelligibility by Picture Identification Test plates. Normative data for the test were obtained from 325 children ages 4 to 9 years. Children in the standardization study fell into three groups: normal achieving, learning-disabled, and teacher concerned with school progress. Results showed that children in the normal group scored substantially better than the other groups. According to Cherry this test is an efficient screening device to help identify children with learning difficulties resulting from an APD for deciding when to administer a lengthy battery of tests. Unfortunately, there are no available data on the sensitivity and specificity of the SAAT, primarily because of the problem of no "gold standard" for definition of APD. According to Cherry the SAAT is appropriate to administer when children appear to be at risk for APD because of behaviors noted by parents or teachers (Cherry, 1980). More recently those behaviors can be quantified using checklists of auditory processing as already discussed.

It appears that a substantial amount of work is needed to develop, standardize, and validate an adequate test battery used for screening of APD. In the meantime educa-

tional audiologists from the Houston area published a set of requirement guidelines for referring for APD evaluations (Kent, 2002). The purpose of the guidelines was to improve the quality of referrals for diagnostic APD testing. According to the guidelines, certain criteria are prerequisite to a referral for an APD evaluation. Students must:

1. Be at least 7 years or older
2. Have passed a hearing screening within the year
3. Have English as their primary language
4. Have an IQ of 85 or higher
5. Have had a recent psychoeducational assessment to determine learning disability, attention deficit, or emotional problems and performance related to cognitive ability
6. Have had a speech and language assessment within the year that examines auditory processing skills
7. Have intelligible speech
8. Be able to follow directions and complete the APD testing

The guidelines also require the referring person to state why the student is being referred for an evaluation and to indicate whether the child is taking medication, which special classes the student attends, what modifications are being made, and what benefit or change in programming/modifications would result from an APD diagnosis. Clearly, requiring that every other possibility be considered before APD assessment is conducted creates restricted access for students. The policies may improve the quality of referrals, and only time will tell whether policies of this type are to the advantage of the student or the system. When brief and validated auditory screening tests are available a better balance may be obtainable.

Diagnostic Testing for Auditory Processing Disorders

According to the ASHA Consensus Conference, categories of behavioral auditory measures that can be used effectively to measure auditory processing disorders includes tests of

- Temporal processing—ordering, discrimination, resolution (e.g., gap detection), and integration
- Localization and lateralization
- Low-redundancy monaural speech (time compressed, filtered, interrupted, competing, etc.)
- Dichotic stimuli including nonsense syllables, digits, words, and sentences
- Binaural interaction (e.g., MLD)
- Electrophysiological procedures may also be useful

For example, some specific tests related to the ASHA list are included in the following:

- Temporal processing—resolution/gap detection
  Auditory Fusion Test (Revised)
  Random Gap Detection Test (RGDT)
- Temporal ordering
  Pitch Pattern Test
  Duration Patterns Test
- Sound localization and lateralization
  Clinical localization of sounds through earphones or speakers
  Median plane localization task
- Low-redundancy monaural speech
  Time Compressed Sentence Test (TCST)
  Filtered Words test from SCAN-C or SCAN-A
  Auditory Figure Ground test from SCAN C or A
  QuickSIN test—for older children
- Dichotic stimuli
  Dichotic Digits Test
  Dichotic Words Test from SCAN-C or SCAN-A
  Staggered Spondaic Word Test
  Competing Sentence Test from SCAN-C or SCAN-A
- Binaural interaction—MLD
- Electrophysiological procedures
  Auditory brainstem response (ABR)
  Middle latency response (MLR)

According to the UTD/Callier Center Consensus Conference (Jerger & Musiek, 2000) the following principles should be considered to improve strategies in APD assessment:

- Compare analogous tasks from multiple sensory modalities
- Control for linguistic variables
- Use contemporary psychological methods
- Minimize memory load
- Employ a simple response mode
- Maximize test efficiency with adaptive computer-controlled psychophysical procedures
- Use a team approach

The UTD/Callier Center Consensus Conference then suggested that a minimal APD test battery include

- Behavioral measures
  Pure tone audiometry
  P-I functions for word recognition
  Dichotic task (digits, words, and/or sentences)
  Duration pattern sequence test
  Temporal gap detection
- Electrophysiological measures
  Immittance audiometry
  Otoacoustic emissions
  ABR
  MLR
  P300 (optional)

One diagnostic battery that includes three of the main requirements for assessment of APD is the SCAN-C Test for Auditory Processing Disorders in Children–Revised (Keith, 2000a, 2000b). The battery includes four subtests, including monosyllabic words that are low-pass filtered at 1000 Hz, auditory figure ground with monosyllabic words presented in speech babble background noise at +8 dB speech-to-noise ratio, competing words, and competing sentences. The two subtests tapping auditory perception of low redundancy speech (filtered words and auditory figure ground) are representative of functional auditory abilities in everyday listening situations. Competing Words and Competing Sentences are dichotic speech tests that demonstrate the development of the auditory system, auditory maturation, and hemispheric specialization. Dichotic tests are also sensitive to the presence of lesions of the auditory system. The test battery requires approximately 25 minutes to administer. SCAN-C is an upward extension of SCAN: Screening Test for Auditory Processing Disorders (Keith, 1986) and was normed on 650 children between 5 and 11 years of age. In addition to mean and standard deviation of subtest and composite test results, the SCAN-C normative data include standard scores, percentile ranks, age equivalents, and standard score confidence levels. Subsequent research has validated the use of the SCAN test in various populations and it is the most frequently used auditory processing test battery currently available (Chermak, Styer, & Seikel, 1995; Chermak, Traynham, Seikel, & Musiek, 1998; Cranford, Kennalley, Svoboda, & Hipp, 1996; Deitrich, Berger, & Keith, 1992; Emanual, 2002; Katbamna, Keith, & Johnson, 1990; Keith, Rudy, Donahue, & Katbamna, 1989; Zarrella, 1995). In addition, when the Random Gap Detection Test (Keith, 2000a) is used with the SCAN-C battery, all of the categories of behavioral tests recommended by the ASHA Consensus Conference are met.

For older children the SCAN-A: Test for Auditory Processing Disorders in Adolescents and Adults (Keith, 1994b) contains four subtests including monosyllabic words low-pass filtered at 500 Hz, auditory figure ground with words presented simultaneously with speech babble background noise at 0 dB S/N ratio, the competing words test, and a competing sentence test. The SCAN-A test battery requires approximately 30 minutes to administer. As with SCAN-C, standardization data include mean and standard deviation of subtests, composite test results, standard scores, percentile ranks, and cutoff scores for normal, questionable, and abnormal performance. The standardization results are also analyzed for content and construct validity.

The Time Compressed Sentence Test (TCST) (Keith, 2002) is another form of a distorted or degraded speech test that provides information on the child's ability to process speech presented at rapid rates. The test indirectly measures temporal processing of rapid acoustic changes of speech format frequencies. It also measures auditory closure because parts of the speech signal are missing and the child is required to interpret the entire sentence. The TCST presents sentences that are time compressed at 40 and 60%. The child simply repeats the sentences. Results are interpreted in terms of percent correct, and normative data are provided for borderline and abnormal performance. In addition, standard scores and percentile rank of performance compared with typical children of the same age are provided.

Temporal ordering or sequencing tasks are potentially valuable screening tests because of the underlying processes they tap. The Frequency Pattern Test (Musiek & Pinheiro, 1987) requires the child to listen to a series of three tones and report the pitch pattern that was heard, such as low-high-low, low-low-high. Conceptually, the tones are initially processed in the nondominant right hemisphere. Interpretation of pitch perception is transferred through the corpus callosum to the language areas of the left hemisphere where a verbal response is sequenced. The test takes approximately 10 minutes to administer. Cut-off scores are available for children from 6 to 12 years. According to Musiek and Pinheiro low scores are associated with auditory dysfunction related to various learning disabilities and to defined lesions of the auditory areas of the cerebrum. Similarly the Duration Patterns Test (Reference) presents three-tone signals of 200 and 500 msec. The child is required to report the pattern that was heard, such as short-long-short, or long-long-short. Results of the pattern recognition tests are said to indicate interhemispheric integration of auditory information and help identify children who experience difficulty using suprasegmental information (stress patterns, intonation, pauses, etc.) when listening to discourse in everyday language; although that relationship is in need of more systematic investigation to verify the relationship between test findings and functional relationships. Unfortunately, as recently as 2002 there were no norms for use of the Durations Patterns Test with individuals suspected of having APD (Medwetsky, 2002).

As a group, behavioral tests of auditory processing all share certain characteristics. They are applicable only after the emergence of language because they require either verbal repetition of syllables, words, or sentences or pointing to pictures that represent the stimulus words. Most of the tests show substantial maturation effects. When given to children at an early age, the results of tests are highly variable, with average performance improving remarkably up to 12 years of age. By about 12 years of age, the auditory system of normal children has matured to the point where their responses approximate those of adult listeners. Most behavioral tests of auditory processing are affected by peripheral hearing loss, even mild conductive and high frequency SNHLs. Children with speech, language, reading, and learning problems have been reported to perform poorly on behavioral tests of auditory processing, although some children with language or reading problems yield normal scores.

Electrophysiological Assessment of Auditory Processing

Both consensus panels discussed in this chapter describe the use of evoked potentials testing in the assessment of auditory processing disorders. For example, the ASHA (1996) panel stated "Electrophysiologic procedures can be used in the diagnosis of APD. The brain stem response is well understood and applied routinely in the detection of lesions of the brain stem. The middle, late, and event-related auditory potentials are still in the developmental stage, but can be of considerable value in certain clinical situations." Because of questions on the efficacy of physiological measures in the assessment of APD, the ASHA panelists recommended that "research priorities for the future include studies to establish the sensitivity and specificity of behavioral and electrophysiologic measures of auditory processing."

The UTD/Callier Center Consensus Conference (Jerger & Musiek, 2000) recommended that the minimal test battery includes "auditory brainstem and middle latency response—key measures of the status of auditory structures at brain stem and cortical levels." In an expression of concern regarding the UTD/Callier Center Consensus Conference recommendations, Katz et al (2002) state that "Research has not substantiated the premise that physiological measures play an important role in typical auditory processing assessment and it does not seem that a positive physiologic finding from . . . auditory brain stem responses and middle latency responses would be beneficial to the remediation of a child diagnosed with APD." Katz et al also state that no suggested readings on MLR are offered to justify its routine use in children seen for APD evaluations. In fact, they cite studies that question its sensitivity and specificity and provide references that contradict the inclusion of MLR in a minimal test battery (Chermak & Musiek, 1997; Musiek, Charette, Kelly, & Musiek, 1999). Their point of view appears to be supported in studies summarized by Cacace and McFarland (Cacace & McFarland, 2002). They summarize that (1) the MLR is not sufficiently sensitive, even in cortical lesion cases, (2) use of the MLR in children under the age of 10 years is problematic because of its variability, (3) the MLR is not widely used in audiology and only rarely with children, and (4) it is not clear how MLR would contribute to making appropriate recommendations if a child "failed" the test procedure.

Clearly, the use of electrophysiological procedures as a routine part of the APD test battery is controversial, and additional evidence is required on the sensitivity and specificity of these measures and their contribution to the management of children with APD. The additional question at the time of writing this chapter is the accessibility of electrophysiological testing to the huge number of children across the country who are candidates for auditory processing assessment. In a reply to Katz et al, Jerger and Musiek (2002) state "another reason for encouraging the use of electrophysiological measures is that, if we are ever going to have a gold standard for APD it will probably be in the form of electrophysiological measures." The answer, therefore, is that electrophysiological measures such as the MLR, late cortical evoked potentials, P-300, and Mismatch Negativity lie in the future and are not feasible for every child in the first decade of the new millennium. It will be up to future research to determine whether these tests will be applied to every child being evaluated for APD, or reserved for special situations.

Designing a School-Based Protocol

Among the many questions regarding APD is that of accessibility of services to large numbers of children in the school setting and, therefore, how to proceed with programs. Among the various issues are the questions of whom to test for APD, what tests should be administered, who will do the testing and design appropriate intervention programs, and who will provide the actual intervention. There are limited educational audiologists in the schools and their broad responsibilities of assessment and management of the hearing-impaired child leaves precious little time for the additional burden of children with APD. Nevertheless, there is increasing pressure to offer services for children with possible APD, and those children are equally deserving of attention as any child with a disability. At least one protocol is published and serves as a model of service; the Colorado Department of Education guidelines for a team approach to screening, assessment, and intervention practices. Written in 1996, the guidelines are reprinted in Appendix 5-C of Johnson, Benson, and Seaton (1997). The guidelines contain three levels:

- Observation procedures
- Assessment procedures
  Screening and preliminary assessment
    procedures

Diagnostic assessment procedures
  Assessment interpretation
  Intervention recommendations
    (classroom management, instructional modifications, therapy, amplification)
Additional diagnostic procedures for
  children with organically based problems or for children who demonstrate poor progress with a variety of interventions

Each level of the guidelines contains procedures for the entire multidisciplinary team including auditory, language, psychological, educational, and other. As stated in the guidelines, they represent the best of what was known at the time, and, although they will continually evolve, they represent one attempt to systematically make "more effective decisions regarding APD in children."

Comment

The sensitivity and specificity of auditory processing measures that are available cannot be determined because there is no gold standard for what constitutes an auditory processing disorder. Without an agreed upon definition there is no way to determine the rate of true-positive and false-positive identifications of APD. Only when professionals agree on definitions of APD can their sensitivity and specificity be determined.

One of the greatest problems with available tests of auditory processing is the lack of normative data on the typical performance of children at each age to include mean, standard deviation, and range of normative values. Several tests include only cut-off scores that are established to separate normal from abnormal performance, and there is no estimate of normal variance information on the population from whom the cut-off scores were obtained (age, gender, socioeconomic status, linguistic background, number of subjects, etc.). Without standardization, results of auditory tests cannot be directly compared to results of speech-language or psychoeducational tests.

Those tests that have a well-established normative database are well suited for the educational setting, whereas cut-off scores may be adequate for medical diagnostic purposes.

The use of tests for auditory processing is increasing, although there is a great deal to learn about interpretation of obtained results. However, well-designed tests of auditory processing abilities reveal some of the following information about the child being tested:

1. The maturation level of the central auditory pathways and, through longitudinal studies on a given child, the development of auditory processing abilities
2. The neurological basis presumed to exist in children with specific learning disabilities
3. The effect of medication on auditory processing abilities
4. Abnormalities of the central auditory pathways that contribute to a language-learning problem
5. Whether appropriate cerebral dominance for language has occurred
6. Whether the auditory channel is "weak" or "strong," and whether classroom, tutoring, or remedial material should be modified to account for auditory processing abilities
7. Specific recommendations for management of the child with an auditory processing disorder

In general, tests of auditory processing are useful in research on auditory processing abilities that will help to increase our understanding of this complex disorder.

Results of auditory processing tests cannot be expected to indicate specific language, learning, or reading deficits. A direct correlation does not always exist. To describe these specific nonauditory problems, the examiner needs to administer tests that are designed for that purpose. The auditory processing test battery does provide information about auditory-specific abnormalities that can be used to develop remedial strategies for auditory processing/language-learning-disordered children.

Remediation

In general, remediation for children with auditory processing disorders falls into three categories:

- Management of the environment, including classroom placement
- Compensatory training to strengthen basic perceptual processes and teach specific academic skills
- Cognitive therapy in which the clinician assists subjects in learning auditory strategies for dealing with their auditory processing disorder

Management of the environment includes altering the psychological environment to modify negative attitudes and habits of the subject and those around the subject. When an auditory figure ground deficit has been identified, recommendations for remediation should be directed toward management of the environment to enhance listening opportunities. Although direct intervention to help achieve better listening skills in noise through cognitive training and focusing of auditory attention may be beneficial, there is no evidence to support the improvement of auditory figure ground perceptual deficits through such training. When auditory figure ground problems are severe, attempts to compensate for the deficit with FM auditory training systems are useful (ASHA, 1991; Chermak & Musiek, 1992; Johnson et al, 1997; Schneider, 1992). However, trials with FM systems should be carefully monitored to be sure that the child, teachers, and parents understand the device, and that real, not imagined, benefits accrue from their use.

Specific recommendations for remediation of auditory processing disorders are beyond the scope of this chapter and can be found in several sources (Bellis, 1996; Johnson et al, 1997; Masters, Stecker, & Katz, 1998) and in Chapter 17 of this book. This author offers one caveat! At the time of this writing there are several "listening programs" and intervention approaches being offered commercially. Most of those programs have no construct validity research, and many appear to be bogus. It is incumbent on concerned parents and professionals to be aware of the entrepreneurial basis of these programs and to proceed with caution.

Finally, diagnosis of an auditory processing disorder and recommendations for remediation/rehabilitation must be made as part of a transdisciplinary team decision to assure that different aspects of the individual's speech, language, auditory, psychological, emotional, and physical function have been evaluated. Only after all these aspects have been examined can an APD be diagnosed and appropriate recommendations for treatment be made. This is especially true when evaluating children and adolescents with learning problems and developing individualized education plans.

Summary

Interest in assessment and remediation of individuals with APDs has grown over the last 40 years. The gradual increase in the understanding of these disorders includes an evolving definition that has yet to achieve consensus. Similarly there is a need for additional tests of auditory processing abilities, including both language-based auditory processing abilities and auditory specific measures. There is an enormous need for standardization of tests with normative data that includes description of the population on whom the data were obtained, descriptive statistics (means and standard deviations), and standard scores and percentiles. The trend appears to be toward development of electrophysiological measures of auditory processing in order to eliminate nonauditory factors in the response and its interpretation. Nevertheless, it is left to the future to determine what mix of behavioral and electrophysiological testing will be required to adequately understand the individual child.

Finally, there is a need to test the remediation models that are currently being promulgated to determine their validity and effectiveness and to identify improved approaches to remediation. Computer-based remediation programs that are in their infancy will be refined and improved with time and hold promise for a partial answer to remediation needs in the future. All approaches to remediation desperately need outcome studies.

Although there are many needs for improved understanding, assessment, and remediation of this complex disorder, a great deal of good is being done to help children and adults with APD. Our current understanding provides us sufficient tools in our armamentarium to provide services and make a significant contribution to children's lives now.

Case Study 6–1   J.M. is a child with a typical auditory processing disorder with poor listening skills; delays in auditory maturation were evidenced by low performance on dichotic listening tasks, and abnormal ear advantage.

History

J.M. is a pleasant, handsome, 10-year-old child who interacts and communicates well with adults. His birth and developmental history are normal. He loves music and has perfect pitch. In conversation he is reported to do better if engaged visually when others are speaking to him. His parents report that since kindergarten he has had difficulty in school, with problems following directions or "listening to instructions." He is beginning to experience difficulty in following multistep instructions and has difficulty completing tasks as instructed. His parents report that he is in fifth grade and is "trying very hard to listen." Results of intelligence testing found no substantial discrepancy between verbal and performance IQs, with a full-scale IQ in the 90th percentile and a standard score of approximately 120. He performs in the 90+ percentile on standardized psychoeducational tests; however his parents report that this has led to his relaxed attitude toward study because much of the material comes naturally. In spite of his intelligence J.M.'s grades are slipping and he recently received some Fs. The SLP has questioned whether he has attention deficit disorder, though the parents feel he does not. He is among the youngest age of children in his class. Finally, he has no obvious problems with coordination or fine motor control, but he dislikes group sports because most other children are better coordinated, and he dislikes physical contact. J.M.'s parents describe his handwriting as "atrocious."

Test Results

Pure tone threshold testing found thresholds at 5 dB for all frequencies with normal tympanometry. Speech reception thresholds were 5 dB HL with 100% word discrimination in quiet.

Results of the SCAN-C Test for Auditory Processing Disorders in Children–Revised were as follows:

Scoring Summary

	Raw Score	Standard Score	% Rank	Confidence Level
Filtered words	34	10	50	7 to 13
Auditory figure ground	35	10	50	6 to 13
Competing words	36	7	16	4 to 10
Competing sentences	13	6	9	3 to 9
Scan composite	33	88	21	78 to 98

Competing Words Ear Advantage

Right Ear First Task		Left Ear First Task	
RE correct	14	RE correct	8
LE correct	5	LE correct	9
Ear advantage	9	Ear advantage	−1
Right ear advantage	Yes	Right ear advantage	No
Left ear advantage	No	Left ear advantage	Yes
Prevalence	2%	Prevalence	15%

Results of Filtered Words and Auditory Figure Ground subtests are in the normal range. The Competing Words Test is "normal" in absolute terms, but the 16th percentile is low for normal processing. The Competing Sentences Subtest results were in the 9th percentile. Moreover, the ear advantage scores found an atypical strong right ear advantage. The same finding was obtained on the Competing Words Subtest, the Competing Sentences Subtest, and the Staggered Spondaic Word Test. Ear advantage scores are powerful indicators of hemispheric dominance for language, and maturational-based language/learning disorders. The right ear advantage indicates that language is appropriately established in the left cerebral hemisphere, but the atypical large right ear advantage in a child approaching 11 years indicates the presence of a developmental delay of the auditory system.

Random Gap Detection Test (RGDT)
The RGDT is a test of temporal processing (auditory timing) ability. Disorders of auditory timing are related to disorders of auditory discrimination, reading, and language. J.M.'s gap detection thresholds of less than 5 msec are normal for his age.

Durations Patterns Test (DPT)
The DPT is a measure of pattern recognition in the time domain, a cortical function reflecting hemispheric interaction between recognition of sound patterns of different duration and providing a linguistic label of what was heard. J.M.'s responses were completely normal.

Frequency Patterns Test (FPT)
The FPT is a measure of pattern recognition in the frequency (pitch) domain, a cortical function reflecting hemispheric interaction between recognition of sound patterns of different pitch and providing a linguistic label of what was heard. J.M.'s responses were 100%.

Staggered Spondaic Word Test (SSW)
The SSW is a dichotic test of binaural separation. The SSW stimuli represent both competing and noncompeting words presented to each ear simultaneously.

Staggered Spondaic Word Test

SSW Conditions	Results (number of errors)	Normative Data (number of errors)
Right ear noncompeting	0	1
Right ear competing	1	3
Left ear competing	12	5
Left ear noncompeting	0	1

The SSW results are abnormal with the number of errors in the left-ear-competing condition more than twice the typical finding for a child this age. When the SSW results are converted to Z scores and percentiles the left competing condition result has a Z score of -4, which is below the 1st percentile. The right competing Z score equals -1.3, which is approximately the 10th percentile.

Observations of behavioral auditory testing
J.M.'s responses to auditory stimuli were characterized by slow responses that occurred at the end of nearly every response time interval allowed during the standardized tests. This delayed latency of response indicated that he was always at the

"threshold" of understanding. The need for additional time to process auditory information indicates that listening under complex acoustic conditions, to rapid or distorted speech, is a difficult task that is frustrating and tiring.

Electrophysiology

A battery of electrophysiological tests was administered. They included

- Auditory Brainstem Evoked Potentials
- Middle Latency Auditory Evoked Potential
- P-100
- P-300

Results of all tests were normal. The P-300 assesses auditory attention at the physiological level. The P-300 response was present with a normal latency and large amplitude, indicating that attention processes as measured by this technique are completely normal.

Speech-Language Evaluation

Results of language testing found a total language standard score of 128. His receptive and expressive language was advanced. On a test of phonological processing he was normal for awareness and memory but low average for rapid naming. Specifically J.M. has difficulty whenever he is required to retrieve specific information or to name things. That is, given freedom to talk freely about the world he appears to be very intelligent. However, when he is required to give specific convergent knowledge his performance is low. He was in the 9th stanine for math and the 7th stanine for reading.

Summary

J.M. was referred for auditory processing testing because of a history of difficulty with listening, missing directions, and doing poorly in school. These difficulties occur even though J.M. is extremely bright, has good language skills, and is reading above grade level. He is a self-admitted dawdler. Results on routine hearing testing found normal hearing thresholds. Tests of auditory processing abilities found normal duration and frequency processing, normal processing in the time domain, and normal auditory processing of minimally distorted speech and speech in noise. Tests of auditory maturation found delays in the development of his central auditory pathways. There are large discrepancies between the standard scores found on intelligence and language testing compared with auditory processing. These findings confirm that learning through the auditory modality may be difficult because J.M.'s listening skills are those of a child who is chronologically younger. In addition, J.M. was slow in responding during behavioral testing. That is, his responses always came at the end of time intervals allowed for response. His responses indicated a need for additional time to process auditory information. His high level of intelligence compensates somewhat for these deficiencies, but may cause him problems because the language closure he utilizes sometimes leads him down the wrong path and causes him to miss basic specific information, assignments, directions, and the like. He was completely attentive throughout testing done on this date, with no evidence of attention deficit. Recommendations for classroom management are discussed following here.

Electrophysiological tests of auditory nervous system function confirm that there is no fundamental physiological central nervous system disorder, that he is "simply" delayed in auditory maturation. The implication is that his auditory system will continue to mature and he will "catch up" with his peers at some time. Finally, the P-300 auditory evoked potential was normal, providing electrophysiological confirmation of behavioral observations that J.M. does not have attention deficit disorder.

Recommendations

Results of this test find normal peripheral hearing, with normal auditory processing for some fundamental perceptual tasks. The delay in auditory maturation found on several tests indicates that J.M.'s listening ability is his poorest academic strength. Because his auditory processing is not strong J.M. may hear some information inaccurately. For example, his auditory analysis and synthesis skills may actually be "harmed" by his cognitive ability. Specifically, J.M. has excellent top-down processing. His world knowledge, knowledge of events, and linguistic knowledge is at a high level. J.M.'s processing is at a low level however, so that auditory subskills processing, short-term memory, and phonological processing skills are comparatively weak. J.M. knows to guess when he misses auditory information, but when he guesses he is sometimes wrong, misses information, and does not get complete or accurate directions. His self-admitted dawdling exacerbates this situation.

Some basic classroom management techniques may help J.M. in classroom activities:

- Provide his teachers with information contained in this report.
- Provide J.M. with preferential seating, close to wherever the teacher does most teaching.
- Identify noise sources, reduce them, and move J.M. away from them.
- Alert J.M. to changes in the topic, and supplement group instructions with individual checks of comprehension.
- Increase one-on-one instruction.
- Monitor his auditory comprehension to be sure he has understood directions, has correct assignments, and understands material covered.
- Break new information into shorter segments.
- Assist J.M. in developing organizational strategies.

J.M. can also help himself by taking responsibility in making the following changes:

- Increase his visual vigilance and watch speakers for information to supplement what is heard
- Increase his vigilance to the task at hand, and reduce the time wasted by dawdling

In addition J.M. needs to begin moving toward an internal locus of control and ask for clarification of auditory information when he is unsure or misses instructional material.

Finally, it was recommended that J.M.'s auditory processing be rechecked in a year to document the rate of change in maturation.

References

Anderson, K. (1989). Screening Instrument for Targeting Educational Risk (SIFTER). Tampa: Educational Audiology Association.

American Speech Language Hearing Association (ASHA). (1996). Central auditory processing: Current status of research and implications for clinical practice. *Am J Audiol*, 51–55.

American Speech Language Hearing Association (ASHA). (1991). Amplification as a remediation technique for children with normal peripheral hearing. Committee on Amplification for the Hearing Impaired. *ASHA, 33* (Suppl. 3), 22–24.

Bellis, T.J. (1996). *Assessment and Management of Central Auditory Processing Disorders In the Educational Setting*. San Diego: Singular.

Benson, P. (1995). Fisher's Auditory Problems Checklist. *Educational Audiology Newsletter, 12*(2), 16.

Brutten, M., Richardson, S.O., & Mangel, C. (1973). *Something's Wrong with My Child*. New York: Harcourt Brace Jovanovich.

Cacace, A.T., & McFarland, D.J. (2002). Middle-latency auditory evoked potentials: Basic issues and potential applications. In: Katz J. (Ed.), *Handbook of Clinical Audiology* (Chap. 19) (5th ed.). Baltimore: Lippincott Williams and Wilkins.

Chelfonte Evans, M. (2001). *Phonological perception, verbal working memory and linguistic peformance: An analysis of propositional complexity and morphosyntactic skills in youngsters with Down syndrome*. Unpublished Ph.D. dissertation, University of Cincinnati, Ohio.

Chermak, G.D., & Musiek, F. (1992). Managing central auditory processing disorder in children and youth. *Am J Audiol*, 1, 61–65.

Chermak, G.D., & Musiek, F. (1997). *Central Auditory Processing Disorders: New Perspectives*. San Diego: Singular.

Chermak, G.D., Styer, S.A., & Seikel, J.A. (1995). Comparing screening tests of central auditory processing. *The Hearing Journal, 48*(5), 29–34.

Chermak, G.D., Traynham, W.A., Seikel, A.J., & Musiek, F. (1998). Professional education and assessment practices in central auditory processing. *J Am Acad Audiol*, 9, 452–465.

Cherry, R. (1980). *Selective Auditory Attention Test (SAAT)*. St. Louis: Auditec.

Cohen, R.L. (1980). Auditory skills and the communication process. *Seminars in Speech, Language and Hearing*, 1, 107–116.

Cranford, J.L., Kennalley, T., Svoboda, W., & Hipp, K. (1996). Changes in central auditory processing following temporal lobectomies in children. *J Am Acad Audiol*, 7, 289–295.

Deitrich, K.N., Berger, S.P., & Keith, R.W. (1992). Lead exposure and the central auditory processing abilities and cognitive development of urban children: The Cincinnati Lead Study Cohort at Age 5 Years. *Neurotoxicol Teratol, 14*, 51–56.

Emanual, D. (2002). The auditory processing battery: Survey of common practices. *J Am Acad Audiol, 13*, 93–117.

English, K. (2001). Assessing auditory processing problems in the school setting. *Journal of Educational Audiology*, 9, 42–46.

Fisher, L. (1976). *Auditory Problems Checklist*. Tampa: Educational Audiology Association.

Gardner, M.F. (1996). *Test of Auditory-Perceptual Skills–Revised*. Hydesville, CA: Psychological and Educational Publications.

Jerger, J., & Musiek, F. (2000). Report of the consensus conference on the diagnosis of auditory processing disorders in school-aged children. *J Am Acad Audiol, 11*, 467–474.

Jerger, J., & Musiek, F. (2002). On the diagnosis of auditory processing disorder: A reply to "Clinical and Research Concerns Regarding Jerger and Musiek APD Recommendations." *Audiology Today, 14*(2), 19–21.

Johnson, C., Benson, P.V., & Seaton, J.B. (1997). *Educational Audiology Handbook*. San Diego: Singular.

Katbamna, B., Keith, R.W., & Johnson, J.L. (1990). Auditory processing abilities in children with learning disabilities: A pilot study. *Hearsay, J Ohio Speech Hear Assoc, Fall/Winter*, 80–87.

Katz, J., & Harmon, C. (Eds.). (1981). *Phonemic Synthesis Testing and Training*. San Diego: College Hill Press.

Katz, J., Stecker, S., & Henderson, D. (1992). *Central Auditory Processes: A Transcisciplinary View*. St. Louis: Mosby Year Book Publishers.

Katz, J., et al. (2002). Clinical and research concerns regarding the 2000 APD consensus report and recommendations. *Audiology Today, 14*(2), 14–17.

Keith, R.W. (1986). *SCAN: A screening test for auditory processing disorders*. San Antonio: Psychological Corporation.

Keith, R.W. (1994a). *The Auditory Continuous Performance Test*. San Antonio: Psychological Corporation.

Keith, R.W. (1994b). *SCAN-A: A test of auditory processing abilities for use with adolescents and adults*. San Antonio: Psychological Corporation.

Keith, R.W. (2000a). *Random Gap Detection Test (RGDT)*. St. Louis: Auditec.

Keith, R.W. (2000b). *SCAN-C: Test for Auditory Processing Disorders in Children–Revised*. San Antonio: Psychological Corporation.

Keith, R.W., & Farrer, S. (1981). Filtered word testing in the assessment of children with central auditory disorders. *Ear Hear, 12*, 267–269.

Keith, R.W., Rudy, J., Donahue, P., & Katbamna, B. (1989). Comparison of SCAN results with other auditory and language measures in a clinical population. *Ear Hear, 10*, 382–386.

Keith, R.W. (2002). Time Compressed Sentence Test, *Examiner's Manual*. St. Louis: Auditec.

Kent, M. (2002). Houston educational audiologists establish guidelines for referring for an auditory processing evaluation. *Educational Audiology Review, Summer*, 3–4.

Lasky, E.Z., & Cox, L.C. (Eds.). (1983). *Auditory Processing and Language Interaction*. Baltimore: University Park Press.

Lindamood, C., & Lindamood, P. (1971). *Lindamood Auditory Conceptualization Test*. Austin: PRO-ED.

Macmillan, D.L. (Ed.). (1993). *Development of Operational Definitions in Mental Retardations: Similarities and Differences with the Field of Learning Disabilities*. Baltimore: Paul H. Brookes.

Masters, M.G., Stecker, N.A., & Katz, J. (1998). *Central Auditory Processing Disorders: Mostly Management*. Needham Heights: Allyn and Bacon.

Medwetsky, L. (Ed.). (2002). *Central Auditory Processing Testing: A Battery Approach* (5th ed.). Baltimore: Lippincott Williams and Wilkins.

Menyuk, P. (Ed.). (1992). *Relationship of Otitis Media to Speech Processing and Language Development.* St. Louis: Mosby Year Book.

Musiek, F., Charette, L., Kelly, T., & Musiek, E. (1999). Hit and false-positive rates for the middle latency resonse in patients with central nervous system involvement. *J Am Acad Audiol, 10,* 124–132.

Musiek, F.E., & Pinheiro, M.L. (1987). Frequency patterns in cochlear, brainstem and cerebral lesions. *Audiology, 26,* 79–88.

Rosenberg, P.D. (1978). Case history: The first test. In: J. Katz (Ed.), *Handbook of Clinical Audiology* (Chap. 7) (2nd ed.). Baltimore: Williams and Wilkins.

Rosner, J., & Simon, D. (1971). The Auditory Analysis Test. *J Learning Disability, 4,* 384–392.

Roush, W. (1995). Arguing over why Johnny can't read. *Science, 267,* 1896–1898.

Schneider, D. (Ed.). (1992). *Audiologic Management of Children with Central Auditory Processing Disorders.* St. Louis: Mosby Year Book.

Semel, E., Wiig, E., & Secord, W. (1995). *Clinical Evaluation of Language Fundamentals* (3rd ed.) San Antonio: Psychological Corporation.

Smoski, W.J., Brunt, M.A., & Tannahill, J.D. (1992). Listening characteristics of children with central auditory processing disorders. *Lang Speech Hear Serv Sch, 23,* 145–152.

Teatini, G.P. (Ed.). (1970). *Sensitized Speech Tests: Results in Normal Subjects.* Odense, Denmark: Danavox Foundation.

VanDyke, J. (1985). Evaluation of classroom listening behaviors. *Rocky Mountain Journal of Communication Disorders, 1.*

Zarrella, S. (1995). Category system, test battery enhances diagnosis and management of CAPD. *ADVANCE for Speech-Language Pathologists & Audiologists,* 6–7.

7

Psychoeducational Assessment of Individuals with Hearing Loss*

Robert E. Kretschmer

Synergy means behavior of whole systems unpredicted by the behavior of their parts.

—Richard Buckminster Fuller, 1895–1983

At the heart of most direct services provided by the school psychologist are the psychoeducational evaluation and the diagnostic prescriptive process. This chapter provides relevant definitions of terms connected with the notions of evaluation and the diagnostic process, and discusses topics related to the assumptions and prerequisites of conducting any evaluation, especially that of a student with hearing impairment. Issues related to the identification, placement process, application of various evaluation materials, as well as results for programming of individual children are also addressed.

The Diagnostic Process

The term "diagnostic process," as used by practicing psychologists, appears to have taken on two meanings in the context of psychoeducational services to children. The first relates to the entire sequence of events that unfold as a child with a disability moves through the educational system, from the point when a disabling condition is suspected to the actual placement and programming for the child. A second, more limited, meaning refers to the sequence of events

whereby individual professionals within this larger framework arrive at their own conclusions about the functional status of the child suspected of having a disabling condition.

When the diagnostic process is thought of as a movement through the educational placement and programming system, the sequence of events generally involves (1) screening individual children to identify those who possibly need special educational consideration; (2) certification by one or more specific professionals with expertise in the disabling condition; (3) verification by a team of individuals, including the parents or their representatives and the child, if appropriate; (4) making and delineating various placement and programmatic decisions, if any are required; and (5) actual implementation of the prescribed program and the subsequent follow-through monitoring evaluations, as required by law (United States Department of Health, Education, and Welfare, 1977; United States Department of Education, Office of Special Education and Rehabilitative Services, 1999). These notions of the diagnostic process, and in particular the notions of *certification* and *verification* of a disability, are considered by many as being the quintessential reflections of an underlying positivistic philosophy (Skritic, 1995). That philosophy,

*"Individuals with hearing loss" refers to those who are classified as hard of hearing and d/Deaf

along with functionalism, has been rejected by a great number of individuals in favor of postmodern, or postpositivistic, philosophies.

Guba (1990) points out that postmodern philosophies exist on a continuum and with certain versions accepting normative testing, a modified objective stance, diagnostic categories, and the like, not as absolute truths, but as regulatory ideals and warranted assertions. Indeed, historically, in many instances this was the case when these notions were developed, though over time they become reified and treated as if they were absolute truths or actual entities [e.g., the notion of an intelligence quotient (IQ)]. When Binet was commissioned to develop a method of identifying individuals who might profit from educational experiences, which eventually led to the development of the Stanford-Binet Test of Intelligence, he cautioned his readers that he had simply developed a heuristic device. It was only later that the notion of intelligence was developed to extend his work, and thereafter became reified and perceived as an "entity" and objective truth.

Furthermore, there is growing recognition that the "verification" process is a socially constructed and negotiated act (Wall, 2000) and, thus, entails the "playing-out" of variously defined social rules unquestioningly as a received review of science and knowledge (Eftekhar, 2002). As a result, care must taken to be constantly aware of these issues and reflect consciously upon them even while engaging in the process itself.

Although many children with severe and profound hearing impairment will have been certified and verified as disabled before they enter school, they typically will still go through the diagnostic process in order to be placed within the educational system. Many children with mild or moderate hearing loss, high frequency hearing loss, and unilateral hearing loss may initially be identified through auditory screening procedures. Other forms of screening commonly used to identify children with a disability are visual screening with such instruments as the Snellen chart, developmental

screening during kindergarten or first grade roundups, and schoolwide achievement testing programs. Thus one definition of screening is the use of any systematic behavioral observation, checklist, rating scale, or objective test to establish initially the possibility of a disability (see Chapter 5).

Once a child has been screened and a potential disabling condition is suspected, a sequence of events is set into motion. Usually, a referral is made to those individuals within the school system who are responsible for ensuring that all the necessary information pertinent to the resolution of the particular child's educational problems is gathered. This would include collecting a social and family history, obtaining informed consent for further diagnostic testing, and scheduling the necessary evaluations with one or more professionals.

The ultimate goal of the diagnostic process is to obtain the necessary information to make warranted decisions regarding placement and subsequent programming of individual children. Ideally and legally, this process should be performed by a team, which would include full participation of the parents and the child. Deciding whether a child is disabled and in need of special educational consideration is a group process and, thus, a socially negotiated act as already noted. Through this dialogic process, a disabling condition is "verified" by the "documented diagnosis" of the disabilities made by a team of various individuals referred to as a multipdisciplinary team (M-team), a transdisciplinary team (T-team), a committee on special education, or some other name adopted by a local educational agency. A diagnosis of disability occurs after all the pertinent background information, observations, and test materials collected on a child have been reviewed and synthesized. Although the team of individuals, including the classroom teacher and the parents, collectively verifies the salient disabling conditions, individual members of the team may certify specific disabilities appropriate to their professional specialties and disciplines.

Individual professionals, at the conclusion of their evaluation, generally present a series of recommendations. The individual education program (IEP), individual family service plan (IFSP), or individualized transition plan (ITP) is the composite of the recommendations of all the M- or T-team members with regard to educational placement and programming. These recommendations should be written as learning outcomes that relate to local, state, and national standards and should address all major aspects of development and the child's specific strengths and weaknesses. In addition to specific recommendations, time frames and performance criteria are to be specified, as well as the person who is to implement each recommendation. At the writing of this text, the President's Commission on Excellence in Education has made certain recommendations to reduce the overwhelming load of paperwork associated with developing and monitoring these IEPs that have not yet been acted upon (United States Department of Education, Office of Special Education and Rehabilitative Services, 2002)

Assumptions Underlying Testing

As already noted, a number of assumptions underlie any evaluation process. Newland (1973), in considering the case of psychological testing, cites six such assumptions. Any violation of these assumptions could yield results of questionable validity and credibility. The first of these assumptions is that the person administering the test is properly trained to do so.

In past years, several national and regional surveys of psychological services for individuals with hearing impairment have been conducted (Levine, 1974; McQuaid & Alovisetti, 1981; Spragins, Schildroth, & Karchmer, 1981; Trott, 1984; Weaver & Bradley-Johnson, 1993). Each survey found that the majority of these service providers did not have formal or special preparation to work with individuals with hearing loss. Although some progress has been made, it seems that the majority of school psychol-

ogists working with youngsters who are d/Deaf or hard of hearing continue to be ill prepared to do so. For example, in a more recent national survey of school psychologists selected from the membership rolls of the National Association for School Psychologists, 54% of all the respondents indicated that they had the responsibility of working with students who are d/Deaf or hard of hearing, but only two individuals reported working full-time with these populations (Weaver & Bradley-Johnson, 1993). Of the 54% who reported working with students having a hearing loss, only 41% reported having had some form of special training, minimal as it might be, and 75% rated themselves as having poor or no sign language proficiency.

The issue of communication difficulty, and the possible test bias resulting from failure to understand the directions of a test, are at the heart of a number of Furth's early studies (1970) and a study by Ray (1980). They note that failure to perform on a task may simply be a function of not understanding the directions, rather than an inherent disability. It is therefore essential that the examiner have experience with clients who have hearing losses and be proficient in all forms of communication used by these individuals. Those tests that have been standardized on persons with hearing loss have usually taken into account the problem of communication and have provided for standardized instructions and procedures. For example, the Hiskey-Nebraska Test of Learning Aptitude (Hiskey, 1966) has two sets of instructions, one verbal and one pantomime, and the Stanford Achievement Test—d/Deaf or hard of hearing, 9th edition, has a series of special instructions and practice items for each battery level (Traxler, 2000). Unfortunately, most of the tests that have not been standardized with people having hearing loss have verbal directions. Some notable exceptions are the Leiter International Performance Scale, and the Chicago Nonverbal Examination, which have essentially pantomime directions. (The references for all of the tests and descriptions of their technical adequacy can be found in either Salvia and Ysseldyke, 2001 or Mitchell, 2001).

Investigations into the influence of various forms of test administration and modification for the Wechsler Intelligence Scale for Children–Revised (WISC-R) Performance Scale have been conducted by Sullivan (1982); Courtney, Hayes, Couch, & Frick (1984); and Ray (1980). Courtney et al (1984) found that when subjects were administered the WISC-R Performance Scale exclusively by means of pantomime gestures, the resulting effect was a decrement of 5 IQ points (resulting IQ = 90) when compared with the Anderson and Sissco (1977) norms for children and youths with hearing impairment. Likewise, Sullivan (1982), in comparing pantomime, visual aids, and total communication test administration modifications (using a residential school sample of children with genetic, questionable, and multiple-disability etiologies), found an even greater decrement when using pantomime gestures (IQ = 88). Although the use of visual aids resulted in slightly better performance, the use of pantomime directions resulted in a performance that was as much as 15 points poorer than when total communication was used. The use of an interpreter as an intermediary for those psychologists not familiar with manual forms of communication did not seem to be an attractive alternative.

Ray (1980) attempted to investigate the possibility that the Performance Scale scatter profile, often associated with the Wechsler Scales for children with hearing impairments, was a function of misunderstanding the task due to certain communication variables. Although not entirely able to demonstrate this, his findings provide the field with a standardized method of administration for the performance section of the WISC-R. As such, the standardized administration can be used with any child with hearing impairment, whether the child relies on oral communication, simultaneous communication, or gestures/pantomime, as well as eliminating the typical overall decrement associated with most forms of test modification. Braden (1992), in reviewing a large body of psychometric data, found that the Ray procedure yielded a significantly higher mean IQ (103.9) than sign and speech, speech alone, or written directions.

The second assumption noted by Newland (1973) is that any test only samples behavior to some statistically satisfactory degree of adequacy and, thus, is but a probability statement. By this, it is meant that the test should be both reliable and valid, but that even in ideal situations they are not "true" measures of ability. These two terms, "reliability" and "validity," are discussed in detail in Chapter 5. In brief, a reliable test is one that yields similar scores over time for individuals after repeated administrations, and that within a postpositivist's perspective can be considered dependable. Validity, on the other hand, is the degree to which a test actually measures what it purports to measure and, thus, might be considered creditable. A valid test by definition must be a reliable test, but the reverse is not true. These notions of reliability and validity refer to both norm-referenced, criterion-referenced tests, observations and interpretations of these events. Even teacher-made tests and observations should demonstrate reliability and validity or their postpositivistic analogs of dependability and creditability.

The third assumption underlying psychological testing is that the individuals on whom a particular test is to be used have been exposed to learning experiences or acculturation comparable to the original norming group. This particular point addresses itself directly to the issue of test bias. That is, a test can only be considered valid in relationship to particular individuals or groups of individuals. What may be valid for one group of individuals may not be valid for another group. This notion of test bias has been the point of much discussion and the source of much litigation, which has finally resulted in certain statements being made within the federal mandate governing the rights of all children with disabilities (United States Department of Health, Education, and Welfare, 1977; United States Department of Education, Office of Special Education and Rehabilitative Services, 1999).

This mandate has stated that information concerning cultural and social background, among a number of other variables, must be taken into account when making placement decisions and when planning for any child with a disability. The manner in which these notions are taken into account will differ according to the philosophical orientation and belief system of the examiner. Those with a positivistic orientation may view it as a set of static and statistical relationships; whereas, those with a more postpositivist orientation may view the issue of testing and the examiner-child/family relationship in a larger cultural and political context.

Newland (1973) has suggested that validity with respect to acculturation is probably not an all-or-nothing matter, but, rather, there are degrees of validity. In addition, the mere fact that a test is normed on a population or that certain subcultures were included in the norming process does not guarantee a nonbiased, valid test. Alternatively, the fact that other subgroups were excluded from the norming process does not automatically invalidate a test's use with these particular subgroups. If the test can be found to perform the same function with a special group as it does with the normed population, then it should he considered valid. In fact, this has been the focus of much of the psychological literature on the population with hearing loss , which will be discussed later in this chapter.

This notion of test bias is complicated not only by the issue of hearing loss but also by the fact that a large percentage of the population with hearing loss consists of individuals from backgrounds other than Northern European descent, whereby the culture may be different and English may not be the language spoken in the home.

The fourth assumption noted by Newland (1973) is that error is associated with all measurement. This means that the instruments used, the conditions under which the individual is examined, and the examiner and examinee are not perfect. This is true even under what are seemingly ideal testing conditions. Because of this implicit error, an individual's performance on any particular test is usually reported as a spread of scores, rather than a single score, which increases the chances of being accurate. The more that the testing situation departs from the ideal, the less accurate the obtained scores on a test become.

Finally, the fifth and sixth assumptions noted by Newland (1973) are that only present behavior is observed and all future behavior, abilities, and disabilities are inferred. For example, when a youngster "fails a test," all that is observed is that the student did not complete the task as expected. Any statements concerning inability to complete the task or future behavior, although educated in nature and based on known relationships (e.g., predictive validity), are considered inferences rather than fact. In discussing the nature of psychoeducational evaluations and the diagnostic–prescriptive process, Salvia and Ysseldyke (2001) advance four additional assumptions that are fairly self-explanatory:

1. Children enter into a teaching situation with identifiable strengths and weaknesses.
2. The strengths and weaknesses are causally related to academic success.
3. Strengths and weaknesses can be reliably and validly assessed.
4. Pupil performance on diagnostic devices interacts with intervention strategies to produce differential instructional gains.

These assumptions are thought to be in operation whether one is concerned with children who have hearing or with children who do not, and are central to the notion of individualized educational programming. Interestingly, despite the fact that psychometric approaches are typically thought to be antithetical to postpositivistic thinking, all but the last four assumptions are not necessarily inconsistent with that perspective as discussed by Phillips (1991). However, for the last four assumptions, postpositivistic thinking, even in its narrowed sense, takes a much more tentative stance. With regard to these issues of causation and the primary focus on just the individual, postpositivists would see them as much more probabilistic and embedded within a cultural/political context.

Identification and Placement

Assessment data are collected for a number of purposes (Salvia & Ysseldyke, 2001). Two of these purposes are for the "classification" and placement of individuals having disabilities in the most appropriate instructional setting possible. Two types of decisions are involved in this process. The first is whether a child should be placed in a special class or within the regular educational setting. The second has to do with choosing specific methodologies, teaching strategies, or communication modes that should be used with a child. The former decision is, in part, determined by the general philosophy and resources of the school system. That is, if the system's organization is highly predicated on ability or homogeneous grouping, the criteria for entrance into or staying within a particular classroom are apt to be very stringent. If, on the other hand, a more heterogeneous grouping emphasizing diversity is adopted, different criteria will be used. Historically, most school systems have adopted a philosophy of homogeneous grouping and, as a result, have developed local plans that include a variety of placement options. In recent years, however, this has been challenged by advocates of inclusion (e.g., Stainback & Stainback, 1992). If the placement decision is to situate the child in a self-contained classroom, another decision must be made as to which classroom, implying further homogeneous grouping, and often decisions as to what communication approach will be used. For the most part, these decisions are based on the use of some form of norm-referenced test. That is, the child will be grouped with other children who perform similarly on a norm-referenced test. In fact, this is one of the uses of such tests. These tests assist in making various classification, selection, and placement

decisions. When used in this manner, in the contexts previously suggested, they can serve a legitimate function.

There are some unfortunate side effects of norm-referenced placement, however, including: (1) once children are classified, they are labeled, and this label then becomes the explanation for all subsequent learning difficulties or behavioral styles; (2) attempts might be made to limit the development of a diagnostic-prescriptive program to specific results or items from these norm-referenced test; and (3) there is not unanimity in the criteria used by various professionals in placing children with hearing impairments within the continuum of possible educational options (Spear & Kretschmer, 1987). The first situation involves reification and is sometimes referred to as nominalism, and the second assumes that certain children, given a particular aptitude or ability, will learn better under one condition than under another. Although it would be highly desirable to use these tests to develop individual programs, the research into "ability by treatment interactions" has not yet provided strong support for this notion (e.g., Speece, 1990).

Domains Assessed

Myklebust, Neyhus, and Mulholland (1962) have suggested a comprehensive evaluation scheme for individuals with hearing impairment in which information is collected in each of the following areas: (1) general background information and developmental history, (2) sensory functioning, (3) cognition or intelligence, (4) language and academic achievement, (5) psychomotor functioning, (6) social maturity and adaptive behavior, and (7) emotional adjustment. Given the comprehensive nature of this scheme, the same general framework will be adopted in this chapter for discussing the psychoeducational evaluation of individuals with hearing losses.

History and Background Information

The first area to be considered in the evaluation of any youngster with a hearing loss is the collection of thorough birth, genetic, developmental, educational, familial, social/emotional, work (if applicable), and previous evaluation (including any previous speech and hearing, educational, medical, or psychological) histories. In addition to these areas of concern, parental expectations, attitudes, observations, judgments, and concerns should be obtained as well. When the referral source is not the parent but another professional, such as the teacher, the professional's expectations, attitudes, observations, judgments, and concerns should be elicited and recorded. The referring agents should feel that their concerns are genuinely recognized and considered when the evaluation process has been completed. Table 7–1 provides a brief overview of some of the major areas to be covered in a life history interview.

Although it is important to obtain a complete history, certain research studies have indicated that not all of these data are equally predictive of academic success or language development, which are often two of the major criteria used in placement decisions for children with hearing loss. There have been conflicting reports about the significance of the age at which a hearing disability is identified, the age at which initial training or admission to school begins, or the age at which amplification is initiated on predictions of academic success. However, Laughton (1976, 1979) and Pressnell (1973) found these variables to have an effect on the achievement of certain oral and written language structures and written language productivity. In terms of family characteristics, family size has been found to be related to academic success for integrated oral children, with children from smaller families having higher levels of achievement than children from larger families as well as having parents who have more positive attitudes, expectations, and child-rearing practices (Pflaster, 1976). In terms of parental attitudes and involvement, Toscano, McKee, and Lepoutre (2002) interviewed a group of college-level-proficiency readers in an attempt to identify factors and characteristics

that students felt positively influenced the attainment of strong academic literacy skills. Their qualitative analysis revealed that heavy parental involvement in early education and educational decisions, extensive family communication regardless of communication modality, early exposure to and intensive experiences with reading and writing, an enjoyment of reading, a relatively limited social life, high parental and secondary school expectations, the positive importance of TV viewing and closed captioning, and positive self-image all contributed to their success. With young children, parental expectations for achievement potential were found to be highly predictive, but as the child became older, the predictive power of parental expectation decreased (Pflaster, 1976). Thus, parental expectation and involvement may be a necessary but insufficient condition for academic success. Interestingly, the parental assessment of the child's athletic or artistic abilities became increasingly more important as a predictor when the child entered adolescence. Neuhaus (1969) also found a definite relationship between the positive and negative attitudes of parents toward their children with hearing loss, and their children's subsequent emotional adjustment, which, in turn, should relate to academic success. Some researchers have noted that parents tend to overestimate the potential and abilities of their children with hearing loss. In addition, some parents tend to have unrealistic future expectations that reflect more their own ambitions than the capacities and abilities of their children (Pflaster, 1976).

It is often generally assumed that hearing parents of children with hearing loss are at risk for psychiatric problems and marital difficulties (Henggeler, Watson, Whelan, & Malone, 1990). However, research conducted in this area does not support these contentions (e.g., Freeman, Malkin, & Hastings, 1975; Henggeler et al, 1990).

It has been found that teacher ratings of intellectual ability correlate well with children's performance on the Leiter International Performance Scale (Birch & Birch, 1956), and a teacher's initial assessment of

Table 7-1. Life History Outline

Medical Genetic, and Developmental	Clinical Evaluation	Family	Educational	Emotional and Social	Vocational	Familial Observations, Expectations, Judgments and Attitudes	Teacher Observations, Expectations, Judgments and Attitudes
Pre-, peri-, postnatal condition of mother and child	When first noticed hearing loss	Genetic basis for hearing loss	When entered school	Method and style of communication and interaction with family members	Vocational and prevocational training	Statement of suspected problem	Statement of suspected problem
Medical history of illness	When began to wear a hearing aid	Other disabling conditions	Type of school	Relationships with peers and neighbors	Work history	Sensory abilities	Sensory abilities
Genetic milestones	Type of hearing aid used	General family structure	How long in school	Relationships with community		Cognitive abilities	Cognitive abilities
Language development	Auditory evaluations	Family milieu	Schools attended	Preference for friends (d/Deaf of hearing)		Language abilities	Language abilities
Language development	Medical evaluations	Ethnic heritage	Academic achievement, adjustment, progress	Leisure time (play) activities and preferences		Academic abilities	Academic abilities
Cognitive development	Psychological evaluations	Extended family		Participation in d/Deaf community		Emotional abilities	Emotional abilities
Emotional development	Educational evaluations	Religious background		Social interests		Social abilities	Social abilities
Social development	Other evaluations	Family values and belief systems		Marital preference and status		Vocational abilities	Vocational abilities
				Social independence			
				Self-evaluation and attitudes toward self, other d/Deaf individuals, and hearing individuals			

the academic potential of children has been cited as a significant predictor of future academic success (Oakland County School District, 1975). However, in considering this, one must entertain the possibility that a self-fulfilling prophecy may be in operation as much as a legitimate predictive relationship.

Finally, in terms of integrating children with hearing loss into a regular classroom, the regular teacher's attitude toward children with a disability in general and children with hearing loss in particular should be considered. Alexander and Sprain (1978) have found that regular teachers often have negative attitudes about and may be less accepting of special education children introduced into their classrooms. The regular teacher's attitude toward the number of children with hearing loss that should be enrolled in a single classroom has been found to be predictive of academic success for oral integrated students (Pflaster, 1976). The sensitivity of administrators to various individual differences and needs of these children is also predictive of academic success for these children (Pflaster, 1976).

Haring, Cruickshank, and Stern (1981) have developed two instruments that may be helpful in determining the attitudes and knowledge of regular education teachers or administrators about various handicapping conditions, including hearing impairment. Berkay, Gardner, and Smith (1995) have developed an Opinions about Deaf People Scale meant to measure hearing adults' beliefs about the capabilities of other adults who are deaf. More recently, Berryman, Neal, and Berryman (1989) revised their Attitudes toward Mainstreaming Scale, which was meant to evaluate educators' attitudes regarding various disabling conditions (particularly low incidence disabilities, including hearing impairment) and aspects of mainstreaming in general. More recent scales that have been developed are the Scale of Attitudes toward Disabled Persons (Antonak, 1982) and the Interaction with Disabled Persons Scale (Gething, 1994; MacLean & Gannon, 1995); both of which are gaining greater acceptance within the special education community.

Since the advent of inclusion, several other scales have been developed but are not yet in wide use. Cochran (1997), for example, specifically targeted teachers' attitudes toward inclusion by developing the Scale of Teachers' Attitudes toward Inclusion, which consists of four subscales called Advantages and Disadvantages, Professional Issues, Philosophical Issues, and Logistical Concerns; and Wilczenski (1995) has developed the Attitudes toward Inclusive Education Scale. Another tack that has been taken is to evaluate the entire program's approach to inclusive education rather than focusing on individuals. Vantre (2001) developed the Marsh Inclusion Scale, which seeks to evaluate the degree to which programs adhere to best practices in implementing inclusion in a reliable and valid way, and Becker, Roberts, and Dumas (2000) developed The Inclusion Inventory, which is meant to survey educators' perceptions of inclusive educational practices in their school.

Sensory Functioning

Although the child possesses five basic senses, only two, and possibly three, are of concern here. These are audition, vision, and possibly the tactile sense, given the increased use of tactile devices (Table 7–2). Obviously, any child who has been identified and certified as hard of hearing will have had an audiometric evaluation. Generally speaking, one would minimally expect an air conduction and (if possible) bone conduction pure tone audiogram (both aided and unaided), speech threshold, discrimination test results if possible, and some statement or objective test results concerning the youngster's candidacy for amplification. In addition, there may be reports of middle ear functioning, as determined by immittance measures, and the results of any special testing that may be warranted by the child's particular case (see Chapter 3).

Although the child with hearing loss should have undergone a thorough audiological evaluation, the child's functional use of residual hearing may still be unknown. To fulfill a need in this area, the Test of Audi-

Table 7–2. Psychoeducational Assessment: Sensory Functioning

Audition	*Vision*	*Taction*

1. Hearing sensitivity
  a) Pure tone
    Audiogram (a/c + b/c)
  b) Speech detection/reception
  c) Word discrimination
  d) Tests of middle ear functioning
  e) Results from hearing aid
    evaluation
  f) Special Test
 	
2. Auditory perception
  a) Test of Auditory
    Comprehension
  b) Developmental Approach to
    Successful Listening, II
	1. Visual acuity
	  a) Snellen chart
	  b) Keystone Telebinocular
	  c) Bausch and Lomb Orthorator
	  d) Titmus Vision Screener
	
	2. Visual motor perception
	  a) Bender-Gestalt Test for Young
	    Children
	  b) Graham and Kendall Memory
	    for Designs Test
	  c) Developmental Test of
	    Visual–Motor Integration
	  d) Rey's Complex Figure Drawing
	
	3. Motor-free tests of visual
	perception
	  a) Embedded Figures Test
	  b) Perceptual Speed Identical Form
	    Test
	  c) Ratner's Test of Visual
	    Perceptual Abilities
	  d) Ratner's Test of Spatial
	    Perception in Sign Language
		No tests available

tory Comprehension (TAC) (Office of Los Angeles County Superintendent of Schools, 1976), and the Developmental Assessment of Successful Listening II (DASL-II) (Stout & Windle, 1992) were developed, each of which includes both a listening curriculum and an evaluation component. Although the Miami Cochlear Implant, Auditory and Tactile Skills Curriculum: CHATS (Serrano-Miranda, 1999) does not have its own assessment battery, the author does review the assessment tools available for children with hearing loss. Additionally, Geers (1994) has discussed techniques for assessing auditory speech perception and lip-reading enhancement in young deaf children. The tests associated with the TAC and DASL-II were designed to evaluate the functional auditory status of children with moderate to profound hearing loss along the continuum of auditory skill development.

More specifically, in the case of the TAC, the test was designed to assess the auditory discrimination of suprasegmentals and segmentals, memory sequencing, story compre-

hension, and figure-ground discrimination of children with hearing impairments ages 4 to 12 years, 11 months. The test was designed to be used as both a criterion-referenced, curriculum-based test in conjunction with its companion auditory training curriculum, as well as a norm-referenced test.

Although there were some technical problems in the selection of a standardization sample, the reliability and validity data presented in the manual suggest that this test and its associated auditory training curriculum may be useful. Additionally, according to the manual, because substantial and positive correlation were obtained between scores on this test and functioning within different types of educational settings, this test may be useful in making placement decisions.

As a part of the DASL-II, a test is provided that has been designed to place a child within the curriculum and, thus, is to be used as a criterion-referenced, not a norm-referenced, test. The curriculum placement test has three parts that correspond to the curriculum against which it is referenced. The three areas evaluated are sound awareness, phonetic listening, and auditory comprehension.

Earlier in the history of the psychology of deafness, Myklebust (1960) proposed the *organismic shift hypothesis* to address whether deaf and hard-of-hearing individuals come to rely on and use their remaining senses, particularly vision, in a compensatory way. Since then, this hypothesis has been debated. Bolton (1978), for example, performed a factor analysis of the Hiskey-Nebraska Test of Learning Aptitude and suggested that the factor patterns were consistent with this hypothesis; whereas others, such as Moores (2001), have rejected the notion of the organismic shift hypothesis and have suggested that individuals with hearing loss are no different than individuals with hearing. More recently, with the increased interest in the visual and neurolinguistic processing of various indigenous signed languages, such as American Sign Language (ASL), there has been renewed interest in the differential use of vision and visual processing and Myklebust's organismic shift hypothesis. Collectively, these studies have suggested that, although no differences exist between individuals who have hearing and those who are congenitally deaf in processing information in central vision, significant differences exist in the sensitivity and range of processing information in the periphery of vision (Swisher, 1993) that cannot be explained on the basis of sign language alone (Proksch & Bavelier, 2002). Differences in visual search patterns (Stivalet, Moreno, Richard, Barraud, & Raphel, 1998), processing of motion (Armstrong, Neville, Hillyard, & Mitchell, 2002), and selectively processing a target while ignoring distracters, in favor of individuals with hearing loss (Bosworth, 2001), have been found as well.

The reported incidence of visual problems among individuals who have hearing losses has ranged from 6% (Wolff & Harkins, 1986) to slightly more than 50% (Lawson & Myklebust, 1970). Although this range is large, there exists general agreement that the inci-

dence of visual problems is greater for individuals with hearing impairment than for individuals with normal hearing.

Many of these visual problems do not appear to be sensitivity problems. Greene (1978), for example, using a sophisticated in-depth optometric clinical screening program, noted that the combined categories of binocularity problems and pathological states were greater than all of the categories of refractive errors. Greene also commented on the inefficiency of the typical screening programs that consist of only the Snellen chart. The Snellen chart could account for the identification of only 23% of his sample of children with visual and hearing impairments. He further noted that other typical vision screening instruments, such as the Keystone Telebinocular, the Bausch and Lomb Orthorator, and the Titmus Vision Screener, although improvements over the simple Snellen chart, are still incomplete. Thus he recommended a complete optometric clinical screening program.

As noted previously, some children failing vision tests might do so not because of acuity problems, but rather because of some form of "perceptual" problem. Essentially, a perceptual problem is one in which the person is unable to be aware of (as opposed to sense), organize, or understand particular stimuli. Thus, although the sense receptor is intact, the individual is unable to understand or has difficulty in processing the visual stimulus. This difficulty apparently can be a function of the individual, the stimulus structure, or the interaction of the two. Occasionally, the term "visual perceptual problem," as used by some psychologists and other special service providers, refers to difficulty in visual–motor integration. That is, this "perceptual problem" manifests itself in the inability to copy specified designs or figures. Actually, the inability to complete such a task may be due either to difficulties in visually analyzing and organizing stimuli or to the execution of the motor act in making a visual motor match. In terms of the former, Locher and Worms (1977) have suggested that visual perceptual difficulties, when they occur, may in fact result from difficulties in focusing or regulating, rather than from an actual visual disability. Such inappropriate scanning of the visual stimulus would not permit the youngster to extract effectively all the necessary information to respond adequately to the task.

Among the most common visual motor tasks used by psychologists in their assessments of children are the Bender-Gestalt Test for Young Children (Bender-Gestalt), the Graham and Kendall Memory for Designs Test, and the Developmental Test of Visual Motor Integration (VMI). Salvia and Ysseldyke (2001) have indicated that most tests of visual motor perception lack the technical adequacy to be used in making important instructional decisions. Despite this, these tests are often used in the evaluation of most children, including children with hearing impairments, and they have been used in various research projects. Generally speaking, when a child is found to have a deficit in this area, it is usually interpreted to mean that the child has either a legitimate visual motor or visual perception problem, possibly symptomatic of "minimal brain damage," or emotional difficulties and anxieties. Unfortunately, there is little empirical evidence to support these claims for most of these tests. This is not to suggest that such "causes" are not possible.

A few of these instruments have been used in research projects with individuals having hearing loss with inconsistent results. Although many individuals with hearing impairment perform poorly on the Bender-Gestalt Test, Keogh, Vernon, and Smith (1970) have found the interjudge reliability scoring of these drawings to be very poor. Interestingly, in contrast to the findings of poor visual motor integration, conflicting results have been reported for these and other such "perceptual" tests, which may be due to the unreliability of the tests themselves. As a result, these tests should probably only be used as a rough screening instrument, and only grossly deviant reproductions should be considered abnormal.

The fact that visual perceptual functioning is difficult to assess does not detract from its possible importance. Sharp (1972) attempted to isolate the visual perceptual correlates of speech-reading in children by comparing the performance of good and poor speech-readers on various measures of visual perceptual and visual perceptual speed tasks. She found that performances on the Porteus Mazes, the Visual Sequential Memory subtest of the Illinois Test of Psycholinguistic Abilities (ITPA), which is a memory task involving geometric designs, and three tests specially designed by the researcher (Rhythm Patterns: A Test of Movement, the Hidden Figures Test, and the Hidden Objects Test) were all related to good speech-reading ability. The latter two tests were essentially figure-ground tests. These results, then, suggest that visual memory for movement, rhythm perception, speed of visual perception, and figure-ground ability are associated with speech-reading ability. To date, there have been relatively few studies investigating the visual perceptual correlates of sign language ability and acquisition. Siple, Hatfield, and Caccamise (1978) in a longitudinal study at the National Technical Institute for the Deaf, investigated the visual perceptual correlates of sign language acquisition by students with hearing loss. Two different sets of predictors were isolated. For the students who were deaf with poor initial sign language scores, improvement in sign language ability was significantly associated with initial scores on a rapid visual perceptual discrimination test (Perceptual Speed Identical Form Test) and the Embedded Figures Test. The predictors of progress for the individuals who used sign language as their primary mode of communication were initial performances on the Flags Test, involving spatial manipulation, and the Visual Closure Speed Test, which assesses the speed at which an individual can recognize or infer a whole from minimal cues. These results suggested to the investigators that the individuals with deafness acquired facility in sign language by attending to details and analyzing the whole, whereas individuals with normal hearing used a process of synthesizing whole patterns and gestalts.

Recently, Ratner (1988) developed two tests designed to evaluate the visual perceptual abilities of children who are deaf as they might relate to the visual processing of sign language. The Test of Spatial Perception in Sign Language (TSPSL) is a 47-item videotaped test designed to evaluate the ability to discern various dynamic features and aspects of signs. The second test, The Test of Visual Perceptual Abilities (TVPA), is divided into two parts: Part I consists of six subtests evaluating various aspects of static visual perception, and Part II consists of six subtests designed to evaluate certain dynamic properties associated with visual perception. Both tests were shown to identify individuals with visual perceptual deficits that interfere with sign language comprehension and that each subtest of the TVPA tapped different visual perceptual abilities and contributed separately and differently to performance on the TSPSL.

Cognition (Intelligence)

The intent of testing in this domain is to obtain general and specific measures of intelligence, creativity, and the mode of internalized mediation. The intelligence tests most widely used with individuals with hearing impairments are shown in Table 7–3.

Only the Hiskey-Nebraska Test of Learning Aptitude was specifically designed for and standardized on the population with hearing impairments. Although a few other scales standardized on individuals with hearing impairments are available, the Hiskey-Nebraska and several tests not standardized on persons with hearing impairments are in much greater use in this country. The Leiter Scale was not standardized on the population with hearing loss, but it does not require verbal instructions. The Leiter-R and some other tests of cognitive functioning of recent vintage have included samples of deaf and hard-of-hearing individuals in the standardization population. As already noted, the fact that certain groups of individuals have been included in the standardization population does not automatically make the test valid for those population of

Table 7–3. Psychoeducational Assessment: Cognition (Intelligence)

Tests Available

1. Wechsler Scales
   Preschool and Primary Scale of Intelligence
   Preschool and Primary Scale of Intelligence-R
   Preschool and Primary Scale of Intelligence III
   Intelligence Scale for Children (WISC)
   Intelligence Scale for Children–Revised (WISC-R)
   Intelligence Scale for Children–III (WISC-III)
   Adult Intelligence Scale (WAIS)
   Adult Intelligence Scale–Revised (WAIS-R)
   Adult Intelligence Scale III (WAIS III)
2. Hiskey-Nebraska Test of Learning Aptitude*
3. Harris-Goodenough Draw-A-Man
4. Leiter International Performance Scales
5. Leiter International Performance Scale–Arthur Adpation
6. Leiter International Performance Scale–Revised
7. Raven's Colored Progressive Matrices
8. Naglieri's Nonverbal Matrix Test
9. Kaufman Assessment Battery Test for Children
10. Learning Potential Assessment Device
11. Torrance Test of Creative Thinking
12. Test for Internal Recoding

*This is the only intelligence test specifically designed for and standardized on individuals with hearing losses.

individuals from which the samples were drawn.

The Wechsler Scales probably have been the most researched instrument used with the population of individuals with hearing loss. Presumably, because of its popularity, norms for individuals with hearing loss were developed for the WISC-R (Anderson & Sissco, 1977). These norms are not applicable to other versions of the Wechsler Scales. Thus, if one wanted to have a direct comparison of an individual's test results with a normative sample of individuals with hearing loss, one is restricted to using the WISC-R.

More recently two new versions of this test have been published, the WISC-III and its successor the WISC-IV. Although the manual of the WISC-III states that 7% of the standardization sample included learning disabled, emotionally disturbed, and physically disabled individuals, no individual with hearing loss was included. Because of its newness, separate norms have yet to be developed for this test, if they will be at all. The WISC-IV version has changed the overall structure of the Wechsler tests in that it has dropped the Picture Arrangement subtest and has made the Arithmetic and Information scales, which are school-based oriented, simply optional rather than mandatory.

The Wechsler tests consist of two scales, each containing a series of subtests. The two scales are a Verbal Scale, in which sets of verbal questions are posed to the examinee, and a Performance Scale involving various manipulation tasks. More precisely, the verbal scales are comprised of the following subtests (see Table 7–4):

1. Information (optional in the WISC-IV), which requires the subject to answer factual, academic-type questions
2. Comprehension, which involves answering open-ended questions concerning various social conventions, institutions, practices, and procedures, requiring one to make explicit one's social and cultural awareness and knowledge of norms within the United States, social problem solving, practical knowledge, and social judgment
3. Similarities, which asks the individual to induce a superordinate term, such as dishes, when given the two subordinate terms, such as cup and saucer, and requires the understanding of semantic, or conceptual, entailments
4. Arithmetic (optional in WISC-IV), requiring the solution of orally presented story problems
5. Vocabulary, which asks the individual to define words, involving verbal preciseness and the understanding of and ability to articulate semantic entailments
6. Digit span (optional), in which the subject has to recall a series of digits presented orally
7. Sentences [only on the Wechsler Preschool and Primary Scale of Intelligence (WPPSI) and the revised WPPSI (WPPSI-R)], in which the subject has to repeat sentences of increasing length and syntactic difficulty
8. Word Reasoning, in which the child is asked to identify the underlying concept when given successive clues
9. Letter-Number Sequencing (WAIS-III and WISC-IV), in which the individual is presented with a mixed series of numbers and letters and is to repeat the numbers back first, in numerical order, and then the letters in alphabetical order, which measures aspects of working memory

The performance scales consist of the following subscales:

1. Picture Completion, requiring the individual to identify missing parts of familiar objects, involving object knowledge and the ability to recognize and distinguish essential from nonessential details
2. Picture Arrangement, requiring the individual to sequence a series of pictures so as to tell a sensible story involving event knowledge, the understanding of social conventions and cause and effect relationships, and the ability to note details (neither the WPPSI, the WPPSI-R, or the WPPSI-III have this subtest and it has been eliminated in the WISC-IV)
3. Block Designs, which requires the individual to copy mosaic designs utilizing a series of multicolored block cubes and involves visual analysis and the ability to note part-to-whole relationships
4. Object Assembly, which is a type of jigsaw puzzle task of familiar objects and involves visual synthesis and the ability to note part-to-whole relationships (neither the WPPSI, the WPPSI-R, nor the WPPSI-III have this subtest)
5. Coding (called Animal House in the WPPSI, WPPSI-R, and WPPSI-III), which is a symbol-association task whereby the individual is, for example, to draw a simple design underneath a series of randomly distributed numbers based on a key that is provided, involv-

Table 7–4. Subtests of the Wechsler Tests

Subtest	WAIS and WAIS-R	WAIS-III	WISC and WISC-R	WISC-III	WISC-IV	WPPSI and WPPSI-R	WPPSI-III
Verbal							
Information	X	X	X	X	X	X	X
Comprehension	X	X	X	X	X	X	X
Similarities	X	X	X	X	X	X	X
Arithmetic	X	X	X	X	X	X	X
Vocabulary	X	X	X	X	X	X	X
Digit Span	X	X	X	X	X		
Word Reasoning					X		
Letter-Number Sequencing		X			X		
Sentences					X	X	X
Performance							
Picture Completion	X	X	X	X	X	X	X
Picture Arrangement	X	X	X	X			
Block Designs	X	X	X	X	X	X	X
Object Assembly	X	X	X	X	X		
Coding	X	X	X	X	X	X	X
Mazes	X	X	X	X		X	X
Symbol Search		X		X	X		
Matrix Reasoning		X		X			X
Picture Concepts					X		X
Cancellation					X		X
Geometric Design						X	X

ing the ability to make rapid symbol associations

6. Mazes (optional), which requires the individual to trace through a series of mazes requiring, impulse control, forethought, and planning ability. (This has been eliminated from the WISC-IV)

7. Symbol Search (WAIS-III, WISC-III, WISC-IV), which requires the individual to determine whether one of two geometric designs is present in an array of four geometric drawings, requiring systematic visual search and speed of processing

8. Geometric Designs (WPSSI, WPSSI-R, and WPPSI only), which requires the individual to copy geometric designs, similar to the Bender Gestalt Test of Visual Perception, requiring visual perceptual analysis and visual motor integration

9. Matrix Reasoning (WAIS-III, WPPSI-III, WISC-IV) in which the child is presented with a partially filled grid and asked to select the item that properly completes the matrix similar to the Raven's progressive matrices

10. Picture Concepts (WISC-IV), in which the child selects objects that go together based on an underlying concept from each of two or three rows of objects that measures fluid reasoning, percep-

tual organization, and categorization, and requires categorical reasoning without a verbal response

11. Cancellation (WISC-IV) measures processing speed using random and structured animal target forms; foils are common nonanimal objects

Because there are two scales and a number of subtests each yielding their own scores, it is possible to have interscale and subtest comparisons on an individual and to engage in profile analyses to determine relative strengths and weakness. Indeed, this practice was and is so pervasive that the author of the WPPSI-III, WISC-III and WISC-IV, and WAIS-III, as a part of the statistical treatment of the normative data, has provided a series of significant difference, frequency, and scatter tables and developed a series of Index Scores based on factor analytic models of the test. These indexes for the WISC-III and WISC-IV are Verbal Comprehension (the composite of Information, Similarities, Vocabulary, and Comprehension); Perceptual Organization (Picture Completion, Picture Arrangement, Block Designs, and Object Assembly); Freedom from Distractibility (Arithmetic and Digit Span); and Speed of Processing (Coding and Symbol Search). Care, however, must be taken when performing such analyses and comparisons, even in the case of the WISC-III and WISC-IV wherein there is much greater technical adequacy, because serious placement and intervention system decisions may be based on unreliable, chance, or error factors. Taking this point into account, however, the Wechsler tests still permit one to observe an individual's performance under several conditions, and it is the only test mentioned in this chapter that permits the comparison of both verbal and nonverbal performances.

For individuals with hearing loss, it has become almost axiomatic that the verbal sections of these tests are considered invalid measures of intellectual abilities because they are assumed to be testing language and language functioning opposed to inherent intellectual or cognitive abilities. (Henceforth, any reference to any of the Wechsler scales will refer to the Performance section only unless otherwise stated.) Although it may be true that failure to perform on the Verbal Scale of these tests might be due to a failure to understand specific questions or other related language factors, rather than a lack of more basic cognitive skills required to acquire the necessary information, the ability to score well on this test is still highly correlated with and related to academic achievement. As a result, it would be very helpful to obtain Verbal Scale scores, whenever and however possible, to assess the ability of persons with hearing impairments to compete verbally with hearing peers. Such scores should properly be treated as verbal achievement scores and reported in the language or academic achievement section of any psychoeducational report. It has been demonstrated that there can be as large as a 16 to 44 IQ point difference between the overall performance scores and verbal scores on these scales for middle childhood to adolescent children who are hard of hearing (Hine, 1970) and adults with congenital deafness (Myklebust, 1960; Ross, 1970). Most recently, in a study using the WISC-III, a group of 30 children with severe to profound deafness in which the verbal section of the Wechsler scale was communicated via ASL or Pidgin Signed English, as warranted, presented a 25.7 IQ point discrepancy between the Verbal and Performance Scales in favor of the latter (Wechsler, 1991). The discrepancy between verbal and performance scores has been noted to be greater for students with congenital deafness than for children who are hard of hearing or who have postlingual deafness (Smith, 1962). It should be pointed out that Hine (1970) found the Picture Arrangement subtest correlated best with the results of the Verbal Scale. This correlation, although low, was positive and statistically significant.

A number of studies have attempted to determine whether youngsters and adults with hearing loss performed as well on the Wechsler performance tests as individuals with normal hearing, and whether a characteristic profile of subtest performance could be identified. The majority of these studies have found little or no difference between the overall performances of the two populations. The composite results of these studies suggest that a characteristic profile of subtest performance for the population with hearing impairments may exist. This composite profile seems to have the following characteristics:

1. Performance on the Picture Completion subtest varies from slightly less than the hearing mean to slightly above it.
2. Performance on the Picture Arrangement subtest varies from no difference to slightly less than the hearing mean.
3. Performance on the Block Designs subtest ranges from no difference to slightly above the hearing mean.
4. Performance on the Object Assembly subtest ranges from the hearing mean to slightly above it.
5. Performance on the Coding subtest ranges from no difference to slightly below the hearing mean.

In a meta-analysis of 25 studies using the Wechsler scales, Braden (1990) derived weighted mean scale scores of 9.4, 9.3, 9.9, 9.9, and 8.8, respectively, for these subtests. As can be seen, these mean scores tend to mirror the relative profile previously suggested, although only the mean scale score for coding was found to be significantly deviant. Thus Braden suggested that only poor performance on this subtest should be considered characteristic of the population with deafness. As Braden noted, however, these weighted mean scores included the results of four studies that used the WISC-R deaf norms that would "wash out" any characteristic profile information and would serve to depress the overall differences. Slate and Fawcett (1995) conducted a factor analysis of the performance scales of the WISC-III. Two factors emerged, Perceptual Organization and Processing Speed, which accounted for 76.5% of the variance in the WISC-III Performance IQ. The WISC-IV is so new it is yet unclear as to whether subtest patterns will emerge because no studies have been conducted. Additionally, as noted earlier, one very useful subtest, Picture Arrangement, has been eliminated, though several new and very promising subscales have been added (e.g., Word Reasoning, Matrix Reasoning, Picture Concepts, and Letter-Numbering Sequencing, in particular).

The previously mentioned profile appears to be more evident with the younger children with deafness and is statistically controlled for in the norms provided by Anderson and Sissco (1977) for the WISC-R. Ray (1980) has challenged the utility of these norms because they were compiled post hoc and no attempt was made to control for standardization of the administration procedures. Sullivan (1982) argued that the previously mentioned profile was an artifact of test administration modifications. Thus norms are available, but they are not standardized. Some investigators have attempted to determine the reliability, validity, and utility of the Wechsler scales with individuals with hearing impairments.

Similarly, scores on the WISC-R performance IQ (PIQ) correlate moderately well and, thus, predict to some degree scores on the Stanford Achievement Test for the Hearing Impaired (SAT-HI) (Kelly & Braden, 1990). Correlations between WISC-R PIQ and percentile ranks on the SAT-HI ranged from 0.33 (spelling) to 0.57 (concept number). Reading Comprehension on the SAT-HI correlated 0.39 with the WISC-R PIQ. It has also been noted that comparable results are obtained when youngsters at the upper age limits of the WISC-R are subsequently evaluated using the WAIS-R (Braden & Paquin, 1985).

The Hiskey-Nebraska Test of Learning Aptitude is the only commonly used test of intelligence designed specifically for the population in this country with hearing loss. Because of this, some individuals have used it as the standard against which other tests are measured. The test has 12 subtests (many of which involve visual memory) and two sets of directions and norms (i.e., verbal directions and hearing norms, and pantomime directions and d/Deaf or hard of hearing norms). Salvia and Ysseldyke (2001), in reviewing the technical adequacy of the test, note several limitations and suggest that the results should be interpreted with caution.

Despite this fact, it has been reported that the Hiskey-Nebraska scores correlate highly with such various measures of academic success as the Stanford Achievement Test, the Gates Reading Test, the Metropolitan Achievement Test, and teacher ratings of academic achievement in the early elementary years, but not during the middle school and adolescent years (e.g., grades 5 to 9) (Giancreco, 1966) and the Peabody Individual Achievement Tests (Watson, Goldgar, Kroese, & Lotz, 1986). Also, the Hiskey Learning Quotient (LQ) score and those subtests stressing visual memory have been found to be moderately predictive of performance on the Test of Language Development and the Reynell Developmental Language Scales administered via total communication (Humphrey, 1976); and it has been noted that the Block Patterns, Paper Folding, Picture Association, and Visual Attention Span subtests, in particular, are predictive of academic achievement with 6- to 12-year-old orally trained children with deafness (Birch, Stuckless, & Birch, 1963).

The Leiter International Performance Scale and its Arthur adaptation have been used to assess the individual with hearing impairment and have been found to be highly predictive of academic achievement, as defined by teacher ratings and performance on tests of reading, despite their technical inadequacy (Salvia & Yssledyke, 2001). This relationship has even held up longitudinally over an 11- to 13-year period (Birch et al, 1963). Bonham (1974) found the Leiter, in combination with the WISC, to be an exceptionally good predictor of success in the reading comprehension subtests of the Metropolitan Achievement Test. The Leiter was designed to be used with individuals with speech and language difficulties, ages 2 to 18 years, and was standardized on a hearing sample. The Arthur adaptation is identical to the original Leiter but is only appropriate for children ages 2 to 12 years. There are no subtests to these tests; instead, they consist of a series of graduated but essentially unrelated tasks. To facilitate test interpretation, Levine, Allen, and Alker, et al (1974) have suggested an item classification scheme. Although the Leiter has been found to be predictive of academic achievement and appears to be sensitive to learning problems, Ratcliffe and Ratcliffe (1979) warn that caution should be exercised in decisions of placement because a few studies using both hearing and youngsters with hearing impairments have found as much as an 11- to 20-point (or greater) discrepancy between scores on this instrument and other tests of intellectual ability, due to technical inadequacies.

Recently the Leiter has been revised and has taken a totally new and different approach than that of its predecessor. The Leiter-R (Roid & Miller, 1997) consists of two groups of subtests: the visualization and reasoning (VR) battery with 10 subtests of nonverbal intellectual ability related to visualization, reasoning, and spatial memory; and the attention and memory (AM) battery with 10 subtests of nonverbal attention and memory function. There are also four rating scales (examiner, parent, self, and teacher), which provide behavioral observation information about the individual. It yields deviation IQ scores rather than a calculated ratio IQ score and permits subtest analysis because separate scores are obtained for each of the subscales and their composite: Reasoning (classification, sequential order, repeated patterns, and design analogies); Visualization (matching, picture context, figure-ground, paper folding, form completion, figure rotation); Memory (memory span, spatial memory, associative memory, immediate recognition, memory span reversed, visual coding, associative delayed memory, and delayed recognition); and Attention (attention sustained and attention divided). As can be seen, many of these subscales are redundant with other tests, such as the WISC-III and the Hiskey-Nebraska. The attention subtests, though, are of interest, particularly the attention-divided subscale.

The Standard Ravens Progressive Matrices and its revision, the Ravens Colored Progressive Matrices, have been used in a few research projects with individuals with hearing impairments, despite the fact that at the time the studies were conducted no norms were available in the United States (only European norms were available). As of 1986, however, norms have been available in the United States (Raven, 1986). In essence, the test involves the pattern completion of a number of items. The Ravens Colored Progressive Matrices have been described as tapping a special aspect of intelligence, and some believe that it measures pure "g" (global or general intelligence). Carlson (1973), however, provides data on children with hearing that suggest that on the Colored Progressive Matrices, sets A and AB evaluate perceptual pattern completion, whereas set B actually evaluates the ability to solve analogies by operations or rules. The composite picture from studies using the Ravens Colored Progressive Matrices with individuals having hearing loss suggests that younger children have difficulty with the test, but that by the time they become young adults, performance improves (Goetzinger, Wills, & Dekker, 1967). Ritter (1976) found essentially normal performance with younger children who are deaf and children with hearing impairments. He also found the Colored Progressive Matrices to correlate well with the Leiter and moderately well with the WISC, and James (1984) found a high correlation with the WISC-R.

In recent years, the Matrix Analogies Test—Expanded Form (RMT-EF), a well-constructed performance test involving the completion of various matrix analogies similar to the Raven Matrices Tests, has been developed (Naglieri, 1985). Unfortunately, few studies have been conducted with this test, although it does seem to hold promise. Naglieri and colleagues have found that for children with severe to profound deafness, performance on this test correlates well with the performance scale of the WISC-R ($r = 0.71$) (Naglieri & Bardos, 1988). For children 11 to 16 years old who are severely and profoundly deaf, performance on this test correlated well with performance on the Standard Progressive Matrices whether using Euro-

pean or U.S. norms (i.e., $r = 0.79$ for both) (Naglieri & Welch, 1991). Additionally, performance on this test did not differ from performance on the Standard Progressive Matrices using U.S. norms but both differed from scores derived from the European norms. Mean average performance results on these tests were as follows: 84.5 (RMT-EF), 84.7 (Raven's U.S. norms), and 89.7 (Raven's European norms). The lower overall performance on these tests is consistent with earlier studies and may be related to difficulty in handling multiple sources of information simultaneously, as suggested by Ottem (1980).

Historically, the use of the Stanford Binet for individuals with hearing loss was considered ill advised, given that it was ostensively a test of verbal knowledge. In addition, like the Leiter, earlier versions of the Binet contained no subtests, but rather were composed of a series of graduated, but essentially unrelated, tasks. The fourth and most recent edition, however, represents a substantial departure from this approach in that it is organized according to a series of verbal and performance subscales. Although no research has been conducted investigating the utility of this instrument with individuals with hearing loss, it does hold promise, given its technical adequacy.

The last three tests of intelligence that have received some attention from researchers are the Harris-Goodenough Draw-A-Man test, the Kaufman Assessment Battery for Children (KABC) and the Test Of Nonverbal Intelligence–2 (TONI-2). Although some early studies using the Draw-A-Man test found that children with hearing loss perform poorly on this test, Myklebust (1960), in an extensive study of deaf children's performance on this test, found that children with hearing losses perform within average limits up to 13 years of age. After this age, decrement of performance to below average was found. As for the KABC, Porter and Kirby (1986) established that children with deafness, who were 7 to 12 years of age, did not differ in their performance from the normative sample, nor was performance affected by the use of pantomime directions or directions communicated via ASL. High correlations have been obtained between KABC scores and performance on the WISC-R, although KABC scores tend to be slightly lower than those on the WISC-R (Phelps & Branyan, 1990; Porter & Kirby, 1986). Moderate correlations have been obtained between KABC scores and those on the Metropolitan Achievement Test (Porter & Kirby, 1986) and on the Wide Range Achievement Test and the KABC reading subtests (Phelps & Branyan, 1990) for students who had hearing losses. Finally, Mackinson, Leigh, and Anthony (1997) established the construct validity of the TONI-2 by finding significant correlations between the TONI-2 and five of six WISC-III subtests; and established its predictive value in determining Stanford Achievement Test, eighth edition, scores in spelling and mathematical problem solving for a group of students who were deaf or hard of hearing.

The Learning Potential Assessment Device (Feuerstein, 1979), although composed of standard instruments or "tools," is not a standard test in the traditional sense. Rather, it is a collection of commercially available tests and some specially designed instruments for which no norms are reported or available. It is one of the newer instruments from the growing trend away from "static" norm-referenced tests toward dynamic measures of learning ability or potential (Andrianopoulos, 2001). The 16 (five verbal and 11 largely performative) instruments are to be used in a Test-Teach-Test paradigm, wherein the "teaching phase" is to follow the tenets of the author's theory of mediated learning, which is similar to and borrows heavily from the work of Vygotsky (1978).

Mediated learning in this context emphasizes that the role of the examiner is one of assisting the child to regulate metacognitively the input, elaboration, and output phases of the child's information processing, and to guide and provoke the use of appropriate learning strategies that will, it is hoped, generalize or transcend to other stimuli and events. (Pedagogically and in

terms of language development, this has been referred to as scaffolding.) The extent to which this can be done is a measure of the child's modifiability and potential for learning. Keane and Kretschmer (1987) reported on the application of this technique and noted its superiority in assessing the learning potential of children with deafness over that of traditional psychometric approaches and even dynamic approaches that provide feedback.

The Torrance Test of Creative Thinking is a test of cognitive functioning. More precisely, it purports to measure an individual's flexibility, fluency, originality, and elaborative skills of thinking. Both verbal and performative tasks are available. Laughton (1988) recommended that the Torrance Thinking Creatively with Pictures, Form A be included with the routine battery used to evaluate children with hearing loss. In her study of children having hearing loss, several scores derived from this measure were found to predict the development of morphological, phrase structure, and transformation rule usage. The originality score in particular predicted usage of all the linguistic structures studied, and the elaboration score aided in the prediction of morphological rule development. Kaltsounis (1970) has demonstrated that children with hearing loss performed as well on this test as did children who can hear, and average to superior performance on the nonverbal form has been supported by other studies (e.g., Silver, 1977).

One of the implicit purposes in formal testing of intelligence and cognition is to gain some insights into the thinking and problem-solving abilities of the examinee. Of particular interest are insights into the examinee's ability to handle symbolic material because they may reveal information about the examinee's mediational processes and capacity to handle symbols in general. Occasionally, the results of some of the more symbolically oriented nonverbal subtests on intelligence tests (e.g., the Picture Arrangement and Coding subtests on the Wechsler tests and the Picture Analogies or Picture

Association subtests on the Hiskey-Nebraska test) are used for this purpose. Although these tests give us insight into the child's ability to deal with symbolically oriented materials, they do not directly assess the mode of internal symbolic representation. Mode of internalized representation must be inferred from behavioral observations and the use of other test materials.

Recently, however, attempts have been made by some researchers to determine empirically the nature of the mediating process. Bellugi, Klima, and Siple (1974) and others have suggested that with children with deafness the mediating process involves the use of signs. Locke and Locke (1971) made the alternative suggestion that children who can hear and many children who are deaf but with intelligible speech tend to recode internally certain visually presented symbolic material phonetically. Children with deafness without intelligible speech have also been found to prefer a dactylic (finger spelling) or visual recording system. Hirsh-Pasek (1987) discussed the relationship between finger spelling and reading achievement. She noted that, although individuals who are deaf may not spontaneously use a finger spelling strategy to decode print, they can be taught such strategies. Recently, Ralston (2002) has developed a videotaped version of his Ralston Test of Fingerspelled Pseudowords (RTFP). In a study of college and postsecondary students, he confirmed that the RTFP subtests in combination with the WAIS-R Digit Span subtest, Peabody Individual Achievement Test–Revised Spelling, and WAIS-R verbal abilities could significantly distinguish the deficient word reader group from high and/or average word reader groups.

Conrad (1979) reported on a series of studies he conducted and argued that the use of a phonetic internal coding system probably is not an all or nothing matter, but rather exists in degrees. The use of a phonetic code by individuals with hearing loss, according to Conrad, is strongly associated with their use of external intelligible speech, a finding that has been supported by the work of Transler, Gombert, and Leybaert (2001). Conrad also

noted that many youngsters who have profound deafness and whose speech would be considered unintelligible use this code form. One possible explanation for this phenomenon is that the individual may have speech gestures for most if not all the phonemes in an oral language such as English, and may use these gestures consistently (Kretschmer, 1982). As a result, these speakers might initially be unintelligible to listeners but be intelligible to themselves. Hauser (2001), using electromyogram recordings of the covert behavior of mouth muscles, concluded that, although deaf American users of ASL are good readers and are relying on English phonemic encoding, they acquire phonetic features of English that are different from those in traditional phonology studies, which supports Kretschmer's contention.

Kretschmer (1982) also suggested that some individuals with hearing loss might be pseudophonetic encoders that are sensitive to the orthographic structure and regularities of print. This finding has been supported by Olson and Nickerson (2001) and Transler, Leybaert, and Gombert (1999)

Lichtenstein's (1985) research suggests that "syntactic skills (proper use of functors) were related to WM [working memory] capacity and to the ability to effectively use a speech-based coding strategy" (p. 113) and that those individuals who failed to recode morphological endings to speech generally demonstrated lowered general knowledge of morphology and had poorer syntactic skills than those who consistently recoded functors. Thus, "although the tendency to be selective in the recoding of free functors may be an adaptive strategy for coping with a limited working memory (WM) it may also effectively limit exposure to English grammatical information so as to cause serious gaps to develop in the student's knowledge of English syntax" (p. 113). Unfortunately, Lichtenstein did not elaborate on these points nor did he publish his stimuli, data, or analyses. However, given this general description, it is entirely possible that among the "functor" and morphological markers not recoded were critical phrase structure markers, cohesion devices, markers of new information, specifiers, modulators, deictic markers, adjuncts and disjuncts, all of which serve to bind text together and give it its richness, and which serve to signal various grammatical and pragmatic functions.

Conrad (1979) developed a testing procedure that he believes can discriminate between children who use a phonetic coding system and those who use a visual coding system. However, his test does not discriminate among individuals who might use other possible coding strategies (i.e., those who might prefer finger spelling, signs, or a combination of all possible internal codes). Kretschmer and Martello (1993) developed a screening test designed to identify the preferred mode of encoding (speech, sign, visual) of young individuals with hearing impairments. Obviously, there is a need for such tests and for further research into what determines mediation preferences. Such knowledge should help in the decision-making process regarding placement and programming for children with hearing impairments.

Language and Academic Achievement

Although this is probably one of the most important areas to be assessed, few studies, ironically, have been conducted using formal assessment techniques with individuals having hearing loss (Table 7–5). As noted in the Cognition (Intelligence) section of this chapter, the verbal scale of the Wechsler test has been used with children and adults with hearing loss under limited circumstances. Although very helpful in providing an index of the child's verbal understanding of the world, the results on this test do not specify more precisely the particular linguistic structures or lexical items (with a few exceptions) that the child knows. Ideally, in a full-language evaluation, all aspects of language functioning should be considered. This would include (1) communication modality preference; (2) articulation skills in terms of speech and signs; (3) knowledge and use of morphological rules of English and ASL, if appropriate; (4) knowledge and use of the syntactic rules of English and ASL, if appro-

priate; (5) vocabulary or semantic aspects of the language used; (6) pragmatic uses of language; and (7) ability to engage in metalinguistic behaviors such as making judgments of grammaticality, being able to paraphrase, dealing with the metaphorical use of language, and in the case of bilingual bicultural youngsters, preferences for, dominance, and abilities in a language other than English or signs.

To review all the possible issues and procedures associated with these topics is beyond the scope of this chapter. As a result, the reader will be referred to other resources when appropriate; for example, Ling (2002) describes in detail a procedure for assessing speech. Two very interesting approaches to assessing speech intelligibility have been developed by Monsen (1981) and Monsen and Moog (1988), which are based on listener responses to speech uttered by individuals who are deaf rather than ratings of intelligibility. Although the technical adequacy of these evaluative procedures has not been fully established, the work that has been done on them is encouraging in that interrespondent reliability is high (i.e., correlations above 0.9) as is concurrent validity (also correlations above 0.9 with a second measure of speech intelligibility).

Unlike English, the assessment of knowledge and use of ASL is still in its infancy. Only one procedure, thus far, has been developed to assess children's understanding and use of ASL, the American Sign Language Proficiency Assessment (ASL-PA) (Maller, Singleton, Supalla, & Wix, 1999). This procedure involves collecting a half-hour ASL sample on video from a child (between ages 6 and 12) across three separate discourse settings that are analyzed and scored by an assessor who is highly proficient in ASL as to the presence of various ASL features. After the language samples are scored, the child is assigned a proficiency rating of Level 1, 2, or 3. Preliminary reliability and validity have been obtained for the ASL-PA using a sample of 80 profoundly deaf children (ages 6 to 12) of varying ASL skill levels.

A number of evaluation instruments and techniques currently are available for the as-

Table 7–5. Psychoeducational Assessment: Language and Academic Achievement

Ability Assessed	Test
Articulation/intelligibility	Ling Speech Articulation Assessment* CID Picture SPINE*

Morphology and syntax	Berko Test of Morphology
	Berry Talbot Exploratory Test of Grammar
	Test of Examining Expressive Morphology
	Northwestern Syntax Screening Test
	Carrow Elicited Language Inventory
	Test of Auditory Comprehension of Language–Revised
	Miller-Yoder Language Comprehension
	Boehm Test of Basic Comprehension
	Bare Essentials in Assessing Really Little Kids—Concept Analysis Profile*
	Grammatical Analysis of Elicited Language*
	    Presentence
	    Simple
	    Complex
	Grammatical Closure Subtest of the Illinois Test of
	    Pyscholinguistic Abilities
	Teacher Assessment of Grammatical Structures*
	Rhode Island Test of Language Structure*
	SKI-HI Reception Language Test*
	Test of Expressive Language Ability*
	Test of Receptive Language Ability*
	Maryland Syntax Evaluation Instrument*
	Test of Syntactic Abilities *
	Clinical Evaluation of Language Fundamentals, 4th edition
	Analysis of Spontaneous Language Sample Procedure
	American Sign Language Proficiency Assessment

Lexical development	Peabody Picture Vocabulary Test–Revised Word Recognition Subtests of Achievement Tests Vocabulary Subtest of the Wechsler Scales Boehm Test of Basic Concepts Bare Essentials in Assessing Really Little Kids—Concept Analysis Profile* SKI-HI Receptive Language Test* Carolina Picture Vocabulary Test* Total Communication Receptive Vocabulary Test* Test of Word Knowledge
Pragmatics	Communication Intention Inventory Dore's List of Primitive Speech Acts Interpersonal Language Comprehension Test Dore's Taxonomy of Conversational Acts Test of Pragmatic Skills
General verbal ability and knowledge	Verbal Scale of the Wechsler Scales Test of Problem Solving

Interactive language	Informal
	    Parent interviews
	    Naturalistic observations
	    Standardized observations
	    Contained observations
	Formal
	    Bales Interactive Process Scales
	    Flanders Interactive Scales
	    Craig and Collins Analysis of Communicative Interaction
	    Cognitive Verbal/Nonverbal Observation Scale

Academic achievement	Stanford Achievement Test Battery Hearing Impaired Edition

*Tests and procedures designed for individuals with hearing losses.

sessment of syntactic and morphological rule knowledge of English. Cooper (1967) successfully administered the Berko test of morphology to a group of children with hearing loss. The Berko test attempts to assess the child's ability to generalize the use of certain inflectional endings and markers, such as the plural [s] or the regular past-tense marker [ed].

The grammatical closure subtest of the Illinois Test of Psycholinguistic Abilities (ITPA), the morphological closure of the ITPA-3, and the Berry Talbot Exploratory Test of Grammar are adaptations of this test and are commercially available. Three other tests that have been used with individuals with hearing loss are the Northwestern Syntax Screening Test (NSST), the Carrow Elicited Language Inventory, and the Boehm Test of Basic Concepts.

The NSST, as the name suggests, is a screening test of receptive and expressive language abilities. Only 40 syntactic structures are used in the test. The Carrow Elicited Language Inventory is meant to evaluate a slightly wider scope of linguistic constructions. The Boehm Test of Basic Concepts was developed to be a criterion-referenced test of certain beginning, academically related concepts (lexical items), and it involves concept identification, statement repetition and comprehension, and pattern awareness. The author of the test made no attempt to specify the linguistic constructions that are being evaluated, but a visual inspection of the items can easily reveal their nature. As might be expected, studies using these instruments have shown that individuals with hearing loss perform more poorly than their hearing counterparts (Davis, 1974; Geers & Moog, 1978; Pressnell, 1973). These tests, and the newest edition of the Boehm Test of Basic Concepts (Boehm Test of Basic Concepts–3), may be used as a type of criterion measure to identify specific language structures with which the individual may be having difficulty. It should be pointed out, however, that these instruments test only a very limited number of possible constructions, and, thus, give only a very narrow picture of the child's linguistic understanding and capacity. Other useful tests might be the Miller-Yoder Language Skills Assessment, the Preschool Language Assessment Instrument, the Test of Auditory Comprehension of Language–Revised, the Test for Examining Expressive Morphology and the Clinical Evaluation of Language Fundamentals, fourth edition, which is a very comprehensive evaluation procedure that evaluates language structure, language content, working memory, phonological awareness, rapid automatic naming, digit span, sequences, and word associations, and provides an observational rating scale and pragmatic profile.

The tests just mentioned have been standardized on individuals that have hearing. In recent years, a number of formal instruments have been developed for the population with hearing loss. As with tests normed on individuals that have hearing, these tests emphasize either receptive abilities or expressive abilities.

Receptive tests/scales include:

1. Bare Essentials in Assessing Really Little Kids—Concept Analysis Profile Summary (Hasenstab & Loughton, 1982), a spoken/signed, criterion-referenced test of certain lexical and semantic relational concepts for children with hearing loss ages 1 year, 6 months to 5 years

2. The Rhode Island Test of Language Structure (Engen & Engen, 1983), a test of receptive understanding of various syntactic constructions designed for d/Deaf or hard-of-hearing individuals ages 3 to 20 years, to be administered via total communication, and youngsters with normal hearing, ages 3 to 6 years

3. SKI-HI Receptive Language Test (Longhurst & Briery, 1975), a criterion-referenced test designed to assess 3- to 6-year-old children with hearing loss for the ability to understand various semantic relationships that increase one element at a time

4. Teacher Assessment of Grammatical Structures (Moog & Kozak, 1983), a series of criterion-referenced checklists

designed to assess the receptive and productive use of various morphological and grammatical structures of children with hearing loss ages 0 to 9 years

5. Test of Receptive Language Ability (Bunch, 1981), a normed, referenced test designed to assess 7- to 12-year-old children with hearing loss for the ability to understand 12 morphological and grammatical structures via print

6. The Test of Syntactic Abilities (Quigley, Steinkamp, Powers, & Jones, 1978), a normed and criterion-referenced paper-and-pencil test designed to screen and test in depth 10- to 19-year-old children with hearing loss for the understanding of nine major areas of syntactic structure in English (i.e., negation, conjunction, determiners, question formation, verb processes, pronominalization, relativization, complementation, and nominalization). From a technical standpoint, this test is the most well constructed of all those normed on those with hearing. Norms for normally hearing youngsters are also available.

Expressive tests/scales include:

1. The Grammatical Analysis of Elicited Language Pre-sentence Level (Moog, Kozak, & Geers, 1983), Simple Sentence (Moog & Geers, 1979), and Complex Sentence Levels (Moog & Geers, 1980), a set of three normed referenced tests on orally taught children with hearing impairments, ages 3 to 5 years, 11 months; 5 to 8 years, 11 months; and 8 to 11 years, 11 months, respectively, with norms available for the Simple Sentence Level when administered via total communication, using a format similar to that of the Carrow Elicited Language Inventory, with the exception that the various activities or tasks are structured so that they are a natural consequence of the object manipulation or pictorial context

2. The Maryland Syntax Evaluation Instrument (White, 1981), a normed referenced test for children who are deaf, ages 6 years to 11 years, 11 months, wherein individuals are to write sentences in response to pictures presented on a filmstrip

3. Test of Expressive Language Ability (Bunch, 1981), a normed referenced test for 7- to 12-year-old children with hearing loss, designed to assess the written control of 13 morphological and grammatical structures

Of these three, the Grammatical Analysis of Elicited Languages tests are the most technically adequate.

Another procedure that has gained acceptance is the use of analysis of spontaneous language samples. In this procedure, a corpus, or sample, of spontaneous language is elicited from the child and a grammatical, semantic, or pragmatic analysis of the production is made using some a priori classification scheme. A number of these schemes are available and are quite powerful in their ability to describe the expressive language abilities of individuals (e.g., Bloom & Lahey, 1978; Kretschmer & Kretschmer, 1978; Tyack & Venable, 1998). Each of these was designed to evaluate the oral English production of children. The only procedure currently available to assess the spontaneous signing ability of students with hearing loss is the ASL-PA (Maller et al, 1999). The procedure offered by Bloom and Lahey has the added advantage that the results can be referenced against a developmental scope and sequence chart that serves as an implicit curriculum, though the information is in need of updating.

Unlike syntax, which is thought to be composed of a finite number of rules that, hypothetically, could be evaluated exhaustively, lexical development is in principle infinite. As a result, it would be virtually impossible to obtain a complete inventory of the child's vocabulary. A number of receptive vocabulary tests that have been standardized on the hearing population are available. One such test is the Peabody Picture Vocabulary Test (PPVT) and its revisions PPVT-R and PPVT-III. All of these tests generally follow the same format. A word is spoken and the examinee is expected to select the appropriate corresponding picture. When administered to individuals with hearing loss in the prescribed fashion, the test becomes as much a test of speech-reading and auditory processing as a test of vocabulary. If a simultaneous form of communication is used, inflated scores may often result, given the iconic nature of the signs that may induce a correct response without actual lexical knowledge of the English word. Similarly, problems arise if the items are administered via finger spelling or presented in a written format because the tests were not intended to be used this way. As a result, tests like the PPVT (-R, -III) have limited value with many individuals with hearing loss. Presumably for this reason, two tests of signed vocabulary following the PPVT (-R, -III) format have been designed for use with children who are deaf: the Carolina Picture Vocabulary Test (Layton & Holmes, 1985), designed for use with children who are deaf, ages 4 years to 11 years, 6 months, and the Total Communication Receptive Vocabulary Test (Scherer, 1981), designed for 3- to 12-year-old children with hearing loss. Of the two tests, the former is more technically adequate.

Yet another index of vocabulary development that does not involve any task modification is the use of word recognition subtests of various achievement tests, such as the SAT-HI. However, such tests tap only one aspect of lexical knowledge (i.e., knowledge of the printed word). A relatively new test on the market, the Test of Word Knowledge (Wigg & Secord, 1993) alternatively attempts to evaluate eight different aspects of word knowledge (Expressive Vocabulary, Receptive Vocabulary, Word Definitions, Word Opposites, Synonyms, Multiple Meanings, Figurative Usages, and the understanding of language structure through the use of Conjunctions and Transition Words).

Interest in pragmatics is of only recent vintage, relatively speaking. Pragmatics has to do with the uses to which language is put and the manner in which it is organized in discourse for social purposes, whereas mathetics has to do with those uses of language for learning about the world.

For the most part, the area of pragmatic assessment is dominated by: (1) various assessment inventories of communicative intent with little attention to assessing the appropriateness of these intents in meeting various felicity conditions, (2) assessments of discourse structure, and (3) the use of cohesion devices as defined by Halliday and Hasan (1976). One problem associated with assessments of discourse structure is that there is a plethora of possible discourse genres that have not been fully explored or developed into various taxonomies or inventories.

With regard to the communication inventories and assessment techniques, the following are most notable: the Communicative Intention Inventory (Coggins & Carpenter, 1981), an inventory designed to assess young children's (8 months to 2 years) nonverbal and verbal intents; Dore's list of Primitive Speech Acts (Dore, 1975); the Interpersonal Language Skills Assessment, designed to assess 8- to 14-year-old children's use of 16 different communication intents during a card game; the Test of Pragmatic Skills–Revised (Sculman, 1985); and, Dore's Taxonomy of Conversational Acts (Dore, 1979).

In terms of mathematics, much interest has focused on metaprocesses. Technically, practically all formal tests involve some form of metacognitive ability in that examinees are usually required to reflect on some aspect of their knowledge. More specifically and with respect to language and culture, this is exemplified in the Vocabulary (defining words), Similarities (inducing superordinate terms), and Comprehension (answering questions about social and cultural conventions) subtests of the Wechsler tests, and with respect to study skills it is exemplified by the work of Peverly and Brobst (1989). Although in name the Test of Problem Solving (Zachman, Jorgensen, Huisingh, & Barrett, 1984) was meant to be a test of problem-solving achievement, it is as much a test of one's ability to understand, solve, and talk about daily social problems and situations.

Language learning, for children with normal hearing and those with hearing losses, at least in part, involves an interactive process, and, as a result, the child's participation in these interactions needs to be assessed. The interactive patterns of the primary caretaker and the child, or the interaction between a classroom teacher and the students, are examples of interactions that could be used for assessment. One could also assess the interaction patterns of a group of children with hearing loss among themselves or in inclusive settings.

The methods used to investigate these interactive patterns are of several types: verbal statements gathered from interviews with parents, naturalistic observation, standardized observation, and containing observation, which is the limiting of one's observation to a specifically prescribed behavior (Ramey, Farran, Campbell, & Finkelstein, 1978). In terms of mother–child, as well as teacher–child interactions, the behaviors of most interest are those that would most promote intellectual development, psychosocial attachment and development, academic achievement, and language development. A good review of strategies used in observing typical mother–child interaction is provided by Ramey et al (1978).

The need for considering these interactions is amply demonstrated by Prezbindowsi (2002) and others who have shown that hearing mothers of children who are deaf respond differently and less effectively as teachers of language than hearing mothers of hearing children. [See Caissie and Cole (1993) and Tanksley (1993) for an alternative consideration of this matter.] Similarly, empirical support has been given for the effectiveness of adopting instructional strategies that are consistent with a social-interaction perspective on language development (Schneiderman, 1995) and deaf mothers of deaf children engage in forms of motherese that are not unlike mothers of children who hear (Masataka, 2000). In the process of simplifying their signing to infants and toddlers, for example, mothers who are deaf use affective facial expression in lieu of the grammatical facial signal (Reilly & Bellugi, 1996), and infants who are either deaf or hearing, respond appropriately to these forms of motherese (Masataka, 2000).

A number of formal interaction scales are available to investigate classroom and teacher–child interactions. Among these are the Flanders Interaction Scales, the Craig and Collins Analysis of Communicative Interaction (Craig & Collins, 1970), and the Cognitive Verbal/Nonverbal Observation Scale (Wolff, 1977), and The Dysfunctional Parent–Child Interactions of the Parental Stress Index.

Earlier studies using these scales have shown that, at least in some classes for students who have hearing losses, the conversations tend to be teacher dominated, with few student-initiated communications (Craig and Collins, 1970); the activities center around memory work as opposed to inference building (Wolff, 1977); and the children find it difficult to ask for information, make suggestions, provide orientations, or clarify others' opinions in group problem-solving situations (Pendergrass & Hodges, 1976), unless forms of scaffolding are used (Schneiderman, 1995).

However, each of these approaches involves the use of some a priori categorization system emphasizing an etic approach to caretaker–child and classroom interaction. A growing trend in the field, however, is the use of ethnographic and microethnographic approaches, which do not specify a priori any categorical system but attempt to induce them by describing the internal emic structure of events and activities. Such an approach might require, however, that the psychoeducational evaluator abandon certain professional orientations and assumptions in favor of a more social psychological perspective.

Historically, there have been several academic tests available that were either normed on students who are deaf or had empirical data available to assist in their interpretation. Only one test presently exists that possesses the technical adequacy to warrant its use. That test is the SAT-HI, which consists of a series of eight graded screening tests to assist the examiner determining which of the eight test batteries is most appropriate for administration, ranging from Primary 1 (typically for grades 1.5 to 2.5) to Advanced 2 (typically for those at grade 8.5 to 9.9). Indeed, it is technically an outstanding test. Not only are norms available for the combined group of individuals who are hard of hearing, but also separate norms for only those with severe to profound losses and a series of specialized norm tables based on degree of loss, type of education program (special schools for the deaf, partial mainstreaming or mainstreaming, mainstreamed), presence or absence of additional handicaps, ethnic background, and region location. One advantage that the Stanford tests have is that they are both norm-referenced and criterion-referenced, and, thus, in principle are amenable to direct translations into an educational program and performance standards (Traxler, 2000) (instructional objectives associated with each item on the screening test and the test batteries themselves are available).

Given that most diagnostic reading tests are phonically based, their utility with the population with hearing loss is limited. Obviously, these tests would be limited to use with children who are hard of hearing or phonically oriented children with deafness. However, Ewoldt (1978) has discussed the application of the Goodman-Burke Reading Miscues Inventory, which is a test of oral reading fluency, to children with hearing loss who used simultaneous communications. Her findings have suggested that children with hearing loss make the same kinds of reading errors as children who hear, and that the reading processes of the two groups are in many ways similar. Gennaoui (1997) has discussed the utility of the Retrospective Miscue Inventory (Goodman & Paulson, 2000), with students who are deaf finding and analyzing their own miscues.

A similar approach to that of the Miscues Reading Inventory has been devised by Mory Clay (1979) and referred to as the running record. Its advantage over the Miscues

Reading Inventory is reportedly its simplicity and adaptability to the teacher's day-to-day activities and routines. In addition to the running record and as a part of the entire diagnostic survey, Clay also developed a letter identification component, an evaluation of young children's concepts about print, a word identification task, and a series of free and dictation writing tasks. Although no literature is known to exist reporting results of using this diagnostic approach with individuals with hearing losses, the approach is being used in the field and it holds promise in providing additional insights into the reading process of children with hearing impairments.

Finally, Reid, Hresko, Hammill, and Wiltshire (1991) developed the Test of Early Reading Ability–Deaf or Hard of Hearing, which was standardized on with hearing loss children from age 3 years, 0 months through 13 years, 11 months to test these youngsters' ability to construct meaning, knowledge of the alphabet and its functions, and awareness of print conventions.

Unfortunately, little research has been done in the area of diagnostic assessment of mathematical ability or the processing of mathematical information in recent years. The reader, however, may find the Sequential Assessment of Mathematics Inventories (Reisman, 1985) to be a useful diagnostic test in this area. This test evaluates the individual in the following areas: Number and Notation, Computation, Math Language, Ordinality, Geometric Concepts, Measurement, Math Applications, and Word Problems. The Key Math and the Test of Early Mathematics Ability (TEMA–3) (Ginsburg & Baroody, 2003) formally and informally evaluate 3 years, 0 months to 8 years, 11 months year olds in the following domains: numbering skills, number-comparison facility, numeral literacy, mastery of number facts, calculation skills, and understanding of concepts. It has two parallel forms. The Wide Range Achievement Test has broad appeal for many evaluators and includes a mathematical section, but it is restricted to computation; overall the test is poor in its technical adequacy, and extreme care should be taken in its use.

Although a great deal of the research on the English language abilities of children who are hard of hearing and deaf has involved the analysis of their written language, few formal tests are available in this area. One notable instrument that has not been reported in the literature for a number of years is the Picture Story Language Test (Myklebust, 1965). Although this instrument attempts to assess syntax in terms of traditional notions of errors of addition, omission, substitutions, and word order, rather than using more sophisticated linguistic analyses (which were not available at the time) it uses an interesting approach to evaluating the ideational component of narratives referred to as the Abstract-Concrete Scale. A story is ranked along a 25-level continuum of ideation ranging from meaningless stories to abstract imaginative stories. Hammill and Larson (1996) created the Test of Written Language–3, which evaluates the children's writing between ages 7 years, 6 months and 17 years, 11 months in a more contemporary fashion. More specifically, the test evaluates two areas: Spontaneous formats (contextual conventions, contextual language, and story construction) and Contrived formats (vocabulary, spelling, style, logical sentences, and sentence combining).

Although they are not yet totally systematized, other considerations need to be taken into account when evaluating the written language of individuals, including the developmental stages and processes that children typically go through (e.g., as described by Calkins, 1994; Applebee, 1978; and others); notions of coherence and cohesion (Halliday & Hasan, 1976); and the role of various forms of writing genres (Applebee, 1978).

Recently, Schirmer, Bailey, and Fitzgerald (1999) developed a rubric to evaluate the writing abilities of students with hearing loss based on many of these writing conventions, which ought to be useful to classroom teachers. This author has also borrowed from the work of Scardamalia (1981), who

Table 7–6. Lexical Matrix to Be Combined into Connected Text

At Harvest	State	
	Michigan	California
Climate	cool	warm
Fruit crop	apples	oranges

investigated the developmental ability of children to integrate a four-by-four matrix in which lexical items appear into a paragraph or sentence (Table 7–6). Scardamalia identified four levels of writing production: A series of simple sentences minimally combining these cells, (e.g., "In the state of Michigan the climate is cool") (p. 86), to a Level 4 performance in which all the elements are considered simultaneously by the child and expressed in a single sentence using various forms of coordination and subordinations. Scardamalia also discusses a parallel task in which the child is to defend a thesis, such as, "Should students be able to choose what things they study in school?" (p. 89), in which the child goes from simply stating a position to defending it, providing counterarguments and, finally, reconciling the two positions. Again such an evaluation is one that can be very useful to classroom teachers in examining and considering the higher-order thought processes of their students.

Finally, the last area to be considered in the assessment of academics is study skills. Although no studies have been conducted in this area with youngsters who have hearing losses, it is an area gaining increasing attention within the psychoeducational literature in general. One promising approach offered by Peverly and Brobst (1989) is to have a student read and study one of a series of graded pieces of expository text. The examinees are asked to summarize what they have read and then are asked some comprehension questions. While reading, examinees are encouraged to use whatever methods they choose to study for this examination, which the examiner notes. Examinees also undergo a structured interview concerning their use of study skills. In evaluating older students who are deaf and hard of hearing, this author includes informal evaluations of their ability to reconstruct a lecture after having taken notes and to synthesize five pieces of seemingly disparate text into a single piece of text with a common theme.

Psychomotor Functioning

Although the psychomotor integrity of the individual may provide the examiner with one more piece of information concerning the total development of the child with hearing impairment, few studies have been performed in this area and few tests of psychomotor ability are available. Myklebust (1960), using the Oseretsky Test of Motor Proficiency, found that some individuals with hearing impairments have difficulties in terms of static balance (standing on one foot) and psychomotor speed (doing a manual task with speed), with lesser but still significant difficulties in maintaining balance while in motion (dynamic balance). Dummer, Haubenstricker, and Stewart (1996), using the Test of Gross Motor Development (TGMD) to assess the fundamental motor skills of children with hearing loss aged 4 to 18 years, found that these youngsters scored lower than those of the TGMD standardization sample of same-aged hearing children on object control and locomotor subscales.

Social Maturity and Adaptive Behavior

Social maturity essentially is the ability to take care of oneself and to assist in the care of others. The related concept of adaptive behavior as defined by the American Association on Mental Deficiency (AAMD) relates to the effectiveness with which an individual copes with the natural and social demands of the environment.

The AAMD further explains that the definition has two major facets: (1) the degree to which the individual is able to function independently, and (2) the degree to which the person meets satisfactorily the culturally imposed demands of personal and social responsibility. The importance of including measures of this kind in a total assessment is emphasized by the official position of both the AAMD and the Office of Civil Rights. Both organizations have stated that an individual can be classified as mentally retarded only if the individual is found to be subnormal in both intelligence and adaptive behavior.

Although a number of adaptive scales are available, only one has been used with individuals with hearing impairments: the Vineland Social Maturity Scale (VSMS) and its most recent revisions the Vineland Adaptive Behavior Scale (VABS), the Survey form, the Expanded Form, and the Classroom form. Both sets of instruments are administered in a structured interview situation with someone who is familiar with the child being rated. The original scale consists of eight clusters of items: self-help general, self-help eating, self-help dressing, locomotion, socialization, occupation, communication, and self-direction; whereas the revised versions contain 11 clusters of items: receptive language, expressive language, written language, personal daily living skills, domestic daily living skills, community living skills, interpersonal relationships, use of play and leisure time, coping skills, gross motor skills, and fine motor skills. These tests were intended to assess the social competency of individuals from birth to adulthood.

Myklebust (1960) and others have used the Vineland Social Maturity Scale with residential school students and have found that in the early years, very little difference existed between youngsters with normal hearing and those that had a hearing loss, except in items directly evaluating communication skills related to English and interacting with society at large. However, as the children matured, the pervasiveness of problems associated with reduced English proficiency and interacting with individuals with hearing at large was found to have serious effects in other areas. So that by age 15 years, the mean social quotient was in the low 80s (the original version calculated a ratio social quotient similar to an IQ in that 100 was considered the average. The revised versions yield standard deviation scores similar to deviation IQ with an average standard score being 100 with a standard deviation of 15. Altepeter, Moscato, and Cummings (1986) studied a small sample of youngsters with hearing loss and found that, although the two versions were positively correlated, a comparison of mean standard scores indicated that the VSMS yielded significantly higher values than the VABS.

Quarrington and Solomon (1975) studied the social maturity of three groups of children with hearing loss, ages 5 to 16 years. The groups studied were day students in a public school setting, students attending a residential school but who had numerous trips home, and residential students who rarely went home. The first two groups had social quotients in the mid 80s, as expected, whereas the latter group had a mean social quotient in the mid 70s, which is distinctly below average.

Although no rationale was given for the procedure, the VABS, the revised version of the VSMS, includes supplemental norms for students with deafness placed in residential facilities. These norms, however, are virtually impossible to interpret and border on being meaningless because an individual's adaptive level is to be judged adequate, above average, or below average based on data collapsed over an age span of 6 years (i.e., 6 years, 0 months to 12 years, 11 months). The survey form of this test, though, has been shown to be useful in classifying persons with hearing impairments according to their ability to acquire independent living skills and, thus, providing some evidence for construct validity when used with adolescents and young adults with hearing loss (Dunlap & Sands, 1990).

Emotional Adjustment

In terms of the child's emotional development, the psychoeducational assessment team needs to be concerned with the child's overall mental health and behavioral functioning and the child's motivation to learn. The need to consider the former is emphasized by the fact

Table 7–7. Psychoeducational Assessment: Emotional Adjustment Tests Available

Rorschach

American Sign Language version of the Rorschach

Make-A-Picture-Story Test

Draw-A-Person Test

Mosaic Test

Id-Ego-Superego Test

Missouri Children's Picture Series

Rotter Incomplete Sentences

Meadow/Kendall Social–Emotional Assessment

Meadow Assessment of Social–Emotional Adjustment in Hearing-Impaired Preschoolers

Hands Test

Sixteen Personality Factor Questionnaire, Form E

Behavior Problem Checklists

Leigh, Robins, and Welkowitz's (1988) adaption of the Beck Depression Inventory, Sociotropy-Autonomy Scale, and the Parental Bonding Instrument

that several surveys have suggested that the incidence of emotional disturbance and behavioral disorders in the population with hearing loss is greater than in the population with normal hearing (Schlesinger & Meadow, 1972). In terms of the latter, the psychoeducational evaluator should also be interested in those behaviors that, although not pathological, do affect learning and functioning within the classroom.

A number of studies have been conducted to examine the personality characteristics of children and adults with hearing loss. Many of these investigations have been based on the use of projective techniques (Table 7–7). Unfortunately, a few of the instruments require extensive verbalization on the part of the examinee, which limits their use to a portion of the population with hearing impairments and calls into question the conclusions derived from the use of such instruments with certain groups of individuals who are deaf or hard of hearing. These criticisms are in addition to those leveled against all projective and most personality tests—that they generally lack the necessary technical adequacy to be considered highly valid or reliable. Despite the technical inadequacy of these tests and the clinical or subjective nature of their interpretations, researchers having access to previous studies tend to come to somewhat similar conclusions regarding certain personality characteristics using different tests (Levine & Wagner, 1974). The fact that these clinical impressions may be socially constructed interpretations in and of themselves may not invalidate them, although care has not always been taken in these cases to authenticate (validate) these findings through some process of corroboration and "triangulation" as required by this approach.

The general pattern of behaviors observed from these studies is emotional immaturity, adaptive rigidity, sociocultural impoverishment, egocentricity, dependency, short attention span, poor impulse control, and aggression. Hogan (1970) has likened these characteristics to an authoritarian personality, whereas Levine and Wagner (1974) have suggested that these characteristics are similar to those of culturally deprived individuals. Although the personality profiles obtained from projective tests give the impression of severe maladaptive behavior, in all probability, they actually reflect good coping skills, considering the impact of the physical disability, the psychosocial reactions to it, and society's reactions to "it" as well. Leigh (1989) showed a higher prevalence of mild depressive symptoms in college students with deafness than in college students who hear, but a lower prevalence of severe depression.

Only recently have attempts been made to address the assessment concerns already expressed in the area of the affective domain. For example, Schwartz, Mebane, and Malony (1990) investigated the effects of the mode of administration (written versus ASL) on the responses elicited on the Rorschach using the Exner's Comprehensive System (Exner, 1986), the current stan-

dard; Brauer (1992) investigated aspects of an ASL version of the Minnesota Multiphasic Personality Inventory (MMPI); Ouellette (1988) successfully investigated the external validity of certain findings obtained on the House-Tree-Person (i.e., aggression, impulsivity, immaturity, egocentricity, and dependency); and Leigh, Robins, and Welkowitz (1988) have developed modified versions of the Beck Depression Inventory, the Sociotropy-Autonomy Scale, and the Parental Bonding Instrument.

The results of the Schwartz et al (1990) study indicated that only a few differences existed between the two administration procedures of the Rorschach (written and signed). In addition, individuals who were deaf tended to score more than one deviation from the mean in terms of perceptual accuracy, perceptual complexity, and self-focus, each of which was interpreted with respect to the biosocial impact of deafness (i.e., the former two being the result of the visual orientation of the deaf clients and the latter the result of normal and expected reactions to societal reactions to deafness). Although a tendency toward "rigidity" was noted, the results were interpreted in terms of qualitative differences with respect to affect expression and modulation. Finally, Brauer (1992) established the possibility of insignificant signer effect on an ASL version of the MMPI.

In recent years, several researchers have investigated various aspects of these personality traits as they relate to the academic setting. More specifically, interest has been expressed in the interrelated notions of impulsivity, external versus internal locus of control, learned helplessness, and the need for achievement. Impulsivity refers to the tendency to make fast decisions with many errors, whereas its opposite, reflection, refers to the tendency to react slowly with relatively few errors. According to Harris (1978) reflectivity is associated with age, reading ability, adjustment, social class, high motivation to achieve, persistence, and long attention spans. Similarly, the bipolar dimensions of external versus internal locus of control have also been associated with several of these variables, as has field dependency (Davey & LaSasso, 1985). For example, locus of control has been associated with greater or lesser information learning, information seeking, academic achievement, and motivation to achieve (Chan, 1979). Some of these ideas have been investigated with individuals with hearing loss. Both Altshuler, Deming, Vollenweider, Rainer, and Tendler (1976) and Harris (1978) have found individuals with hearing loss to be less reflective and, thus, more impulsive than their counterparts who hear. Harris (1978) also found children with deafness of parents with deafness to be more reflective than children who were deaf born to parents with hearing.

Apparently, the nature of the home environment in terms of the quality of the parent–child interactions and communication patterns has a bearing on the extent of the child's reflectivity or impulsivity. Similarly, Stinson (1978) found that the motivation of children with hearing loss to achieve, their persistence, and their actual achievement were a function of the mother's interaction with her child in a learning/teaching situation; Kampfe (1985) found that children's reading achievement may be related to the signing skill levels of mothers who used manual communication. Thus the quality of the mother–child interaction and the extent of the actual external (locus of) control placed on the child has an effect on immediate achievement and probably on the child's eventual perception of locus of control. To the extent that children with hearing loss are actually overprotected, controlled, and directed, they may not learn to take responsibility for their behavior, and, thus, develop what McCrone (1979) has identified as learned helplessness. [See Caissie and Cole (1993) for an alternative consideration of the role of directiveness in mother–child interactions.] Learned helplessness is characterized by (1) an external locus of control, (2) underachievement, and (3) reduced performance when faced with failure. These are characteristics that are common in many children with hearing loss.

Table 7–8. Psychoeducational Assessment: Measures of Impulsivity and Locus of Control

Materials available

  Matching Familiar Figure Test

  Timed Draw-A-Person Test

  Porteus Mazes

  Wechsler Mazes

  Id-Ego-Superego Test

  Rotter Test of Internal/External Control

Because these behaviors appear to be modifiable (e.g., Feuerstein, 1979; Keane & Kretschmer, 1987; Kozulin, 2000), it would seem important to include various measures of impulsivity and locus of control within a standard battery, if possible. Some instruments that could be used are shown in Table 7–8.

Specific Criteria for Integration

This chapter has described instruments and procedures that have been used in identifying and programming for the academic and language needs of the child with hearing impairments. No attempt was made to discuss minimal competencies needed to integrate or include children in a regular classroom either on a full- or part-time basis. There are few studies of this issue. Reich, Hambelton, and Houldin (1977), on the basis of a study of "integrated" children with hearing losses, suggested several sets of minimal criteria that depend on the type of program and the age of the child. Criteria were derived for elementary age children who were candidates for either full integration (EFI) or integration with itinerant help (EIH), and secondary age children who were candidates for full integration (SFI), integration with itinerant help (SIH), or partial integration (SPI). The minimum requirements for full integration at the elementary level were:

1. No greater than a moderate (70 dB HL) pure tone average hearing loss

2. No greater than a severe (90 dB HL) high frequency average (the average of the thresholds at 4000 and 8000 Hz)
3. Aural functioning of 62% or better correct response to a specially designed test of sentence and paragraph understanding
4. Oral functioning of 78% or better on a test similar to that used to assess aural functioning
5. An English language background
6. Parents who had no less than a high school education
7. Parents who had aspirations for their child of high school graduation or college
8. Some degree of help at home, and good parental contact with the school
9. An IQ of no less than 90
10. Diagnosis of hearing impairment no later than age 7 years; a hearing aid being fitted no later than age 8 years

Almost identical criteria for the other four groups were reported, with the exception of permitting:

1. Severe hearing losses in the case of pure tone averages for the EIH and the SPI children
2. Profound high frequency average losses for all four groups
3. Slightly lower aural functioning (58%) for the EIH children
4. Slightly higher oral functioning (86%) for all the secondary groups
5. Slightly lower intelligence for the EIH children, but slightly higher intelligence for the SIH and SPI children (IQs of 97 and 95, respectively)
6. Slightly later age of diagnosis (9 years) for the SIH and SPI children
7. Slightly younger age (5.5 years) for a hearing aid fitting for the EIH children, but slightly older for all the secondary children (age 9 years)

Rudy and Nance (1973) also have developed criteria whereby an individual's candidacy for integration can be estimated. The procedure is based on ratings in the areas of intelligence, academic achievement, social adjustment, and degree of loss. These ratings yield a composite score that can be compared with a decision-making cutoff point provided by the researchers to determine eligibility for integration. Although these minimal criteria can be very useful, it should be remembered that they have not been tested beyond the initial populations studied. Thus they should only be used as guidelines.

Assessment of Transition Competence

There has been long-standing interest in the adult population with deafness and the transition from school to the work world in the field of deafness. Given recent legislation, increased attention is being paid to this critical event of transition in the lives of individuals with disabilities. Although a number of approaches have been taken to assess transition skills, the approaches often do not effectively address certain crucial skills needed by individuals with hearing impairments or the content necessary to succeed independently at work or in the community (Bullis, Reiman, Davis, & Thorkildsen, 1994). As a result, the Transition Competence Battery for Deaf Adolescents and Young Adults was developed, which, according to Bullis et al (1994) was designed to be a "language-appropriate, content-relevant and psychometrically sound measure of transition skills for deaf persons" (p.13), standardized on adolescents and adults with deafness from both mainstream and residential settings. The two multiple-choice versions of the test, a written and a signed version, consist of six subtests covering various aspects of Job-Seeking, Work Adjustment, Job-Related Adjustment, Money Management, Health and Home Skills, and Community Awareness. An interesting feature of this test is its attention to assessing subtle aspects of the examinee's conscious (meta) awareness of social and work ethic conventions, in general, and as it relates to adult deafness issues in particular (e.g., where an interpreter should sit during a job interview). Another interesting point is that, based on pilot data and feedback from their examinees, the videotape version was signed in Pidgin English rather than ASL. Although difficulties exist with the norming sample, the instrument does hold some promise, particularly if the psychometric properties and norms could be enhanced and further demonstrated.

Future Directions and Needs

Psychoeducational assessment is or should be moving in a number of directions that have to do with the diagnostic process, in general, and with assessment, in particular.

Currently, there seem to be two parallel, but seemingly contradictory, trends occurring. The first trend has to do with the consequences of certain sociopolitical acts that have resulted in a heuristic, overly bureaucratized approach to the evaluation process that emphasizes reliance on strict adherence to static measures. The second trend is more academic and theoretically oriented and involves the movement toward ecological, process-oriented, and dynamic assessment procedures. The former trend seems to be a reaction to the increasing regulations (real, imagined, or interpreted) associated with current legislation, mounting litigation, and fears thereof. It may also reflect the ongoing tradition of the positivist's philosophical orientation within school psychology. This has been of such great concern that in 2002 the Presidential Commission on Excellence in Special Education was established, and it recommended, among a great number of other things, the reduction of the "paper work" and bureaucracy associated with special education placements and instruction (United States Department of Education, Office of Special Education and Rehabilitative Services, 2002). Although well-intentioned and of merit, PL94–142, PL99–457, and the Americans with Disabilities Act have produced some profound unintended consequences in many situations, most notably an overreliance on rigid, minimal, norm-referenced batteries of tests; the restriction of psychological services to evaluative functions for purposes of placement and moni-

toring; and the trivialization of the individual education, family plan, and transition planning process and products themselves.

The alternative trend operating out of a (social) constructivist philosophical orientation is more theoretically oriented and views teaching, learning, comprehension, intervention, and decision making (even about placement of disabled children) as dynamic processes. As a result, various models and approaches to process testing have been devised that operate out of various social psychological or information processing models [e.g., Feuerstein's (1979) Learning Potential Assessment Device; Brown, Campione, Weber, & McGilly's (1992) dynamic assessment approaches in terms of cognitive function; Ewoldt's (1978) and Clay's (1979) approaches in terms of reading processes and comprehension; Garrison, Dowaliby, and Long's (1992) work in terms of reading comprehension test item difficulty; and Locher and Worms's (1977) work in terms of visual–motor functioning]. Indeed, this trend toward putting theory into practice is reflected in various aspects of the reform movement and, interestingly enough, in the professional literature in that a special section of the *Journal of School Psychology* has been created entitled the "Scientific Practitioner."

Consistent with this approach has been the growing trend and interest in the nature and construction of knowledge, including social knowledge and social competence (Bye & Jussim, 1993); various metaprocessess and thought processes, including those relating to the affective domain as discussed within the framework of rational emotive therapy (Bernard, 1990); social psychological processes (Tingstrom & Little, 1990); and attributional processes. Even within the framework of traditional testing, the impact of this approach has been felt in that school psychologists are increasingly using testing the limits procedures and are incorporating various types of informal testing techniques based on various theoretical notions and constructs when the working conditions are conducive to it. Additionally, traditional methods of interpreting test results are being augmented by what we know about learning in general, language, and culture (e.g., the interpretations associated with the Comprehension, Similarities, and Vocabulary tests of Wechsler tests as discussed earlier, which differ from those originally proposed by Wechsler). Finally, this approach advises and encourages more ecologically oriented approaches examining actual behavior and learning in real contexts (e.g., school, the workplace, the home).

Another trend, which was only touched on in this chapter, is and will be of interest in the future: the assessment of infants and toddlers and those in transition from school to work.

As for the needs within the field, the following are cited:

1. Large-scale studies investigating the various components of successful mainstreaming/inclusion of successful learners who are deaf or hard of hearing, including family, social, and cultural variables

2. Large-scale studies of language and literacy acquisition and intervention, including English, ASL, and other languages, and learning strategies and characteristics of successful learners

3. Large-scale studies of the psychometric properties of various cognitive, linguistic, academic, social, and emotional evaluative techniques, taking into account the pluralistic and heterogeneous nature of the population with hearing impairments

4. Continued research into the specifics of the structure of knowledge within various domains

5. Better accounts of the structure of emotions and the affective domain as it relates to personal well-being, literature, and the understanding of others

6. Continued work in understanding the relationship between thought, language, social behavior, and affect

7. The pre- and in-service preparation of psychologists to work with individuals with hearing losses, with a firm foundation in information processing and social psychological approaches to knowing, comprehension, learning, and instruction

References

Alexander, C., & Sprain, P.S. (1978). A review of educators' attitudes toward handicapped children and the concept of mainstreaming. *Psychol in the School, 15,* 390–396.

Altepeter, T.S., Moscato, E.M., & Cummings, J.A. (1986). Comparison of scores of hearing-impaired children on the Vineland Adaptive Behavior Scales and the Vineland Social Maturity Scale. *Psychol Rep, 59,* 635–639.

Altshuler, K.Z., Deming, W.E., Vollenweider, J., Rainer, J.D., & Tendler R. (1976). Impulsivity and profound early deafness: A cross cultural inquiry. *Am Ann Deaf, 121,* 331–345.

Andersen, R.J., & Sissco, F.M. (1977). *Standardizations of the WISC-R Scale for Deaf Children.* Washington, DC: Gallaudet College Press.

Andrianopoulos, L.P. (2001). *The perceived utility of traditional and dynamic psychoeducational assessment recommendations by teachers of the deaf.* Unpublished doctoral dissertation, Columbia University, New York.

Antonak, R.F. (1982). Development and psychometric analysis of the Scale of Attitudes Toward Disabled Persons. *Journal of Applied Rehabilitation Counseling, 13,* 22–29.

Applebee, A.N. (1998). *The Child's Concept of Story: Ages Two to Seventeen.* Chicago: The University of Chicago.

Armstrong, B.A., Neville, H.J., Hillyard, S.A., & Mitchell, T.V. (2002). Auditory deprivation affects processing of motion, but not color. *Cognitive Brain Research, 14,* 422–434.

Becker, H., Roberts, G., & Dumas, S. (2000). The Inclusion Inventory: A tool to assess perceptions of the implementation of inclusive educational practices. *Special Services in the Schools, 16,* 57–72.

Bellugi, U., Klima, E.S., & Siple, P. (1974). Remembering in signs. *Cognition, 3,* 93–125.

Berkay, P.J., Gardner, J., & Smith, P.L. (1995). The development of the Opinions about Deaf People scale: A scale to measure hearing adults' beliefs about the capabilities of deaf adults. *Educ and Psychol Meas, 55,* 105–114.

Bernard, M.E. (1990). Rational-emotive therapy with children and adolescents: Treatment strategies. *School Psychology Review 19,* 294–303.

Berryman, J.D., Neal, W.R., & Berryman, J.E. (1989). *Attitudes toward Mainstreaming Scale–Revised.* Athens, GA: University of Georgia.

Birch, J.R., & Birch, J.W. (1956). Predicting school achievement in young deaf children. *Am Ann Deaf, 101,* 348–352.

Birch, J.R., Stuckless, E.R., & Birch, J.W. (1963). An eleven-year study of predicting school achievement in young deaf children. *Am Ann Deaf, 108,* 236–240.

Bloom, L., & Lahey, M. (1978). *Language Development and Language Disorders.* New York: John Wiley & Sons.

Bolton, B. (1978). Differential ability structure in deaf and hearing children. *Appl Psychol Meas, 2,* 147–149.

Bonham, S.J. (1974). Predicting achievement for deaf children. *Psychol Serv Cntr J, 14*, 35–44.

Bosworth, R.G. (2001). *Psychophysical investigation of visual perception in deaf and hearing adults: Effects of auditory deprivation and sign language experience.* Unpublished doctoral dissertation, University of California, San Diego.

Braden, J.P. (1990). Do deaf persons have a characteristic psychometric profile on the Wechsler Performance Scales? *J of Psychoed Assess, 8*, 518–526.

Braden, J.P. (1992). Intellectual assessment of deaf and hard-of-hearing people: A quantitative and qualitative research synthesis. *School Psychology Review, 21*, 82–94.

Braden, J.P., & Paquin, M.M. (1985). A comparison of the WISC-R and WAIS-R Performance Scales in deaf adolescents. *Journal of Psychoeducational Assessment, 3*, 285–290.

Brauer, B.A. (1992). The signer effect on MMPI performance of deaf respondents. *Journal of Personality Assessment, 58*, 380–388.

Brown, A., Campione, J.C., Weber, L.S., & McGilly, K. (1992). *Interactive Learning Environments: A New Look At Assessment and Instruction.* Berkeley: University of California, Commission on Testing and Public Policy.

Bullis, M., Reiman, J., Davis, C., & Thorkildsen, R. (1994). Structure and videodisc adaptation of the Transition Competence Battery (TCB) for deaf adolescents and young adults. *Exceptional Children, 61*, 159–173.

Bunch, G.O. (1981). *Test of Receptive Language Ability.* Toronto: G.B. Services.

Bye, L., & Jussim, L. (1993). A proposed model for the acquisition of social knowledge and social competence. *Psychology in the Schools, 30*, 143–161.

Caissie, R., & Cole, E.B. (1993). Mothers and hearing-impaired children: Directiveness reconsidered. *Volta Review, 95*, 49–59.

Carlson, J.S. (1973). A note on the relationship between Raven's Colored Progressive Matrices Test and operational thought. *Psychology in the Schools, 10*, 211–214.

Chan, K.S. (1979). Locus of control and achievement motivation-critical factors in educational psychology. *Psychology in the School, 15*, 104–110.

Clay, M.M. (1979). *The Early Detection of Reading Difficulties.* Birkenhead, New Zealand: Heinemann.

Cochran, H.K. (1997). *The development and psychometric analysis of the Scale of Teachers' Attitudes toward Inclusion.* Unpublished doctoral dissertation, University of Alabama, Birmingham.

Coggins, T.E., & Carpenter, R.L. (1981). The communication intention inventory: A system for observing and coding children's early intentional communication. *Appl Psycholing* (2), 235–351.

Conrad, R. (1979). *The Deaf School Child.* London: Harper and Row.

Cooper, R.L. (1967). The ability of deaf and hearing children to apply morphological rules. *J Speech Hear Res, 10*, 77–86.

Courtney, A.S., Hayes, F.B., Couch, K.W., & Frick, M. (1984). Administration of the WISC-R performance scale to hearing-impaired children using pantomimed instructions. *Journal of Psychoeducational Assessment, 2*, 1–7.

Craig, W.N., & Collins, J.L. (1970). Communication patterns in classes for deaf students. *Except Child, 37*, 283–289.

Davey, B., & LaSasso, C. (1985). Relations of cognitive style to assessment components of reading comprehension for hearing-impaired adolescents. *Volta Review, 87*, 17–27.

Davis, J. (1974). Performance of young hearing-impaired children on a test of basic concepts. *J Speech Hear Res, 17*, 342–351.

Dore, J. (1975). Holphrase, speech acts and language universals. *J Child Lang, 2*, 21–40.

Dore, J. (1979). Conversational acts and the acquisition of language. In: E. Ochs & B.B. Schiefelin (Eds.), *Developmental Pragmatics* (pp. 339–362). New York: Academic Press.

Dummer, G.M., Haubenstricker, J.L., & Stewart, D.A. (1996). Motor skill performances of children who are deaf. *Adapted Physical Activity Quarterly, 13*, 400–414.

Dunlap, W.R., & Sands, D.I. (1990). Classification of the hearing impaired for independent living using the Vineland Adaptive Behavior Scale. *Am Ann Deaf, 135*, 384–388.

Eftekhar, B.L. (2002). *Communicative Ethics in Early Childhood Special Education: The Professional–Parent Relationship.* Unpublished Ph.D. Dissertation, Teachers College, Columbia University, New York.

Engen, E., & Engen, T. (1983). *Rhode Island Test of Language Structure.* Baltimore, MD: University Park Press.

Ewoldt, C. (1978). Reading for the hearing or hearing impaired: A single process. *Am Ann Deaf, 123*, 945–948.

Exner, J.E. (1986). *The Rorschach: A Comprehensive System.* New York: Wiley-Interscience.

Feuerstein, R. (1979). *The Dynamic Assessment of Retarded Performers.* Baltimore, MD: University Park Press.

Freeman, R.D., Malkin, S.F., & Hastings, J.O. (1975). Psychosocial problems of deaf children and their families: A comparative study. *Am Ann Deaf, 210*, 391–405.

Furth, H.G. (1970). A review and perspective on the thinking of deaf people. In: J. Hellmuth (Ed.), *Cognitive Studies* (pp. 291–338). New York: Brunner/Mazel.

Garrison, W., Dowaliby, F.J., & Long, G. (1992). Reading comprehension test item difficulty as a function of cognitive processing variables. *Am Ann Deaf, 137*, 22–30.

Geers, A.E. (1994). Techniques for assessing auditory speech perception and lipreading enhancement in young deaf children. *Volta Review, 96*, 85–96.

Geers, A.E., & Moog, J.S. (1978). Syntactic maturity of spontaneous speech and elicited imitations of hearing-impaired children. *J Speech Hear Disord, 43*, 380–391.

Gennaoui, M. (1997). *Retrospective miscues analysis: A tool for readers to discover and evaluate their own reading.* Paper presented at the International Reading Association 42nd Annual Convention, Atlanta, Georgia.

Gething, L. (1994). The Interaction with Disabled Persons Scale. *Journal of Social Behavior and Personality, 9*, 23–42.

Giancreco, C. (1966). The Hiskey-Nebraska Test of Learning Aptitude (revised) compared to several achievement tests. *Am Ann Deaf, 111*, 556–577.

Ginsburg, H.P., & Baroody, A.J. (2003). Test of Early Mathematics Ability (TEMA–3) Third Edition. Austin, TX: PRO-ED.

Goetzinger, C.P., Wills, R.C., & Dekker, R. (1967). Non-language IQ tests used with deaf pupils. *Volta Review, 69,* 500–506.

Goodman, Y., & Paulson, E.J. (2000). *Teachers and Students Developing Language about Reading through Retrospective Miscue Analysis.* Urbana, IL: National Council of Teachers of English.

Greene, H.A. (1978). Implications of a comprehensive vision-screening program for hearing-impaired children. *Volta Review, 80,* 467–475.

Guba, E. (Ed.). (1990). *The Paradigm Dialog.* Newbury Park: Sage.

Halliday, M.A.K., & Hasan, R. (1976). *Cohesion in English.* White Plains, NY: Longman.

Hammill, D., & Larson, S. (1996). Test of Written Language (TOWL-3). Austin, TX: PRO-ED.

Haring, N., Cruickshank, W.M., & Stern, G. (1981). *Attitudes of Educators toward Exceptional Children.* Syracuse: Syracuse University Press.

Harris, R.I. (1978). The relationship of impulse control to parent hearing status, manual communication, and academic achievement in deaf children. *Am Ann Deaf, 123,* 52–67.

Hasenstab, M.S., & Loughton, J. (1982). Bare essentials in assessing really little kids: An approach. In: M.S. Hasenstab & J.S. Horne (Eds.), *Comprehensive Intervention with Hearing-Impaired Infants and Preschoolers.* Rockville, MD: Aspen Park Publishers.

Hauser, P.C. (2001). *Deaf readers' phonological encoding: An electromyogram study of covert reading behavior.* Unpublished doctoral dissertation, Gallaudet University, Washington, DC.

Henggeler, S.W., Watson, S.M., Whelan, J.P., & Malone, C.M. (1990). The adaptation of hearing parents of hearing-impaired youths. *Am Ann Deaf, 135,* 211–216.

Hine, W.D. (1970). The abilities of partially hearing children. *Br J Educ Psychol, 40,* 171–178.

Hirsh-Pasek, K. (1987). The metalinguistics of fingerspelling: An alternate way to increase reading vocabulary in congenitally deaf readers. *Read Res Q, 22,* 455–474.

Hiskey, M. (1966). *Hiskey-Nebraska Test of Learning Aptitude.* Lincoln, NE: Union College Press.

Hogan, H.W. (1970). Authoritarianism among white and black deaf adolescents: Two measures compared. *Percept Mot Skills, 31,* 195–200.

Humphrey, J.M. (1976). *Performance of Deaf Children on Tests of Cognitive, Linguistic, and Academic Achievement.* Houston: University of Houston.

James, R.P. (1984). A correlational analysis between the Raven's Matrices and WISC-R Performance Scales. *Volta Review, 86,* 336–341.

Kaltsounis, B. (1970). Comparative study of creativity in deaf and hearing children. *Child Study J, 1,* 11–19.

Kampfe, C.C. (1985). *Reading comprehension of prelingually deaf adolescents and its relationship to maternal use of manual communication.* Unpublished doctoral dissertation, University of Arizona, Tempe.

Keane, K.J., & Kretschmer, R.E. (1987). Effect of mediated learning intervention on cognitive task performance with a deaf population. *J Educ Psychol, 79,* 49–53.

Kelly, M.D., & Braden, J.P. (1990). Criterion-related validity of the WISC-R Performance scale with the Stanford Achievement Test—Hearing-Impaired Edition. *J Sch Psychol, 28,* 147–151.

Keogh, B.K., Vernon, M., & Smith, C.E. (1970). Deafness and visuo-motor function. *J Spec Educ, 4,* 41–47.

Kozulin, A. (2000). The diversity of instrumental enrichment applications. In A. Kozulin, Y. Rand (Eds.), *Experience of Mediated Learning: An Impact of Feuerstein's Theory in Education and Psychology* (pp. 257–273). Advances in Learning and Instruction Series. Elmsford, NY: Pergamon.

Kretschmer, R.E. (1982). Reading and the hearing impaired individual: Summation and application. *Volta Review, 84,* 107–122.

Kretschmer, R.R., & Kretschmer, L.W. (1978). *Language Development and Intervention with the Hearing Impaired.* Baltimore: University Park Press.

Kretschmer, R.E., & Martello, A. (1993). *Developing a screening test and follow-up procedure for identifying encoding preference.* Paper presented at the Convention of American Instructors of the Deaf, Baltimore, MD.

Laughton, J. (1979). Nonlinguistisc creative abilities and expressive syntactic abilities of hearing-impaired children. *Volta Review, 81,* 409–420.

Laughton, J. (1988). Strategies for developing creative abilities of hearing-impaired children. *Am Ann Deaf, 133,* 258–263.

Laughton, J.W. (1976). *Nonverbal creative thinking abilities as predictors of linguistic abilities of hearing impaired children.* Unpublished doctoral dissertation, Kent State University, Kent, Ohio.

Lawson, L.I., & Myklebust, H.R. (1970). Ophthalmological deficiencies in deaf children. *Exceptional Children, 37,* 17–20.

Layton, T.L., & Holmes, D.W. (1985). Carolina Picture Vocabulary Test. Tulsa, OK: Modern Education Corporation.

Leigh, I.W. (1989). Towards greater understanding of depression in deaf individuals: An investigation. *Am Ann Deaf, 134,* 249–254.

Leigh, I.W., Robins, C.J., & Welkowitz, J. (1988). Modification of the Beck Depression Inventory for use with a deaf population. *J Clin Psychol, 44,* 728–732.

Levine, E.S. (1974). Psychological tests and practices with the deaf: A survey of the state of the art. *Volta Review, 76,* 298–319.

Levine, E.S., & Wagner, E.E. (1974). Personality patterns of deaf persons: An interpretation based on research with the Hand Test. *Percept Mot Skills, 39,* 1167–1236.

Levine, M.N., Allen, R., Alker, L., et al. (1974). Clinical profile for the Leiter International Performance Scale. *Psychological Service Center Journal, 14,* 45–51.

Lichtenstein, E. (1985). Deaf working memory processes and English Language Skills. In: D.S. Martin (Ed.), *Cognition, Education, and Deafness* (pp. 111–114). Washington, DC: Gallaudet University Press.

Ling, D. (2002). *Speech and the Hearing-Impaired Child* (2nd ed.). Washington, DC: Alexander Graham Bell Association.

Locher, P.J., & Worms, P.I. (1977). Visual scanning strategies of neurologically impaired, perceptually, impaired, and normal children viewing the Bender Gestalt Designs. *Psychol in the School, 14,* 147–157.

Locke, J.L., & Locke, V.L. (1971). Deaf children's phonetic, visual, and dactylic coding in a grapheme recall task. *J Exp Psychol, 89,* 142–146.

Longhurst, T.M., & Briery, D. (1975). SKY-HI Receptive Language Test. Logan, UT: Department of Communication Disorders, Utah State University.

Mackinson, J.A., Leigh, I.W., & Anthony, S. (1997). Validity of the TONI-2 with deaf and hard of hearing children. *Am Ann Deaf, 142,* 294–299.

MacLean, D., & Gannon, P.M. (1995). Measuring attitudes toward disability: The Interaction with Disabled Persons Scale revisited. *J Soc Behav Pers, 10,* 791–806.

Maller, S.J., Singleton, J.L., Supalla, S.J., & Wix, T. (1999). The development and psychometric properties of the American Sign Language Proficiency Assessment (ASL-PA). *Journal of Deaf Studies and Deaf Education, 4,* 249–269.

Masataka, N. (2000). The role of modality and input in the earliest stage of language acquisition: Studies of Japanese sign language. In: C. Chamberlain, J.P. Morford, & R.I. Mayberry (Eds.), *Language Acquisition by Eye* (pp. 3–24). Mahwah, NJ: Lawrence Erlbaum.

McCrone, W.P. (1979). Learned helplessness and level of underachievement among deaf adolescents. *Psychology in the Schools, 16,* 430–434.

McQuaid, M., & Alovisetti, M. (1981). School psychological services for hearing-impaired children in the New York and New England Area. *Am Ann Deaf, 126,* 37–42.

Mitchell, J. (Ed.). (2001). *Fourteenth Mental Measurement Year Book.* Lincoln: Buros Institute of Mental Measurement, University of Nebraska Press.

Monsen, R.B. (1981). A usable test for the speech intelligibility of deaf talkers. *Am Ann Deaf, 126,* 845–852.

Monsen, R.B., & Moog, J.S. (1988). *CID Picture SPINE.* St. Louis: Central Institute for the Deaf.

Moog, J.S., & Geers, A.E. (1979). Grammatical Analysis of Elicited Language Simple Sentence Level (GAEL-S). St. Louis: Central Institute for the Deaf.

Moog, J.S., & Geers, A.E. (1980). Grammatical Analysis of Elicited Language: Complex Sentence Level (GAEL-C). St. Louis: Central Institute for the Deaf.

Moog, J.S., & Kozak, V.J. (1983). *Teacher Assessment of Grammatical Structures.* St. Louis, MO: Central Institute for the Deaf.

Moog, J.S., Kozak, V.J., & Geers, A.E. (1983). Grammatical Analysis of Elicited Language, Pre-sentence Level. St. Louis: Central Institute for the Deaf.

Moores, D.F.P. (2001). *Educating the Deaf: Psychology, Principles, and Practices* (5th ed.). Riverside, CA: Houghton Mifflin.

Myklebust, H.R. (1960). *Psychology of Deafness.* New York: Grune and Stratton.

Myklebust, H.R. (1965). *Picture Story Language Test.* New York: Grune and Stratton.

Myklebust, H.R., Neyhus, A., & Mulholland, A.M. (1962). Guidance and counseling for the deaf. *Am Ann Deaf, 107,* 370–415.

Naglieri, J.A. (1985). Matrix Analogies Test–Expanded Form. New York: The Psychological Corporation.

Naglieri, J.A., & Bardos, A.N. (1988). Canadian children's performance on the Matrix Analogies Test. *School Psychol International, 9,* 309–313.

Naglieri, J.A., & Welch, J.A. (1991). Use of Raven's and Naglieri's Nonverbal Matrix Test. *J Rehabil Deaf, 24,* 98–103.

Neuhaus, M. (1969). Parental attitudes and the emotional adjustment of deaf children. *Exceptional Children, 35,* 721–727.

Newland, T.E. (1973). Assumptions underlying psychological testing. *Journal of School Psychology, 11,* 316–322.

Oakland County School District. (1975). *Hard of Hearing Child in the Regular Classroom* (No. Eric Number ED 145646). Pontiac, MI: Oakland County School District.

Office of Los Angeles County Superintendent of Schools. (1976). Test of Auditory Comprehension. North Hollywood, CA: Foreworks.

Olson, A.C., & Nickerson, J.F. (2001). Syllabic organization and deafness: Orthographic structure or letter frequency in reading? *Q J Exp Psychol A, 54,* 421–438.

Ottem, E. (1980). An analysis of cognitive studies with deaf students. *Am Ann Deaf, 125,* 564–575.

Ouellette, S.E. (1988). The use of projective drawing techniques in the personality assessment of prelingually deafened young adults: A pilot study. *Am Ann Deaf, 133,* 212–218.

Pendergrass, R.A., & Hodges, M. (1976). Deaf students in group problem solving situations: A study of the interactive process. *Am Ann Deaf, 121,* 327–330.

Peverly, S., & Brobst, K. (1989). *Inventory and Assessment of Study Skills.* New York: Teachers College, Columbia University.

Pflaster, G. (1976). *A factor analytic study of hearing impaired children integrated into regular schools.* Unpublished doctoral dissertation, Teachers College, Columbia University, New York.

Phelps, L., & Branyan, B.J. (1990). Academic achievement and nonverbal intelligence in public school hearing-impaired children. *Psychology in the Schools, 27,* 210–217.

Phillips, D.C. (1991). Postpositivistic science: Myths and realities. In: E. Guba (Ed.), *The Paradigm Dialog* (pp. 31–45). Newbury Park, CA: Sage.

Porter, L.J., & Kirby, E.A. (1986). Effects of two instructional sets on the validity of the Kaufman Assessment Battery for Children–Nonverbal Scale with a group of severely hearing impaired children. *Psychology in the Schools, 23,* 37–43.

Pressnell, L. (1973). Hearing-impaired children's comprehension and production of syntax in oral language. *Journal of Speech and Hearing Research, 16,* 12–21.

Prezbindowski, A.K. (2002). *The quality of mother–child interaction and social competence of deaf and hearing preschoolers: A longitudinal study.* Unpublished doctoral dissertation, Georgia State University, Atlanta.

Proksch, J., & Bavelier, D. (2002). Changes in the spatial distribution of visual attention after early deafness. *J Cogn Neurosci, 14,* 687–701.

Quarrington, B., & Solomon, B. (1975). A current study of the social maturity of deaf students. *Can J Behav Sci, 7,* 70–77.

Quigley, S.P., Steinkamp, M.W., Powers, D.J., & Jones, B. (1978). Test of Syntactic Abilities. Beaverton, OR: Dormac.

Ralston, F. (2002). *Use of the videotaped Ralston Test of Fingerspelled Pseudowords (RTFP) in exploring reading among deaf adults in college and postsecondary training programs.* Unpublished doctoral dissertation, Gallaudet University, Washington, DC.

Ramey, C.T., Farran, D.C., Campbell, F.A., & Finkelstein, N.W. (1978). Observation of mother–infant interactions: Implications for development. In: F.D. Minife & L.L. Lloyd (Eds.), *Communicative and Cognitive Abilities: Early Behavior Assessment* (pp. 349–376). Baltimore: University Park Press.

Ratcliffe, K.J., & Ratcliffe, M.W. (1979). The Leiter Scales: A review of validity findings. *Am Ann Deaf, 124,* 38–44.

Ratner, V. (1988). Test of Visual Perceptual Abilities–Revised. South Salem, NY: Visual Perceptual Abilities.

Raven, J.C. (1986). *Manual for Raven's Progressive Matrices and Vocabulary Scales.* London: H.K. Lewis.

Ray, S. (1980). *An adaptation of the Wechsler Intelligence Scales (Performance) for Children–Revised for the deaf.* Unpublished Ed.D., University of Tennessee, Knoxville.

Reich, C., Hambleton, D., & Houldin, B.K. (1977). The integration of hearing-impaired children in regular classrooms. *Am Ann Deaf, 122,* 534–543.

Reid, K.D., Hresko, W., Hammill, D., & Wiltshire, S. (1991). Test of Early Reading Ability–Deaf or Hard of Hearing (TERA-D/HH). Austin, TX: PRO-ED.

Reilly, J.S., & Bellugi, U. (1996). Competition on the face: Affect and language in ASL motherese. *J Child Lang, 23,* 219–239.

Reisman, R.K. (1985). *Sequential Assessment of Mathematics Inventories.* San Antonio: Psychological Corporation.

Ritter, D.R. (1976). Intellectual estimates of hearing-impaired children: A comparison of three measures. *Psychol in the Schools, 13,* 397–399.

Roid, G.H., & Miller, L.J. (1997). Leiter International Performance Scale, Revised. Wood Dale, IL: Stoelting Company.

Ross, D.R. (1970). A technique of verbal ability assessment of deaf adults. *Journal of Rehabilitation for the Deaf, 3,* 7–15.

Rudy, J.P., & Nance, J.G. (1973). A transitional instrument. In: W.H. Northcott (Ed.), *The Hearing Impaired Child in a Regular Classroom* (pp. 128–133). Washington, DC: The Alexander Graham Bell Association.

Salvia, J.A., & Ysseldyke, J.E. (2001). *Assessment.* Boston: Houghton Mifflin.

Scardamalia, M. (1981). How children cope with the cognitive demands of writing. In: C.H. Frederiksen & J.F. Dominic (Eds.), *Writing: The Nature, Development, and Teaching of Written Communication* (Vol. 2, pp. 81–104). Hillsdale, NJ: Lawrence Erlbaum.

Scherer, P. (1981). *Total Communication Receptive Vocabulary Test.* Northbrook, IL: Mental Health and Deafness Resources.

Schirmer, B.R., Bailey, J., & Fitzgerald, S.M. (1999). Using a writing assessment rubric for writing development of children who are deaf. *Exceptional Children, 65,* 383–397.

Schlesinger, H.S., & Meadow, K. (1972). *Sound and Sign Childhood Deafness and Mental Health.* Berkeley: University of California Press.

Schneiderman, E. (1995). The effectiveness of an interactive instructional context: Principles from the parent–child interaction literature. *Am Ann Deaf, 140,* 8–15.

Schwartz, N.S., Mebane, D.L., & Malony, H.N. (1990). Effects of alternate modes of administration on Rorschach performance of deaf adults. *J Pers Assess, 54,* 671–683.

Sculman, B.B. (1985). Test of Pragmatic Skills–Revised. Tucson, AZ: Communication Skill Builders.

Serrano-Miranda, A. (1999). *Lismar House: Early intervention program for the prevention of emotional and behavioral problems in deaf children.* Unpublished doctoral dissertation, Miami Institute of Psychology of the Caribbean Center for Advanced Studies, Miami, Florida.

Sharp, E.Y. (1972). The relationship of visual closure to speechreading. *Exceptional Children, 38,* 729–734.

Silver, R.A. (1977). The question of imagination, originality, and abstract thinking by deaf children. *Am Ann Deaf, 122,* 349–354.

Siple, P., Hatfield, N., & Caccamise, F.F. (1978). The role of visual perceptual abilities in the acquisition and comprehension of sign language. *Am Ann Deaf, 123,* 852–856.

Skritic, T. (Ed.). (1995). *Disability and Democracy: Deconstructing (Special) Education for Postmodernity.* New York: Teachers College Press.

Slate, J.R., & Fawcett, J. (1995). Validity of the WISC-III for deaf and hard of hearing persons. *Am Ann Deaf, 140,* 250–254.

Smith, C.S. (1962). The assessment of mental abilities in partially deaf children. *Teacher of the Deaf, 60,* 216–224.

Spear, B.S., & Kretschmer, R.E. (1987). The use of criteria in decision making regarding the placement of hearing impaired children. *Special Services in the Schools, 4,* 107–122.

Speece, D.L. (1990). Aptitude by treatment interactions: Bad rap or bad idea? *Journal of Special Education, 24,* 139–149.

Spragins, A.B., Schildroth, A.N., & Karchmer, M. (1981). Profile of psychological service providers to hearing-impaired students. *Am Ann Deaf, 126,* 94–105.

Stainback, S., & Stainback, W. (1992). Schools as inclusive communities. In: W. Stainback & S. Stainback (Eds.), *Controversial Issues Confronting Special Education: Divergent Perspectives* (pp. 29–43). Boston: Allyn and Bacon.

Stinson, M. (1978). Effects of deafness on maternal expectations about child development. *Journal of Special Education, 12,* 75–81.

Stivalet, P., Moreno, Y., Richard, J., Barraud, P.-A., & Raphel, C. (1998). Differences in visual search tasks between congenitally deaf and normally hearing adults. *Cogn Brain Res, 6,* 227–232.

Stout, G.G., & Windle, E.V.J. (1992). *The Developmental Approach to Successful Listening, II.* Houston, TX: Houston School for the Deaf.

Sullivan, P.M. (1982). Administration modifications on the WISC-R Performance scale with different categories of deaf children. *Am Ann Deaf, 127,* 780–788.

Swisher, M.V. (1993). Perceptual and cognitive aspects of recognition of signs in peripheral vision. In: M.D.C.E. Marc Marschark (Ed.), *Psychological Perspectives on Deafness* (pp. 209–227). Hillsdale, NJ: Lawrence Erlbaum.

Tanksley, C.K. (1993). Interactions between mothers and normal-hearing or hearing-impaired children. *Volta Review, 95,* 33–47.

Tingstrom, D.H., & Little, S.G. (1990). School consultation from a social psychological perspective: A review. *Psychology in the Schools, 27,* 43–50.

Toscano, R.M., McKee, B., & Lepoutre, D. (2002). Success with academic English: Reflections of deaf college students. *Am Ann Deaf, 147,* 5–23.

Transler, C., Gombert, J., & Leybaert, J. (2001). Phonological decoding in severely and profoundly deaf children: Similarity judgment between written pseudo words. *Applied Psycholinguistics, 22,* 61–82.

Transler, C., Leybaert, J., & Gombert, J.-E. (1999). Do deaf children use phonological syllables as reading units? *Journal of Deaf Studies and Deaf Education, 4,* 124–143.

Traxler, C.B. (2000). The Stanford Achievement Test, 9th edition: National norming and performance standards for deaf and hard-of-hearing students. *Journal of Deaf Studies and Deaf Education, 5,* 337–348.

Trott, L.A. (1984). Providing school psychological services to hearing-impaired students in New Jersey. *Am Ann Deaf, 129,* 319–323.

Tyack, D., & Venable, G.P. (1998). *Language Sampling, Analysis, and Training: A Handbook* (3rd ed.). Austin, TX: PRO-ED.

United States Department of Health, Education, and Welfare. (1977). *Rules and regulations for implementation of the Individual Disabilities Education Act of 1975.* Unpublished manuscript.

United States Department of Education, Office of Special Education and Rehabilitative Services. (1999). *Assistance to the States for the Education of Children with Disabilities: Final Rule, 64*(121), 34048– 34100.

United States Department of Education, Office of Special Education and Rehabilitative Services. (2002). *A New Era: Revitalizing Special Education for Children and Their Families.* Washington, DC: Education Publications Center, U.S. Department of Education.

Vantre, E.M. (2001). *Evaluating the presence of best practices for inclusion: The Marsh Inclusion Scale.* Unpublished doctoral dissertation, Temple University, Philadelphia, Pennsylvania.

Vygotsky, L.S. (1978). *Mind in Society.* Cambridge: Harvard University Press.

Wall, A.D. (2000). *The IEP staffing. The road to collaboration or litigation: A qualitative study of highly effective special education staffing teams.* Unpublished doctoral dissertation, University of Denver, Colorado.

Watson, B.U., Goldgar, D.E., Kroese, J.M., & Lotz, W. (1986). Nonverbal intelligence and academic achievement in the hearing impaired. *Volta Review, 88,* 151–158.

Weaver, C.B., & Bradley-Johnson, S. (1993). A national survey of school psychological services for deaf and hard of hearing students. *Am Ann Deaf, 138,* 267–274.

Wechsler, D. (1991). Wechsler Intelligence Scale for Children–III. San Antonio: Psychological Corporation.

White, A.H. (1981). *Maryland Syntax Evaluation Instrument.* Sanger, TX: Support Systems for the Deaf.

Wigg, E.H., & Secord, W. (1993). Test of Word Knowledge. New York: Psychological Corporation.

Wilczenski, F.L. (1995). Development of a scale to measure attitudes toward inclusive education. *Educational and Psychological Measurement, 55,* 291–299.

Wolff, A.B., & Harkins, J.E. (1986). Multihandicapped students. In: A.N. Schildroth & M.A. Karchmer (Eds.), *Deaf Children in America* (pp. 276–293). San Diego, CA: College Hill Press.

Wolff, S. (1977). Cognition and communication patterns in classrooms for deaf students. *Am Ann Deaf, 122,* 319–327.

Zachman, L., Jorgensen, C., Huisingh, R., & Barrett, M. (1984). Test of Problem Solving. Moline, IL: LinguiSystems.

8

Psychoeducational Assessment of Children with Auditory Language Learning Problems

R. RAY BATTIN

Auditory space has no point of favored focus. It's a sphere without fixed boundaries, space made by the thing itself, not space containing the thing.
—Carpenter (1960)

Auditory verbal language disturbances can range from the severely involved, as seen in children with aphasia, auditory agnosia, or autism, to the more mildly involved children with auditory imperceptions or learning disabilities. For the child with severe auditory–verbal language problems, psychoeducational assessment will, by necessity, consist of a modified test battery tailored to the perceptual and communicative skills of the child. Test instruments typically used for evaluating the severely hearing impaired are also applicable to this population (see Chapter 7).

Children with auditory language-learning problems are more difficult to identify than those with peripheral hearing loss or impaired vision. Their behaviors may be misunderstood. As a result, these children are frequently labeled immature or inattentive. Their performance in school worsens each year, and by grades 3 or 4 they are either making failing grades or significantly underachieving for their level of abilities. At this point, the teacher or parent may seek further evaluation of these children.

The child is referred to the educational diagnostician, counselor, or school psychologist because of school or behavioral difficulties. It is the responsibility of the examiner to assess the child's general abilities, how the child learns, and how he or she perceives and deals with new situations. The examiner must also present an extensive analysis of independent responses and test scatter. Specific test data, if properly analyzed, may delineate the child with an auditory processing problem.

This chapter deals with the selection and interpretation of psychoeducational tests and their use in evaluating the child with an auditory–verbal processing or perceptual disturbance. It also demonstrates how the child's test profile can be used in educational planning and in establishment of a remedial program directed to specific deficits.

Validity and Reliability

Care must be taken when choosing an assessment instrument. With the proliferation of tests (they sprout like leaves on a tree), the examiner must know how to choose appropriately.

Standards, as recommended by the Committee on Standards of the American Psychological Association, apply to any published test used in evaluation, diagnosis, or prognosis. Each test should have data available on validity and reliability, directions for administration and scoring, and qualifications required to administer and properly interpret the test (Turner, DeMers, Fox, & Reed, 2001).

Informal versus Formal Testing

Increasing criticism has been directed toward formal testing. Intelligence tests have come under critical review because they have been used to classify children for placement in classes for the mentally retarded. It was found that blacks tended to score lower on the Wechsler Intelligence Scale for Children (WISC) and the Stanford-Binet tests, and thus were overrepresented in these classes. As a result, a moratorium on the use of formal psychological testing for special education placement has been declared in many school districts (Jackson, 1975; Mercer, 1971; Zimmerman & Woo-Sam, 1978). To discontinue the use of generalized intelligence tests, however, is to throw out the good with the bad. The error comes when examiners use such tests as the Wechsler Intelligence Scale for Children–III (WISC-III), the Wechsler Preschool and Primary Scale of Intelligence–III (WPPSI-III), or the Stanford-Binet Intelligence Scale, fourth or fifth edition, to compute a single composite score, rather than analyzing the components. As will be pointed out in later sections of this chapter, the WISC-III, WPPSI-III, and the Stanford-Binet Intelligence Scale, fourth or fifth edition, can provide information on auditory–verbal and visual–motor skills.

Informal assessment may provide insight into the child's problems, but with the present concern over accountability, it does not provide an adequate base on which to build a treatment or educational program. The generalized assessment utilizing well-standardized tests provides the examiner with more reliable and valid data against which treatment gains versus maturational gains may be checked. By using the child as the control, a learning and abilities profile can be plotted and used to determine if significant strengths and weaknesses exist and whether therapeutic intervention is indicated. Classification can be made according

to independent learning skills, as opposed to a more global labeling.

Unimodal, Bimodal, or Multimodal Assessment

It is extremely difficult to dissect learning by modality. Jastak and Jastak (1976) theorize that the three sensory modalities, hearing, vision, and kinesthesia (touch), are "involved in the formation of lexigraphic and other linguistic communication codes."

With increasing specialization, learning disorders are divided into discipline-specific disabilities. As each specialty tests the child and identifies problems based upon that specialty's training, it becomes like the proverbial blind men describing the elephant. Rarely is a child with a learning disability depressed in only a single modality. Furthermore, if one is looking only at a single modality when assessing a child's capabilities, it is possible to label as deficient areas in which the child falls below what is expected according to chronological age, when in fact, the child is depressed in all modalities and thus performing within his abilities level. To reemphasize, a child must be used as his or her own control for the examiner to understand the learning potential as well as the disabilities of that child.

History as a Part of the Assessment

A detailed birth, health, family, social, educational, and behavioral history is a critical part of any comprehensive assessment. A preinterview questionnaire, which the parents can complete at home with the help of the baby book, and which is returned prior to the testing, allows the examiner some insight into the problems presented by the child. A comparison of the behaviors described in the questionnaire with test behavior and performance provides the examiner with some support for the interpretation drawn from the assessment.

In addition to specific questions, the questionnaire should contain several open-ended questions that allow the parents to describe the child's behavior and personality. Methods of discipline used by the parents should also be explained in detail. The examiner will want to review the responses to questions on birth, health, and development carefully, as well as scrutinize the behavioral responses.

Behaviors that point to a disturbance in the auditory–verbal area include inattentiveness, short attention span, daydreaming, and a tendency to play with younger children. The child may also be withdrawn, unable to follow directions, and forgetful. The child may misunderstand instructions or directions, be disruptive in school and at home, fail to complete homework, or be unable to remember assignments. For example, the child might know spelling words or other material at home, but fail a test on the material at school. Teachers may label the child as a "smart aleck" or one who "refuses to conform."

Specific Test Instruments

A comprehensive psychoeducational test battery for children suspected of an auditory–verbal learning disturbance should include tests that fall under five general categories: general abilities, auditory–verbal behavior, visual–motor behavior, academic behavior, and personality. Table 8–1 summarizes the psychological tests that should be considered for assessment in these five areas.

General Abilities Assessment

The most widely used tests of general abilities are the Stanford-Binet and the Wechsler scales. The first scale of intelligence, the Binet, was published by Binet and Simon in 1905. It was developed to help separate the uneducable from the educable in the schools of Paris. In 1916, while at Stanford University, Terman revised the Binet test; thus the name Stanford-Binet (Terman & Merrill, 1937). Since that time, it has gone through several additional revisions. In 1960, the best items from the L and M forms of the 1937 scale were combined into a single scale (Terman & Merrill, 1962). This revision was re-standardized in 1972. Thorndike, Hagen, and Sattler (1986) introduced the fourth edition and Roid (2003) introduced the fifth edition.

The fourth and fifth revisions cover the same age range, and require the examiner to establish a basal age with many of the same types of test items. All other aspects of the test differ significantly from previous editions. Items of the same type are grouped into 15 tests in the fourth edition, with each test tapping different cognitive skills and different funds of information.

Four broad areas, Verbal Reasoning, Abstract/Visual Reasoning, Quantitative Reasoning, and Short-Term Memory, are assessed by the 15 tests. The tests provide a composite standard age score of general reasoning ability and standard age scores for the four areas. Standard age scores are also available for any combination of the four areas as well as for individual test scores for the 15 tests. This edition was constructed to better identify individuals who are mentally retarded, have specific learning disabilities, or are gifted. Once examiners become familiar with this test, they find it is much more flexible than earlier editions. This edition can be more readily adapted to the child undergoing the test, and provides information in both the auditory–verbal and visual–motor modalities. This information can then be used in the development of a treatment program (see Case Study 8–1).

The complete battery consists of 8 to 13 tests and takes 1 hour to 90 minutes to administer. A screening battery composed of the Vocabulary, Bead Memory, Quantitative, and Pattern Analysis can be administered in 30 to 40 minutes. A six-subtest battery, which requires less testing time than the complete battery, can be assembled by adding Memory for Sentences and Comprehension to the original screening test. The authors recommend that assessment of students experiencing difficulty in school include tests that have the greatest diagnostic value and a balance of verbal and abstract/visual reasoning tests. The test manual provides recommendations for abbreviated batteries (Thorndike, Hagen, & Sattler, 1986).

Table 8–1. Psychoeducational Test Battery

Type of Assessment	Sequence of Tests
	Appropriate instruments
I. General abilities	1. Stanford-Binet Intelligence Scale: Fourth or Fifth Edition
	2. Wechsler Intelligence Scale for Children–III (WISC-III)
	3. Wechsler Preschool and Primary Scale of Intelligence–III (WPPSI-III)
	4. Kaufman Assessment Battery for Children (KABC)
	5. Kaufman Brief Intelligence Test (KBIT)
	6. Test of Nonverbal Intelligence–Second Edition (TONI-2)
	7. Comprehensive Test of Nonverbal Intelligence (CTONI)
	8. The Leiter International Performance Scale–Revised (Leiter-R)
	9. NEPSY
	10. Raven Progressive Matrices–R
II. Auditory–verbal behavior	1. Illinois Test of Psycholinguistic Abilities– Third Edition (ITPA-3)
	2. Detroit Tests of Learning Aptitude–Fourth Edition (DTLA-4)
	3. Comprehensive Test of Phonological Processing (CTOPP)
	4. Swanson Cognitive Processing Test
	5. Peabody Picture Vocabulary Test–III
	6. Expressive Vocabulary Test
	7. Expressive One-Word Picture Vocabulary Test–2000 Edition
	8. Receptive One-Word Picture Vocabulary Test–2000 Edition
	9. Children's Memory Scale (CMS)
	10. Goldman-Fristoe-Woodcock Test of Selective Attention (GFW)
III. Visual–motor behavior	1. Detroit Tests of Learning Abilities–4 (DTLA-4)
	2. Swanson Cognitive Processing Test
	3. Children's Memory Scale
	4. Bender-Gestalt Test
	5. Slosson Drawing Coordination Test for Children
	6. Primary Visual Motor Test
	7. Goodenough-Harris Draw-A-Person Test
	8. Developmental Test of Visual–Motor Integration–Fourth Edition
IV. Academic behavior	1. Woodcock Johnson Tests of Achievement–III (WJ-III)
	2. Wechsler Individual Achievement Test–II (WIAT-II)
	3. Peabody Individual Achievement Test–R/NU (PIAT-R/NU)
	Selected tests
V. Personality	1. Rorschach Test
	2. Thematic Apperception Test (TAT)
	3. Children's Apperception Test (CAT)
	4. Incomplete Sentences Test
	5. Kinetic Family Drawing Test
	6. House-Tree-Person Test
	7. Others as needed

The organization of the fifth edition is broken into two domains (nonverbal and verbal) and five factors; fluid reasoning, knowledge, quantitative reasoning, visual–spatial processing and working memory. The normative sample for the fifth edition closely matched the education level based on the 1999 U.S. Census data and was gathered from 4800 individuals between the ages of 2.0 and 85 years (Roid, 2003).

The revised, restandardized WISC-III (Wechsler, 1991) (see Case Study 8–2) was developed for use with children between 6 and 16 years, 11 months. The lower limit overlaps with the WPPSI-III and the upper limit with the WAIS-III. In addition to the 12

Case Study 8–1   S.R., a kindergartner who is 5 years, 9 months of age, was tested at the request of the parents to rule out possible dyslexia due to a strong family history of dyslexia. S.R. had been enrolled in day care since he was 2 years of age. He was described as having poor work habits, not paying attention, and not listening.

Birth history reflected a birth weight of 7 pounds, 8½ ounces at 2 weeks past due date. No complications were reported at the time of the delivery. Motor development was on the slow side of average, with significant speech and language development delay.

Neither childhood diseases nor a history of chronic middle ear disease was reported. He had received a hearing screening at the beginning of the school year.

S.R. was described as easily embarrassed, sensitive to criticism, very stubborn, and exceptionally quiet.

During the testing, S.R. exerted good effort but became frustrated when items became difficult, and, consequently, he needed to be placed on a reward system in order to perform adequately. S.R. experienced some difficulty with understanding the intent of questions and directions and would mumble when he was not sure of an answer. There were two items he failed on the Pattern Analysis subtest of the Stanford-Binet due to time limit and could not solve any math calculation problems. In addition, he failed to cross the midline on the Visual Attention subtest. On Imitating Hand Positions and Fingertip Tapping, he did mirror patterning. He could not recall any story on the Narrative Memory subtest of the NEPSY, but recalled some facts on the cued recall questions.

Gross and fine coordination fell within normal limits, and S.R. had a good pencil grip. He was left-handed, left-footed, and left-eyed for near- and far-point vision; there was a family history of sinistrality.

Pure tone threshold audiometry documented normal hearing sensitivity for both ears. A pure tone average of 3 dB for both the left and right ear with speech reception thresholds of 5 dB and word recognition scores of 100% at 35 dB HL presentation level were reported. Impedance audiometry results suggested type A tympanograms bilaterally; indicating normal middle ear function.

The Goldman-Fristoe-Woodcock Test of Selective Attention was administered as a binaural speech-in-noise test. S.R. performed at the 91% correct level in quiet, and dropped to 7% when competing messages were introduced. He had extreme difficulty when a steady-state noise was used as the competing sound, and mild to moderate difficulty when a voice was used as the competing sound. His performance was in the low end of average when a random noise was present. Clinical experience has suggested that when a steady-state noise is the lowest subtest, emotional issues are present.

The Goldman-Fristoe-Woodcock Test for Sound Symbolization, also administered, showed that S.R. had problems associating sounds to individual letters. On the Katz Phonemic Synthesis Picture Test, performance fell one standard deviation below the mean for his age; the greatest number of errors was on the first ordered response where he used substitution for the initial phoneme.

Because S.R. was difficult to understand at times, the Templin-Darley Tests of Articulation were administered and showed that articulation development was age appropriate. However, a /f/ substitution for the voiceless /th/ and a /v/ substitution for the voiced /th/ was observed. He substituted a /s/ for the final /ch/. Examination of the oral peripheral mechanism revealed no contributing structural or functional deviations. Diadochokinesis was age appropriate.

Performance on the Stanford-Binet Intelligence Scale: Fourth Edition was in the average range of abilities with stronger nonverbal than verbal skills. Verbal reasoning ability fell in the average range, somewhat on the low side, with verbal fluency and word comprehension in the low average range. Practical knowledge and social judgment as well as understanding absurdities in pictures fell in the average range. Abstract/visual reasoning tested in the high average range of abilities. Quantitative reasoning ability fell in the average range, somewhat on the low side, with short-term memory falling in the average range overall. Visual sequential memory was in the average range with auditory memory for sentences falling in the low average range of abilities.

S.R.'s performance on the NEPSY, a developmental neuropsychological assessment instrument, showed attention/executive function in the average range with visuospatial skills falling in the high average range of abilities. Language skills were in the low average range as were sensorimotor skills. Memory was in the borderline slow learner range of abilities. He had extreme difficulty with narrative memory and memory for names, and with processing kinesthetic information effectively. Language skills fell in the low average range overall, with phonological processing, which assesses his capacity to identify words from segments and to form an auditory gestalt, falling somewhat on the low side of the average range. Speeded Naming was in the low average range as was his ability to process and respond to verbal instructions of increasing complexity.

He demonstrated appropriate visuospatial and eye–hand coordination on the Bender-Gestalt and the Goodenough-Harris Drawing Test.

Academically, S.R. was performing at beginning kindergarten level in word attack skills and at midkindergarten level in reading comprehension. Math calculation fell at beginning kindergarten level, with applied problems at end of kindergarten level. His ability to write from dictation was at midkindergarten level, with writing samples falling at first-grade level. Overall, broad reading and broad math skills were at beginning kindergarten level, with broad written language skills falling at end of kindergarten level.

Emotionally, S.R. expressed positive feelings about himself, and although he expressed some fear of the dark, he was comfortable with his intellectual, physical, and personal self. S.R. believed he was a helpful individual who was accepted by his peers

In summary, the testing results placed S.R. in the average range of abilities with stronger nonverbal than verbal skills. He was experiencing difficulty in auditory memory, selective attention, and verbal fluency. Strengths were observed in abstract/visual reasoning and visuospatial skills. Academically, S.R.'s strongest areas of performance were in math reasoning and writing, with the weakest areas in math calculation and word attack skills.

S.R.'s problems with auditory processing might lead to later problems with reading and it was recommended that he be placed on a program to help develop better auditory processing and selective attention skills. In addition, S.R. needed to work on math calculation and to learn the language of math.

Case Study 8–2 J.N. was enrolled in the second grade, and testing was requested by J.N.'s parents in order to assess his behavior and the decline in his reading grade. He had been retained in the first grade and had participated in reading tutorials at school. Grades were described as inconsistent, ranging from As to Cs. Previous testing by an educational specialist placed J.N.'s intellectual abilities in the high average range with verbal skills in the average range and performance skills in the high average range of abilities. Academic skills fell in the average to very superior range.

J.N. was delivered 2 weeks past due date by cesarean section, with a birth weight of 6 pounds, 12 ounces. Motor development was within normal limits.

J.N. contracted whooping cough, chicken pox, and pneumonia as a youngster, and developed a mild reflux problem at 2 years of age. He had allergies and was mildly asthmatic. No history of early middle ear problems was present. J.N. lives with his brother, mother, and stepfather. Social adaptation skills were described as easily embarrassed, sensitive to criticism, and at times overly neat and particular. He was also described as very stubborn, bossy, and irritable.

The Battin Clinic Auditory Processing and Attention Survey as well as the Fisher's Auditory Problems Checklist were completed by J.N.'s mother. Both were significant for attention and central auditory processing problems. J.N. demonstrated poor ability to pay attention, remember routine tasks, recall what was heard in the immediate past, and respond to verbal directions and instructions. He frequently asked for things to be repeated, and often misunderstood what was said. He had difficulty with phonics and trouble recalling a sequence and would forget what was said in a few minutes.

J.N. was a friendly, quiet young man who was cooperative, had good eye contact, exerted good effort, but needed encouragement when items became difficult. On math tests, J.N. used his fingers to help in solving the problems. On the Speeded Naming subtests of the NEPSY, J.N. had trouble recalling the label (square) in the middle of the task.

Gross and fine coordination fell within normal limits. Responses to the Reitan Finger Oscillation Test were on the slow side of average with no significant difference between the sides. Bilateral presentation was slow and mildly dysynchronous. J.N. was right-handed, right-footed, and right-eyed for near and far point vision.

Results from the audiological evaluation were consistent with normal hearing; pure tone average of 0 dB for both the right and left ears, speech reception thresholds of 0 dB, and word recognition scores of 100% obtained at 30 dB HL presentation level. Impedance audiometry suggested type A tympanograms bilaterally with clearly present otoacoustic emissions testing for both the right and left ears. Masking level difference results, which looks at the integrity of the lower brainstem and its ability to process subtle interaural time and amplitude differences, fell within normal limits.

The Phonemic Synthesis Test, which requires the individual to fuse words presented one phoneme per second, revealed performance above age level for both quantitative as well as qualitative scoring. However, responses to the Staggered Spondaic Word Test were greater than four standard deviations below the mean for his age with a significant low/high ear effect and a low/high order effect.

The Goldman-Fristoe-Woodcock Test of Selective Attention was administered as a binaural speech-in-noise test. J.N.'s high score on the quiet subtest indicated that he knew the vocabulary, but a subsequent 20th percentile score occurred when competing messages were introduced. He was able to handle a steady-state noise as well as a voice as the competing message but had significant difficulty when a random noise, such as that found in the classroom, was used. This suggests that J.N. will experience difficulty handling classroom noise and would benefit from preferential seating so that competing messages are behind him rather than between him and the primary sound source (teacher).

J.N. performed in the average range of abilities with stronger performance than verbal skills as reflected on the WISC-III. He performed in the superior range in processing speed skills whereas perceptual organization and freedom from distractibility fell in the average range. Verbal comprehension skills fell in the average range, somewhat on the high side. There was a significant spread between subtests. He performed within the very superior range on a task that involved scanning for the appropriate symbol. Average ability was observed in alertness to visual detail, learning a meaningless code and rapidly transferring it to paper, visual praxis, the ability to copy an abstract design from a pattern, visual gestalt, object assembly, practical knowledge, and social judgment. However, performance was somewhat on the low side of average in understanding social situations when presented through pictures and auditory recall for numbers. Low average ability was observed in general fund of information, verbal reasoning, word knowledge, and verbal fluency.

Average ability in visuospatial skills and eye–hand coordination was reflected on the Bender-Gestalt and the Goodenough-Harris Drawing Test.

J.N.'s performance with the NEPSY, a developmental neuropsychological assessment instrument, was in the average range on the attention/executive core domain. He was above expected level in planning, strategizing, self-monitoring, and problem solving; at expected level for his age in simple and complex auditory attention; and slightly below expected level in simple and complex visual attention and inhibition. In contrast, J.N. performed in the low average range on the language core domain and fell slightly below expected level in conceptualization of changing speech-sound patterns, which underlies decoding and spelling. He also performed slightly below expected level in speeded access to language labels, which research has shown is critical to reading, but was at expected level for his age in comprehension of instructions.

Performance for the sensorimotor core domain was in the borderline range, and at expected level for his age in handling simple and complex sequential fine motor movements. However, performance was well below expected level in integration of visual-static fine motor position, poor performance on this subtest is indicative of problems with handwriting (dysgraphia). J.N.'s performance was well below expected level in immediate and delayed memory for faces and below expected level in name learning and delayed memory for names. He performed slightly below expected level for his age in free and cued recall of a narrative story.

Academically, J.N. performed at his intellectual abilities level and grade level in math while performing somewhat below his abilities level and grade placement in reading and writing.

Emotionally, J.N. was experiencing some anxiety and sadness. He saw support as coming from his parents, and he also used avoidance as a coping mechanism to deal with emotional situations. Although he wanted to achieve, he didn't associate effort with achieving one's goals.

In summary, J.N. was performing in the average range of abilities overall with somewhat stronger performance than verbal skills. He demonstrated significant problems with central auditory processing, which would interfere with performance in the classroom. In addition, he experienced difficulty with selective attention when a random noise was present in the environment. It was recommended that he receive preferential seating and a visual cue prior to the presenting of verbal information. It was also recommended that J.N. be placed in a therapy program directed to improving his auditory processing skills.

subtests that made up the WISC (1949) and WISC-R (1974), the publishers added a new optional subtest, Symbol Search. Six subtests make up the Verbal Scale and seven subtests constitute the Performance Scale. As with earlier editions, 10 of the WISC-III tests are considered mandatory; the Digit Span, Symbol Search, and Mazes subtests are supplementary tests and were not included in establishing the IQ tables. In addition to the verbal, performance, and full-scale IQ scores, four factor based scores can be calculated for verbal comprehension, perceptual organization, freedom from distractibility, and processing speed.

The WISC-III (Wechsler, 1991) has improved subtest content, administration, and scoring rules. An effort was made to minimize content bias and to refine and update the artwork. Easier as well as more difficult items were added to various subtests. Although many of the test items were retained and unchanged in the verbal subtests, other items were modified and new items were added. On the performance scale, the pictures have been redrawn, color has been added, and there is an increase in the number of items. The Picture Completion subtest has been increased from 26 to 30 items. There are 12 items instead of 11 on the Block Design subtest and a new item has been added to both the Object Assembly subtest and the Mazes subtest. Symbol Search is a new optional subtest with levels A and B.

The new order for presenting subtests, plus the improved artwork with the addition of color, makes the test more interesting and less tiring, for both the child and the examiner. Subtests most relevant to auditory–verbal dysfunction are the verbal ones; however, they only reveal a disturbance within a particular child when they are compared with that child's scores on the performance subtests.

Analysis of a child's performance on the individual subtests of the WISC-III will indicate whether further testing in specific modalities is needed. The Information subtest indicates how well the child stores information gained from education and experience and how well this information can be retrieved on command. By comparing responses on the Information, Arithmetic, and Digit Span subtests, the examiner can observe the effectiveness of the child's delayed recall as opposed to immediate recall, auditory attention, and mental control. The ability to provide practical solutions to everyday problems and social concerns may be seen through the Comprehension subtest, with the Vocabulary subtest providing an estimate of verbal fluency, word knowledge, and expressive skills. The Similarities subtest provides information on the child's logical and abstract verbal reasoning ability.

By careful observation of the child's behavior during the verbal subtests, an understanding of how the child processes auditory stimuli emerges. Questions that indicate auditory processing function include:

1. Does the child need frequent repetitions or restatement of questions?
2. Does the child tend to reauditorize the material or are there long response latencies?
3. How are the numbers on the Digit Span subtest retrieved?
4. Are the problems on the Arithmetic subtest forgotten before they can be solved?
5. Are there difficulties in perceiving the questions or following directions on the Information, Comprehension, and Similarities subtests?
6. Does the child appear to confuse words (e.g., pail for nail) on the Vocabulary subtests?

Similar analysis of the subtests of the Performance Scale can pinpoint problems in visual closure, gestalt, praxis, short-term memory, scanning, and left–right tracking. Problems with delayed visual recall, visual problem-solving, and fine motor control can also be delineated.

The fourth revision of the WISC (WISC-IV) (Wechsler, 2003) was published in the fall of 2003. The format has been changed to specific cognitive domains: Verbal Comprehension Index, Perceptual Reasoning Index, and Working Memory Index. It also provides a composite score that represents general intellectual ability. Subtest content and administration and scoring procedures have been changed. New subtests have been added and Picture Arrange, Object Assembly, and Mazes have been dropped. Block Design, Similarities, Digit Span, Coding, Vocabulary, Comprehension, Symbol Search, Picture Completion, Information, and Arithmetic have been retained. Picture Concepts, Letter-Number Sequencing, Matrix Reasoning, Cancellation, and Word Reasoning have been added. The Core Test is composed of 10 subtests with Information, Word Reasoning, Picture Completion, Arithmetic, and Cancellation serving as supplemental subtests.

The WPPSI-III (Wechsler, 2002) was published to replace the WPPSI-R (Wechsler, 1989). Like the WPPSI-R, the revision is an individually administered test of intelligence for children. The age range has been extended to cover children age 2 years, 6 months through 7 years, 0 months. Nonverbal and verbal fluid reasoning, receptive vocabulary, and processing speed are measured by new subtests, which include Picture Naming, Receptive Vocabulary, Matrix Reasoning, Picture Concepts, Symbol Search, and Coding. Testing is divided into two age groups: 2 years, 6 months through 3 years, 11 months; and 4 years, 0 months through 7 years, 3 months. Although the upper age range overlaps the WISC-III (Wechsler, 1991), the possibility of practice effect has been reduced. Validity studies with the Wechsler Individual Achievement Test–II (WIAT-II) as well as other test instruments have been conducted. In addition, ongoing studies are being conducted on such special groups as those with mental retardation, developmental delay, expressive-receptive language delay, attention deficit/hyperactivity disorder (ADHD), English as a second language, gifted and autism disorder or Asperger's syndrome. The WPPSI-III (Wechsler, 2002) can be either hand scored or computer scored by using a computer software program that includes an individualized written report.

The Kaufman Assessment Battery for Children (KABC) (Kaufman & Kaufman, 1983) was published as an individually ad-

ministered measure of intelligence and achievement for children 2 years, 6 months thorough 12 years, 6 months of age. Administration time is approximately 45 minutes for preschool children and 75 minutes for school-age children. The test is made up of the following 16 subtests: Hand Movements, Number Recall, Word Order, Magic Window, Face Recognition, Gestalt Closure, Triangles, Matrix Analogies, Spatial Memory, Photo Series, Expressive Vocabulary, Faces and Places, Arithmetic, Riddles, Reading/Decoding, and Reading/Understanding. Seven subtests are administered to 2 years, 6-month-old children, nine subtests to 3-year-old children, and the maximum (13) to children 7 years old and older. It provides standard scores (mean 100, standard deviation 15) in four areas: Sequential Processing, Simultaneous Processing, Mental Processing Composite (obtained from Sequencing Processing and Simultaneous Processing, which provides an IQ equivalence), and Achievement. Supplemental sociocultural norms assist in interpreting the tests of children from minority groups. In addition, a nonverbal scale made up of selected subtests that can be administered and responded to through gestures provides assessment of the general abilities level of children with auditory processing problems, speech and language delay, or hearing impairment.

The KABC was developed from neuropsychological theory but does not claim to be a neuropsychological test. However, those examiners who look at brain dysfunction as it relates to performance and developing a therapy plan will find the test fits well into their assessment battery.

An estimate of cognitive skills may be useful if an examiner is evaluating central auditory processing or language-learning ability, or if a standard test of intelligence has been administered by another agency and the examiner wants a more current assessment of function. The Kaufman Brief Intelligence Test (KBIT) (Kaufman & Kaufman, 1990) was published as an excellent instrument for an individually administered test that measures both verbal and nonverbal intelligence. Verbal and crystallized abilities are measured by a vocabulary test, and nonverbal and fluid abilities are measured by a matrices subtest. The KBIT (Kaufman & Kaufman, 1990) has an age range of 4 to 90 years and is easy to administer. The authors state that it may be administered by technicians or allied health professionals not licensed in standard intelligence test administration. The test takes from 15 to 30 minutes to administer and was developed as a screening instrument that provides an estimate of intelligence. Care must be taken to avoid using this test for diagnosis, placement, or neuropsychological evaluation.

The Test of Nonverbal Intelligence, second edition (TONI-2) (Brown, Sherbenou, & Johnsen, 1990), was developed for use with individuals who require a language-free, motor- and culture-reduced test format (Brown, 1990). It was revised in 1997 (TONI-3) (Brown, Sherbenou, & Johnsen, 1997) and measures intelligence, aptitude, abstract reasoning, and nonverbal problem-solving ability. The age range is from 6 years through 90 years. It takes approximately 15 minutes to administer and has no reading, writing, listening, or speaking requirement. Gestures are used for giving instructions and there are six training items for which examinees indicate their response by pointing. School psychologists have used the TONI-3 to qualify a student for services when standard intelligence tests fail to provide the required discrepancy between achievement and IQ.

The Comprehensive Test of Nonverbal Intelligence (CTONI) was developed by Hammill, Pearson, and Wiederholt (1997) as an unbiased measure of nonverbal intelligence. Depending upon instruction presentation (i.e., oral or pantomime), the CTONI (Hammill, Pearson, & Wiederholt, 1997) can be either a performance or a nonlanguage, nonverbal intelligence test. It is made up of six subtests, which measure high order cognitive abilities. A sample of 2901 individuals (of which 772 were adults) from 30 states and the District of Columbia was used in norming the CTONI. The age range is from 6 years, 0 months through 89 years, 11 months. The authors recommend using the pantomime directions for individuals who

are hearing impaired or non–English speaking. They do not recommend translating the oral instructions into sign language or another language because this would create a variation in difficulty.

The Leiter International Performance Scale (Leiter, 1969), a standard for testing the hearing impaired, has been revised (Roid & Miller, 2002) and nationally standardized with revisions of the original Visualization and Reasoning Domain for measuring IQ and a new Attention and Memory domain. The new domain can be used to identify children with ADHD as well as for neuropsychological assessment. It has an age range of 2 years, 9 months through 20, years 11 months.

Other intelligence tests that test special abilities are the Hiskey-Nebraska Test of Learning Aptitudes (Hiskey, 1966), Naglieri Nonverbal Ability Test–Multilevel Form (Naglieri, 1996), Slosson Intelligence Test for Children and Adults–R (Nicholson & Hibpshman, 1990), Raven Progressive Matrices–P (Raven, 2000a, b), and the Columbia Mental Maturity Scale (Burgemeister, Blum, & Lorge, 1972).

The NEPSY (Korkman, Kirk, & Kemp, 1997), a developmental neuropsychological assessment instrument based on Luria's Theories of Brain Organization, was published by the Psychological Corporation. The NEPSY has proven to be an excellent test for assessing children with language-learning problems as well as ADHD. It is divided into five domains, the first of which addresses attention/executive function with three of six subtests required for the standard battery under this domain. However, there are four subtests that are favored under this first domain: the Tower, Auditory Attention and Response Set, Visual Attention, and Knock and Tap. The latter assesses the child's ability to self-regulate and to inhibit immediate impulses created by visual stimuli that are in conflict with a verbal direction. Under the language core domain, there are seven subtests, four of which are critical to the standard battery: Body Part Naming, Phonological Processing, Speeded Naming, and Comprehension of Instructions. If one is looking specifically at the language-learning problem, the additional subtests of Verbal Fluency and Oral Motor Sequencing, which taps the ballistic movements for speech, are recommended. The sensorimotor domain has five subtests; three are critical to the standard battery. Under visuospatial processing, there are four subtests; two are critical to the standard battery. There are five subtests in the memory and learning domain. It is recommended that consideration be given to administering all five of the subtests. The age range for the NEPSY is 3 years, 0 months through 12 years, 11 months, with an administration time of approximately 90 minutes. According to the authors, the NEPSY was "developed with four interrelated purposes in mind": to "create a reliable and valid instrument that would be sensitive to subtle deficiencies within and across the five functional domains that interfere with learning in preschool and school-age children"; to "create an instrument that would contribute to understanding the effects of brain damage in young children as a result of congenital or acquired brain damage"; "to create an instrument that would be used for long-term follow-up"; and "to create a reliable and valid instrument for the study of normal and atypical neuropsychological development in preschool and school-age children" (Korkman, Kirk, & Kemp, 1997, pp. 2–3; see Case Study 8–2).

Phonological Processing and Speeded Naming are considered critical skills for the development of reading and written language. Although the NEPSY (Korkman, Kirk, & Kemp, 1997) taps these skills, some examiners may not have that assessment available to them or may not meet the qualifications for using the NEPSY. Another option is the Comprehensive Test of Phonological Processes (CTOPP), which has been developed to look at an individual's phonological processing strengths and weaknesses (Wagner, Torgesen, & Rashotte, 1999). The authors designed their test to tap three aspects of phonological processing: phonological awareness, phonological memory, and rapid naming. It is based on a belief that a deficit in one or more of these phonological

processing abilities is the most common cause of learning disabilities, particularly reading disabilities. There are two versions of the test; the first version covers individuals 5 and 6 years old, the second version covers ages 7 through 24 (second grade through college). Testing time is approximately 30 minutes.

Although memory skills are assessed to some degree by the cognitive tests, the examiner may want to look more in depth at immediate and delayed auditory and visual memory skills. The Children's Memory Scale (CMS) (Cohen, 1997) compares memory and learning ability. It is linked to the WISC-III and the WPPSI-R and allows comparisons of memory and intellectual ability. It tests 5- through 16-year-olds for attention and working memory, verbal and visual memory, immediate and delayed recall, and recognition and learning characteristics. The CMS is considered to be an excellent addition to test batteries geared for those children who fall above the upper age level of the NEPSY.

The Swanson Cognitive Processing Test (S-CPT) (Swanson, 1996) measures different aspects of mental processing ability and potential for ranges from 5 years to adulthood. The test can be individually administered as a complete (11 subtests) or abbreviated (five to six subtests) form. The normative sample was made up of 1611 individuals residing in four geographic regions of the United States and two regions in Canada. The author believes that "to understand an individual's processing potential, one must separate the current state of functioning from that which is influenced by instruction" (Swanson, 1996, p. 1). To accomplish this, the individual's performance is compared before and after the examiner provides cues to assist performance. The subtests require the examiner to store some information while processing other information. Swanson sets forth the rationale for his test that all major information processing models show working memory to be highly correlated with performance on language-related and academic tasks. As a consequence, the test assesses a passive short-term memory system and a dynamic working memory system. The author states, "The purpose of the S-CPT is to measure the sensitivity of a test-related intervention that is sufficiently brief to administer within a normal testing period" (Swanson, 1996, p. 4). To better understand the premise for the S-CPT, the reader should review the extensive research that provided a base for the test.

Auditory–Verbal Behavior Assessment

The Illinois Test of Psycholinguistic Abilities–Third Edition (ITPA-3) (Hammill, Mathers, & Roberts, 2001) has replaced the ITPA-R (Kirk, McCarthy, & Kirk, 1968) with an instrument that assesses various linguistic abilities considered important to "scholastic success." The original ITPA (McCarthy & Kirk, 1961) was a test of cognitive functioning whereas the present test addresses linguistic abilities in both oral and written language. All of the subtests of the third edition measure aspects of language, with none of the subtests directed to visual–motor performance. The age range of the ITPA-3 has been broadened to include 5 years, 0 months through 12 years, 11 months, and has an enlarged normative sample that better reflects the U.S. population. The test is a composite of the 12 subsets. These are divided into a general language composite quotient, spoken language composite quotient, and written language composite quotient. The general language composite quotient is considered the best predictor of achievement. The spoken language composite quotient is made up of 6 subtests that measure semantics, grammar, and phonology. The written language composite is also made up of 6 subtests that measure reading comprehension, written vocabulary, phonics, and orthographic ability. In addition to the three main quotients, eight specific composite quotients can be obtained for semantics, grammar, phonology, comprehension, word identification, spelling, sight-symbol processing, and sound-symbol processing. For clinicians engaged in remediation of language, learning, and auditory processing skills, the ITPA-3 would be an excellent instrument for monitoring progress.

The Detroit Tests of Learning Aptitude were revised in the second edition (DTLA-2) (Hammill, 1985), in the third edition (DTLA-3) (Hammill, 1991), and more recently in the fourth edition (DTLA-4) (Hammill, 1998). Like its predecessors, the DTLA-4 is a flexible, comprehensive test containing 10 subtests that assess interrelated mental abilities. The test takes from 50 minutes to as much as 2 hours to administer to children ages 6 through 17 years. The test was normed on 1350 individuals from 37 states. The author describes the fourth edition as "a battery that measures a variety of developed abilities. Depending on the orientation or need of the test user, DTLA-4 results can be used to estimate general cognitive functioning (intelligence), predict future success (aptitude), or show mastery of particular content and skills (achievement)" (Hammill, 1998, p. 9). It can be used to verify areas of difficulty and to supplement the WISC-III (Wechsler, 1991) and Stanford-Binet: Fourth Edition (Thorndike, Hagen, & Sattler, 1986). In addition to providing a general mental ability quotient and three domain composites (linguistic, attentional, and motoric), the DTLA-4 provides an optimal composite and a theoretical composite. The optimal composite is acquired by combining the individual's four largest standard scores and is an important feature for evaluating children with auditory processing problems.

Individual assessment places the child in an optimum testing learning situation. Children who have problems with auditory figure-ground or selective attention may do well in the one-to-one situation, but have extreme difficulty attending in the classroom. The Revised Goldman-Fristoe-Woodcock (GFW-R) Test (Goldman, Fristoe, & Woodcock, 1974), or discrimination tests presented both in quiet and with competing noise, should be given. Clinically, it has been found that children who have difficulty selectively attending in the classroom are depressed on the Cafeteria and/or Voice Noise subtests of the GFW-R. Children who are depressed on the Fan Noise subtest but who fall at or above the 50th percentile on the other two subtests (Cafeteria and Voice Noise), would be considered to have emotional rather than auditory perceptual problems.

Of course, the ideal situation is for the child to have an audiological evaluation including threshold testing for pure tones and speech, word recognition testing, and impedance prior to or during the psychoeducational evaluation. Otoacoustic emissions testing and masking level differences should be included. It is also this author's preference to use the speech-in-noise test, phonemic synthesis test, and staggered spondaic word test from Katz's central battery (Katz, 1998).

Picture vocabulary tests are often used to assess receptive and expressive language. The most frequently used vocabulary test, the Peabody Picture Vocabulary Test–Third Edition (PPVT-III) (Dunn, 1970), provides age-based standard scores, percentile ranks, and age equivalents for 2 years, 6 months through 90-year-old individuals. It is described as a screening test of verbal ability and a wide-range measure of receptive vocabulary for standard English. It takes 10 to 15 minutes to administer. The Expressive Vocabulary Test (EVT) is co-normed with the PPVT-III and measures expressive vocabulary and word retrieval of Standard American English (Williams, 1997). Like the PIAT-III, it is appropriate for a wide range of ages.

Standard scores ($M = 100$; $SD = 15$) obtained from the PPVT-III are not interchangeable with either the WISC-III or the Stanford-Binet Intelligence Test: Fourth Edition, IQ scores. The PPVT is useful in measuring extensiveness of vocabulary and degree of cultural assimilation of children. Costello and Ali (1971) described the PPVT as a screening instrument for children who have a limited expressive vocabulary or are verbally inhibited. It should not be used in measures of general abilities.

Two other vocabulary tests used by speech pathologists and educational diagnosticians are the Expressive One-Word Picture Vocabulary Test–2000 Edition (Gardner, 2000) and the Receptive One-Word Vocabulary Test–2000 Edition (Brownell, 2000). Both are individually norm referenced for use

with individuals ages 2 years, 6 months through 18 years, 11 months with a 15- to 20-minute administration for each test.

Visual–Motor Behavior Assessment

A complete evaluation should include one or more tests of visual perception, integration, and execution. The Bender-Gestalt Test has been widely used since it was developed by Loretta Bender in 1938. Koppitz revised the scoring system in 1963 and again in 1975. This objective scoring system, normed for children 5–0 through 11–11 years, has been adopted by many individuals administering the Bender-Gestalt Test (Koppitz, 1963). In addition, the scoring allows delineation indicators of brain injury for children ages 5 through 11 years. The Watkins Bender-Gestalt Scoring System is an alternative scoring system (Watkins, 1976) that has been standardized on over 33,000 individuals and is useful in identifying children with a visual learning disability.

Three other tests of visual perception and eye–hand coordination are the Slosson Drawing Coordination Test for Children (Slosson, 1975), the Primary Visual Motor Test (Haworth, 1970), and the Developmental Test of Visual–Motor Integration: Fourth Edition (Berry, 1996).

The Draw-A-Person Test (Harris, 1963) allows the examiner to compare the youngster's spatial, size, and shape orientation as well as sequencing ability when drawing freehand without a pattern, as opposed to copying designs. The youngster is asked to draw a picture of a person, then a picture of the opposite sex, and then a self-drawing. This exercise provides insight into a child's body imagery and emotional state. New norms were established for the test in 1970 for ages 6 to 11 years by the U.S. Department of Health, Education, and Welfare (*Intellectual Maturity*) (1970). Naglieri, McNeish, and Bardos (1991) normed the Draw-a-Person as a screening test on 2260 students age 6 to 17. The test is nonthreatening and serves as a good introduction to the total test battery. Care should be taken to observe which hand the youngster uses to write and draw as well as how the pencil is held.

Academic Assessment

Some estimate of academic performance should be made during the comprehensive evaluation. This allows the examiner to observe how well the child handles academic material in a one-to-one testing situation as opposed to the group timed achievement test administered in the classroom. The report of results should describe how the child handles different types of problem solving, as well as areas in which there are difficulties. All difficulties should be analyzed in light of deficits observed in auditory, verbal, and visual motor areas. For example, one might report the results of testing as follows: "The memory problems did not overly hamper academic achievement. She worked slowly in reading; however, performance fell in the same range as her intellectual ability. The youngster seemed to perform better when given ample time to consider responses. The memory problems did not interfere with spelling, but did appear to hamper long-term retention of academic facts."

A popular individual achievement test used by school psychologists and educational diagnosticians is the Woodcock Johnson Tests of Achievement–III (Woodcock, McGrew, & Maither, 2001) (Case Study 8–3) that contains 22 tests and two auxiliary writing subtests. These 22 tests are combined into clusters. There are two forms, A and B, with each form divided into two parts: a standard battery and a supplementary battery. The standard battery is made up of 12 tests that measure basic reading skills, reading comprehension, reading fluency, basic mathematics skills, mathematical reasoning, mathematical fluency, basic writing skills, writing fluency, and written expression. In addition, broad cluster scores in reading, mathematics, writing, and knowledge skills are provided. Most examiners use 9 of the 12 tests when administering the Woodcock Johnson Tests of Achievement–III. The raw scores are entered into a computer program

that provides age level, grade level, and age and grade standard scores and percentiles.

With the exception of the Written Expression subtest, the Peabody Individual Achievement Test–Revised/NU (PIAT-R/NU) (Markwardt, 1998) is an untimed power test of achievement. The "NU" stands for normative data update. The test takes approximately 60 minutes to administer. Some children will take less time to complete the test; however, the examiner must not make the subject feel hurried. It is advised to give the test in one uninterrupted session. The test instructions should be followed precisely. The examiner may repeat an item when requested by the child being tested or if the child does not respond. However, the items must be repeated in their entirety without any change in the wording. An item cannot be readministered once a response has been given. The examiner must note carefully whether the child seems to misperceive the instructions or does not know the material.

The order of subtest administration was changed in the revised version to increase interest and motivation. General Information is administered first, followed by Reading Recognition, Reading Comprehension, Mathematics, Spelling, and Written Expression. The total test score does not include the Written Expression subtest, allowing the examiner the option to omit it from the test battery. A computer scoring system available for the PIAT-R/NU provides the examiner with a printout of age- and grade-level standard scores and percentiles. In addition to providing scores for the individual subtests, the PIAT-R/NU provides a total reading, total test, and written language composite score.

A new individual achievement test was published by the Psychological Corporation (WIAT, 1992) and revised in 2001 (WIAT-II, 2001). The Wechsler Individual Achievement Test–II (WIAT-II, 2001) consists of a screening test that evaluates basic reading, mathematics reasoning, and spelling, and a comprehensive test that evaluates reading comprehension, numerical operations, listening comprehension, oral expression, and written expression in addition to the items

Case Study 8–3 J.T. was referred for comprehensive evaluation when he was 13 years, 9 months of age because of behavior problems at school that resulted in his frequently getting into trouble. He was in detention hall for talking, being late, and fighting with students both on and off campus.

Behavior during the evaluation revealed a quiet youngster who was somber, cooperative, and had fair eye contact. He was inconsistent in his effort and became frustrated when tasks became difficult. Questions had to be repeated throughout the session. Gross and fine coordination skills fell within normal limits.

Audiological findings were within normal limits with pure tone averages of 3 dB for the left ear and 0 dB for the right, speech reception thresholds of 5 dB for the left ear and 0 dB for the right, and word recognition scores of 100%, bilaterally. Impedance audiometry were consistent with normal middle ear function (type A tympanograms) bilaterally.

Performance on the Staggered Spondaic Word Test was consistent with a moderate to severe disturbance in central auditory processing, with a significant ear as well as a significant order effect. He experienced his greatest difficulty when the competing message was in the right ear, suggesting involvement in the auditory reception area of the left temporal lobe.

Administration of Clinical Evaluation of Language Fundamentals–Revised resulted in J.T. failing the test at five points below the criterion score for his age. Most notably, he had problems in auditory association and reconstructing sentences.

This young man was performing in the average to low average range of abilities, with performance skills in the average range and verbal skills in the low average range. He showed severe auditory processing problems and mild to moderate auditory memory problems. Academically, he was performing at the level of his ability, with the exception of mathematical computation, which fell below grade placement. Emotionally, he showed a poor self-concept and poor coping skills. His responses to the Rorschach indicated a thought disorder, although not of the bizarre type. Responses to the Thematic Appreciation Test were constricted with anxiety, sadness, anger, and an indication of a parting of the ways between mother and son. In addition, he was concerned about his father's alcoholism. He was somewhat guarded and distant in regard to what precipitated his suicidal thoughts; the suicide potential was still present and needed to be explored further. It was recommended that he receive therapy for the severe auditory processing disturbance. The problem in processing what he received auditorily may have been a contributing factor to the observed thought disorder.

J.T. met the criteria for 296.22 Major Depression, 300.40 Dysthymia, and 313.81 Oppositional Defiant Disorder.

on the screening test. Results are reported as standard scores and percentiles. The WIAT-II assesses children in grades prekindergarten through college and ages 4 through adults. The test was normed on a sample equivalent to that used in standardizing the WISC-III (Wechsler, 1991) and the WAIS-III (Wechsler, 1997).

An estimate of ability-achievement discrepancies can be calculated when the WIAT-II is used with the Wechsler scales. The test is a useful tool in evaluating for learning disabilities, including the child with an auditory learning disability.

The Wide-Range Achievement Test–3 (WRAT-3) (Wilkensen, 1993) has returned to a single-level format with an age range of 5 to 75 years. The revised test has two scales that cover the entire age range. The two forms can be used together or individually and may take 15 to 30 minutes each to complete. Academic skills are measured by converting the raw scores into standard scores, grade scores, absolute scores, and percentiles. As with the revised WRAT (Jastak & Jastak, 1986), the new edition measures basic skills in reading, spelling, and arithmetic. The time limit on the Arithmetic subtest has been extended to 15 minutes. As with the earlier edition, additional information can be obtained if the examiner records what the child has completed at the 15-minute limit and then allows the youngster to continue until he or she can no longer work the problems.

Both the WRAT-3 (Wilkensen, 1993) and the PIAT-R/NU (Markwardt, 1998) tend to overestimate when the results are compared with teacher-administered achievement tests. Williamson (1979) questioned whether this was due to the diagnostician, who tests on a one-to-one basis, being in a more supportive role and thus obtaining much higher scores. It may be that group (classroom) testing underestimates the ability of the child with a learning disability. It would also tend to punish the child that is easily distracted or has problems in selective attention or attention span. Therefore, the individually administered achievement test may give a more accurate estimate of academic achievement of a child with auditory–verbal problems.

Personality Assessment

Whether or not children are disabled, they will acquire a distinct manner of handling different situations and dealing with their environment and people. They are individuals with distinct personalities. Personality tests (Murstein, 1965) provide information about the inner workings of individuals, their perceptions of their world, how they cope, their social skills, their self-concept, and their frustration tolerance level (see Case Study 8–3). Such tests give the examiner some understanding of individuals' attitudes toward self, family, and the outside world, and how they perceive that they "fit into the scheme of things." Personality assessment utilizes projective tests and personality inventories (Molish, 1972). Many

test instruments are available, and each examiner has favorites. The most popular are the Rorschach Test (Exner, 2001; Rorschach, Lemkan, & Krononberg, 1942); the Thematic Apperception Test and Children's Apperception Test (Bellak, 1971); the Rotter Incomplete Sentences Test (Rotter, Lah, & Rafferty, 1992); the House/Tree/Person Test (Buck, 1948); the Children's Self-Report and Projective Inventory (Ziffer & Shapiro, 1992); and the Kinetic Family Drawings (Burns & Kaufman, 1972).

One or two personality tests should be a part of the comprehensive evaluation. Only a qualified examiner should administer and interpret projective instruments. It is important that information on the perceptual disabilities be available at the time of interpretation of the projective tests. When a child's misperceptions of the environment result from an auditory perceptual disturbance, the child's responses to the projective instrument will be affected. If a child constantly misperceives what is said by improper coding, or if the child cannot hold information in short-term memory long enough to rescan it and interpret and act on the message, or if selective attention is disturbed, the child's environment will be constantly punishing. Frustration, poor self-worth, and a sense of failure, as well as feelings of anger, aggression, and hostility, are bound to develop. These feelings are secondary to the primary disorder of disturbed auditory perception and processing. Clinically, it has been found that when specific deficits are remediated, the emotional components tend to resolve themselves. When an emotional disturbance does remain beyond specific treatment of deficits, it responds quickly to psychotherapy.

Educational Planning and Remediation

The primary purpose of a comprehensive psychoeducational evaluation is to provide the parents, school, and remediation specialists with a better understanding of the child and the child's general abilities, disabilities, and academic strengths and weaknesses. Test results should also provide an explanation of nonconforming behavior and allow for the development of an individualized educational, behavioral, and remediation plan. The test profile may dictate such things as:

1. Modifications in the home and school environment to allow the child to attend selectively to what is being said
2. Preferential seating close to the primary sound source
3. Reinforcement of auditory instruction by visual and kinesthetic means
4. Allowing the child to record written work on a tape recorder and then transcribe from his or her own dictation
5. Use of a "Study Buddy" to assist in getting assignments
6. Modifying the length and sequence of orally presented material
7. Placement in a resource program
8. Individualized therapy directed to remediating specific deficits (Bradley, Battin, & Sutter, 1979)

The case evaluations in this chapter show how information relating to intellectual, academic, and behavioral factors is obtained from the history and how this information may be interpreted.

Case Study 8–4 D.F. was tested to assess progress following completion of the Fast ForWord-Language Program (Fast ForWord, 1997). He had attended a private school, and initial testing was accomplished through that facility. Supplemental testing accomplished at the Battin Clinic revealed severe problems with central auditory processing. He experienced difficulty with auditory figure-ground, auditory closure, handling competing words, and understanding language as represented by the Test of Auditory Reasoning and Processing Skills (TARPS) (Gardner, 1993).

D.F. separated easily from his mother and came willingly with the examiners. He was friendly and cooperative but did lose interest in the testing situation and laid on the couch to "nap" in order to avoid testing that he felt was difficult. He was manipulative, and encouragement and a reward system had to be used to maintain his attention. Some tangential language was observed but observation revealed nice growth over previous language behavior.

Pure tone threshold audiometry suggested D.F. was hearing within normal limits; with a pure tone average of 0 dB for both the right and left ears. Speech reception thresholds were noted at 5 dB with word recognition scores of 100% for both ears. Impedance audiometry was consistent with normal middle ear function (type A tympanograms) bilaterally.

D.F. had made significant gains over previous testing that were observed not only on formalized tests but on informal assessment as well. He was more equipped to handle his communication environment, which should allow him to perform better in the classroom and be less frustrated. He continued to show mild problems and it was recommended that consideration be given to placing him on the next level of the Fast-ForWord-Language to Reading Program (Fast ForWord, 1998). Test results were as follows:

SCAN	Present		Previous		Gain	
	SS	%ile	SS	%ile	SS	%ile
Filtered words	10	50	3	1	+7	+49
Auditory figure-ground	14	91	<3	<1	>11	>90
Competing words	9	37	5	5	+4	+32
SCAN Composite	99	47	65	1	+34	+46

Summary

A comprehensive psychoeducational assessment of auditory language-learning problems should use each child as his or her own control. It should evaluate general abilities as well as specific auditory, language, and learning areas. The examiner should be concerned with the child's optimum performance level at the time of testing as well as abilities when the child is under stress or fatigued, and in a variety of learning situations. Examiners should also look to specific deficits, as well as strengths, in the auditory, visual, haptic-kinesthetic, and language areas. It is important to determine how the child performs in a quiet, nonstimulating environment, as well as when distractions or competing messages are introduced. Some understanding of family health issues should be a part of the assessment, as should a comprehensive history that explores birth, health, behavior, developmental milestones, academic performance, and peer and family relationships. Furthermore, the examiner must be an astute observer of behavior, noting how a child perceives questions, whether the child asks for repetition, whether restatement is necessary, how environmental noises affect the child, and what type of response latency is present.

A profile of the child should be drawn to show strengths as well as deficits so that an individualized educational plan and a comprehensive remediation program can be developed. Each child's strengths should be utilized for ego building, while deficits are being remediated, thus improving function in the classroom, at home, and with peers (Case Study 8–4).

References

Bellak, L. (1971). *The Thematic Apperception Test and the Children's Apperception Test in Clinical Use, ed 2.* New York: Grune & Stratton.

Berry, K. (1996). Developmental Test of Visual–Motor Integration–Fourth Edition. Columbus: Modern Curriculum Press.

Bradley, P.E., Battin, R.R., & Sutter, E.G. (1979). Effects of individual diagnosis and remediation for the treatment of learning disabilities. *Journal of Clinical Neuropsychology, 1,* 23–35.

Brown, L., Sherbenou, R.J., & Johnsen, S.K. (1990). Test of Nonverbal Intelligence–Second Edition: A Language-Free Test of Cognitive Ability. Austin: PRO-ED.

Brown, L., Sherbenou, R.J., & Johnsen, S.K. (1997). Test of Nonverbal Intelligence–Third Edition. New York: Psychological Corporation.

Brownell, R. (2000). Receptive One-Word Picture Vocabulary Test–2000 Edition. Wilmington: Wide Range, Inc.

Buck, I.N. (1948). The HTP Technique: A Qualitative and Quantitative Scoring Manual. *J Clin Psychol, 4,* 317–396.

Burgemeister, B.B., Blum, L.H., & Lorge, I. (1972). *Columbia Mental Maturity Scale, ed 3.* New York: Harcourt, Brace, Jovanovich.

Burns, R.C., & Kaufman, S.H. (1972). *Actions, Styles, and Symbols in Kinetic Family Drawings: An Interpretive Manual.* New York: Brunner/Mazel.

Carpenter, E., & McLuhan, M. (1960). *Explorations in Communication* (p. 67). Boston: Beacon Press.

Cohen, M. (1997). Children's Memory Scale. San Antonio: Psychological Corporation.

Costello, J., & Ali, F. (1971). Reliability and validity of Peabody Picture Test scores of disadvantaged preschool children. *Psychol Rep, 28,* 755–760.

Dunn, L.M. (1970). *Peabody Picture Vocabulary Test–Revised Manual.* Circle Pines, MN: American Guidance Service.

Exner, J.E., Jr. (2001). *The Rorschach: A Comprehensive System–Fifth Edition.* New York: John Wiley & Sons.

Fast ForWord-Language Program. (1997). Berkeley: Scientific Learning.

Fast ForWord-Language to Reading Program. (1998). Berkeley: Scientific Learning.

Gardner, M.F. (1993). Test of Auditory Reasoning and Processing Skills (TARPS). Hydesville, CA: Psychological and Educational Publications.

Gardner, M.F. (2000). Expressive One-Word Picture Vocabulary Test–2000 Edition. Wilmington: Wide Range.

Goldman, R., Fristoe, M., & Woodcock, R.W. (1974). GFW Auditory Selective Attention Test. Circle Pines, MN: American Guidance Service.

Hammill, D.D. (1985). Detroit Tests of Learning Aptitude–2. Austin: PRO-ED.

Hammill, D.D. (1991). *Detroit Tests of Learning Aptitude, Third Edition, Examiner's Manual.* Austin: PRO-ED.

Hammill, D.D. (1997). *Comprehensive Test of Nonverbal Intelligence: Examiner's Manual.* Austin: PRO-ED.

Hammill, D.D. (1998). Detroit Tests of Learning Aptitude–Fourth Edition. San Antonio: The Psychological Corporation.

Hammill, D.D., Mathers, N., & Roberts, R. (2001). Illinois Test of Psycholinguistic Abilities–Third Edition. Austin: PRO-ED.

Hammill, D.D., Pearson, N.A., & Wiederholt, J.L. (1997). Comprehensive Test of Nonverbal Intelligence. Austin: PRO-ED.

Harris, D. (1963). *Children's Drawings as Measures of Intellectual Maturity: A Revision and Extension of the Goodenough Draw-A-Person Test.* New York: Harcourt, Brace & World.

Haworth, M.R. (1970). *The Primary Visual–Motor Test.* New York: Grune & Stratton.

Hiskey, M. (1966). Hiskey-Nebraska Test of Learning Aptitude. Lincoln: Union College Press.

Jackson, GD (1975) On the report of the Ad Hoc Committee on Educational Uses of Tests with Disadvantage

Students: Another psychological view from the Association of Black Psychologists. *Am Psychol, 30,* 88–92.

Jastak, J.F., & Jastak, S.R. (1976). The Wide Range Achievement Test: 1976 Revised Edition. Wilmington: Guidance Associates of Delaware.

Jastak, J.F., & Jastak, S.R. (1986). The Wide Range Achievement Test. Wilmington: Guidance Associates of Delaware.

Katz, J. (1998). *Central Test Battery.* Vancouver: Precision Acoustics.

Kaufman, A.S., & Kaufman, N.L. (1983). Kaufman Assessment Battery for Children. Circle Pines, MN: American Guidance Service.

Kaufman, A.S., & Kaufman, N.L. (1990). *Manual for the Kaufman Brief Intelligence Test.* Circle Pines, MN: American Guidance Service.

Kirk, S.A., McCarthy, J.J., & Kirk, W.D. (1968). The Illinois Test of Pyscholinguistic Abilities–Second Edition. Austin: PRO-ED.

Koppitz, E.M. (1963). *The Bender-Gestalt Test for Young Children.* New York: Grune & Stratton, p. 195.

Korkman, M., Kirk, U., & Kemp, S. (1997). *NEPSY.* San Antonio: Psychological Corporation.

Leiter, R.G. (1969). *General Instructions for the Leiter International Scale.* Chicago: Stoelting Company.

Markwardt, F.C., Jr. (1998). Peabody Individual Achievement–Revised–Normative Update. Circle Pines, MN: American Guidance Service.

McCarthy, J.J., & Kirk, S.A. (1961). Illinois Test of Psycholinguistic Abilities: Experimental Edition. Urbana: University of Illinois, Institute of Research on Exceptional Children.

Mercer, J. (1971). Sociological factors in labeling mental retardates. *Peabody Journal of Education, 48,* 188–203.

Molish, H.B. (1972). Projective methodologies. *Annu Rev Psychol, 23,* 577–614.

Murstein, B.I. (Ed.). (1965). *Handbook of Projective Techniques.* New York: Basic Books.

Naglieri, J.A. (1996). Naglieri Nonverbal Ability Test–Multilevel Form. San Antonio: Psychological Corporation.

Naglieri, J.A., McNeish, T.J., & Bardos, A.N (1991). *Draw-a-Person: Screening Procedure for Emotional Disturbance.* Austin: PRO-ED.

Nicholson, C.L., & Hibpshman, T.L. (1990). Slosson Intelligence Test for Children and Adults–R. East Aurora, NY: Slosson Educational Publications.

Raven, J.C. (2000a). *Guide to Using the Colored Progressive Matrices–P.* San Antonio: Psychological Corporation.

Raven, J.C. (2000b). *Guide to Using the Standard Progressive Matrices–P.* San Antonio: Psychological Corporation.

Roid, G.H. (2003). *Stanford-Binet Intelligence Scales, ed. 5 (SB5).* Chicago: Riverside Publishing.

Roid, G.H., & Miller, L.J. (2002). Leiter International Performance Scale–Revised. Sacramento: Psychological Assessment Resources.

Rorschach, H., Lemkan, P., & Krononberg, B., trans. (1942). *Psychodiagnostics, ed 2.* Berne: Huber.

Rotter, J.B., Lah, M.I., & Rafferty, J.E. (1992). Rotter Incomplete Sentences Blank–Second Edition. San Antonio: Psychological Corporation.

Slosson, R.L. (1975). Slosson Drawing Coordination Test for Children and Adults. East Aurora, NY: Slosson Educational Publications.

Swanson, H.L. (1996). *Swanson Cognitive Processing Test (S-CPT): A Dynamic Assessment Measure.* Austin: PRO-ED.

Terman, L., & Merrill, M. (1937). *Measuring Intelligence.* Boston: Houghton-Mifflin, p. 461.

Terman, L., & Merrill, M. (1962). *Stanford-Binet Intelligence Scale: Manual for the Third Revision Form L-M.* Boston: Houghton-Mifflin, p. 362.

Thorndike, R.L., Hagen, E.P., & Sattler, J.M. (1986). *The Stanford-Binet Intelligence Scale, ed 4.* Chicago: Riverside Publishing.

Turner, S.M., DeMers, S.T., Fox, H.R., & Reed, G.M. (2001). APA's Guidelines for Test User Qualifications: An Executive Summary. *Am Psychol, 56,* 1099–1113.

United States Department of Health, Education, and Welfare, Public Health Service. (1970). *Intellectual Maturity of Children as Measured by the Goodenough-Harris Drawing Test.* National Center for Health Statistics Series 11, No. 105.

Wagner, R.K., Torgesen, J.K., & Rashotte, C.A. (1999). *The Comprehensive Test of Phonological Processing: Examiner's Manual.* Austin: PRO-ED.

Watkins, E.O. (1976). *Watkins Bender-Gestalt Scoring System.* San Rafael, CA: Academic Therapy Publications.

Wechsler Individual Achievement Test Manual. (1992). San Antonio: Psychological Corporation.

Wechsler Individual Achievement Test–Second Edition. (2001). San Antonio: Psychological Corporation.

Wechsler, D. (1989). *Manual for the Wechsler Preschool and Primary Scale of Intelligence–R.* San Antonio: Psychological Corporation.

Wechsler, D. (1991). *Manual for the Wechsler Intelligence Scale for Children–III.* San Antonio: Psychological Corporation.

Wechsler, D. (1997). Wechsler Adult Intelligence Scale–Third Edition. San Antonio: Psychological Corporation.

Wechsler, D. (2002). Wechsler Preschool and Primary Scale of Intelligence–Third Edition. San Antonio: Psychological Corporation.

Weschler, D. (2003). *Manual for the Wechsler Intelligence Scale for Children–IV.* San Antonio: Psychological Corporation.

Wilkensen, G.S. (1993). *WRAT-3: Administration Manual.* Wilmington: Wide Range.

Williams, K.T. (1997). Expressive Vocabulary Test. Circle Pines, MN: American Guidance Service.

Williamson, W.E. (1979). The concurrent validity of the 1965 Wide Range Achievement Test with neurologically impaired and emotionally handicapped pupils. *J Learn Disabil, 12,* 201–202.

Woodcock, R.W., McGrew, K.S., & Maither, N. (2001). Woodcock-Johnson Tests of Achievement–III. Itasca, IL: Riverside.

Ziffer, R.L., & Shapiro, L.E. (1992). *Children's Self-Report and Projective Inventory.* Bala Cynwyd, PA: Psychological Assessments.

Zimmerman, I.L., & Woo-Sam, J.M. (1978). Intellectual testing today: Relevance to the school-age child. In: L. Oettnger & L.V. Majowski (Eds.), *The Psychologist, the School and the Child with MBDILD* (p. 51). New York: Grune & Stratton.

SECTION III

Remediation

9

Family and Early School Intervention for the New Era Child

KAREN A. CLARK AND DIANA L. TERRY

Learning and teaching . . . embark on a journey together.
—Loris Malaguzzi (1920–1994)

What Defines a New Era

Welcome to the future of early intervention. Even as this chapter is being read, the parameters of early intervention for children with hearing loss are changing. Change agents include widespread implementation of newborn hearing screening, rapidly evolving technology for amplification and cochlear implants, and the role of family as an increasingly active habilitation partner, seeking information from a burgeoning Internet and from multiple service providers. In addition, the growing number of young children served by early intervention programs is allowing researchers to obtain data that has significant implications for the profession. The professional who plans to journey into this new early intervention arena will do well to consider the short- and long-term effects of these changes.

New Era Influences

Universal Newborn Hearing Screening

In 1993, the National Institutes of Health Consensus Conference recommended that all infants be screened for hearing loss. At that time, only two states were universally screening newborns for hearing but in less than 10 years the numbers jumped significantly, with all states reporting some level of universal newborn hearing screening (UNHS). Today at least 32 states have legislation requiring screening (National Center for Hearing Assessment and Management, 2003). Comprehensive data management systems are being established in many states to track infants from screening through identification to intervention. If early UNHS data are an indicator of national numbers, as many as 16,000 infants with hearing loss will be identified and referred for early intervention each year (Arehart & Yoshinaga-Itano, 1999).

Technological Advances

In past decades access to sound was not an option for many infants who were born deaf or with significant hearing loss. However, recent and continuing advances in amplification and cochlear implants are changing this dynamic. Although technology is not a simple solution for a complex issue, it is most assuredly changing the landscape of early intervention. The most significant of all parameters of hearing technology is the knowledge that it is never static. Answers to family questions that are true one month or year may well be outdated the next. Providing current, accurate information for families requires having a reliable means of updating one's own technology information.

Information Access

There is more information currently available than at any other point in time. Families can access information through a variety of sources including the Internet and television. Mainstream newspapers and magazines have discovered reader interest in topics such as the use of American Sign Language (ASL) with infants and cochlear implants that "restore" hearing. Families, as well as their friends, neighbors, and relatives, all want to learn about these new developments, so they are reading, researching, and sharing information. The professional is no longer the only and most trusted source of information and must, in fact, spend significant amounts of time to keep abreast of consumer knowledge of current information and even more time to understand and analyze this information.

New Era Participants

The Children

UNHS has redefined the meaning of "early" and expanded the population of infants referred for intervention services. Prior to UNHS, infants who were identified early were often those with multiple disabilities; even those referred as toddlers most typically had severe to profound bilateral hearing loss. Today the youngest candidates for habilitation are as young as 4 to 5 weeks of age and may include infants with bilateral or unilateral hearing loss ranging in degree from mild or moderate to profound. Whereas many infants have multiple disabilities, others have no other apparent disabilities. With the right combination of early identification and intervention, it is possible for children to develop language equal to their cognitive ability. Research is demonstrating that this combination of factors includes identification and intervention by age 6 months and a high level of family partici-

pation in the intervention process (Moeller, 2000; Yoshinaga-Itano, 1995; Yoshinaga-Itano, Sedey, Coulter, & Mehl, 1998).

Earlier identification programs will also have a major impact on needs and services for the preschool and school-aged child. Examples may include less need for self-contained classes for children who are deaf and hard of hearing and greater need for support services to children whose typical language development allows them to enter mainstream and inclusion programs. Early identification and intervention may offer unwanted surprises as well. Some children with hearing loss may not meet qualification guidelines for special education services at age 3, even when these services might be desirable as a way of ensuring later school success.

The Families

Every public education law, including the current law, Individuals with Disabilities Education Act (IDEA, 1997) has recognized the family's importance in the early intervention process. The laws are periodically revised, but the importance of the family has been reaffirmed and strengthened with each renewal. More importantly, families are increasingly aware of their rights and those of their children under federal and state laws. Recent research has also validated what most interventionists knew to be true, parental involvement is one of the key factors in language growth for young children who are deaf and hard of hearing (Moeller, 2000).

The combination of early identification and enhanced technology already mentioned are giving families ever-increasing options. Greater access to information is ensuring that more families are aware of these options. Societal recognition of individual and cultural differences is facilitating professional awareness that intervention choices may be appropriately guided by family culture, individual difference, and personal choice.

Today's family may be one parent and a baby or may include uncles, aunts, grandparents, siblings, and step-versions of all these. The family members may be from a cultural background similar to the early interventionist, or they may be from a vastly different background with different beliefs and values.

The Professionals

Early interventionists and aural habilitation therapists familiar with working "catch up" with children and families now have the opportunity to assist with facilitating typical development for many of these early-identified babies. Understanding typical child development has always been important but today's early interventionist cannot hope to succeed without a thorough understanding of infant development. Because learning and development constitute an integrated process, knowledge must extend beyond that of language and speech to encompass all aspects of social–emotional, cognitive, and physical development. The importance of early relationships to emotional well-being and language development, as well as the interplay of these factors with parental feelings and reactions to hearing loss, must be key components of the intervention process.

Most child learning and development will occur between professional visits or therapy sessions. The role of the early interventionist is primarily one of supporting the family and other caregivers in helping these children to develop their full potential. Professionals must learn to work successfully and sensitively with a wide range of family situations and to provide support for family values and choices as well as information and guidance to assist families in helping their children.

Although the early interventionist may be the only professional involved with the family, it is more likely that the intervention partners will be multidisciplinary and include audiologists, speech-language pathologists, therapists, health care workers, child care providers, and preschool teachers. When the educational needs of the earlier identified infants and children are more varied, early interventionists who specialize in aural habilitation may need to develop less

direct ways to provide support for children with hearing loss. These may include identifying child communication strengths and needs for the intervention team, observation of children in their learning environments with suggestions for modification and support, and consultation with and training for other professionals.

A Framework for Intervention in the New Era

An ultimate goal for the education of young children who are deaf is the development of their full potential as happy, healthy individuals who are responsible members of society, confident and capable in their ability to communicate with others. Speech, language, and listening are each important dimensions of the communication process, but it is the spontaneous, appropriate, and integrated use of this communication within all aspects of life that are the true measures of success. When intervention is viewed in this context, it can only be considered effective when designed to facilitate communication that is relevant and integral to the lives of children and families, utilizing strategies that support total child development within the context of the family. This comprehensive approach to intervention is best achieved through the combined efforts of many people, beginning with the assessment process and continuing through early intervention and the preschool years. This model for intervention incorporates some basic assumptions about child learning and communication development.

Understanding Typical Development

Influence of Biology and Environment

Researchers today recognize that both biological and environmental influences have a significant impact on development (National Research Council & Institute of Medicine, 2000). The role of genetics in human development is becoming more precisely known as science continues to sort through the complexities of the genetic code. This research has provided further knowledge of the relationship of genetics and deafness. Based on current knowledge, estimates indicate that approximately 50% of congenital hearing loss is linked to a genetic cause, with approximately 70% of these cases classified as nonsyndromic. The other 50% of congenital hearing loss is linked to environmental factors, which include cytomegalovirus, meningitis, rubella, prematurity, neonatal icterus, ototoxicity, and other infections (American College of Medical Genetics Statement, 2002).

Beyond these causal factors of hearing loss, biology and environment continue to interact throughout development. Because of these complex interactions, the genetic and biological traits of each individual child may result in very different outcomes even for two children who live within the same home and have the same caregivers. For example, the inherent traits of one child may cause a caregiver to respond differently to that child than to a sibling, which in turn may result in different experiences for each child. The understanding of the interrelationship between biology and experience contributes to a better understanding of developmental disorders and the effects of early intervention. "Hereditary vulnerabilities establish probabilistic, not deterministic, developmental pathways that evolve in concert with the experiential stressors, or buffers, in the family, the neighborhood, and the school" (National Research Council & Institute of Medicine, 2000, p. 55). For a detailed yet highly readable review of research related to early development, refer to *From Neurons to Neighborhoods: The Science of Early Childhood Development* (National Research Council & Institute of Medicine, 2000).

How Children Learn

Young children who are deaf, like all young children, learn through interactions with their immediate world and with the people who live in that world. For young children, learning is an interactive, cyclical process through which they become aware, explore, inquire, and ultimately begin to utilize new

ideas and abilities (Bredekamp & Rosegrant, 1995). The best opportunities for learning occur during play and through daily routine experiences. As children develop, they are at different stages of the learning cycle as they experience the same daily events. As they begin to explore one concept more fully, they may concurrently become aware of another. Taking a bath provides an opportunity to learn that water can feel hot or cold, that slapped water splashes, that soap doesn't taste good, and that you sit in the water but your toy duck sits on the water. Each experience of the young child provides more information.

Communication and language development occur concurrently and as an integral part of the process of overall child development. During the early stages of development, children begin to learn first words as they are heard repeatedly in connection with experiences that are important to them and that happen frequently. At later stages, language itself becomes a tool for learning more about the meaningful events occurring in their lives. At all times, language and communication connect children with their world and with the people in their lives.

Experiences that are mediated by involved caregivers can be heightened to provide even more information and a scaffold to the next level of learning. Adults set the stage and provide the environment in which learning and development will take place. At times, adults take the lead and at times they respond to actions and ideas initiated by the child. Adult and child interactions, both verbal and nonverbal, significantly influence all aspects of development, including physical, cognitive, social, emotional, and language.

Legislative Mandate for Early Intervention

The Individuals with Disabilities Education Act (IDEA) Amendments of 1997, Part C, outline the requirements for early intervention services for infants and toddlers. One of the most significant aspects of the federal law is the importance of the family within all aspects of early intervention. In addition, the need for a multidisciplinary team for assessment and for the development of an individualized family service plan (IFSP) is emphasized. The information found in subsequent sections of this chapter, Models of Early Intervention, Importance of Partnerships, and Assessment Process, are all congruent with the mandates of IDEA, Part C.

Individualized Family Service Plan

The IFSP outlines child strengths and needs, family strengths and needs, intervention outcomes that are desired by the family, strategies designed to facilitate these desired outcomes, and the criteria for determining if the outcomes have been achieved. As the title of the plan implies, the needs of the child are considered within the context of the family. Outcomes and strategies chosen for an IFSP encompass a wider range of issues and are written in broader terms than behavioral objectives. For example, if the parent needs child care, locating a quality child care provider may be included in the IFSP as a desired outcome. Strategies for this outcome would outline the methods to be used in finding child care, including ways to ensure that the caregivers would work with and be receptive to the needs of a child who is deaf.

Models of Early Intervention

A large body of research on systems of early intervention and the best practice interrelationships of interventionists and families within these models has emerged from the work of Carl Dunst and his colleagues (Dunst, 2000; Dunst & Trivette, 1996). Whereas traditional intervention utilizes professionally centered models in which families are the clients of professionals, depending on professionals to solve their problems, newer intervention paradigms focus on family-centered models in which professionals are the agents of families, creating opportunities for families to utilize existing capabilities and develop new ones. In family-centered models, families determine the outcomes they hope to achieve and professionals work with families to support these outcomes and goals. At times this support may help families establish new goals through a broader understanding of the options that are available. The most recent of the Dunst models (2000) places the learning and development of the child at the heart of the model with all other support components functioning as an interrelated whole to support the family and community in facilitating the development of the child.

For many professionals, engaging in truly family-centered practices is difficult. Professionals may state that they agree with the concept but have difficulty when it comes to implementation. The discrepancy between verbal agreement with the model and actual practice is most apparent when there is a values conflict between what the parent wants and what the professional believes to be the best approach to intervention (Mertens, Sass-Lehrer, & Scott-Olson, 2000; Roush, Harrison, & Palsha, 1991).

In aural habilitation an example of values conflict might be one created when the parent desires a different mode of communication for the child than the one that would be the recommended choice of the professional. Working within a family-centered arena, the professional in this example would support the parents' choice, acknowledging that a method can be successful only when supported by the parents, that the parents may be correct in their belief that this method will be successful, or that with ongoing assessment and intervention the parents may come to a different decision about communication mode.

A model of early intervention that applies the principles of family-centered practice to work with families of infants and toddlers who are deaf and hard of hearing is the SKI-HI Model (Watkins, 2004). This model involves working in partnership with parents, establishing goals based on family-desired outcomes, gathering ongoing observational assessment data, building on parent strengths and resources, sharing additional resources, and determining the topics that are appropriate as parents integrate new information and learn new skills.

Importance of Partnerships

Professional Partnerships within Early Intervention

The mandates of IDEA, as well as the complex needs of families, often result in families being served by more than one professional. For services to be most beneficial, team members must work together in realizing family-determined outcomes. For the young child with hearing loss, professional team members may include audiologists, speech-language pathologists, educators with a specialization in deafness and/or early intervention, as well as additional professionals selected to meet specific needs such as occupational or physical therapists and vision specialists. The role of each may vary but collectively the professional team members will provide the services needed for the development and implementation of the intervention plan. These include an ongoing determination of hearing levels and management of recommended technology, initial and ongoing assessment of development with a special emphasis on all aspects of early communication, and implementation of the intervention strategies that have been agreed upon by the team. With many professionals involved in the intervention process, the door is open to the possibility of miscommunication, misinformation, and confusion for the family. Each IFSP team designates a service coordinator who has the responsibility to ensure that all program components work together to meet the needs of the family and child.

Family Partnerships within Early Intervention

One of the first collaborative partnerships in the education of young children who are deaf is that of the parent/primary caregiver and professional. Even if the early interventionist is providing service more than once a week, there is no way the professional can hope to have direct significant influence on the development of the child. It is the parent who best understands what is meaningful for the child, who observes and interprets communication signals from the child, and who is in the best position to provide the consistency of interaction on a daily and routine basis. The professional must find ways to support parent-generated outcomes and to recognize the role of the professional as one of enhancing the interactions of parent and child. The first and most important role of the professional is to listen to what parents want for their children. By actively listening to parents and designing intervention that will support their goals and dreams for their children, professionals will foster the development of trust, rapport, and mutual respect within the partnership. The professional contributes a vast amount of technical knowledge about communication, language, hearing aids, and auditory development to the partnership. The professional can help parents access a variety of resources and services. These professional contributions help to form a framework or plan in which the parental contributions can be directed and enhanced.

The Assessment Process

There are four main purposes for assessment of individual children and families within the early intervention process: determining eligibility for the program, helping the family determine their priorities and concerns, assisting in establishment of specific goals and outcomes for intervention, and guiding the programming during intervention. In an effective early intervention program, the purposes for assessment will mesh with the similar phases of early intervention.

Determining Eligibility for the Program

For children who have a hearing loss the determination of eligibility is often more straightforward than for many other types of developmental delays, and the diagnostic audiological assessment will generally provide the documentation that is needed for services. Although it is important to gather information in other developmental areas, it is the audiological information that most frequently provides the basis for eligibility.

Helping the Family Determine Their Priorities and Concerns

Assisting families to identify their concerns and priorities is a significant and complex aspect of the assessment process. Surveys and questionnaires are often utilized as a framework in helping the professional and family as they work to specify the family and child needs and outcomes. More extensive and individualized information can be obtained through open discussion or personal family interviews. Information that is relevant to establishing needs may include functional assessment of family needs as well as information in related areas, such as family members' roles and support systems, critical life events, and family environments. The value of determining family needs is in utilizing that knowledge to enhance services to the family. Frequent discussions and attentiveness to parent concerns will ensure that the services remain congruent with family needs over time.

Assisting in Establishment of Specific Goals and Outcomes for Intervention

Identification of child competencies in communication, listening, and other areas of development is a significant responsibility of the habilitation specialist. Effective, useful assessment involves families in a significant manner, utilizes multiple sources and contexts, and emphasizes information gathering as an ongoing process.

In planning assessments that identify children's abilities and needs, information is gathered in communication/language, auditory development (including hearing aid or implant use), and cognitive, physical, social, and emotional development. Because communicative competence is a goal, diagnostic measures selected should be varied and provide a multidimensional picture of the child's development. It is not enough to know how an infant or toddler responds to a word or a sound in an isolated setting; it is also important to know how the child responds at home, in the park, or at the babysitter's. Traditional, professionally administered, norm-referenced tests generally record what a child does in one setting with a certain set of materials at a given moment in time. Measures that incorporate parental reporting provide a broader view but do not necessarily give the professional an opportunity to observe directly the way in which these children use communication within their daily life. Interview-type assessments also provide little information about the communicative interaction between parent and child so additional observational data are needed to help round out the picture of the child as communicator. Observational data, when utilized effectively, can provide a broader picture of the child's system of communication. The child's auditory abilities are measured quantitatively during audiological assessment to provide aided hearing levels and, eventually, speech reception and discrimination abilities. Again, observational data in a variety of settings are needed to supplement and give information about children's ability to use their early hearing in meaningful ways. For a comprehensive overview of assessment practices and measures for young children with hearing loss, refer to *Assessment in SKI-HI* (Clark, Abraham, Lambourne, & Madsen, 2004).

Guiding Programming during Intervention

Currrent models view assessment as ongoing and interrelated with intervention. When outcomes are established for an early intervention plan, there should always be an indication of how the progress toward achieving those outcomes will be monitored. Curriculum-based assessments are one excellent method of ensuring that ongoing assessment will be an accurate reflection of the intervention plan.

Whatever method is utilized, ongoing data gathering through observation and documentation allow both the family and the service provider the opportunity to observe progress and to make adjustments when necessary in the intervention plan. When family members are active participants in both the intervention and the ongoing assessment, they are often more able to see when a change in intervention strategies or methods is needed. For example, a family who has helped to establish the criteria for progress in an auditory communication program and has been active in the documentation of that progress may readily understand when new options such as a cochlear implant or the addition of signs to the communication system must be considered.

Intervention Strategies— the Early Years

Early identification alone will not result in improved communication development for infants and toddlers with hearing loss. Early identification must be combined with high-quality, comprehensive early intervention. Research in the early intervention arena with infants with hearing loss is just beginning to emerge and early interventionists who work with this population must learn as much as possible about issues of family intervention and strategies related to early communication development.

Family Matters

The two factors that best correlate with increased vocabulary and verbal reasoning skills for children with hearing loss at age 5 are age of enrollment and family involvement in the early intervention program (Moeller, 2000). Of these two indicators, family involvement is the most significant single factor and children who have the combination of family involvement and early enrollment demonstrate the best language skills.

This research-based confirmation of the importance of family reaffirms the need to find better ways to support family involvement in early intervention. Work with infants as young as 4 to 5 weeks poses new challenges that include understanding the effect of identification on the early attachment process, recognizing the importance of early emotional development and its relationship to early communication development, and developing better ways to support early development within the contexts that are natural for individual families.

Much of communication and language development emerges from the interaction of caregivers and infants. These interactions are more successful when babies and parents are in tune with each other. The term "emotional availability" (Emde & Easterbrooks, 1985) has been used to describe the sensitivity of mothers and babies to each other. Some of the characteristics associated with emotional availability include warmth, responsiveness, and providing a supportive framework for the child's development. Recent research seems to indicate that greater emotional availability may be linked with better language development. "When mothers are emotionally available, their children who are deaf or hard of hearing make stronger language gains than when the mother is not emotionally available" (Pressman, Pipp-Siegel, Yoshinaga-Itano, Kubicek, & Emde, 2000, p. 271).

Emotional Impact of Hearing Loss for Families

Most parents of children who are deaf are hearing people who never expected to be the parents of a child with a hearing loss. It is important that service providers understand as clearly as possible the emotional impact that may be experienced by some parents as they attempt to deal with this new direction in their life. The research on emotional availability and its possible link to language development makes it more important than ever that the early interventionist be skilled in understanding and responding to the emotions of parents in the grief process.

An attitude of acceptance of parents' emotions and empathy for the range of their feelings are perhaps the most effective responses that service providers can have. Listening to families, establishing rapport and trust, offering both ongoing support and unbiased information when requested, and recognizing when referral for additional counseling might be needed are all significant aspects of early intervention.

The advent of UNHS programs and their impact on parental feelings and reactions is another factor to consider. The effects of earlier identification on parental reaction to hearing loss are not fully known and research in this area is evolving. One pilot study of 16 families looked at grief resolution of families of children with hearing loss (Siegel, 2000). The mean age of identification of hearing loss of children in families who had resolved their grief was 8.1 months whereas that of children whose families had not resolved their grief was 16 months. Additional research in this area is needed.

Cultural Considerations

Individual family values as well as cultural differences have a significant impact on the partnership. Cultural diversity between the family and the service provider is present when the service provider attributes different meaning or value to events and behaviors than does someone from the family's environment (Barrera, 1996). Basic parent and child communication patterns, child care practices, family structure and roles, and expectations for children may vary across cultures. Assumptions and decisions based on the cultural background and family values of the professional, rather than that of the family, are rarely successful.

A major source of cultural misunderstanding can be found within the communication process. The styles in which individuals exchange information and converse may differ widely for various cultural groups and these differences may include the manner of greeting, norms for initiating and ending conversations, the degree of eye contact, the directness of approach, the level of formality, the value of silence, the ways in which information is gathered, and the views on disability (Lynch & Hanson, 1998; Wyatt, 1998). Although an early interventionist should never assume information about a family's culture from merely knowing race, language, or ethnic background, it is important to be aware of differences that may exist.

Professionals who do not have sufficient information on cultural differences in communication styles may find themselves alienated from the family without understanding why. Research and homework prior to the first family contact as well as an overall awareness of existing differences in communication and culture are needed. For additional information, early interventionist and preschool professionals are referred to Lynch and Hanson (1998). Their work, designed specifically for early intervention professionals, provides a conceptual framework as well as more in-depth information on various cultural groups.

Working with families who speak a different language than the habilitation specialist poses special problems, and simply utilizing an interpreter does not solve all the inherent challenges. Barrera (1996) uses the term "culture-language mediator" to describe a person who goes beyond the role of a traditional interpreter. Mediators have a dual responsibility to assist service providers in becoming aware of any unfamiliar values, beliefs, language, or rules that are part of the family's environment and to assist the family with awareness of those areas within the early intervention arena.

Families who are culturally Deaf and who use ASL bring an additional dimension to the professional family partnership. Considerations for the use of an interpreter and a respect for the communication and lifestyle values of the family remain applicable. Language assessments based on English will not provide an accurate assessment of the language of a child whose first language is ASL, and interpretations must reflect the limitation of the process. Families who are culturally Deaf may also place a different value on the importance of listening and speech development than families who are part of the hearing culture. Based on these parameters, it is important that interventionists not make assumptions in either direction and respect the family's role in determining outcomes.

Early Communication Development

With the very real possibility that a baby may enter early intervention as early as 1 month of age, it is imperative that the early interventionist understand the process of early communication development in in-

Table 9–1. Helping Families Encourage Infant Communication

Techniques That Support Both Auditory and Visual Communication
- Understand that daily routines such as feeding, changing, and comforting are effective situations for encouraging infant communication development.
- Watch closely for communication "signals" such as points, gestures, gazes, and facial expressions and respond to them.
- Think about what the infant's signal is meant to convey and give the words/signs for that person, object, or action.
- Talk/sign to the infant about what is happening.
- Use lots of facial expression when communicating and be certain that your expression matches your words/signs.
- Use natural gestures in combination with words/signs.
- Use reciprocal, or "back and forth" communication, pausing where the infant's turn should be and encouraging the infant to take a turn.

Techniques That Support Early Listening and Speech
- Encourage the infant to wear his or her hearing aids or cochlear implant during all waking hours.
- Point out interesting or meaningful sounds and show what is making the sound.
- Be certain that sounds are loud enough to be heard (30 to 50 dB above threshold) and vary them to maintain interest.
- Get close when you talk. This provides a more audible signal and minimizes interference from other noises in the room.
- Remember that infants like listening to speech. Make your voice as interesting as possible by using lots of intonation (up or down inflection) when talking.
- Encourage vocalization and use of voice for communication. Show how happy and excited you are when the infant vocalizes in return.
- Respond to all vocalizations as if they were communication.
- Using vowels and consonants, focus on specific speech sounds by associating them with activities such as rocking or toy movement.

Techniques That Support Early Visual Communication
- Pay attention to hand movements and respond positively to this "manual babbling" in the same way you might respond to vocalization.
- Pay close attention to what the infant is looking at and provide the sign. Make the sign close to the object or bring the object into the infant's line of vision.
- Make visual communication interesting by using gestures, facial expressions, and whole body movements along with signs.
- Wait to be certain that you have the infant's attention before signing. You may need to wait patiently or touch the child's shoulder.
- Make signs easy to see by positioning yourself at the infant's eye level.

fants. For communication development to flourish early interventionists and caregivers must recognize potential infant communication signals and respond to them as communication. They must recognize and utilize daily routines as opportunities to encourage communication development. The role of the early interventionist is to help families recognize and respond to the infant's signals using the best techniques possible, initiate communication in ways that are interesting and effective, and create environments that encourage communication (Table 9–1).

Federal law and common sense both support the use of natural environments for this process. For infants the home often provides one of the best locations for service delivery. Excellent opportunities for learning and communication arise from the family's daily routines, and the early interventionist needs to become familiar with these routines and the contexts for communication that may be specific to that family. For families who have not made a decision about method of communication, it's important that the early interventionist reinforce the idea that what's most important is communication and that many techniques encouraging early communication are effective for both early auditory and early visual communication.

Speech Development

Development of spoken language has always been an area of discussion, focus, and sometimes controversy in the field of deaf education. Those who have worked in the area of early intervention know that when asked to state outcomes for the IFSP, hearing parents often select "I want my child to talk." There are many routes to achieving this outcome and the challenge for the interventionist is to take this starting place and devise strategies that are appropriate for a particular family. Recent and continuing research is providing information to help families establish reasonable expectations for speech development and to make decisions on what methods and strategies are best for their family.

One finding is that babbling levels in the first year of life do not predict later speech intelligibility and that in the first year of life, even with early identification and intervention, there is no differentiation in speech production by degree of hearing loss (Wallace, Menn, & Yoshinago-Itano, 2000). The authors hypothesize that this may be due to a threshold of in utero hearing necessary for normal speech development in the first year of life. Another finding of Wallace et al mitigating this potential concern is that children with hearing loss may develop speech skills even if these skills are not present in the first few years of life. Of even greater importance is the finding that, after controlling for age and cognitive ability, the primary predictors of speech outcomes in children from 12 to 60 months are expressive language for both spoken and signed forms and amount of hearing loss. When the data on amount of hearing loss are further analyzed, they suggest that the speech development of children with mild through severe loss is similar by older age levels whereas that of children with profound loss remains poorer (Yoshinaga-Itano & Sedey, 2000).

These findings reinforce the focus on communication and language development as most important in an early intervention program. When language development occurs, through either spoken or signed forms, speech may develop throughout the early years. Speech can and should be encouraged as an important part of communication development. Encouraging and reinforcing the infant's vocalizations, making vocalizations a part of early turn-taking activities, using varied vocalizations and intonation, and focusing on specific sounds by associating them with activities such as rocking, toy movement, or touch such as tracing an imaginary line on the baby's arm, will all help to encourage vocalization.

Auditory Development

Earlier identification makes early access to sound possible for infants and with this opportunity come added challenges for families and professionals. Feedback and ear molds are two of these challenges. Feedback occurs when amplified sound leaks from around the ear mold; this can happen when growth overtakes the ear mold replacement schedule. Rapid growth may mean that ear molds need to be replaced monthly during infancy. Feedback also results from head contact of the baby against the caregiver's body or against the bed. Switching off the aid on the contact side can alleviate the need to constantly put hearing aids on and off. Problems inherent in the amplification of infants can be frustrating for families and also affect the amount of time that hearing aids are worn. This may have an effect on auditory development and true listening age, which is the length of time that a child has had access to sound.

Another challenge of early intervention is helping families to provide appropriate auditory experiences for their baby. Yoshinaga-Itano (2000) summarizes the intervention implications of numerous studies of auditory development in infants who are hearing, deaf, or hard of hearing. Some of her suggestions for families and interveners include using sounds in the environment that are between 30 dB and 50 dB above threshold when attempting to condition a response to sound and using different auditory stimuli for each attempt to get a response because newborns and infants tend to adapt quickly to repeat sounds. Also noted are a baby's preference for speech to other types of sounds and a recommendation for using both vowels and consonants—vowels for suprasegmentals and consonants because infants respond at levels closer to their threshold for high frequency sounds than for low frequency sounds.

Perhaps even more important than the focus on getting just the right sound is the parents' enjoyment of the interaction with the baby during auditory activities. Whereas parents and other family members may enjoy selecting toys with auditory interest, it should also be remembered that there are many potentially meaningful sounds found within the daily routine. When using speech, the early communication techniques mentioned earlier are applicable and parents should be encouraged to warmly reinforce all auditory responses from the infant. The best auditory development activities are those integral to daily routines and that emerge from enjoyable parent–child interactions.

Putting It All Together

Case Study 9–1 provides an opportunity to review the many components of early intervention and the way in which they can come together to provide a successful outcome for a child and family.

Intervention Strategies— the Early School Years

Comprehensive Communication Purposefulness

To understand language as a versatile, multidimensional system that facilitates interaction with people and acquisition of information during the early school years, one must understand its various components. It is generally accepted that language develop-

ment can be observed within three dimensions: content, form, and use. Content, the meaning of language, reflects knowledge of objects and people and the relationship among these objects, people, and events in the environment. Form involves word order, or syntax, as well as the sounds of spoken language and the configuration of signed language. Use includes reasons for speaking or signing and knowledge of the situation or other person that helps one determine the form of the message.

Each component of language may begin developing separately in early infancy and emerge in the form of early words around age 1. Communication purposefulness depends on the continued integration and interconnection of these three aspects of language as children mature. Communication is an integration of social and individual factors that encompass syntax, cognitive knowledge, and social context. In each communication interaction or event, variables that influence communication might include the environment or setting, the communication partner, experiential history, current knowledge constructs, current needs, personal motivation, and expectation of results.

Every aspect of language and true competence in its use reflects its dynamic and fluid nature. One might best take a "kaleidoscopic" view of communication in which each of the factors described above represents a bit of colored glass within the kaleidoscope and each communicative interaction finds those factors rearranged in a different relationship and presenting a different picture. For early school-age children to be considered competent in language, they must adapt to the ever-changing patterns; they must be able to use language spontaneously and appropriately in a wide variety of contexts and with a wide variety of communication partners. For therapists to be effective in facilitating this competence, the parameters of therapy must be expanded beyond a single therapy setting. Children need opportunities to acquire and practice skills throughout the day rather than having all language facilitation compressed into small amounts of isolated time. Communi-

Case Study 9–1

Part 1

Cliff and Maria were thrilled that they were having a baby and, because there were no complications with pregnancy or delivery, were very surprised to learn that baby B.R. was referred for diagnostic audiological assessment following her newborn hearing screening. No words could describe their shock when, within the next month, they learned that she had a permanent hearing loss. Somehow the word "moderate" did nothing to alleviate the fears and sadness over this new direction their life was taking. The early intervention program contacted them within 2 days of the audiologist's referral. The intake and IFSP passed by in a haze of "not me" and "this can't be true."

Part 2

B.R. at 10 months is bright and inquisitive. She doesn't seem to notice her hearing aids much and wears them all her waking hours. Cliff and Maria are getting more used to putting the aids on and dealing with the feedback; they are even starting to feel comfortable with the curious stares they get from people in the grocery store. Their early interventionist, Eva, introduced them to several other parents who had children with hearing loss. She demonstrated the best ways to help B.R. get experience with listening to and understanding all the sounds in her world. Eva reinforced all the ways they responded to B.R.'s attempts to communicate such as pointing, reaching, or making speech sounds. She gave suggestions on ways they could create even more opportunities for listening and communication throughout the day. Maria told Eva that the very most important things she did was listen to them, honestly try to answer their questions, and help them to understand that the everyday things they did made a difference.

Part 3

Prior to B.R.'s third annual IFSP at age 21 months, Cliff, Maria, and Eva worked together to complete the assessment. Because many things are documented on an ongoing basis, this is an opportunity to pull together information on vocabulary development, interactive communication in various settings (including child care), listening skills (including the most recent audiological), and overall development. B.R.'s progress continues to show month for month development.

Postscript

B.R.'s story of early identification, parental involvement, and support from competent, caring professionals demonstrates the best of early intervention.

cation skills must be embedded into the times when a child needs the skill. It is important that therapy be designed to help children use important skills purposefully in settings where they are needed.

Continued Partnership and Collaboration

When communication purposefulness throughout the day is the recognized goal for the child, then homes, playgrounds, and preschool classrooms are all potential therapy settings. Parents, teachers, and day-care providers are all potential language facilitators. The ultimate goal of language development is enhanced when this group works together as a comprehensive communication enhancement team, adhering to principles of contextually relevant learning opportunities, integrated learning, and programmed generalization. Communication purposefulness is effectively addressed when there is recognition among all team members that pooling talents and resources of everyone who is a part of the child's environment is mutually advantageous, that naturalistic settings are appropriate contexts for language intervention, that language change can be implemented in a variety of ways, and that effectively addressing the child's needs merits an expenditure of time, energy, and resources. All team members feel ownership within the process because they are actively involved in identifying the needs, generating the plans, and participating in collaborative decisions. This type of collaboration requires participant interaction, appreciation of diverse expertise, development of creative solutions, mutually defined goals, shared responsibilities for implementation and documentation, as well as continued parent education.

Identifying Family and Child Needs— the Early School Years

When children enter a school program, the focus of needs identification continues to include the family, the child, and the professionals who work with them. Parents should be encouraged to provide information about family and community culture, contexts for meaningful communication, and changes in their child and the child's environment. Parents also continue to be important in the assessment process as observers, informers, describers, evaluators, and interpreters of information. They should be encouraged to ask as many questions as necessary to find out what is being assessed and how the outcome of each assessment will be used in their child's education. Parents should also be encouraged to become as knowledgeable as possible about developmental milestones and the typical age spans in which they occur.

During the early school years, the diagnostic process continues to rely on collaborative input and thus is individualized to meet the specific needs of the child, family, and professionals. Before utilizing specific diagnostic measures for speech, language, and listening skills of preschoolers, it is impor-

tant to have an overall plan for assessment. The plan for assessing the child's skills is defined by a combination of who is to be involved, why the skills are being assessed, what information is being assessed, in which contexts the skills are to be assessed, how the skills will be assessed in the various contexts, and how that information will be utilized.

When considering who is to be involved in the assessment, it is advisable to consider anyone who has questions to be answered or issues they want resolved as part of the collaborative assessment plan. Most often, the child's family and the professionals who are providing their services are the ones who are involved in the assessment process.

The selection of assessment methods and tools is often influenced by the reason for the assessment. The overall purposes continue to be those addressed earlier in the chapter: determining eligibility, identifying priorities, establishing goals and objectives for intervention, and guiding programming. There will be variations in these purposes as children get older. Perhaps the assessment is necessary to determine eligibility for services as the child transitions from early intervention to school-based programming. Perhaps the habilitation specialist and teachers need information to determine additional steps to take in the intervention plan or to document progress for that plan. Sometimes assessment is needed to document that the child is maintaining expected skills, or to gather more information for a decision on communication methodology or class placement.

The reasons for the assessment will also be a factor in determining if standardized, norm-referenced measures should be used or if more informal, organized observation systems and interview type assessments are appropriate. Standardized tests are designed and published by various test-making companies and yield number scores based on comparison of the individual child to a very large sample of children from across the country. Nonstandardized tests may include formal interview/observation measures as well as materials designed by a teacher or therapist to enable team members to record and organize their observations of the child in his or her environment. Because assessment should always have the goal of helping team members fit instruction to the child's needs, the assessment that yields a richer description of the child's abilities and weaknesses is more valuable than one that simply yields a number. For this reason, a portfolio approach to assessment is becoming more widely used (Flexer, 1994).

In the assessment plan it is important to discuss how the observance or nonobservance of skills will be documented and who will be responsible for that documentation. A decision also needs to be made as to whether qualitative judgments are appropriate or whether the documentation needs to follow standardized guidelines. Additional considerations include whether the skills are to be assessed in isolated settings such as a therapy room or in naturalistic settings, including the home environment. Inventories and checklists that are completed by more than one person in the child's environment provide a wider range of information than that obtained from one isolated setting. For example, completion of listening and speech skill development checklists by the habilitation specialist, parent adviser, classroom teacher, and parent provide a more complete picture of the child's skill development in a variety of settings than a single measure in only one environment. The focus is not on who is "right," but rather on which behaviors are seen in different environments and how they might be generalized to all settings (Crais, 1993).

The manner in which the assessment results are interpreted and utilized is partially dependent on the purpose of the assessment. The information will be used differently if the purpose is to determine additional steps to take in the intervention plan than if the information is being used to evaluate the educational placement for the child. A variety of assessment team members may bring their perspectives and competencies to the interpretation process. These perspectives provide related and overlapping information that will help to ensure that a child's specific needs are accurately assessed and that an intervention program is relevant to the child's language and learning environment across contexts. These varied perspectives allow for focus on establishing meaningful skills and outcomes for parents, caregivers, professionals, and the child.

Communication Methodology Decisions

To understand a team approach to methodology decisions, it may first be helpful to apply the principles of professional-centered and family-focused program philosophies to the communication methodology issue. In a traditional, professional-centered model, the recommendation for communication methodology is the responsibility of the professional. The professional reviews child assessment data that include amount of hearing loss, age at identification, additional handicapping conditions, and other factors. The resulting recommendation is usually heavily influenced by the educational philosophy of the professional or the program making the recommendation. The recommendation often conveys to the family, either directly or through implication, that there is a "right" choice. The role of the family is to accept or reject the recommendation.

In a family-centered program, the family is the primary decision maker in determining the choice of communication methodology. Family values and experiences, child and family needs and strengths, and information and resource availability may all be factors in the decision. The approach still recognizes the need for professional input, but also recognizes the importance of a wider range of family, community, and cultural issues. The professional continues to want what is best for the child but understands that there may be more than one right answer. The role of the professional shifts from the supplier of the right answer to the supplier of information and information resources. The range of information resources may be broader than in the past, encompassing varied mixes of communication professionals as well as adults who are deaf and other families with children who are deaf. Ongoing availability of information presented in many formats in a nonbiased manner is recommended. Listening and following the family's lead will allow the professional to have information resources available when the family is ready. Available resources for the family might include (1) opportunities to read about or discuss a wide variety of aural and sign-based methods, including auditory–verbal, auditory–oral, and total communication using manually coded English and ASL; (2) opportunities to meet older children and adults who are deaf, and who, collectively, have a wide variety of opinions about and experiences with the various methodologies; (3) opportunities to explore fully and understand the advantages and limitations of new technologies that support auditory methodologies; (4) opportunities to explore fully and understand the concept of bilingualism as it applies to children who are deaf; (5) opportunities to meet parents who have selected various methodologies for their children; and (6) opportunities to visit school programs that offer various methodologies.

An additional role of the professional is to gather ongoing child information through the assessment and documentation process described earlier in this chapter. This information is also shared with the parents so that they, in making their decisions, have the opportunity to reflect on what is known about the development of their child's communication and language system over time. A family's decision about communication methodology is often a process rather than a single decision. Early choices about communication systems may be based on parents' personal or family experiences, their dreams for themselves and their children, and currently available information. New information, including assessment data, as well as increased experiences and changing perspectives may influence parents' subsequent choices.

Parents, teachers, and therapists need to see themselves as a team in which each member respects the needs, questions, fears, and ideas of the others, with all members working toward the best for the child. The parent is the key decision member of the team and needs to be informed of all the options available and of their child's developmental level and knowledge base. Communication between and among the members of the team is essential and all must guard against being less than open with one another. It is possible for members of the team to hold differing philosophies about what is best for the child, and as long as these are not profoundly oppositional, the parent can learn from the differing philosophies. When there is too wide a difference, though, the parent will need to make decisions that could result in a new team with new members (Flexer, 1994).

Providing Services to Children and Families—the Early School Years

During the early school years, intervention plans continue to rely on input from team members that is responsive to both home and classroom needs. The goal of those working with young children who are deaf or hard of hearing is to get them ready for school while at the same time remembering that children with and without deafness learn at different rates. All language work must be meaningful. Being aware of the child's developmental level as well as understanding the normal ranges of development for particular skills within language acquisition can help parents, teachers, and therapists decide when to target particular skills and when to sit back and wait awhile. For those children in aural/oral programs, it is important to remember to base speech, language, and listening acquisition milestones on the listening age of the child rather than on chronological age alone. Understanding the ranges associated with skill acquisition also allows team members to identify when a child is falling behind, thus signaling a need for a change in intervention strategies. Objectives are selected to focus on responding to the child's needs, allowing shared educational roles, emphasizing the child's strengths, providing real-life success, developing communicative competence, and promoting a child- or student-centered approach. Needs are generally identified in the areas of auditory processing, speech or sign communication, pragmatics, semantics, and syntax. Early school objectives that focus on communication purposefulness and real-life success might include skills such as requesting objects, help, or information; answering questions; negotiating rules for play or games; participating in show and tell; attending to directions; relaying messages; or expressing a desire or problem.

The teacher's task during the early school years is one of identifying where the child is and then either continuing the process of closing the gap in language development or maintaining skills in relation to the student's peers with normal hearing and language development. Some children may have particularly large gaps and others may have no gaps at all or very small ones. The school curriculum needs to be one that is functional and satisfies each student's needs. Teachers, therapists, and parents must continually assess where the child is and what needs are next. Modifications and enhancements in curriculum should be commonplace and designed to meet the needs of individual children. Team members who recognize that language learning is variable for different children are less likely to insist that all children learn the same material the same way and at the same time, regardless of their knowledge base. Classroom settings allow children to discover how the students around them are using language and stimulate language growth in a variety of ways.

Objectives can be provided in educational environments in three ways: within the context of existing classroom routines; as a concurrent activity imposed on, but consistent with, the context of existing classroom routines; as a separate activity apart from the context of existing classroom routines. Team members first consider development, needs,

and interests of the child and then purposefully construct opportunities that allow the child to participate actively in and ultimately utilize the targeted objectives. One significant aspect of the intervention process is defining who is to be involved in the process and where the intervention strategies will be implemented. To some extent, anyone in contact with a child in need of speech/language/listening intervention can share in the responsibility for providing input or opportunities for interaction in contexts in which those skills can be used and learned. In the school setting, intervention may include implementation by the habilitation specialist and the teacher; by the educator or parent, with the habilitation specialist providing consultation; by the habilitation specialist outside the classroom setting; or a combination of these. Within a purposefully prepared environment, the child, parent, habilitation specialist, or teacher may appropriately initiate learning experiences.

Providing appropriate organization of the school environment to target objectives first requires several observations of the child to determine the level of play and interaction. It is necessary to observe the child as a part of both the social and the physical environment. These observations provide an understanding about how the child gives and receives information and interacts with his or her environment. The new information or target objective is then provided so that it is contextually relevant and conforms to the child's social and physical behaviors. Successful intervention strategies involve creating real needs to communicate through routine situations in which the child is motivated to signify communicative intents, such as requesting, possession, imperative, location, desire, or problem. Adults provide support for the child's choices and may best respond to the child's initiative by extending and encouraging rather than by directing.

Isolated settings such as therapy rooms can be altered to be more like the natural environments of the child by rearranging the physical attributes of the therapy setting and re-creating events that occur naturally in the home or classroom. Therapy becomes more functional when conducted in a variety of settings other than the therapy room, such as the playground, lunchroom, classroom, hallway, or bus room, and when using materials that are real, functional, everyday objects. Moving from one-on-one settings to interactive small group settings enhances variety in therapy environments. An understanding that it is easiest for a child to learn new skills if the routine is familiar and predictable should be a component of intervention strategy planning. Repetition, routine, and consistency are important in the understanding and development of new skills. Learning experiences are the most beneficial when organized in a continuous and sequential order so that the child can relate one learning experience with another, day after day.

Documentation of skill acquisition in a variety of settings is an essential component of the intervention process. Table 9–2 provides an example of a weekly speech, language, and listening intervention summary showing the various settings where each objective was targeted. Table 9–3 shows a tool for specific skill development over a longer period of time.

Least Restrictive Environment and Its Implications for the New Era Child

The concept of least restrictive environment is defined in IDEA, Part B, which outlines services for children ages 3 to 21 years. IDEA (1997) maintains that, to the maximum extent appropriate, children with disabilities, including children in public or private institutions or other care facilities, are educated with children who are nondisabled, and that special classes, separate schooling, or other removal of children with disabilities from the regular educational environment occurs only if the nature or severity of the disability is such that education in regular classes with

Table 9–2. Objectives Targeted This Week: In These Settings

Objective	Music	Group	Centers	Play	Pullout	Snack/ Meal	Other
Shows awareness to environmental sounds	x	x	x	x	x	x	
Looks for source of sounds		x		x		x	
Turns when name is called	x	x		x	x		
Attempts to imitate pitch, rhythm, duration, volume of an adult vocal model	x	x		x			
Imitates vowel and consonant sounds on request		x			x		
Imitates spoken words on request/ spontaneously	x	x	x	x	x	x	
Follows familiar directions presented without gestures/signs	x			x	x	x	
Spontaneously imitates and uses meaningful speech	x		x			x	
Indicates familiar people, objects, activities in environment when asked	X		X				
Uses words to signify communicative intents	x		x		x	x	

Table 9–3. Auditory Awareness, Attention, and Perception

Use this form to track auditory progress over time. For each item, write the date when the child consistently utilizes the skill within the indicated setting.

Therapy Classroom

1. ____ ____ Wears amplification most of the day/shows some awareness to sound
2. ____ ____ Shows awareness of loud environmental sounds when directed
3. ____ ____ Attends to or has a "listening" facial expression whenever a sound occurs
4. ____ ____ Associates a specific sound with an object or happening in the environment
5. ____ ____ Communicates an interest in sound
6. ____ ____ Vocalizations increase when amplification is on and decrease when off

LOCALIZATION AND DISTANCE HEARING

1. ____ ____ Begins to look for source of certain sounds
2. ____ ____ Begins to turn when name is called
3. ____ ____ Attends to close environmental and speech sounds
4. ____ ____ Attends to distant environmental and speech sounds

AUDITORY COMPREHENSION AND DISCRIMINATION

1. ____ ____ Cooperates for structured listening tasks and responds to an auditory stimulus
2. ____ ____ Indicates presence or absence (on/off) of sounds
3. ____ ____ Discriminates between sounds differing in length, loudness, pitch
4. ____ ____ Begins to attempt to imitate vowel and consonant sounds on request
5. ____ ____ Attempts to imitate pitch, rhythm, duration, and volume of a model
6. ____ ____ Understands that sound has meaning and is used for communication
7. ____ ____ Identifies and recognizes the meaning of some environmental sounds
8. ____ ____ Uses a few functional words such as bye-bye and all gone
9. ____ ____ Recall words or sounds associated with a situation
10. ____ ____ Consistently imitates speech sounds on request
11. ____ ____ Spontaneously imitates and use meaningful speech

AUDITORY MEMORY, SEQUENCING, AND PROCESSING

1. ____ ____ Vocabulary is increasing steadily
2. ____ ____ Comprehends single words indicating familiar people, objects, activities in environment
3. ____ ____ Consistently imitates labeling people, objects, actions in environment without prompt
4. ____ ____ Uses the words he knows spontaneously to communicate
5. ____ ____ Comprehends a few short phrases in his natural environment
6. ____ ____ Comprehends two details in a message during structured task
7. ____ ____ Speaks in single words
8. ____ ____ Speaks using short phrases

the use of supplementary aids and services cannot be achieved satisfactorily. In considering educational placement decisions, the IFSP and individual educational plan (IEP) teams must first identify the educational environment where the child would be educated if he or she were not eligible for special services, and then determine if special services can be delivered in that setting with the use of modifications and supplementary assistance. The challenge of identifying and providing the least restrictive environment

(LRE), originally associated with school-age children, now also extends to school programs for very young children. In all situations, the challenge is to identify the most natural environment possible in which the child will experience optimal development. Case Study 9–2 illustrates the challenges associated with determining the child's optimal school environment.

Providing LRE services for preschool children who are deaf or have other special needs is especially challenging for public schools because general education programs for children typically do not begin until prekindergarten at age 4 years or kindergarten at age 5 years. Because there is no general definition of natural environments for children younger than prekindergarten, a wide variety of programs and approaches have developed for

this population. As discussed earlier in this chapter, the home environment is often utilized effectively as a natural environment with infants. With children 3 and older, school programs may rely on coordination with a wide variety of community-based programs, including private preschool programs.

School programs generally have varying degrees of flexibility and must be diligent in ensuring their program's educational settings are designed to encompass a broad range of child skill levels. Classroom modifications, curriculum adaptations, and direct or consultative services of an aural habilitation specialist may be offered as support to children in the various educational settings. In this new era the approach to education of children with hearing loss is a commitment that, to the maximum extent appropriate, all

---

Case Study 9–2   J.S. is 6 years old and was diagnosed with a profound bilateral sensorineural hearing loss at age 14 months. He participated in an early intervention, home-based program until he was 3 years old, at which time he transitioned to an integrated school-based program. That program utilized an approach that was highly dependent on the collaborative efforts of many professionals and parents. In his integrated class 30% of the children had a hearing loss and the rest of the class were children with hearing and typical language development. J.S.'s class was team taught by a deaf educator and a regular early childhood educator. The deaf educator ensured that J.S.'s IEP objectives were addressed during all of his activities throughout the day. J.S. made significant gains in both receptive and expressive language skills while enrolled in the preschool program and successfully completed the targeted IEP objectives. However, he still showed a delay of 18 months in his overall language development and school readiness skills. School personnel recommended that J.S. attend the integrated kindergarten class team taught by a regular kindergarten teacher and an educator of the deaf similar to his preschool setting. The school staff felt that J.S. still required specific strategies and curriculum modifications to meet his needs. This class was at an elementary school several miles from J.S.'s home. His parents, however, wanted him to attend his neighborhood school. The challenge of the individual education plan committee was to identify the most natural environment possible in which J.S. would experience optimal development. It was decided that a team consisting of J.S.'s parents, his regular early childhood educator, his preschool deaf educator, and his speech therapist would first visit the school where the kindergarten class was team taught by an educator of the deaf so they could identify and observe the strategies, curriculum adaptations, and support services that were utilized. Following that visit, they would then visit his neighborhood school kindergarten program to see if those same components could be provided there. They would report back at the ARD meeting and make an informed decision on placement.

children will have the opportunity to be in preschool and early elementary settings similar to those available to them if there were no special needs.

A key element to successful programming is adherence to a philosophy of developmental appropriateness. A developmentally appropriate program incorporates knowledge about the predictable growth and sequence of typical child development (age appropriateness); recognizes the individual uniqueness of each child in learning style and rate, and pattern of development (individual appropriateness); and incorporates knowledge of the social and cultural contexts in which children live (cultural appropriateness) (National Association for Education of Young Children Position Statement, 1996). This type of program provides an environment in which individual needs of children are a significant part of the planning process.

The concept of least restrictive may also be influenced to some extent by the communication mode of the child. For a child to benefit most fully from peer interactions, the optimal situation will provide the opportunity for shared linguistic communication. Programs that have the capability of providing instruction via total communication for all children eliminate some of the barriers to inclusive education for young children who are deaf.

Summary

Infants who are deaf or hard of hearing enter intervention programs as early as 1 month of age. To ensure language development equal to cognitive potential, the aural habilitation specialist must understand current hearing technology, utilize intervention practices based on recent research, and work in partnership with families and other professionals to support outcomes established by families. Effective early identification and intervention programs have a major impact on services for preschool-aged children with fewer children enrolled in self-contained classes and more children in need of support services within an inclusion setting. Comprehensive communication purposefulness is the goal for children in all settings, and to achieve this, working collaboratively with families and other professionals remains essential throughout the preschool years and beyond.

References

American College of Medical Genetics Statement. (2002). Genetics evaluation guidelines for the etiologic diagnosis of congenital hearing loss. *Genet Med, 4,* 162–171.

Arehart, K.H., & Yoshinaga-Itano, C. (1999). The role of educators of the deaf in the early identification of hearing loss. *Am Ann Deaf, 144,* 19–23.

Barrera, I. (1996). Thoughts on the assessment of young children whose sociocultural background is unfamiliar to the assessor. In: S.J. Meisels & E. Fenichel (Eds.), *New Visions for the Developmental Assessment of Infants and Young Children* (pp. 67–84). Washington, DC: Zero to Three National Center for Infants, Toddlers, and Families.

Bredekamp S., & Rosegrant, T. (1995). Reaching potentials through transforming curriculum: Introduction. In: S. Bredekamp and T. Rosegrant (Eds.), *Reaching Potentials: Transforming Early Childhood Curriculum and Assessment,* Vol. 2 (pp. 1–4). Washington, DC: National Association for the Education of Young Children.

Clark, K., Abraham, H., Lambourne, M., & Madsen, M. (2004). Assessment in SKI-HI. In: Watkins, S. (Ed.), *The SKI-HI Resource Manual.* Logan, UT: SKI-HI Institute.

Crais, E. (1993). Families and professionals as collaborators in assessment. *Topics in Language Disorders, 14,* 29–40.

Dunst, C.J., & Trivette, C.M. (1996). Empowerment, effective help-giving practices and family-centered care. *Pediatr Nurs, 22,* 334–343.

Dunst, C.J. (2000). Revisiting "Rethinking Early Intervention." *Topics in Early Childhood Education, 20,* 95–104.

Emde, R.N., & Easterbrooks, M.A. (1985). Assessing emotional availability in early development. In: W.K. Frankenburg, R.N. Emde, & J.W. Sullivan (Eds.), *Early Identification of Children at Risk: An International Perspective* (pp. 70–101). New York: Plenum.

Flexer, C. (1994). *Facilitating Hearing and Listening in Young children.* San Diego, CA: Singular.

Individuals with Disabilities Education Act (IDEA), Pub.L.No. 105–17 (1997). *Federal Register,* June 4.

Lynch, E.W., & Hanson, M.J. (1998). *Developing Cross-Cultural Competence.* Baltimore: Paul H. Brookes.

Mertens, D.M., Sass-Lehrer, M., & Scott-Olson, K. (2000). Sensitivity in the family-professional relationship: Parental experiences in families with young deaf and hard of hearing children. In: P.E. Spencer, C.J. Erting, & M. Marschark (Eds.), *The Deaf Child in the Family and at School* (pp.133–150). Mahwah, NJ: Lawrence Erlbaum.

Moeller, M.P. (2000). Early intervention and language development in children who are deaf and hard of hearing. *Pediatrics, 106,* E43.

National Association for Education of Young Children. (1996). Position statement. In: S. Bredekamp, & C. Copple (Eds.), *Developmentally Appropriate Practice in Early Childhood Programs* (rev. ed., 1997) (pp. 3–30) Washington, DC: National Association for Education of Young Children.

National Center for Hearing Assessment and Management. (2003). Web site: http://www.infanthearing.org.

National Research Research Council and Institute of Medicine, Committee on Integrating the Science of Early Childhood Development. (2000). Rethinking nature and nurture. In: J.P. Shonkoff & D.A. Phillips (Eds.), *From Neurons to Neighborhoods: The Science of Early Childhood Development* (pp. 39–56). Washington DC: National Academy Press.

Pressman, L.J., Pipp-Siegel, S., Yoshinaga-Itano, C., Kubicek, L., & Emde, R.N. (2000). A Comparison of the links between emotional availability and language gain in young children with and without hearing loss. In: C. Yoshinaga-Itano & A.L. Sedey (Eds.), *Volta Review Monograph* (pp. 251–277). Washington DC: Alexander Graham Bell Association for the Deaf and Hard of Hearing.

Roush, J., Harrison, M., & Palsha, S. (1991). Family-centered early intervention: Professionals' perceptions. *Am Ann Deaf, 136*, 360–366.

Siegel, S. (2000). *Resolution of grief of young children with hearing loss.* Unpublished manuscript. Cited in: E. Kurtzer-White & D. Luterman (Eds.), *Early Childhood Deafness* (pp. 13–28). Baltimore: York Press.

Wallace, V., Menn, L., & Yoshinga-Itano, C. (2000). Is babble the gateway to speech for all children? A lon-gitudinal study of children who are deaf or hard of hearing. In: C. Yoshinaga-Itano & A.L. Sedey (Eds.), *Volta Review Monograph* (pp. 121–148) Washington DC: Alexander Graham Bell Association for the Deaf and Hard of Hearing.

Watkins, S. (Ed.). (2004). *The SKI-HI Resource Manual.* Logan, UT: SKI-HI Institute.

Wyatt, T. (1998). Assessment issues with multicultural populations. In: D. Battle (Ed.), *Communication Disorders in Multicultural Populations*. Boston: Butterworth-Heinemann.

Yoshinaga-Itano, C. (1995). Efficacy of early identification and intervention. *Seminars in Hearing, 16*, 115–120.

Yoshigna-Itano, C. (2000). Development of audition and speech: Implications for early intervention with infants who are deaf or hard of hearing. In: C. Yoshinaga-Itano & A.L. Sedey (Eds.), *Volta Review Monograph* (pp. 213–234). Washington, DC: Alexander Graham Bell Association for the Deaf and Hard of Hearing.

Yoshinaga-Itano, C., & Sedey, A. (2000). Early speech development in children who are deaf or hard of hearing: Interrelationships with language and hearing. In: C. Yoshinaga-Itano A.L. Sedey (Eds.), *Volta Review Monograph* (pp. 213–234). Washington DC: Alexander Graham Bell Association for the Deaf and Hard of Hearing.

Yoshinga-Itano, C., Sedey, A., Coulter, D., & Mehl, A. (1998). Language of early- and later-identified children with hearing loss. *Pediatrics, 102*, 1161–1171.

10

Contribution of Mild Hearing Loss to Auditory Language Learning Problems

MARION P. DOWNS

It is only with the heart that one can see rightly; what is essential is invisible to the eye.

—Antoine de Saint-Exupery, 1900–1944

Views regarding what is an educationally handicapping hearing loss have undergone dramatic changes. Traditionally, if a child passed a school hearing screening test at the usual 25 dB hearing level (HL), that hearing would be considered adequate for educational purposes. However, there has been documented evidence that pure tone screenings with an intensity criterion of 25 dB HL have resulted in missed ear disorders. Approximately 2 to 5% of children who are screened at a 15 dB level can be expected to have educationally handicapping conductive hearing losses (Hoffman, MacTurk, Gravel, Chiu, & Cosgrove, 1999; Jerger, Jerger, Alford, & Abrams, 1983; Jordan & Eagles, 1961). Educators, school nurses, health service personnel, physicians, and school administrators have expressed an immediate concern with the changing criteria for the term "handicapping loss."

Although sensorineural loss is considered a more distressing handicap, it occurs less frequently than conductive loss in school children. Often caused from active ear disease, conductive hearing loss is a more widespread concern because of its connection with many language disorders and school failures seen in the school population. Children may arrive at school with developmental language dysfunction caused by early re-

current ear disease. Recognition of this fact will make a difference in the educational approaches used with such children.

What kind of a hearing loss caused by ear disease would result in educational handicap? How prevalent is the disease in the school-age child? What intensity level should be used as the criterion to define the educationally handicapping condition? Why do mild losses from common ear disease become learning handicaps? What evidence suggests that ear disease in early life results in language learning disorders? On the basis of new information, what change should schools make in their identification and remediation program of hearing loss? These questions are thoroughly covered in this chapter because they represent a revolutionary change in the way of looking at hearing loss in school children. In addition, other forms of environmental deprivation affecting the auditory language learning process are explored; after all, almost all language is learned through audition.

Prevalence of Otitis Media in the School-Age Child

Definitive data collected in the Third National Health and Nutrition Examination Survey of 1988–1994 (Hoffman et al, 1999)

233

are finally available on the prevalence and epidemiology of hearing loss and otitis media in school age children. After screening 4445 children aged 6 to 19, with both audiometry and tympanometry, the following prevalence of childhood otitis media with effusion (OME) by age has been documented:

Age 6: 5.1%
Age 7 to 10: 4.5%
Age 11 to 14: 3.3%
Age 15 to 19: 2%

There was an increased prevalence of OME noted for Hispanic and African American children when compared to their Caucasian cohorts.

These prevalence data are particularly significant for all professionals with the responsibility of planning hearing screenings in the school. Suggestions concerning those specific concerns in school screenings are also covered here.

The Handicap of Conductive Hearing Loss

Just for a moment, perform a little experiment: with index fingers extended, press the tabs in front of each ear into the earcanals, occluding the earcanals completely. If firmly occluded, a 25 dB HL average hearing loss will be achieved (Fig. 10–1). Carrying on a normal conversation or listening to a conversation in a crowd will cause a great deal of strain and disruption in communication. Yet, this kind of hearing loss would have passed the traditional school screening tests consisting of only three frequencies (1000, 2000, and 4000 Hz) at an intensity level of 25 dB HL. Often this kind of loss is from an extremely common ear disorder called otitis media. Table 10–1 shows the approximate prevalence of ear disease in children (20% on the average) reported by the National Academy of Sciences (Kessner, Snow, & Singer, 1974).

However, for the benefit of some medical professionals, it is important to reiterate which kind of otitis media is the culprit in

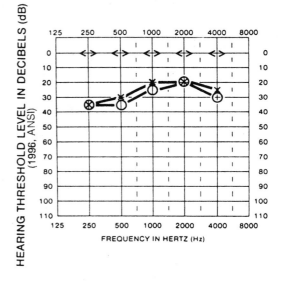

Figure 10–1. Simulation of conductive-type hearing loss obtained when occluding ears with fingers.

hearing losses. As detailed in Chapter 4 there are three main types of otitis media:

1. Acute suppurative otitis media, characterized by fever, pain, redness of the drum, and a significant conductive hearing loss (Fig. 10–2). These symptomatic episodes of acute otitis media are easily recognizable. Because this disease is caused by bacteria, it may yield readily to antibiotics, so it is easily medically treated.

2. Chronic otitis media, usually characterized by a perforated eardrum accompanied by purulent (puss-filled) drainage. There may be some pain and potentially severe hearing loss associated with it. Children between the ages of 5 and 10 are quite likely to suffer the onset of this problem.

3. Serous otitis media (also called secretory otitis media), with the exception of an occasional conductive hearing loss, is an almost completely asymptomatic disease.

Figure 10–3 shows the mean conductive hearing loss of serous otitis described by (Bluestone, Beery, & Paradise, 1975). There is

Table 10–1. Distribution of Otologic Examination Results in Children Age 6 Months to 11 Years*

Otologic Examination Results[†]	6 mo–3 yr (%)	4–5 yr (%)	6–7 yr (%)	8–9 yr (%)	10–11 yr (%)	All Ages (%)
Bilaterally normal	68.8	74.3	72.2	81.2	78.8	74.6
Small fibrotic scarring only	3.6	4.6	8.0	5.6	6.7	5.7
Ear pathological condition	27.6	21.1	19.8	13.2	14.4	19.7
Total percent	100.0	100.0	100.0	100.0	99.9	100.0
Total number	499	411	451	407	390	2158[‡]

*Community sample, selected areas in Washington, D.C., 1971.
[†]Total chi square (4 df) = 34.132, $p < 0.001$: regression with chi square (1 df) = 30.401, $p < 0.001$.
[‡]Excludes 22 children who could not be examined.
Reprinted with permission from Kessner, Snow, & Singer (1974).

no pain, no fever, no drainage, no bulging drum, and only a thin fluid behind the eardrum that may be difficult to see in a cursory examination. This ear disease is a particular concern for both infant and school child because the resulting hearing loss may be a great deal more educationally handicapping than previously thought (Friel-Patti & Finitzo, 1990).

When present, serous otitis media usually affects both ears (see Chapter 4). It may cause a constant or recurrent or fluctuating hearing loss. Even when fluctuating, serous otitis media handicaps the overall language learning situation of the child; acoustic in-

formation will be heard sporadically and differently from time to time and cause confusion in the child's learning strategies. Various intensities of speech sounds heard in relation to the mild conductive hearing loss found with otitis media are demonstrated in Figure 10–4. It can be seen that, although the voiced vowel and consonant sounds may be heard at around 40 dB HL on the audiogram, a great many of the unvoiced consonant sounds may be heard faintly or not at all with a mild conductive hearing loss. It is important to understand the relevance of audi-

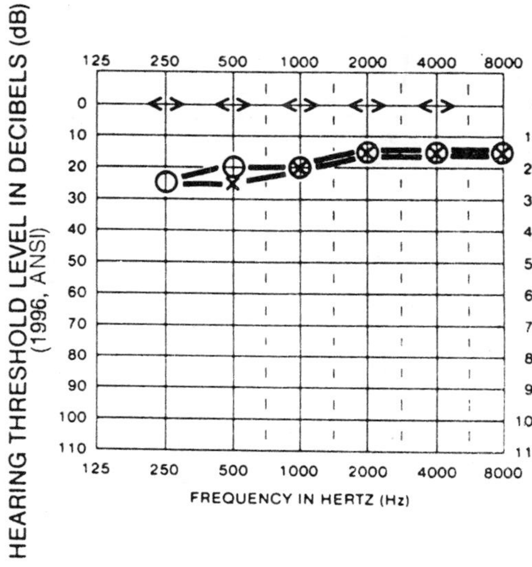

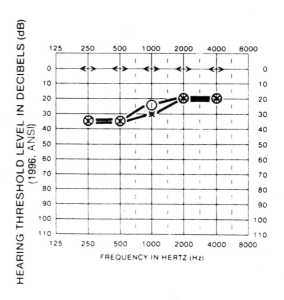

Figure 10–2. Mild conductive hearing loss characteristic of acute suppurative otitis media.

Figure 10–3. Mean conductive hearing loss characteristic of serous otitis media (Bluestone, Beery, & Paradise, 1975).

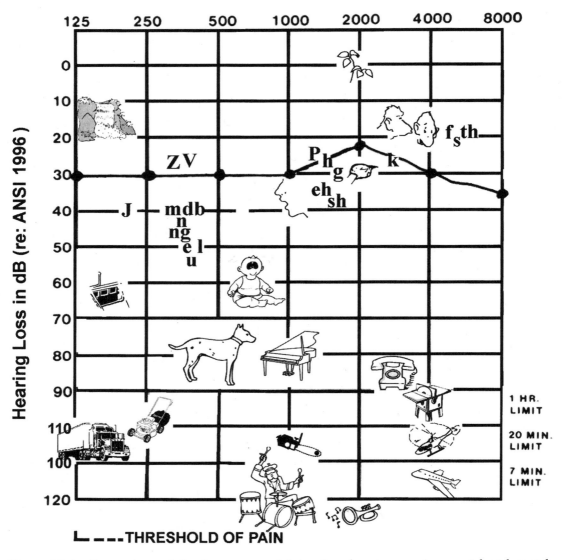

Frequency in Cycles per Second

Figure 10–4. Comparison of the frequency and intensity of various environmental and speech sounds in relationship to the mild conductive hearing loss of otitis media (Northern & Downs, 2002).

bility of speech sounds in terms of learning strategies for children.

When both ears are occluded (as in the preceding exercise), it is clearly possible to understand ordinary conversation, though it will sound considerably muffled. However, there are some speech sounds that are not audible at all or are not heard distinctly. Due to the familiarity of utilizing strategies for understanding speech through contextual clues, listeners occluding their ears will have no conscious effort in predicting those missing segments of the missed sounds. What if the above experiment were conducted on a

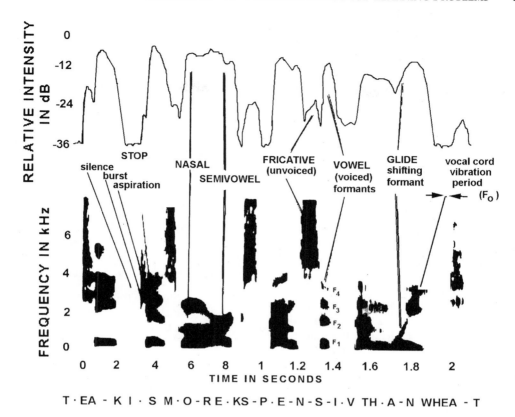

Figure 10–5. Spectrographic analysis and relative intensity of a speech sample showing why some acoustic cues may not be perceived when mild hearing loss is present (Skinner, 1978).

first grader who was learning a variety of words for the first time? It is exceedingly more important for a first grader to hear all of the speech sounds in a new word than it is for an experienced listener. Figure 10–5 illustrates why some of the acoustic sounds may be missed by a child with a mild hearing loss. In some of the examples the voiceless stop (e.g., /p/ as in pay, /t/ as in to, and /k/ as in key) and voiceless fricative consonants (e.g., /f/ as in for, /s/ as in see, /th/ as in thin, and /sh/ as in she) can be 30 dB less intense than vowels or other consonants. For example, the word "teak" (see Fig. 10–5) contains the /e/ sound that is almost 29 dB more intense than /k/.

For the child who is still learning language, a mild conductive hearing loss may place an unbearable strain on coping abilities. Only the rare child—one with unusu-

ally high intellectual abilities—can surmount this learning hazard without being affected in some way. Thus, when speech sounds are missed entirely or not heard distinctly, or are heard differently from one time to another, the usual learning strategies of the child become disorganized and ineffective.

Moreover, the normal background noise level found in present-day environments can be a most destructive liability to educational processes, especially when a conductive hearing loss co-occurs. Stop for a moment and do another experiment in hearing. Sit back and listen to the ambient noise levels within the immediate environment. Perhaps there will be audible noise from air conditioning, fluorescent lights, heating blowers, people talking, etc. According to Skinner (1978), this background noise is usually 10 to 15 dB below the level of speech, giving a + 10 to + 15 dB signal-to-noise (S/N) ratio (see Chapters 12 and 13). This S/N ratio is not difficult for the normal-hearing adult to communicate in because an adult is able to fill in contextual clues and predict the missed acoustic signals. However, if children are to hear all of the acoustic clues clearly, the noise should be 30 dB below the level of speech. Unfortunately, our classrooms do not get a clean bill of health as far as S/N ratio is concerned. Chapters 12 and 13 describe the studies that have shown the detrimental effects of unfavorable S/N ratios found in most school classrooms.

Environmental noise problems in the schools have been exacerbated by open-plan or open-area classrooms, air conditioning and heating systems, and the lack of good acoustic treatment of most classrooms. Even the normal-hearing child may be affected by this rising ambient noise level. Cohen (1970) was able to document that groups of children who lived in high environmental noise backgrounds tended to have more reading difficulties than their cohorts who lived in lower (quieter) background noise levels. Methods to remedy the background noise situation in the classrooms are described in Chapters 12 and 13. One method involves amplifying the teacher's voice through loudspeakers and also using amplification for pupil recitation. These remedies appear to be beneficial for both the child with conductive hearing loss as well as the normal hearing child.

Dobie and Berlin (1979) were able to provide dramatic support that confirmed Skinner's (1978) theory regarding the acoustic liabilities of mild conductive hearing loss. Knowing that a child with hearing thresholds at 20 dB HL loss would pass a screening test using a criterion intensity level of 20 dB HL, Dobie and Berlin (1979) investigated what kind of speech perception problems a child with a very mild hearing loss would have in a language-learning situation. Recorded speech sample utterances were subjected to attenuation and filtering in order to more closely simulate acoustic signals re-

ceived at the ear with a mild conductive hearing loss.

When comparing unattenuated with attenuated utterances, the following two observations were reported: (1) there was a potential loss of transitional information, especially plural endings and related final position fricatives; and (2) brief utterances or high frequency information could conceivably either be distorted or degraded if S/N conditions were less than satisfactory (remember that the S/N ratios in almost all schools are inadequate).

Dobie and Berlin (1979) reasoned that, on the basis of their findings, a child with a 20 dB hearing loss from otitis media might be handicapped acoustically in the following ways:

1. Morphological markers might be lost or sporadically misunderstood; for example, "Where are Jack's gloves to be placed?" might be perceived as "Where Jack glove be place?"
2. Very short words that are elided often in connected speech (see "are" and "to" in the preceding example) will lose considerable loudness because of the critical relationship between intensity, duration, and loudness.
3. Inflections, or markers, carrying subtle nuances such as questioning and related intonation contouring can at the very best be expected to come through inconsistently.
4. Due to the variability in the acoustic input, markers for the beginnings and endings of words and ideas could be inconsistently noted.

From these studies, some would predict that (1) conductive loss is more devastating to the educational activity of the school child than had previously been suspected, and (2) children who have a history of recurrent otitis media with mild conductive hearing loss might be expected to have central-like symptoms masquerading as auditory processing disorders, language-learning problems, and attention difficulties. There is a great deal of evidence indicating that such is the case. The following text summarizes some of the studies that have demonstrated these conditions.

Sequelae of Conductive Hearing Losses

A large number of reports have appeared in the literature describing the effect of otitis media on the language functioning of children. The retrospective nature of many of the studies has been severely criticized by Ventry (1980), who believes that only prospective studies will reveal the pathophysiological effects of otitis media on language development in children. However, more recently, prospective as well as retrospective studies have appeared indicating that otitis media cannot be overlooked when considering this problem.

A careful review of the literature as shown in Table 10–2 will reveal several critical conclusions:

1. When highly discriminating tests are used to identify differences in language skills, school-age children who have had histories of otitis media show significant deficiencies. It is only when standard global tests are used that no differences are found because, by the time school age is reached, speech and language have become so highly redundant, so highly socialized, and so highly global, that it is difficult to see differences in the wide range of normalcy found in these tests. However, special distinguishing tests revealed deficiencies in those children with otitis media histories in the following areas: morphological ending production; proportional use of compound or complex sentences and prepositional phrases; word production; speech-sound production and auditory perception; ratings of independence, task orientation, attentional skill, and patterns of verbal performance discrepancies in intellectual development; social behavior; phonological process tests; and pitch pattern perception.
2. A recurrent theme, and one that has never been negated, is that attention skills are markedly impaired in chil-

dren with otitis media. This point was first noted by Feagans, Sangal, Henderson, Collier, and Applebaum (1986) who used rating scales to show that those children with otitis media histories had twice the amount of distractibility and inattention as children who were normal while in the classroom. This same phenomenon has consistently been repeated using the Classroom Behavior Inventory (Roberts, Burchinal, & Henderson, 1993; Roberts, Burchinal, Koch, Footo, & Henderson, 1990). The reason for this problem was originally demonstrated (Jerger et al, 1983) in children with otitis media from 2 to 4 years of age who had difficulty discriminating words in the presence of background noise (competing sentences). Evidently, the habits formed during periods of mild hearing loss due to otitis media produce listening habits that persist well beyond the episodes of active ear disease. Whether these faulty habits can be remediated is yet to be determined, but it is clear that the mere presence of ear infections may be considered presumptive evidence that a hearing disability exists. It follows that it is urgent to establish effective programs to identify middle ear disorders in school screening programs (see Chapter 5).

3. The most significant deficits from otitis media are found in middle-class children. Klein, Teele, and Pelton (1992) and others (Black & Sonnenschein, 1993; Robb, Psak, & Pan-Ching, 1993), have shown that children in low socioeconomic groups have significant deficiencies in their language and developmental status, and any effects from otitis media will be completely hidden by the fundamental inadequacies of their speech and language. It is the middle-class children, who have high expectation of accomplishment, that are most affected by the sensory deprivation caused by otitis media. These children are labeled "normal" or "aver-

Table 10–2.   Studies on the Language Sequelae of Recurrent Otitis

Study	L/R	No.	Ages	Tests	Results	P/N
Schilder et al (1993)	L	47	7–9 yr	Reynell, language, reading, spelling	The association between OME and language at preschool was no longer present	N
Harsten et al (1993)	L	113	B–7 yr	Phoniatric and linguistic examinations— auditory discrimination	Recurrent acute aero otitis media by 3 years: no difference	N
Robb et al (1993)	L	1	11–21 mo	Phonetic inventory analyses of child with recurrent otitis media	Consonants fewer; lack of phonetic complexity in speech	P
Klein et al (1988)	L	498	B–3 yr	PPVT, Fischer-Logeman, Goldman-Fristoe, language structure test, articulation scores	Significant association between time with middle ear effusions and language tests	P
Klein et al (1992)	L	207	B–7 yr	WISC, Metropolitan Achievement, Articulation, Morphological markers	Difference persisted in all areas tested: intelligence, school achievement, speech and language	P
Updike and Thornburg (1992)	R		6–7 yr	Auditory perception reading ability	OM group: lower scores on all tests	
Gravel and Wallace (1992)	L		B–4 yr	Language and cognitive— Pediatric Speech Intelligibility	No difference in groups, OM in 1st year: needed better S/N ratio	N P
Freeark et al (1992)	R	56	3–4 yr	Video parent–child interactions: McCarthy Verbal Scale: verbalizing	Active verbalization with parents buffered the bad effects of OM	P
Roberts et al (1993)	L	30	4½–6 yr	Standard tests and language sample	No relationship between OME and language	N
Knishkowy et al (1991)	L	233	B–3 yr	Development quotient: Stanford-Binet	All significantly lower with recurrent OM	P
Teele et al (1984)	L	207	B–7 yr	WISC-R: Metropolitan Achievement, Articulation, Morphological Markers	Significant differences in all tests for OM before 3 years; after 3 years, no difference	P
Friel-Patti et al (1993)	L	213	B–21 mo	SICD, audiometry	Hearing is related to bouts of OM; hearing is related to lower scores both expressive and receptive	P

Table 10–2. **Studies on the Language Sequelae of Recurrent Otitis** *(continued)*

Study	*L/R*	*No.*	*Ages*	*Tests*	*Results*	*P/N*
Whiteman et al (1986)	R	30	Down's Syndrome	Adolescent Basic Skills, Receptive and Expressive Language	Tubed: 100% above mean No OM: 65% above mean OM: 18% above mean	P
Webster et al (1989)	R	10	7–11 yr	Auditory, educational and psychological measures	Matched OM group: lower educational and psychological scores	P
Clarkson et al (1989)	R		5 yr	Perception of voice onset time (VOT)	OM groups: deficits in identifying and discriminating speech patterns	P
Pearce et al (1988)	L	43	B–6 yr	SICD, Bayley, McCarthy scales at 3 and 6 years	Receptive language and cognitive tests significantly worse in OM group at both 3 and 6 years	P
Rach et al (1991)	R	65	Preschool	Reynell Developmental	Expressive language significantly lower in OM group	P
Roberts et al (1993)	L	55	2½–8 yr	Standardized tests of speech	Number of phonological processes lower for OM occurring before 3 years	P
Wright et al (1988)	L	210	B–2 yr	Speech and language tests	No language delays in the OM children	N
Wallace et al (1993)	L	27	12 mo	Bayley, SICD	Lower expressive language in OM children	P
Lous et al (1988)	L	463	3–8 yr	Silent Reading Word Test, PPVT, Verbal WISC	No differences between groups but greater variability in OM group	P
Wallace et al (1988)	L	74	B–2 yr	SICD, videos of parent interaction and the Peterson and Sherrod scale	OM group with good parent language had better language	P
Brookhouser & Goldgar (1987)	L	1864	9–59 yr	Language battery and development tests	Wide range of disabilities attributable to OM	P
Hall & Hill (1986)		10		Language developmental tests	Wide range of disabilities attributable to OM	P
Van Cauwenberge et al (1985)	R	1512	2–7 yr	Language, IQ, manual skills, social behavior, tympanometry	All showed negative influence, greatest under 47 months in speech and language: greatest over 47 months in IQ and activity	P
Fischler et al (1985)	L	167	B–8 yr	Battery of language battery	No difference between groups	N

Table 10–2.   Studies on the Language Sequelae of Recurrent Otitis *(continued)*

Study	*L/R*	*No.*	*Ages*	*Tests*	*Results*	*P/N*
Schlieper et al (1985)	R	26	3–5 yr	Auditory Comprehension of Language test, Northwestern Syntactic Development	Highly significant differences between matched groups; retests a year later showed the same except for Auditory Comprehension	P
Hasenstab (1993)	R	60	6 yr	Nonsense Syllable test, Phonological process test, pitch pattern perception, Kaufman, McCarthy	OM group showed problems in processing; immediate recall, problem-solving strategies, memory, and sequential tasks	P
Roberts et al (1990)	L	55	3–8 yr	IQ, achievement scores; Classroom Behavior Inventory	Only Classroom Behavior showed differences: poor and attentional skills and Verbal Performance discrepancies	P
Friel-Patti et al (1993)	L	213	B–3 yr	SICD on OM and non-OM children in 1. Home Care 2. Sitters home 3. Day care center	Number of bouts related to number of children in care; children in sitter's home had best language (small groups, stimulated)	P
Black and Sonnenschein (1993)	L	31			An inner-city group, low SES, experienced significant decline in their language and developmental status regardless of their history of OM	P
Gravel et al (1993)	L	39	B–4 yr	Adaptive pediatric speech intelligibility scores	Significant association between percent visits for OM in 1st year of life	P
Lous (1993)	R	387	2 yr	Silent word reading between type of tympanogram and reading	Significant correlation	P
Wendler-Shaw et al (1993)		105	B–2 yr	PPVT, sound discrimination, sentence repetition, and sentence comprehension	Frequency of OM in 1st year of life and perception of production of words and morphemes	
Luloff et al (1993)	L	138	1–3 mo	Speech sound repertoire	Number of episodes of OM in 1st year equaled reduction in number of consonants	P

Table 10–2. Studies on the Language Sequelae of Recurrent Otitis *(continued)*

Study	L/R	No.	Ages	Tests	Results	P/N
Roberts et al (1999)	L	55	3 mo–8 yr	IQ, academic performance, ratings of attention, task orientation, verbal performance discrepancies	No differences found for academic performance; early OM predicted all ratings for attention and verbal performance	

L/R, longitudinal (L) or retrospective (R); P/N, P indicates those studies that found significant differences between otitis groups and nonotitis groups; N indicates those studies in which no differences were found between groups on the measures used; B, birth; OM, otitis media; OME, otitis media with effusions; PPVT, Peabody Picture Vocabulary Test; WISC, Wechsler's Intelligence Scale for Children; S/N, signal-to-noise ratio; SICD, Sequenced Inventory of Communication Development; SES, socioeconomic status.

age," but should be achieving in the superior ranges. This fact is particularly poignant for some children: those who hold bright promises for the future, who will not reach their highest potential in productivity. What is particularly significant about all of these reports is that the children studied may be classified as having "auditory processing deficits, auditory perceptual problems, language-learning problems, auditory language deficits, etc." Yet many of these deficits may be developmental in origin, caused by early deprivation in a sensory avenue. This calls for a reconsideration of the entire question of labeling children as having auditory perceptual problems.

4. A meta-analysis of all prospective studies on otitis media sequelae has been performed by Roberts and cohorts (Roberts, Rosenfeld, Ziesel, & Derbenwick, 1999). Their findings showed "a modest but statistically significant association of OME to language, particularly expressive language." This study did not break down the potential differences between middle-class and lower-income children. That variable might have accentuated the association in the middle-class group as suggested by previous investigations.

Degraded language input in the home can be identified as auditory deprivation. Reports have indeed demonstrated that early exposure to low-quality language or reduced opportunities for listening have the same effect on language skills as does auditory sensory deprivation. Infants raised in slum environments reportedly will show significantly slower development at a much earlier age than previously suspected (Uzgiris, 1970; Wachs, Uzgiris, Hunt, & Hunt, 1971). These differences appear as early as 11 months and increase from 18 months and older. Indeed, 13-month-old children in lower-income groups vocalize less than their middle-class peers and are also less mobile in the playroom (Messer & Lewis, 1970). It appears that understimulation produces apathy and reduced language skills. These are the children who end up in language-learning classes.

Not only will lack of language stimulation victimize children, but high intensity stimulation and exposure to an excessive variety of circumstances can also be responsible for lower levels of cognitive development (Uzgiris, 1970; Wachs et al, 1971). When using an infant psychological development scale, there was evidence that stimulus bombardment actually resulted in developmental problems (Uzgiris & Hunt, 1966).

Other studies have shown that children raised in noisy environments do not respond as well in a distractive situation as do their peers from quiet homes (Bellussi, Mezzedimi, Psalli, & Psalli, 1999; Vernon-Feagans, Yont, & Hurley, 1999). Thus these environmental conditions, in effect, may constitute sensory deprivation just as devastating as hearing loss; they are societal problems.

Demographic Implications of Otitis Media

The need for remediation may become increasingly widespread if the present trends in the demography of otitis media continue. In the general population, 71% of children have had at least one episode of acute otitis media by 3 years of age, and 33% have had three or more such episodes (Teele, Klein, Rosner, & Group, 1984). However, this percentage escalates in day care centers, where 80% of the children have three or more episodes of acute otitis media by age 3 years (Denny, 1984). With the proliferation of such centers caring for the children of working mothers, the incidence of recurrent serous otitis will continue to increase alarmingly.

The peak occurrence of otitis media in day care centers is now at 6 months of age, and studies show that such early occurrence places a child at risk for persistent recurrence of the disease (Wendler-Shaw, Menyuk, & Teele, 1993). In fact, it seems that the longer the disease process for serious otitis in infants 6 to 12 months of age, the worse the language levels of the children later on (Teele et al, 1984). Thus school systems can expect an escalation of language-learning problems with the predicted increased incidence in early otitis.

Unless otitis media is treated vigorously, it can recur or also occur anew into the school years, resulting in a growing problem for school health departments. Consequently, it could be rationalized that frequent school hearing screenings will ultimately facilitate the educational process of all children. An in-depth study reported from New Zealand emphasizes the problem. One hundred children 7 to 8 years old were given audiometry and tympanometry tests every 2 to 3 weeks throughout a school year. An average prevalence of 62% for some ear abnormality was found, with a mean duration of 6 weeks for an episode. A correlation between educational tests and threshold audiometric results was reported, showing that the children with poorer hearing had poorer scores on language and achievement tests. It was concluded that one audiometric test per school year was not adequate to identify hearing loss and ear disease. They suggested that tympanometry tests three times per year will be the most cost-effective program to detect ear disease, with threshold audiometry once per year. That recommendation was subsequently adopted by the New Zealand Public Health Department for all its schools.

The effects of escalation of otitis media may be felt in the schools within a short time. Feagans and Blood (1993) followed a group of school-age children with histories of recurrent otitis media beginning at 6 months of age. They were found to have lowered narrative and discrimination skills mediated by problems in attentional processes. These children had difficulty in attending to a stimulus, probably due to poor hearing during early critical years. Another significant finding within a special subcategory of school-age children, talented and gifted, having histories of early recurrent otitis was a misperception of lower functioning (poorer) school performance by some children (Uzgiris, 1970). Yet, when given in-depth testing, these same children were found to be highly gifted. Again, deficits in attending seem to be responsible, along with marked weaknesses in sequential processing. It is conceivable that these problems may result from many of the auditory processing deficits that are seen (Downs, 1985).

Schools should also expect to find behavioral problems increasing as a result of early hearing deficits. Silva (1985) followed a group of children with early recurrent otitis media through the age of 11 years. In addition to persistent reading and articulation problems, the behavior ratings by teachers were also lower in the otitis group than in the normal controls, with significant effects seen at 3, 5, 7, 9, and 11 years of age.

It seems clear that the schools may see a growing number of children with deficits described (Deutch, 1964) as attributable to early mild hearing losses or present hearing losses from otitis media. Remediating these problems as basic language delays and attending disorders is the road to follow.

Unilateral Hearing Loss

Hearing loss in only one ear was formerly considered to involve no handicap as long as preferential seating was given in the classroom (i.e., sitting near and with the good ear toward the teacher). However, this long-held philosophy has now been challenged and schools are cautioned not to be sanguine about children with unilateral hearing losses. Bess (1986) documented the effects of unilateral hearing loss in 60 children, 6 to 13 years old, who had normal hearing in one ear, and sensorineural hearing losses of more than 45 dB in the other ear. Despite classroom preferential seating, 35% had failed one or more grades in school, and another 13% were in need of special resource assistance— a total of almost 50% with educational problems. Further testing and analysis showed that:

1. Children with unilateral hearing loss exhibited greater difficulty than children with normal hearing in understanding speech in the presence of a competing noise background. This difficulty occurred even when the good ear was on the side of speech and the bad ear was on the side of the competing noise. Thus preferential seating in the classroom is not an adequate solution to the problem.
2. Those children who had severe to profound unilateral hearing loss (greater than 61 dB) exhibited significantly lower full-scale IQs than those children with milder losses (45 dB to 60 dB). Thus, the degree of loss made a difference in the severity of the effect on the IQ.

3. Children with unilateral hearing impairment were consistently rated by teachers as having greater difficulty in peer relationships and social confidence, as well as a greater likelihood of acting-out behavior or withdrawal from social situations, greater frustration, increased need for dependence on the teacher, and more frequent distractibility.
4. Common factors among children with unilateral hearing impairment with greater educational problems include early age of onset of the hearing loss; perinatal (e.g., prematurity) or postnatal (e.g., meningitis) complications; severe to profound sensorineural impairment (greater than 61 dB); and right ear impairment. Of the children who failed one or more grades, 63% had right ear hearing losses, and a large mean difference was found between verbal IQ scores of 108 and 99 in children with, respectively, left ear and right ear hearing impairments.

Bess (1986) concluded that it is no longer appropriate to assume that preferential seating will solve the problems of the child with unilateral hearing loss. Innovative solutions must be devised for these children. Some possible interventions that schools can use include applying FM wireless systems to the good ear; use of infrared systems; or simply amplifying the entire classroom to improve the S/N ratio. Special resource assistance is another alternative but is an after-the-fact remedy. Whatever is done for the child with unilateral hearing loss, it must go beyond the traditional recommendations.

Suggestions for Educators and Professionals

On the basis of new findings reported, schools might consider some changes in dealing with the identification and remediation of hearing loss. The following suggestions are offered:

1. Screening
   - Audiometric screening intensity level should be set no higher than 20 dB HL, and at 15 dB HL whenever acoustic environments permit.
   - For students entering first grade, screening should include tympanometry. The report of the Third National Health and Nutrition Examination Survey of 1988–1999, showed otitis media is most prevalent at 6 years of age (5.1%). The purpose of tympanometry is to identify active ear disease that can be treated immediately. Children at this age who fail either the audiometric screening or the tympanometry must be referred for medical intervention as soon as possible. Periodic telephone follow-up checks with the parents should be made to determine that the child has received medical attention; often parents can be slow to follow through on these requests.
   - The additional use of otoacoustic emissions (OAE) screening would be useful in identifying children who have auditory neuropathy (see Chapters 5 and 17). A child who fails the auditory screen yet shows normal cochlear hair cell function on OAE would be at high risk for this difficulty and should be thoroughly evaluated by experts.

2. Unilateral Hearing Loss
   - Children identified through hearing screening programs to have unilateral hearing losses should receive special treatment. In addition to being considered for hearing aid use and special remediation, they should be given yearly audiometric tests to monitor hearing status of both ears. A recent study of babies who are found at birth to have unilateral hearing loss showed that as many as 17% develop a progressive hearing loss in the good ear within 2 years of life (Sedey, Elfenbein, Schum, & Bentler, 2002). Although progressive hearing loss has only been documented during the first years of life, there may still be a prevalence of progressive hearing loss in school-age children.

Summary

Among school children, mild hearing losses of any type or cause result in language deficits, lowered academic performance, reduced cognitive skills, or behavioral problems. Many of the problems are due to otitis media, whether incurred in infancy or at school age. Such hearing losses must be zealously identified and remediated, both medically and educationally. The language problems that are found can best be remediated by the comprehensive therapy described in Chapter 17.

References

Bellussi, L., Mezzedimi, C., Psalli, G., & Psalli, D. (1999). *Long-term sequelae of otitis media with effusion on linguistic and cognitive development.* Paper presented at the 7th International Symposium on Recent Advances in Otitis Media, University of Pittsburgh.

Bess, F. (1986). Special issue: Unilateral sensorineural hearing loss in children. *Ear Hear, 7,* 3–54.

Black, M., & Sonnenschein, S. (1993). Early exposure to otitis media: A preliminary investigation of behavioral outcome. *J Dev Behav Pediatr, 14,* 150–155.

Bluestone, C., Beery, Q., & Paradise, J. (1975). Audiometry and tympanometry in relation to middle ear effusion in children. *Laryngoscope, 83,* 594–604.

Brookhouser, P., & Goldgar, D. (1987). Medical profile of the language-delayed child: Otitis prone versus otitis-free. *Int J Pediatr Otorhinolaryngol, 12,* 237–271.

Clarkson, R., Eimas, P., & Marean, G. (1989). Speech perception in children with histories of recurrent otitis media. *J Acoust Soc Am, 85,* 926–933.

Cohen, S. (1970). Cause vs. treatment in reading achievement. *J Learn Disabil, 33,* 163–166.

Denny, F. (1984). Article on otitis media. *Pediatr News, 18,* 1, 38.

Deutch, C. (1964). Auditory discrimination and learning: Social factors. *Merrill-Palmer Q Behav Dev, 10,* 277–296.

Dobie, R., & Berlin, C. (1979). Influence of otitis media on hearing and development. *Ann Otol Rhinol Laryngol, 88* (Suppl. 60), 48–53.

Downs, M. (1985). Effects of mild hearing loss on auditory processing. *Otolaryngol Clin North Am, 18,* 337–344.

Feagans, L., & Blood, I. (1993). Language and behavioral sequelae of otitis media in infants and young children attending day-care centers. In: D. Lim (Ed.), *Recent Advances in Otitis Media* (pp. 521–522). Toronto: Decker Periodicals.

Feagans, L., Sangal, M., Henderson, F., Collier, A., & Applebaum, M. (1986). The relationships of middle ear disease in early childhood to later narrative and attention skills. *J Pediatr Psychol, 12*, 581–594.

Fischler, R., Todd, N., & Feldman, C. (1985). Otitis media and language performance in a cohort of Apache Indian children. *Am J Dis Child, 139*, 355–360.

Freeark, K., Frank, S., Wagner, A., Lopez, M., Olmsted, C., & Girard, R. (1992). Otitis media, language development, and parental verbal stimulation. *J Pediatr Psychol, 17*, 173–185.

Friel-Patti, S., & Finitzo, T. (1990). Language learning in a prospective study of otitis media with effusion in the first two years of life. *J Speech Hear Res, 33*, 188–194.

Friel-Patti, S., Finitzo, T., Chinn, K., & Lindgren, M. (1993). Effects of day-care setting on incidence of OME and language development in a cohort of children followed prospectively. In: D. Lim (Ed.), *Recent Advances in Otitis Media* (pp. 569–572). Toronto: Decker Periodicals.

Gravel, J., Wallace, I., & Ruben, R. (1993). Auditory capabilities of preschoolers with and without a history of otitis media. In: D. Lim (Ed.), *Recent Advances in Otitis Media* (pp. 543–546). Toronto: Decker Periodicals.

Gravel, J., & Wallace, I. (1992). Listening and language at 4 years of age: Effects of early otitis media. *J Speech Hear Res, 35*, 588–595.

Hall, D., & Hill, P. (1986). When does secretory otitis media affect language development? *Arch Dis Child, 61*, 42–47.

Harsten, G., Nettelbladt, U., Schallen, L., Kalm, O., & Prellner, K. (1993). Language development in children with recurrent acute otitis media during the first three years of life: Follow-up study from birth to seven years of age. *J Laryngol Otol, 107*, 407–412.

Hasenstab, M. (1993). Auditory processing and cognitive performance of five- and six-year-old children with recurrent otitis media with effusion. In: D. Lim (Ed.), *Recent Advances in Otitis Media* (pp. 549–551). Toronto: Decker Periodicals.

Hoffman, H., MacTurk, R., Gravel, J., Chiu, M., & Cosgrove, C. (1999). Epidemiological risk factors for otitis media and hearing loss in school-age children based on NHANES III, 1988–1994. *7th International Symposium on Recent Advances in Otitis Media* (p. 317). University of Pittsburgh, Pennsylvania.

Jerger, S., Jerger, J., Alford, B., & Abrams, S. (1983). Development of speech intelligibility in children with recurrent otitis media. *Ear Hear, 4*, 138–145.

Jordan, R., & Eagles, E. (1961). The relation of air conduction audiometry to otologic abnormalities. *Ann Otol Rhinol Laryngol, 70*, 819–927.

Kessner, D., Snow, C., & Singer, J. (1974). *Assessment of Medical Care for Children* (Vol. 3). Washington DC: National Academy of Sciences.

Klein, J., Teele, D., & Pelton, S. (1992). New concepts in otitis media: Results of investigations of the Greater Boston Otitis Media Study Group. *Adv Pediatr, 39*, 127–156.

Luloff, A., Menyuk, P., & Teele, D. (1993). Effect of persistent otitis media on the speech sound repertoire

of infants. In: D. Lim (Ed.), *Recent Advances in Otitis Media* (pp. 531–533). Toronto: Decker Periodicals.

Lous, J. (1993). Secretory otitis media and reading score in the first grade. In: D. Lim (Ed.), *Recent Advances in Otitis Media* (pp. 537–539). Toronto: Decker Periodicals.

Lous, J., Fiellau-Nikolajsen, M., & Jeppesen, A. (1988). Secretory otitis media and language development: A six-year follow-up study with case-control. *Int J Pediatr Otorhinolaryngol, 15*, 185–203.

Messer, S., & Lewis, M. (1970). *Social class and sex differences in the attachment and play behavior of the year-old infant.* Presented at the Annual Meeting of the Eastern Psychological Association, Atlantic City.

Northern, J., & Downs, M. (2002). *Hearing in Children* (4th ed.). Baltimore, MD: Lippincott Williams and Wilkins.

Pearce, P., Saunders, M., Creighton, D., & Sauve, R. (1988). Hearing and verbal–cognitive abilities in high-risk preterm infants prone to otitis media with effusion. *J Dev Behav Pediatr, 9*, 346–351.

Rach, G., Zielhuis, G., Van Baarle, P., & Van Den Broek, P. (1991). The effect of treatment with ventilating tubes on language development in preschool children with otitis media with effusion. *Clin Otolaryngol, 16*, 128–132.

Robb, M., Psak, J., & Pan-Ching, G. (1993). Chronic otitis media and early speech development: A case study. *Int J Pediatr Otorhinolaryngol, 26*, 117–127.

Roberts, J., Burchinal, M., & Henderson, F. (1993). Otitis media and school age outcomes. In: D. Lim (Ed.), *Recent Advances in Otitis Media* (pp. 561–564). Toronto: Decker Periodicals.

Roberts, J., Burchinal, M., Koch, M., Footo, M., & Henderson, F. (1990). Otitis media in early childhood and its relationship to later phonological development. *J Speech Hear Disord, 53*, 424–432.

Roberts, J., Rosenfeld, R., Ziesel, S., & Derbenwick, E. (1999). Does otitis media contribute to language sequelae? A meta-analysis of prospective studies. *7th International Symposium on Recent Advances in Otitis Media* (p. 320). University of Pittsburgh, Pennsylvania.

Schlieper, A., Kisilevsky, H., Mattingly, S., & Yorke, L. (1985). Mild conductive hearing loss and language development: A one-year follow-up study. *J Dev Behav Pediatr, 6*, 65–68.

Schilder, A., Van Manen, J., Zielhuis, G., Grievink, E., Peters, S., & Van Den Broek, P. (1993) Long-term effects of otitis media with effusion on language, reading and spelling. *Clin Otolaryngol, 18*, 234–241.

Sedey, J., Elfenbein, J., Schum, R., & Bentler, R. (2002, July). Report on Unilateral Hearing Loss Project. *Colorado Infant Hearing Symposium.* Denver, Colorado.

Silva, P. (1985). Some long-term psychological, educational, and behavioral characteristics of children with bilateral otitis media with effusion. In: J. Sade (Ed.), *Proceedings of the International Symposium on Acute and Secretory Otitis Media* (pp. 217–220). Jerusalem.

Skinner, M. (1978). The hearing of speech during language acquisition. *Otolaryngol Clin North Am, 11*, 631–650.

Teele, D., Klein, J., & Rosner, B. (1984). Otitis media with effusion during the first three years of life and development of speech and language. *Pediatrics, 74*, 282–287.

Updike, C., & Thornburg, J. (1992). Reading skills and auditory processing ability in children with chronic otitis media in early childhood. *Ann Otol Rhinol Laryngol, 101,* 530–537.

Uzgiris, I. (1970). Sociocultural factors in cognitive development. In: H. Haywood (Ed.), *Social–Cultural Aspects of Mental Retardation* (pp. 231–264). New York: Appleton-Century.

Uzgiris, I., & Hunt, J.M. (1966). *An instrument for assessing infant psychological development.* Prepared for the Psychological Development Laboratory, University of Illinois.

Van Cauwenberge, P., Van Cauwenberge, K., & Kluyskens, P. (1985). The influence of otitis media with effusion on speech and language development and psycho-intellectual behaviour of the preschool child: Results of a cross-sectional study in 1,512 children. *Auris Nasus Larynx, 12* (Suppl. 1), S228–S230.

Ventry, I. (1980). Effects of conductive hearing loss: Fact or fiction. *J Speech Hear Res, 45,* 143–156.

Vernon-Feagans, L., Yont, K., & Hurley, M. (1999). The effects of otitis media on children's bookreading at 4 years of age. *7th International Symposium on Recent Advances in Otitis Media* (pp. 156–158). University of Pittsburgh, Pennsylvania.

Wachs, T., Uzgiris, I., Hunt, I., & Hunt, J.M. (1971). Cognitive development in infants of different age levels and from different environmental backgrounds: An exploratory investigation. *Merrill-Palmer Q Behav Dev, 17,* 288–317.

Wallace, I., Gravel, J., Ganon, E., & Ruben, R. (1993). Two-year language outcomes as a function of otitis media and parental linguistic styles. In: D. Lim (Ed.), *Recent Advances in Otitis Media* (pp. 114–128). Toronto: Decker Periodicals.

Wallace, I., Gravel, J., McCarton, C., Stapells, D., Bernstein, R., & Ruben, R. (1988). Otitis media, auditory sensitivity, and language outcomes at one year. *Laryngoscope, 98,* 64–70.

Webster, A., Bamford, J., Thyer, N., & Ayles, R. (1989). The psychological, educational and auditory sequelae of early, persistent secretory otitis media. *J Child Psychol Psychiatry, 30,* 529–546.

Wendler-Shaw, P., Menyuk, P., & Teele, D. (1993). Effects of otitis media in the first year of life on language production in the second year of life. In: D. Lim (Ed.), *Recent Advances in Otitis Media.* Toronto: Decker Periodicals.

Whiteman, B., Simpson, G., & Compton, W. (1986). Relationship of otitis media and language impairment in adolescents with Down syndrome. *Ment Retard, 24,* 353–356.

Wright, P., Sell, S., McConnell, K., Sitton, A., Thompson, J., Vaughn, W., & Bess, F. (1988). Impact of recurrent otitis media on middle ear function, hearing, and language. *J Pediatr, 113,* 581–587.

11

Maintenance of Personal Hearing Aids

CAROLYN H. MUSKET

An ounce of prevention is worth a pound of cure.

—Bracton, *De legibus,* 1240

Background

Hearing aids are a most important resource for the rehabilitation of children with hearing impairments. However, the instruments are prone to physical and electroacoustic breakdowns. Common defects include clogged earmolds, weak batteries, intermittent controls, cracked tubing, poor frequency response, and excessive distortion. The need for vigilance in hearing aid maintenance is always present. Case Study 11–1 clearly demonstrates the need for regular hearing aid maintenance.

Professionals were first alerted to the need for regular hearing aid maintenance in the schools by a study that evaluated hearing aids worn by children in regular school programs. In 1966, after examining hearing aids used by children with hearing impairments, Gaeth and Lounsbury reported that over two thirds of the aids were inadequate (Gaeth & Lounsbury, 1966). Subsequent studies throughout the following decades confirmed that this situation was prevalent (Bess, 1977; Coleman, 1972; Potts & Greenwood, 1983). During a summer program for children, Elfenbein, Bentler, Davis, and Niebuhr (1988) reported that hearing aids presented an almost constant problem. The implication of all these findings is important for those educational approaches that assume the child's own hearing aid is an integral part of rehabilitation, whether in the classroom or in the home. These studies highlighted the fact that having consistent, optimal hearing aid performance is a continuing issue of major concern. Today, the need for daily, ongoing monitoring and maintenance of children's hearing aids is an accepted fact (Johnson, Benson, & Seaton, 1997).

One important reason for the repeated high incidence of malfunctioning hearing aids is a generalized lack of knowledge about all aspects of wearable amplification. Many children with hearing loss are educated in regular school settings; however, classroom teachers, public school nurses, and speech-language pathologists have been found to possess limited information about the operation and care of hearing aids (Johnson, Stein, & Lass, 1992; Lass, Tecca, & Woodford, 1987; Lass et al, 1989). The educators are not alone. Parents, also, know very little about a hearing aid and its care (Blair, Wright, & Pollard, 1981; Elfenbein, 1994). This chapter strives to meet the crucial need for practical, applicable information about hearing aids for those persons in direct daily contact with them—teachers, other school professionals, and parents.

Case Study 11–1   T.P., a 5-year-old, was seen at a university center for communication disorders. T.P., who has been wearing a monaural hearing aid since the age of 2 years, has a severe, flat, bilateral sensorineural hearing loss. Figure 11–1 shows his unaided response to warble tones presented through a loudspeaker in the test suite. His average minimal response level was 77 dB hearing level (HL). However, when wearing a hearing aid his aided responses to these same warble tones occurred at an average of 45 dB HL. His aided speech threshold was 40 dB HL. This child has a hearing loss so severe he cannot hear conversational speech at all. With a hearing aid, however, conversational speech is audible, except for sounds in the octave band centered at 4000 Hz. This is a crucial factor for T.P. as he strives to acquire speech and language.

One week later, T.P. returned to explore his performance with binaural amplification. At the start of the session, the aided results from the week before were rechecked. This time, however, his aided speech threshold was 90 dB HL, not 40 dB HL, and his aided responses to warble tones agreed with this new finding. T.P. was not receiving any help whatsoever from the hearing aid. Figure 11–2 displays these second test results. The audiologist soon determined that these discrepancies occurred because T.P.s earmold was completely occluded by earwax. Even though the hearing aid was working, the amplified sound could not pass through the earmold into his ear because of the blockage from earwax. Once the earmold was cleaned, his aided scores agreed with those of the previous week.

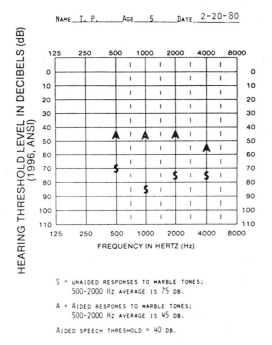

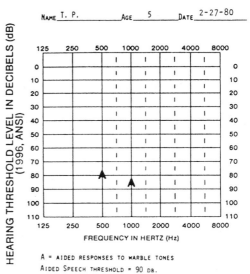

Figure 11–1. Unaided (S) and aided (A) responses to sound field warble tones for T.P. (see Case Study 11–1).

Figure 11–2. Aided sound field responses for T.P., 1 week after the results shown in Figure 11–1 were obtained (see Case Study 11–1).

The Hearing Aid

No one hears perfectly all of the time. In everyday life, even persons with normal hearing experience difficulty in certain listening situations, such as a large meeting where the speaker addresses a group from some distance away. It would not be possible for those in the audience to hear well without the help of amplification. Some device must be used to intensify the speaker's voice to make it audible to the listener who may be out of normal conversational range. Fortunately, amplification with a public address system is available. The speaker talks into a microphone; this signal is then carried to an amplifier where it is intensified greatly and directed to loudspeakers strategically placed around the meeting room. From these loudspeakers the magnified voice is delivered to the audience. In addition, this system uses some source of electrical power. The amplification arrangement just described is an accepted feature of auditoriums, stadiums, and theaters.

It is helpful to know that a wearable electronic hearing aid really is a miniature public address system. As shown in Figure 11–3, it has the same components that were just described: microphone, amplifier, loudspeaker (receiver), and power source. Basically, it is designed to accomplish the same goal. The purpose of a hearing aid is to amplify speech so someone with a hearing loss will hear it comfortably. This increased intensity is needed not because a great distance exists between speaker and listener, but because the impaired ear has a loss in hearing sensitivity. In hearing aids, the recognizable parts of a public address system are not easily discernible because they are extremely small and packaged together in the unfamiliar form of a hearing aid case. Therefore, instead of being in front of the speaker, the microphone is worn at the ear of the person with a hearing loss (the listener) as a built-in part of the hearing aid. This explains why hearing aids work most effectively in quiet, structured surroundings, where the speaker is at a conversational distance of 3 to 4 feet. When greater distances are involved, the speaker is not within the range of the microphone. When noise is present, it reaches the microphone too, and is amplified, making it difficult for the listener to separate the desired speech signal from this interference.

Hearing Aid Components

MICROPHONE

Sound travels through the air by movement of air molecules. This acoustic transmission is cumbersome and difficult to magnify, although it can be done. When one cups a hand behind the ear, more sound waves are collected and directed into the ear, thus enlarging the original signal. An old-fashioned ear trumpet took advantage of this fact. However, the increase in intensity that may be obtained this way is minimal. If the acoustic transmission of sound is converted into electric energy, a much greater increase is possible. This desired energy conversion—acoustic energy into electric energy—is the function of the hearing aid microphone. As the sound waves strike the diaphragm of the microphone, their acoustic energy causes it mechanically to move back and forth. The vibrating motion of the diaphragm in turn causes a change in electric voltage that varies with the type of microphone used. Variations in the sound waves impinging on the microphone create corresponding changes in an electric signal flowing from it.

The microphone itself is housed inside the hearing aid case and can be located by look-

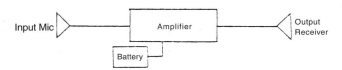

Figure 11–3. A simple block diagram of a hearing aid.

ing for a small opening in the case. It is important to identify this sound inlet because it should not be occluded by debris or obstructed when the instrument is worn.

Some hearing aids have microphones that are directional. The most typical directional microphone receives signals from two locations; it has both a front-facing and a rear-facing opening. Another design combines two microphones to achieve directionality. With directional microphones, sounds occurring from the rear are attenuated, thereby giving emphasis to sounds occurring in front of the hearing aid user.

AMPLIFIER

As the electric current from the microphone passes through the amplifier, it is selectively processed and amplified. This is accomplished through various stages of complex circuitry. In all hearing aids, the amplifier is contained within the case of the hearing aid. It is an extremely small component.

RECEIVER (EARPHONE)

The part of a hearing aid that corresponds to a loudspeaker is usually referred to as a receiver. The function of the receiver is to convert the amplified electric energy back into acoustic energy. Through magnetic action, the electric current from the amplifier causes physical movement of the diaphragm of the receiver. This movement disturbs the adjacent air molecules, thereby creating sound waves again. However, the converted sound waves are of much greater magnitude than those that originated at the diaphragm of the microphone.

An air conduction receiver is almost always housed internally inside the hearing aid; however, it is possible for it to be a separate part connected to the aid by a cord. For both types, the amplified sound will eventually be directed into the child's earcanal. For a small number of hearing aid users, such a fitting is not advisable due to draining ears or a malformed or absent earcanal. These children use a bone conduction oscillator for a hearing aid receiver. An oscillator is a small, boxlike device attached to the hearing aid by a cord; a headband holds it against the prominent bone behind the external ear. Mechanical vibrations from the side of the oscillator's case transmit sound to the inner ear through the skull.

BATTERY

Also contained within the hearing aid case is a small battery, which provides the power for the instrument. The battery is a reservoir of stored chemical energy that is converted into electric energy when used in the hearing aid. Zinc air batteries combine air, through holes in the battery case, with contents inside the battery. The adhesive tab on a zinc air battery, which covers the tiny holes, is removed when the battery is to be used because air must enter the battery for it to function. A zinc air battery is the most common type of hearing aid battery. It is environmentally safe as well as long lasting. Specifications from the manufacturer indicate the size and type of battery recommended for use in a particular aid, as well as the voltage it should supply.

Hearing Aid Arrangements

Wearable hearing aids are available in styles that are named according to their location on the user. They are pictured in Figure 11–4.

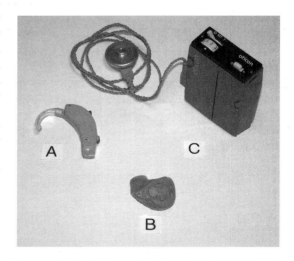

Figure 11–4.   Styles of hearing aids. (A) Behind-the-ear. (B) In-the-ear. (C) Body-worn.

BEHIND-THE-EAR

In this hearing aid style, all components of the system—microphone, amplifier, receiver, and battery—are contained within a small, slightly curved case. It is designed to fit behind the ear of the wearer. Behind-the-ear (BTE) hearing aids are widely used with children. This style has the advantage of being easily connected to assistive listening devices. Also, powerful BTE models are available if needed, in addition to the mild- and moderate-gain BTE instruments that have been available for some time.

IN-THE-EAR

All parts of an in-the-ear (ITE) hearing aid, including the battery, are contained within a custom plastic shell that fits entirely into the outer ear itself. An in-the-canal (ITC) aid is an even smaller version of this style. ITE aids are not often used with young children because of tiny controls and the fact that the hearing aid casing must be modified continually as the size of the earcanal changes. As a group, BTE, ITE, and ITC instruments are referred to as ear-level hearing aids. They all provide the advantage of locating the microphone in a natural position at the ear.

BODY-WORN

The term "body-worn" refers to a small, rectangular instrument that is worn on the chest. It is clipped to an article of clothing, such as a shirt pocket, or, with young children, inserted into a cloth carrier or harness, which is strapped around the chest. The microphone, amplifier, and battery on a body-worn aid are all within the case; an external button-sized receiver is connected to the aid by a cord. There has been a definite decline in the use of body-worn hearing aids. With children, they are primarily reserved for the very young or for those whose physical disabilities necessitate the use of a more durable body aid. In most other instances, children may be fit appropriately with BTE instruments. The body-worn instruments often seen in the classroom on school children today are most likely assistive listening device receivers, which may also have the potential to function as hearing aids (see Chapter 13).

MONAURAL, BINAURAL

In a monaural hearing aid arrangement, the output from a single hearing aid is directed into only one ear of the wearer. A binaural fitting refers to the use of an ear-level hearing aid for each ear.

Hearing Aid Controls

A conventional hearing aid is controlled through dials, switches, and screw adjustments. Figure 11–5 depicts a conventional BTE instrument to help clarify the descriptions of hearing aid controls in this section. A programmable hearing aid has a microchip, contained within the hearing aid itself, which stores desired settings in digital memory. One may select or program various settings for this type of instrument by connecting the hearing aid (having a microchip) via a cable to a handheld programming device or a computer. After digital storage of the settings, the cable is removed. Programming technology also offers the user a choice of electroacoustic settings to compensate for different listening environments.

ON–OFF SWITCH

The switch that turns on the aid may be found in various locations, depending on the design of the aid. It may be incorporated into the swing-out battery compartment; snapping the plastic battery tray completely shut turns on the aid. This switch also may be combined with the rotary volume control, so the first click when this dial is advanced indicates the aid has been turned on, or the aid may have a separate on–off switch with a plus (+) sign indicating when it is functioning. Finally, in some aids this switch may be combined with the input control where "O" indicates the aid is off and not operating.

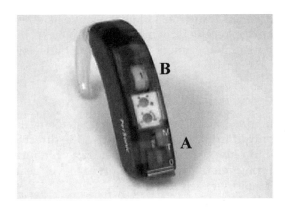

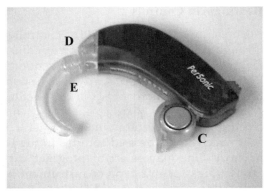

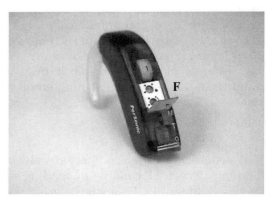

Figure 11–5. View of a conventional behind-the-ear hearing aid. A, input control; B, gain (volume) control; C, battery compartment; D, microphone port; E, receiver port and earhook; F, panel open to reveal screw settings.

INPUT CONTROL

The input control determines what signal is being transmitted to the amplifier. The choices available for input on a specific hearing aid include: *M*, which means the microphone is picking up airborne signals; *T*, which shows the aid will interact with a telephone or other device emitting a magnetic signal; *MT*, which indicates both the microphone and magnetic inputs are functional; and -⊙ or *E*, which denotes that the aid may be coupled to an external audio source. Although these latter symbols are advocated by the International Electrotechnical Commission to indicate audio-input entry, some manufacturers may use other markings.

When the control is on *T*, the microphone of the aid is turned off. Instead, an induction coil, commonly referred to as a telecoil, inside the case of the hearing aid receives and transmits a magnetic signal that comes from the telephone handset, which is held in close proximity to the hearing aid. This signal continues through the circuitry of the hearing aid amplifier to the receiver. When the telephone switch is in use, the only signal amplified comes from the message emitted over the telephone, and it is not the actual acoustic sound of the voice itself that enters the hearing aid, but rather a magnetic signal that exists simultaneously with it. Other sounds, such as room noise and the user's own voice, are not amplified because the microphone of the aid is not functioning.

Also of interest is the fact that in the *T* position, the hearing aid will pick up magnetic signals emanating from an induction loop. An induction loop is created by connecting both ends of a loop of wire to an amplifier whose input is usually a microphone. Sound from the microphone is carried through this loop as electric current, which also produces an electromagnetic field; the electromagnetic field, in turn, induces current in the telecoil of the hearing aid when in the *T* position. A neckloop is a small induction loop and may be used to couple a hearing aid with various assistive listening devices. A large induction loop might encircle an entire room to provide an assistive listening system (see Chapter 14). The advantage of an *MT* setting is that, with input from both the microphone and the telecoil, users may monitor their own voice and respond to the voices of others while receiving the signal from the telecoil.

A direct audio input (DAI) option is available on some BTE instruments. When set for this mode of operation, the hearing aid may be connected directly to an external audio source via an auxiliary cord. In this way, it is possible for a child's hearing aid to receive input from an assistive listening device, such as a personal FM receiver (see Chapter 13), or a remote microphone. An alternative input setting may exist that allows use of both the hearing aid's microphone and the external audio input source at the same time.

GAIN (VOLUME) CONTROL

This rotary dial on a conventional hearing aid allows the user to adjust the sound of the hearing aid from minimum to maximum amplification. Most often, it is continuously adjustable and operates much like the volume control on a radio. The dial also may be numbered or color-coded to assist the user in finding the desired setting. Some programmable hearing aids have no user-operated gain control; other models regulate this function via a remote control.

DIRECTIONAL–OMNIDIRECTIONAL SWITCH

On some hearing aids, the use of a directional microphone is optional. A standard omnidirectional microphone may be changed to one with directional capabilities when a selector switch is placed in a certain position.

TONE CONTROL

With the tone control, the relative strength of the high frequency and low frequency sounds that are amplified may be changed. A tone control appears either as a selector switch available to the user or as a screw adjustment or programming option that is determined when the aid is dispensed. Usually, the high frequency range is emphasized by suppressing amplification of low frequencies when the tone control is set on S or H. On L, the opposite occurs; the low frequency sounds are emphasized because high frequencies are suppressed. The position N denotes the standard or normal frequency response for a particular instrument. Tone control markings are not standardized and should be verified by consulting performance data from the manufacturer for each model of hearing aid.

OUTPUT CONTROL

This screw adjustment or programming choice imposes a limit to the maximum amount of sound the hearing aid will transmit. It sets a ceiling—the hearing aid will not produce a more intense sound than this limiting level no matter how great the input to the microphone. This output limiting may be achieved in the aid's circuitry through either peak clipping or compression; the latter is also referred to as automatic gain control.

Earmolds

In BTE hearing aid arrangements, it is necessary to couple the hearing aid to the user's ear with an earmold. An earmold is a piece of plastic with a channel called the sound bore running through the center; the earmold is attached to the hearing aid and inserted into the wearer's ear. Its purpose, of course, is to deliver the amplified sound directly from the receiver into the earcanal. In addition, modifications to the earmold may affect the transmission of sound. For example, a sound bore of constant diameter transmits low frequencies well; however, when the sound bore flares at the end like a horn, and is a certain length, it actually enhances output in the high frequencies.

There are many different types of earmolds. The National Association of Earmold Laboratories uses standard nomenclature to classify them (Valente, Valente, Potts, & Lybarger, 2000). Only a few are mentioned here. For BTE instruments, sound from the internal receiver is directed through a rigid plastic hook or elbow; then a piece of flexible plastic tubing carries sound from this hook to the earmold, which is usually either a shell earmold or a skeleton earmold, as seen in Figure 11–6. A receiver earmold, which also is referred to as a standard or regular earmold, has a solid base with a snap to be used with an external button receiver. Today

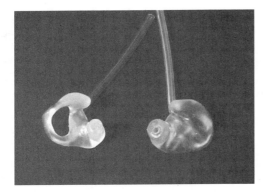

Figure 11–6. Sample styles of earmolds. Left, a skeleton earmold; right, a shell earmold.

a standard earmold is used more often with some assistive listening devices than with body-worn hearing aids. With ITE aids, a separate earmold is not needed because the casing or shell of the hearing aid itself fulfills this function.

Each earmold is custom-made. An impression is taken of the user's ear to exactly reproduce the contours of the canal and bowl-like portion of the ear. This is accomplished by packing these areas with a soft impression material. After this substance has set, it is carefully removed, packaged, and mailed to an earmold laboratory with an order describing the type of earmold desired. The laboratory fabricates the actual earmold following these specifications. Earmolds may be made from a variety of materials, which include acrylic, vinyl, silicone, and polyethylene substances. Depending on the material, the result may be either a hard earmold or a soft one. The more pliable earmolds are used with children because they are less likely to cause injury as a result of any boisterous activity. An earmold must fit comfortably and securely in order to retain the hearing aid in the ear. In addition, a snug fit ensures that amplified sound from the hearing aid receiver will actually arrive at the eardrum. A properly fitting earmold, which prevents sound from leaking out at the sides of the canal, often is of concern when powerful hearing aids are used on children with severe losses. Special materials or earmold styles may be needed to obtain a mold with

a tight enough seal. However, conversely, for some children with certain audiometric configurations, special earmolds or earmolds with certain modifications are recommended to provide a pathway for amplified sound to escape. This is usually done to alter the output of the hearing aid in some way. The special earmolds are described as nonoccluding earmolds. The modification frequently made to other earmolds is termed a vent, which is also used for pressure equalization in the ear.

Because the outer ear grows as the child matures, it is expected that new earmolds will be needed periodically to maintain a proper fit. Children less than 4 years of age may require a new earmold as often as every 3 to 6 months; older youngsters may need to exchange their earmolds yearly until the age of 8 or 9 years.

Electroacoustic Characteristics

A hearing aid is described and compared with other hearing aids according to the way it amplifies sound. Such information about a hearing aid indicates how sound coming from the receiver (output) differs from what entered the microphone (input). These measures of various input–output functions of a hearing aid are referred to as electroacoustic characteristics. The way in which these performance measurements are made and expressed is mandated in a standard from the American National Standards Institute: ANSI S3.22–1996, Specification of Hearing Aid Characteristics (ANSI, 1996). This standard was first approved in 1976 and has been revised several times, most recently in 1996. The intent of such a standard is to enable measurements of hearing aid performance obtained at different facilities to be compared with one another. It is noteworthy that this standard became law in this country in 1977 when the Food and Drug Administration's Rules and Regulations Regarding Hearing Aid Devices: Professional and Patient Labeling Conditions for Sale went into effect (U.S. FDA, 1977). As part of this FDA document, it was specified that the performance characteristics of hearing aids be determined in accordance with the existing ANSI standard. Thus, the ANSI standard for hearing aid characteristics for the first time became enforceable. The FDA regulation has been updated periodically to require adherence to each revision of ANSI S3.22. At the time of this writing, hearing aids designed and manufactured after March 17, 2000, must adhere to ANSI S3.22–1996. Hearing aids in current production that were originally designed and manufactured prior to March 17, 2000, using ANSI S3.22–1987 may continue to use the 1987 revision of the standard. A 2003 revision of ANSI S3.22 is pending (K. Frye, personal communication, January 28, 2003).

Another significant feature of ANSI S3.22 is that it stipulates tolerance limits for each characteristic measured. The reason for having a tolerance limit, or range of acceptable deviation, is to improve quality control. Because of these requirements, each hearing aid of a particular model should perform within the tolerance limits allowed by the standard when measured accurately. Some of these measurements will be summarized.

GAIN

Gain refers to the amount in decibels by which the hearing aid amplifies or intensifies sound. If a sound of 70 dB sound pressure level (SPL) enters the hearing aid microphone and a sound of 115 dB SPL is measured coming from the receiver, then the gain of this hearing aid, or the additional intensity supplied by the amplifying circuit, is 45 dB. The amount of gain a hearing aid offers varies with the frequency of the entering signal; that is, a hearing aid does not amplify all incoming sounds by the same amount. ANSI S3.22 specifies that the gain present at 1000, 1600, and 2500 Hz be averaged; under certain conditions, a manufacturer may select three other frequencies. This average is obtained with the gain (volume) control rotated to the full-on position; the resulting gain is referred to as the high frequency average full-on gain. Manufacturers often repeat this measure with the gain control rotated to a specific setting more nearly

simulating use conditions (less than full-on); they report this value as reference test gain.

OUTPUT

"OSPL-90" is the term used in ANSI S3.22–1996 to describe the maximum output SPL that a hearing aid is able to produce at its receiver with an input signal of 90 dB SPL. The same measure is referred to as saturation SPL (SSPL-90) in ANSI S3.22–1987. Procedures call for the output of a hearing aid to be measured with the gain control full-on, and with an input signal of 90 dB SPL applied to the hearing aid microphone. The output for frequencies from 200 to 5000 Hz is recorded. Again, the values at 1000, 1600, and 2500 Hz are averaged, and the resulting number is reported as the high frequency average OSPL-90 or SSPL-90 for the hearing aid. In addition, the maximum decibel output present for a single frequency is noted and reported, along with the frequency at which it occurred.

FREQUENCY RESPONSE

The frequency response refers to descriptive information about the way in which a hearing aid amplifies various frequencies because it does not increase all frequencies equally. A frequency response curve is a graph that illustrates how the output of the aid changes as the frequency progresses from low to high. It is possible, then, to use this graph to determine the frequency range, or that band of frequencies from low to high for which the aid provides enough amplification to be potentially useful.

HARMONIC DISTORTION

Distortion is present in an amplifying system when the acoustic parameters of the input sound at the microphone are not reproduced exactly in the output at the receiver. One form of such distortion is harmonic distortion. This occurs when new frequencies, which are whole-number multiples of the input frequency, appear. The standard states that this should be reported in terms of percentage of total harmonic distortion at 500 Hz, 800 Hz, and 1600 Hz.

EQUIVALENT INPUT NOISE LEVEL

This measurement pertains to the internal noise present in the hearing aid similar to the on noise found in many electrical devices. It is calculated according to a formula given in the standard.

SIMULATED TELEPHONE SENSITIVITY

In the 1996 revision, a hearing aid having a telecoil is exposed to a magnetic field produced by a telephone magnetic field simulator (TMFS). The aid's input switch or program must be on *T* and the gain control is in reference test position. Measures are taken throughout the frequency range; the high frequency average is computed and compared to gain in this position. The resulting simulated telephone sensitivity (STS) value tells how much adjustment must be made when the aid is switched from microphone to telecoil mode. The 1987 revision is less precise and measures only whether or not the telecoil is working.

Hearing Aid Maintenance

A maintenance program to ensure continued maximum performance of a hearing aid should be composed of (1) a daily visual inspection and listening check, and (2) periodic electroacoustic measurement. Through a daily monitoring program, obvious causes of hearing aid malfunction may be identified quickly and are often resolved. A few supplies should be assembled to simplify this inspection. The electroacoustic measurements, which require more elaborate equipment, provide information of a different type about the way the hearing aid amplifies sound.

Hearing Aid Maintenance Kit

To implement the first step of this program, it is recommended that several items be kept in the classroom and in the home of each hearing aid user. These articles will fit into a

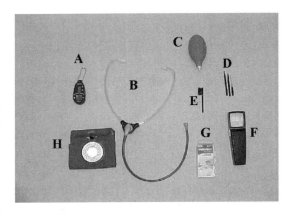

Figure 11–7. Hearing aid maintenance kit. See text for description of contents.

small utility box or zippered case; having access to them facilitates the task of caring for a hearing aid. Some suppliers and organizations offer a hearing aid maintenance kit already assembled; there are hearing aid manufacturers who include a maintenance kit with the purchase of new hearing aids for a child. For further information, consult the Appendix. The suggested contents are listed below and appear in Figure 11–7.

A. *Battery tester*. The battery tester is used to ascertain whether a battery supplies the necessary voltage. It may have colored areas or lights to differentiate acceptable batteries (green) from poor ones (red).

B. *Hearing aid stethoscope and adapter*. Use of a hearing aid stethoscope enables one to listen only to sounds amplified by the aid because both ears of the listener are occluded. It may be used with any style of hearing aid.

C. *Air blower.* This device is used to remove moisture from earmolds and tubing after they have been cleaned. It is helpful, too, in determining if there is an obstacle to the passage of sound through an earmold.

D. *Wax pick or pipe cleaners.* These are useful for removing earwax from an earmold sound bore and vent. Pipe cleaners may also be used to dry out the sound bore after an earmold has been washed. These items should not be used with an ITE aid; a wax loop is more appropriate.

E. *Small, soft brush.* This brush helps in clearing dust and lint from hearing aid switches and the opening to the microphone.

F. *Small, lighted magnifying glass*

G. *Extra batteries*

H. *Plastic bag or jar with dehumidifier.* The hearing aid may be stored in a plastic bag or jar, especially during humid periods, with a chemical that will remove moisture from the air and dry out the aid. However, zinc air batteries, once the tab is removed, should not be placed in such a container because this would shorten rather than prolong battery life; they should be removed before the hearing aid is placed in the container.

Visual Inspection

BATTERY

First on any maintenance list should be inspection of the battery. Initially, one should determine that the correct battery is used. Both the desired battery size and the voltage are specified in information supplied with the aid by the manufacturer. The battery size and maximum voltage available in each cell will be labeled on a battery package. Battery voltage should be checked with a battery tester; decreased battery voltage is a significant factor in the unsatisfactory electroacoustic function of hearing aids. Generally, a battery voltage of 1.1 volts is accepted as the minimum level needed for optimal hearing aid operation (Preeves & Curran, 2000). However, most button cell battery testers used today do not yield an actual voltage reading; instead, they indicate if a battery is dead and if the voltage is acceptable or low.

One should observe whether the battery and the battery contacts in the aid yield evidence of corrosion. Corrosion on battery contacts may cause a hissing sound in the aid. If minimal corrosion is present, the white powdery substance that forms on the battery contacts may be wiped away with a soft cloth or an alcohol swab. Sometimes, it may be necessary to rub battery contacts with a pointed eraser to remove all traces of corrosion. Only gentle pressure should be applied, so that any coating covering the battery contacts will not be damaged. A battery that is extensively corroded should not be used. To minimize the possibility of corrosion, the battery should be removed from the aid overnight.

Finally, one should observe if the battery is installed properly in the aid. The plus (+) side of the battery should be aligned with the plus (+) marking in the battery compartment. Instead of this marking, most aids have battery compartments that will only accept placement of a battery in the correct position. If the battery compartment will not close, it is likely that the battery has not been inserted correctly.

EARMOLD

The earmold should be examined both alone and coupled to the ear of the child. Note whether the earmold is cracked or chipped because any rough edge will cause discomfort to the wearer. It is vital that the sound bore of the earmold not be occluded with earwax. Such an accumulation in this opening may be removed with a wax pick and the channel cleaned out with a pipe cleaner. Care must be taken not to push earwax back into the mold, where it is more difficult to remove. When the earmold is inserted into the child's ear, it should fit comfortably; a whistling sound, known as acoustic feedback, should not occur when the aid is in use.

To remove an earmold from a BTE aid, gently slip the tubing from the earhook. The tubing must not be pulled from the earmold itself because it is permanently secured there. With the earmold separated from the aid, it is possible to use the air blower to demonstrate that there is, indeed, a clear passageway through the earmold (and tubing) for amplified sound. Position the bulb at one end of the mold (or tubing), squeeze it, and feel the flow of air at the other end. The earmold may be washed in warm water and mild soap provided it is detached from the hearing aid; dry it and use a pipe cleaner and the air blower to remove moisture from the sound bore. Make sure the earmold is completely dry before joining it again to the hearing aid. Moisture will damage the hearing aid. The earmold should be cleaned periodically, but unless the child accumulates an unusual amount of earwax, it should not be necessary to wash the earmold daily. Detaching an earmold by slipping the tubing off the earhook eventually will stretch the tubing somewhat. When this connection becomes loose, the amplified sound passing through it can escape and cause acoustic feedback. An earmold may be separated from an external button receiver of a body-worn instrument simply by unsnapping it.

TUBING

Any tubing that forms a loose connection, has yellowed, or is hardened and brittle needs to be replaced by an audiologist or a hearing aid specialist. Check to see that moisture has not collected inside the tubing to block the passage of sound. If moisture problems persist, consider the use of special tubing designed to absorb and exhaust moisture as it accumulates. When the aid is in place on the child, the tubing should not be twisted, thereby obstructing sound.

EXTERNAL RECEIVER AND CORD

If the hearing aid has an external button receiver, look to see if it is cracked or damaged in any way. Often a washer of thin plastic film is placed around the nubbin of the receiver to ensure a tight seal when it is snapped onto the earmold. Determine if any sections of the cord connecting the receiver to the aid appear to be frayed. The cord should be firmly attached.

SETTINGS AND CONTROLS

The input switch should be on *M* unless the telecoil (*T,TM*) or direct auditory input is being used with a classroom listening system. The gain control settings should be that recommended for the child.

HEARING AID CASE

If necessary, the case itself should be cleaned with a soft cloth. A brush from the maintenance kit may be used to clean crevices and around controls.

Listening Check

It is important to listen to the hearing aid to obtain information about the function of the switches and controls and to monitor, as much as possible, the quality of sound reproduction. If parents begin this practice when their child's instrument is new, they will establish a reference for future listening checks.

STANDARD LISTENING CHECK

The listener may attach the hearing aid to a hearing aid stethoscope. The external receiver of a body-worn aid may be snapped onto the stethoscope. Figure 11–8A shows an adapter in use with a BTE aid that has an internal receiver; the nozzle of a connecting tube is slipped over the aid's earhook, and the other end of the tube is snapped onto the stethoscope. Still another alternative is to place the nozzle end of the tubing extension over the canal portion of an earmold or ITE aid, as seen in Figure 11–8B. In this way, one may listen to the combined system of any hearing aid and earmold together or to an ITE aid. This latter method, especially, offers some practical advantages in daily listening checks of BTE aids by teachers and parents. Because the nozzle may be fastened directly over the end of the earmold, it does not necessitate routinely separating the tubing from the earhook; thus, fewer problems would be likely to develop at this point. In a school program, where several aids are to be checked, the outside of each earmold should be sanitized by wiping it with Cetylcide, or a similar product, before it is inserted into the end of the adapter. Cetylcide is an antibacterial instant earmold cleaner available from a supplier of hearing aid products.

The input switch of the aid should be set on *M*, the aid should be off, and the gain control should be turned down. Because it is

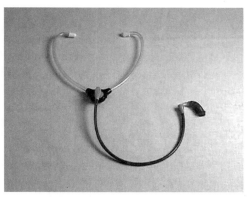 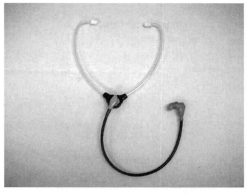

A   B

Figure 11–8. (A) Attachment of a hearing aid stethoscope adapter to a behind-the-ear hearing aid. (B) Attachment of a hearing aid stethoscope adapter to an in-the-ear hearing aid.

difficult to talk and listen simultaneously, one may want to listen to speech on a tape recorder or radio during this check. While the tester is listening, the aid should be turned on and the gain control rotated slowly back and forth to note if there is a smooth change in intensity, if there is a constant signal, and if the control operates quietly. The various switches should be moved to determine if they are functional. The cord, if the aid has one, should be rolled gently between the fingers in several places; an intermittent incoming sound would identify a defective cord that should be replaced. Finally, the case should be rotated slightly to ascertain whether this causes interruption of the sound.

Such a listening check will identify faulty controls. Judging the quality of sound reproduction is more problematic because the tubing of the stethoscope alters the signal (Thibodeau, DeLaRosa, & Champlin, 2000). Moreover, deterioration in the quality of sound may occur gradually over a period of time and not be readily apparent on a day-to-day listening basis. Another consideration is the intensity of the speech input. When the gain control is set in the position used by the child, the hearing aid normally responds to conversational speech input from about 3 feet away and to the child's own voice at a distance of about 8 inches. When the person making the listening check

uses his or her own voice, as so often happens, input to the aid reflects the intensity of the user's own voice, but does not assess how the aid responds to speech at other input levels. Finally, it must be recognized that those with normal hearing may find it uncomfortable to listen to the high output levels of the more powerful hearing aids at gain control settings used by the child. This discomfort precludes careful listening at such a setting. Although distortion of sound may be present for the child, it may not be detected at the lower gain control setting preferred by the adult performing the listening check.

TELECOIL

An informal listening check of the telecoil (*T*) function may be performed using the magnetic field present in a corded or cordless telephone handset as the input.

LING SIX-SOUND TEST

This technique uses sounds representing the various octave bands of speech to monitor the frequency response of a hearing aid. One listens to six speech sounds—*oo*, *ah*, *ee*, *sh*, *s*, and *m*—as they are transmitted by the aid. If parents or caregivers do this daily, they will become familiar with how these sounds are reproduced by the child's hearing aid and be able to identify a change with confidence. In the classroom, this test may be given while the aid is worn to observe any deviation from the child's usual response. The teacher or aide presents the six sounds, one at a time, without visual clues. The child claps after hearing each sound, and, if capable, repeats the sound.

BONE CONDUCTION HEARING AIDS

There is not a satisfactory way to perform an adequate listening check on a bone conduction hearing aid. When the instrument is in actual use, the tension with which the oscillator is held against the head is very important. If the headband does not have sufficient tensile strength, being placed repeatedly on an adult's head for a listening check eventually might stretch it. Also, the listener would have to occlude both ears with earplugs or by pressing them shut to hear only through the bone conduction oscillator. It is possible for an audiologist or hearing aid specialist to check the integrity of the aid's controls and switches after substituting an appropriate air conduction receiver. Such persons should provide frequent routine maintenance for these aids. Daily checks may include testing the battery and inspecting the aid visually.

Acoustic Feedback

"Acoustic feedback" refers to the high-pitched whistling sound so annoying to those in the company of hearing aid users. Many times the hearing aid user does not hear this sound because of hearing loss. Acoustic feedback occurs whenever there is a clear pathway between the output from a hearing aid receiver and the microphone of the same hearing aid. Ordinarily, this whistling interaction is avoided because the output of the receiver is directed through the earmold into the earcanal and away from the hearing aid microphone. However, if the earmold does not fit snugly in the earcanal, the amplified sound waves may escape around the sides of the mold and be reproduced as feedback when they reach the aid's microphone. This happens most often with a powerful ear-

level instrument. The amplified sound might also leak through a crack or pinhole in the tubing or earhook of a BTE aid or through the sides of tubing if it is too thin.

Preventing acoustic feedback, then, becomes a matter of determining where the sound leakage is occurring by the process of elimination. Once the trouble spot is identified, the cause may be corrected. The following procedures tell how to check for the source of feedback in a BTE aid:

1. Remove the hearing aid, with the earmold attached, from the child.
2. Place your thumb over the earmold sound bore opening, turn the aid on, and rotate the gain control to its maximum. If whistling is heard, quickly turn the gain control down and detach the earmold by slipping the tubing from the end of the earhook.
3. Place your thumb over the end of the earhook. Increase the gain control to maximum for only a short time. If the feedback is gone, it must have been present due to damage to the earmold or tubing. If the whistling continues, it must be caused by a leak in the earhook or a problem internal to the aid. Consult an audiologist or hearing aid specialist for replacement of the earhook or repair of the aid.

It may be that feedback occurs when the hearing aid is on the child, but not during this check. In such cases there are two considerations: (1) this may be an indication of a middle ear problem, and immittance measurements should be obtained to investigate this; or (2) a new earmold may be needed. The latter cause is frequent with growing children. Once the other causes of feedback have been eliminated, a new earmold should be obtained.

Caring for a Hearing Aid

BATTERIES

Batteries should be stored in a dry location at room temperature in their original protective package. Keep spare batteries in their original dial package; this will prevent them from touching metal, such as when carried loosely in a pocket with change and keys or in a purse. Contact with metal can cause batteries to discharge or short circuit. A magnetic battery retriever tool is available to assist with placing a battery in the battery compartment. One manufacturer of zinc air batteries packages each battery with a long tab on it that serves as a handle to assist in removing the battery from the package and placing it in the hearing aid. Remove the battery from the hearing aid at night; this will prolong its life and decrease the possibility of corrosion. Extra batteries should be kept at school.

BATTERY DISPOSAL

Keep used batteries away from children. Zinc air batteries may be disposed of in a routine manner with household waste.

BATTERY INGESTION

Button batteries, which power ear-level hearing aids as well as other items such as watches, present a potential health hazard because they may be swallowed easily. Their popularity and availability have resulted in increasing instances of battery ingestion, especially among children who are attracted to loose or discarded batteries within their reach, or who remove batteries from hearing aids and other products. Litovitz (1983) reviewed cases of battery ingestion and found 78% occurred in children less than 5 years of age. Hearing aids were the most common intended use of these batteries. In the majority of cases reviewed, Litovitz found that ingested batteries the size of those used in ear-level hearing aids passed spontaneously through the gastrointestinal system without complications. However, serious injuries may result from caustic chemicals, toxicity, and constant pressure if the battery becomes lodged in the esophagus for any length of time; the small size of ear-level hearing aid batteries makes this unlikely in children 18 months and older. Zinc air batteries pose less of a toxic threat than other batteries, al-

though the possibility of electrolyte leakage does exist. Consequently, it is of paramount importance that parents, caregivers, and teachers be counseled regarding the inherent dangers of button batteries to children. These small batteries may also cause injury if placed in the nose or ears.

Prevention of battery ingestion and other misuses must be stressed at all times. Some hearing aid manufacturers offer the option of a tamper-resistant closure on the battery compartment of a hearing aid. Battery manufacturers are printing warning statements on product packages. Clinicians and educators should give the following precautions in verbal and written form to all hearing aid users and those working with children:

1. Keep extra batteries and hearing aids not in use out of children's reach.
2. Dispose of batteries properly away from children.
3. Do not dispose of batteries in incinerators or fires because they can rupture and explode.
4. Dispose of any batteries that show signs of leakage.
5. Never change batteries in front of children.
6. Never put batteries in the mouth for any reason, as they are slippery and easy to swallow accidentally. A child may mimic you.
7. Whenever possible, secure the battery drawer from casual access by children (may use tape, a tamper-resistant compartment, or a hearing aid retainer).
8. Always check medications; batteries have been mistaken for tablets.
9. *If a battery is swallowed*:
   a. Find another battery exactly like the one swallowed, or the package from which the battery came, to obtain the identification number.
   b. Promptly seek medical advice from a physician.
   c. For battery contents and recommended treatment protocol, telephone, collect, the National Button Battery Ingestion Hotline. The number is (202) 625–3333 (voice) or (202)

362–8563 (TTY). This hotline is operated by the National Capital Poison Center at Georgetown University Hospital in Washington, D.C.

HEARING AID

Keep the hearing aid away from excessive heat and humidity. During especially humid times of the year, place a hearing aid overnight in a plastic bag or jar with a drying agent. Avoid dropping the hearing aid. Keep the aid turned off when it is not in use, and never open the case of the hearing aid in an attempt to repair it yourself. For body-worn aids with top-mounted microphones, food guards may be purchased; a food guard is a cover designed to protect the microphone opening from food spills.

Consult an audiologist or hearing aid specialist promptly if you have any questions or concerns about the function of the hearing aid.

HEARING AID RETAINERS

It is often difficult to secure a BTE aid on a small child, and some dispensers have advocated the use of toupee tape in such situations. However, retainers for BTE hearing aids are available. Retainers have two plastic bands that fit around each end of the hearing aid. They are connected to either a plastic loop that encircles the ear or a cord that clips to clothing. Retainers have the possible added advantage of preventing tampering with the aid's gain control and battery compartment. Other styles of retainers are designed for bone conduction receivers, for holding aids to the heads of difficult-to-fit children who have absent or deformed ears or misshapened heads, and for the external button receivers of body-worn aids and assistive listening devices. For more information, consult the Appendix.

MOISTURE AND DUST PROTECTION

There are at least two alternatives for protecting a BTE aid from moisture, dirt, and dust. These options may be especially helpful during some recreational activities. A protective cover of a specially designed fabric may be slipped over the entire instrument; this casing is loose enough to allow adjusting of the aid's controls. Also, a nonallergenic latex sheath is available, which must be applied with a special tool. It results in a snug fit that makes it difficult for young children to manipulate the aid's controls when it is in place. For more information, consult the Appendix.

Electroacoustic Analysis

An effective hearing aid maintenance program must include monitoring the electroacoustic performance of a hearing aid. Although a visual inspection and listening check will contribute to an aid's optimal operation, with the possible exception of the Ling Six-Sound Test, they will not reveal problems in electroacoustic performance unless the aid is grossly malfunctioning. Electroacoustic measurements may be made with a standard or portable hearing aid analyzer. A commercially available hearing aid test system is pictured in Figure 11–9. A test system has the following components.

TEST CHAMBER

Measurements must be performed with the aid in a sound-free environment. This is accomplished by placing the aid in an insulated chamber. Spaces around the sides and the lid of the chamber are filled with sound-absorbent material to minimize standing and reflected sound waves and to reduce the effects of room noise in the test environment. A test point is indicated in the chamber where the hearing aid microphone should be placed.

LOUDSPEAKER

A loudspeaker is situated in the test chamber oriented toward the test point. A sweep of pure tones at a given intensity is directed from the loudspeaker to the microphone of the hearing aid to obtain measures according to ANSI S3.22. A broadband composite signal is also included in the analyzer to have a stimulus available that reflects the in-

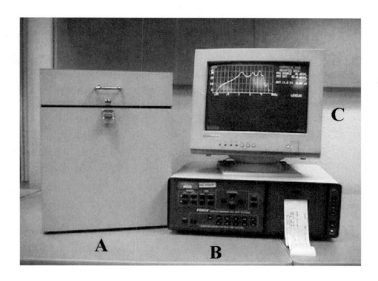

Figure 11–9. Hearing aid analyzer. A, test chamber; B, electronics module; C, monitor. (Courtesy of Frye Electronics.)

tensity and spectral shape of the long-term value for speech.

REGULATORY SYSTEM

Some system is used to ensure that input from the loudspeaker does not vary from the desired intensity as it enters the hearing aid microphone. This uniformity is achieved by the use of a predetermined and stored correction curve that compensates for the effects of the test chamber

2 CC COUPLER

Output from the receiver of the hearing aid is sent into a stainless steel cylinder containing a cavity with a volume of 2 cc. This size was selected as the standard because it was thought to approximate the space between the tip of an earmold and the eardrum in an adult ear.

MEASURING MICROPHONE

A microphone is inserted into the opposite end of the 2 cc coupler to pick-up the amplified signal from the hearing aid receiver. The diaphragm of this microphone forms the bottom boundary of the 2 cc space. Thus sound leaves the hearing aid receiver, passes through the 2 cc hard-walled cavity, and activates this measuring microphone.

TELEPHONE MAGNETIC FIELD SIMULATOR

A TMFS is required to measure telecoil performance according to ANSI S3.22–1996. It is a wand, similar in size to a telephone handset, that produces a magnetic field that complies with the standard.

ELECTRONICS MODULE

The signal from the measuring microphone is fed into components that analyze this output from the hearing aid. Data resulting from these various measurements appear visually in a graphic display, which may be recorded permanently in printed form.

Educational programs should take advantage of the availability and ease of operation of hearing aid analyzers. Measurement procedures were developed explicitly for the purpose of maintaining quality control and product uniformity. In this way, analyzers may also meet the needs of rehabilitative programs. Routine electroacoustic monitoring should be used to verify that the amplification characteristics of hearing aids are consistent over time and in agreement with those that the aids had when they were originally selected for the child.

How often a child's aids should be evaluated depends realistically upon the accessibility of the hearing aid analyzer and the number of children it must serve. A recommendation is that aids receive at least an annual electroacoustic evaluation. The need for this monitoring varies with the age of the child. Small children lead more active lives; consequently, it may be beneficial to check the performance of younger children's aids more frequently. In addition, such measurements should be made whenever there is a change in a child's aided abilities without apparent reason, or whenever a problem in the aid's electroacoustic performance is suspected on the basis of the daily listening check.

The manufacturer's printed performance specifications for the various instruments worn by children in the school must be on file. Only then may measurements made with the test set be used to determine if an aid is functioning as originally designed. As additional information, it would be ideal to include in each child's records an electroacoustic analysis obtained with the aid adjusted to the use settings recommended when the aid was fit. Then the aid could be monitored periodically with this information as a reference. The difficulty lies in coordinating this exchange of information between those fitting and dispensing the aids and those monitoring their function. Finally, in this monitoring, the limits of acceptable variation must be somewhat arbitrary until the relationship between these electroacoustic characteristics and speech intelligibility and hearing impairment in children is more clearly defined.

TESTING REPAIRED HEARING AIDS

Many problems detected with an electroacoustic analysis of children's hearing aids are repairable. Therefore, a hearing aid test set is an asset to a maintenance program in yet another way. Measurements may be made when aids are returned from repair to ascertain if, indeed, they received adequate service before the aids are used.

TESTING LOANER HEARING AIDS

A hearing aid test set may be used with loaner hearing aids. Because a child's personal hearing aids may be an integral component of the amplification arrangement used in the classroom, the child needs instruments in good working order. Accordingly, some schools supply loaner aids to students whose personal aids are being repaired. With a hearing aid test set, the performance characteristics of a loaner aid may be verified before the aid is issued to a child.

Hearing Aid Maintenance Program

There can be no doubt that the need to establish a viable hearing aid maintenance program for children is of the utmost importance. Teachers, other school professionals, parents, and the children themselves, when they are old enough, must share this responsibility. Such maintenance was actually mandated in 1977 in regulations for PL-94–142, Education for All Handicapped Children Act, which subsequently has been renamed and reauthorized, most recently as PL 101–497, Individuals with Disabilities Education Act–Reauthorization (IDEA, 1997). According to the regulations, "Each public agency shall ensure that the hearing aids worn in school by children with hearing impairments, including deafness, are functioning properly" (34 CFR §300.303). Consequently, schools must be engaged in hearing aid maintenance on a routine basis. Schools should plan hearing aid maintenance programs that foster student participation. The tools and techniques of simple hearing aid monitoring and troubleshooting may be introduced through demonstration sessions that include the preschool child. Then, when older, the child may begin to assume responsibility for hearing aid performance, which increases as the child matures. In fact, age-appropriate goals for hearing aid maintenance should become part of an individualized educational plan (IEP) for the child with hearing impairment. A training program for students that combines hands-on instruction, criterion-referenced IEP goals, troubleshooting skills, and knowledge of problem-solving resources and personnel at school is advocated (Elfenbein et al, 1988; Flexer, 1999; Johnson et al, 1997).

Parental involvement in hearing aid maintenance should not be overlooked. When parents are provided with information about hearing loss and amplification along with training in maintenance procedures, the occurrence of hearing aid malfunctions significantly declines (Diefendorf & Arthur, 1987; Foust & Wynne, 1991).

The American Speech-Language-Hearing Association (ASHA) recently approved new *Guidelines for Audiology Service Provision in and for Schools* (2002). These guidelines make recommendations for appropriate cost-effective audiology services in the schools, whether school-based or contracted, and recognize the unique role of audiologists in educational settings. One rehabilitative service for audiologists in these guidelines is described as follows:

> Ensure appropriate functioning of the student's hearing aids ... by directly providing or training and supervising school staff to conduct daily visual and listening checks and troubleshooting of common causes of malfunction and provide for daily visual and listening checks of students' hearing aids ... and troubleshooting of common causes of malfunction. (p. 118)

Indeed, ensuring the proper functioning of hearing aids is an important and vital segment of comprehensive services for children with hearing impairments. The immediate result will be more consistent, functional amplification for the child. The additional benefits may be even more far-reaching as children actually experience this improved auditory input in their rehabilitative programs.

Summary

This chapter addresses the need for regular maintenance of children's hearing aids. A basic review of a hearing aid and its electroacoustic performance is presented. Then, the various components of a hearing aid maintenance program—visual inspection, listening check, and electroacoustic analysis—are discussed. Information about the care of a hearing aid and resources are included.

Appendix

Hearing Aid Maintenance Resources

Items for hearing aid maintenance may be obtained from: (1) Hal-Hen Co., 180 Atlantic Avenue, Garden City Park, NY 11040–5028, phone, 800–242–5436, www.halhen.com; and (2) Westone Labs, Inc., 2235 Executive Circle, PO Box 15100, Colorado Springs, CO 80935, phone, 800–525–5071, www.earmold.com. An assembled kit is available from A.G. Bell Assoc., 2000 M Street, N.W., Suite 310, Washington, D.C. 20036, phone, 202–337–5220, www.agbell.org. Hearing aid retainers are available from: (1) Huggie Aids, LDT, 838 NW Tenth St., Oklahoma City, OK 73106, phone, 405–232–7848, www.members.aol.com/huggieaids; and (2) Westone Labs, Inc., which offers animal-theme retention clips. For moisture protectors: (1) the Hearing Aid Sweat Band may be obtained from VanB Enterprises, 9905 Rock Springs Road, West Valley, NY 14171, phone, 716–942–6313, www.vanbent.com; and (2) Super Seals are manufactured by Just BeKuz Products Co., 5629 E.Tabor Dr., Castle Rock, CO 80104–9719, phone, 800–795–5153, www.superseals.com.

References

American National Standards Instiutute (ANSI). (1987). Specification of hearing aid characteristics (ANSI S3.22–1987). New York: Acoustical Society of America.

American National Standards Institute (ANSI). (1996). Specification of hearing aid characteristics (ANSI S3.22–1996). New York: Acoustical Society of America.

American Speech-Language-Hearing Association (ASHA). (2002). *Guidelines for Audiology Service Provision in and for the Schools*. Rockville, MD: ASHA.

Bess, F.H. (1977). Condition of hearing aids worn by children in a public school setting. In: F.B. Withrow (Ed.), *The Condition of Hearing Aids Worn by Children in a Public School Program*, Report No. (OE)77- 05002 (Chap. 2). Washington, DC: U.S. Dept. of Health, Education, and Welfare, Public Health Service.

Blair, J.C., Wright, K., & Pollard, G. (1981). Parental knowledge and understanding of hearing loss and hearing aids. *Volta Review*, 83, 375–382.

Coleman, R.E. (1972). *Stability of Children's Hearing Aids in an Acoustic Preschool*. Final Report, Project No. 522466, Grant No. OEG-4–71–0060. Washington, DC: U.S. Dept. of Health, Education, and Welfare, Office of Education.

Diefendorf, A.O., & Arthur, D.A. (1987). Monitoring children's hearing aids. *Volta Review*, 89, 17–26.

Elfenbein, J. (1994). Monitoring preschoolers' hearing aids: Issues in program design and implementation. *Am J Audiol, 3,* 65–70.

Elfenbein, J.L., Bentler, R.A., Davis, J.M., & Niebuhr, D.P. (1988). Status of school children's hearing aids relative to monitoring practices. *Ear Hear, 9,* 212–217.

Flexer, C. (1999). Technological management of hearing and hearing loss. In: C. Flexer (Ed.), *Facilitating Hearing and Listening in Young Children* (pp. 107–176). San Diego: Singular.

Foust, T.E., & Wynne, M.K. (1991). Effectiveness of supplemental parent training in hearing aid checks. *J Am Acad Rehab Audiol, 24,* 85–96.

Gaeth, J.H., & Lounsbury, E. (1966). Hearing aids and children in elementary schools. *J Speech Hear Dis, 31,* 283–289.

Individuals with Disabilities Education Act–Reauthorization (IDEA). (1997). 20 (USC §§ 1400 et seq.).

Johnson, C.D., Benson, P.V., & Seaton, J.B. (1997). *Educational Audiology Handbook.* San Diego: Singular.

Johnson, C.E., Stein, R.L., & Lass, N.J. (1992). Public school nurses' preparedness for a hearing aid monitoring program. *Lang Speech Hear Serv Sch, 23,* 141–144.

Lass, N.J., Tecca, J.E., & Woodford, C.M. (1987). Teachers' knowledge of, exposure to, and attitudes toward hearing aids and hearing aid wearers. *Lang Speech Hear Serv Sch, 18,* 86–95.

Lass, N.J., Woodford, C.M., Pannbacker, M.D., Carlin, M.F., Saniga, R.D., Schmitt, J.F., & Everly-Myers, D.S. (1989). Speech-language pathologists' knowledge of, exposure to, and attitudes toward hearing aids and hearing aid wearers. *Lang Speech Hear Serv Sch, 20,* 115–132.

Litovitz, T.I. (1983). Button battery ingestions. *JAMA, 249,* 2495–2500.

Potts, P.L., & Greenwood, J. (1983). Hearing aid monitoring: Are looking and listening enough? *Lang Speech Hear Serv Sch, 14,* 157–163.

Preeves, D., & Curran, J. (2000). Hearing aid instrumentation and procedures for electroacoustic testing. In: M. Valente, H. Hosford-Dunn, & R. Roeser (Eds.), *Audiology Treatment* (pp. 1–58). New York: Thieme.

Thibodeau, L.M., DeLaRosa, M.A., & Champlin, C.A. (2000). Acoustic consequences of evaluating hearing aids via stethoscopes and listening tubes. *Volta Review, 102,* 25–33.

U.S. Food and Drug Administration (FDA). (1977). Rules and regulations regarding hearing aid devices: Professional and patient labeling and conditions for sale, Part IV. *Fed Reg, 42* (February 15), 9294–9296.

Valente, M., Valente, M., Potts, L.G., & Lybarger, E.H. (2000). Earhooks, tubing, earmolds, and shells. In: M. Valente, H. Hosford-Dunn, & R. Roeser (Eds.), *Audiology Treatment* (pp. 59–104). New York: Thieme.

12

Classroom Acoustics

CARL C. CRANDELL AND JOSEPH J. SMALDINO

My eyes are dim with childish tears,
My heart is idly stirred,
For the same sound is in my ears
Which in those days I heard.

—William Wordsworth, *The Fountain*

Accurate perception and processing of speech are fundamental for academic achievement in the classroom environment. In a classroom setting, speech perception can be influenced by many acoustic, linguistic, and cognitive variables. Acoustic variables include the reverberation time (RT) of the classroom, the power of the teacher's voice relative to the level of ambient noise in a room, and the distance from the teacher to the student. Some of the more salient linguistic and cognitive factors consist of the articulation abilities and dialect of the speaker or listener, completeness of knowledge concerning the rules of language, context of the message, memory processes, length of utterance, ability to listen and attend, word familiarity, and vocabulary size of the listener. This chapter considers the acoustic factors that can influence speech perception in the classroom environment. For additional information on linguistic, articulatory, and cognitive factors, the reader is directed to Crandell and Smaldino (1992).

Reverberation

One of the most important variables that define the acoustic climate of a classroom is the reverberant characteristics of that enclosure (Bolt & MacDonald, 1949; Lochner & Burger,

1964). "Reverberation" refers to the prolongation, or persistence, of sound waves within a room as they are reflected off of surfaces in the classroom. Operationally, reverberation time (RT) refers to the amount of time it takes for a sound at a specific frequency to decay 60 dB (or to one millionth of its original intensity) following termination of the signal (ANSI, 1976). For example, if a 100 dB sound pressure level (SPL) signal at 1000 Hz took 1 second to decrease to 40 dB SPL, the RT of that enclosure at 1000 Hz would be 1 second. RT can be expressed via the following formula (Sabine, 1964):

$$RT = 0.05 \, V/a$$

where "V" is the volume of the room, "a" is the total sound absorption in the enclosure, and 0.05 is a constant. Room reverberation increases as a function of the volume of the classroom and is inversely related to the amount of sound absorption in an environment. Consequently, larger classrooms tend to exhibit higher RTs than classrooms with more traditional quadrilateral dimensions because of the interactions of the reflected sound.

Classrooms with bare cement walls, floors, and ceilings tend to exhibit higher RTs than classrooms that contain absorptive surfaces, such as carpeting, draperies, and acoustic ceiling tile. A useful index in determining the reverberant characteristics of a classroom is the absorption coefficient. The absorption coefficient is the ratio of unreflected sound energy to incident sound energy present in a room (Nabelek & Nabelek, 1985). A surface with an absorption coefficient of 1.00 would technically absorb 100% of all reflections, whereas a surface structure with an absorption coefficient of 0.00 would reflect all of the incident sound. Absorption coefficients, which are typically indicated from 125 to 4000 Hz, are frequency dependent. Most surface materials in a classroom do not absorb low frequency sounds as effectively as higher frequencies. Due to these absorption characteristics, classroom reverberation is often shorter at higher frequencies than in lower frequency regions.

Measurement of Reverberation

RT in a classroom is measured by presenting a high intensity stimulus, such as ⅓ octave bands of noise, into an unoccupied room and measuring the amount of time required for that signal to decay 60 dB. Instruments to measure RT vary from inexpensive compact battery units that will allow the audiologist to do rudimentary measures of reverberation to highly technological, computer-based devices that can measure and record numerous aspects of the acoustic decay properties of an environment. RT can also be approximated using well-established formulae such as the one previously presented. Because the primary energy of speech is between 500 and 2000 Hz, RT is often reported as the mean decay time of 500, 1000, and 2000 Hz. Unfortunately, such a measurement paradigm may not adequately describe the reverberant characteristics of a classroom because high RTs may exist at additional frequencies. Thus it is recommended that RT be measured at discrete frequencies from 125 to 4000 Hz whenever possible. This more detailed information can significantly aid the audiologist or acoustic engineer in determining the appropriate degree and type of absorptive materials needed for that environment. The reader is directed to additional sources for further details concerning the measurement of reverberations (ANSI, 1976; Bolt & MacDonald, 1949; Knudsen & Harris, 1978; Kurtovic, 1975; Lochner & Burger, 1964; Nabelek & Nabelek, 1985).

Effects of Reverberation on Speech Perception

One way reverberation compromises speech perception is through the masking of direct sound energy by reflected energy. In a reverberant classroom, the reflected speech signals reaching the child are temporally delayed and overlap with the direct signal, resulting in masking of speech. Specifically, reverberation typically causes a prolongation of the spectral energy of the vowel phonemes, which tend to mask consonant information (particularly word final consonants). These effects of reverberation are to be expected because vowels are more intense in sound energy than consonants. In highly reverberant environments, words may actually overlap with one another, thus causing reverberant sound energy to replace, or fill in, pauses between words. Reverberation can also alter the temporal relationships between acoustic elements important to speech perception. This alteration can produce a mismatch between the acoustic signal received and a child's acoustic knowledge of language, leading to misperception of the speech signal.

In general, speech perception scores decline with increasing RT. For example, Moncur and Dirks (1967) examined the monosyllabic word recognition ability of adult listeners in four levels of reverberation (RT = 0.0, 0.9, 1.6, and 2.3 seconds). Speech recognition scores gradually declined as the RT of the environment increased. Binaural recognition scores were far superior to monaural perceptual abilities in the reverberant listening conditions. This finding has important implications for listeners with unilateral hearing loss. Gelfand and Silman (1979) examined consonant perception in a reverberant (RT = 0.8 seconds) and nonreverberant (RT = 0.0 seconds) listening environment. In the reverberant listening condition, errors for initial and final consonants increased by 5% and 9%, respectively.

Numerous investigators have shown that the speech perception of listeners with sensorineural hearing loss experience more deleterious effects in reverberation than individuals with normal hearing. Finitzo-Hieber and Tillman (1978), for example, examined monosyllabic word recognition at various RTs. Subjects included 12 children (ages 8 to 12 years) with normal hearing and 12 children with sensorineural hearing loss. Children with hearing impairment obtained poorer recognition scores at each listening condition. Moreover, differences in perception scores between the two groups increased as the listening environment became more adverse. Specifically, in a nonreverberant listening condition (RT = 0.0 seconds), the performance difference between the groups was approximately 12%. In a highly reverberant condition (RT = 1.2 seconds), differences in speech perception increased to 32%.

Data from additional studies have indicated that several populations of children with normal hearing sensitivity experience greater difficulties understanding reverberated speech than adult listeners. These listeners (see Table 12–1) include children with fluctuating conductive hearing loss, learning disabilities, articulation disorders, central auditory processing deficits, language disorders, minimal degrees of sensorinueral hearing loss [pure tone sensitivity from 15 to 25 dB hearing loss (HL)], and unilateral hearing loss. Children for whom English is a second language are also included in this group. Nabelek and Donahue (1984), for example, reported that, although native and nonnative English-speaking adult listeners (Chinese, Japanese, and Spanish) obtained essentially identical perception scores in a nonreverberant (RT = 0.0 seconds) environment (100% for native English-speaking listeners; 99% for nonnative English-speaking listeners), significant differences were noted between the groups (97% for native English-speaking listeners; 88% for nonnative English-speaking listeners) when listening to reverberant speech (RT = 0.8 seconds). Boney

Table 12–1. Populations of Listeners with "Normal Hearing"

Young children (less than 15 years)

Conductive hearing loss

History of otitis media

Articulation and/or language disorders

Learning disabled

Nonnative English

Central auditory processing deficits

Minimal, or borderline, degrees of SNHL (16 to 25 dB HL)

Unilateral hearing loss

Developmental delays

Attentional deficits

Reading deficits (dyslexia)

HL, hearing loss; SNHL, sensorineural hearing loss.

and Bess (1984) demonstrated that children with minimal degrees of sensorineural hearing loss (pure tone thresholds from 15 to 30 dB HL from 500 to 2000 Hz) experience greater difficulty understanding speech degraded by reverberation than children with normal hearing sensitivity. Specifically, speech perception scores were obtained in nonreverberant (RT = 0.0 seconds) and reverberant environments (RT = 0.8 seconds). Results from this investigation indicated that the children with minimal hearing loss performed more poorly than the control group, particularly in the reverberant listening condition.

Surprisingly, an additional group of normal hearers who experience more difficulty understanding speech in the classroom than has traditionally been suspected are younger children (less than 15 years of age). Investigators have demonstrated that young pediatric listeners require better acoustic environments than older children to achieve equivalent recognition scores (Crandell & Bess, 1987). Adultlike performance on speech perception tasks is typically not obtained until the child reaches approximately 13 to 15 years of age. It is thus reasonable to assume that commonly reported classroom reverberation levels have the potential of adversely affecting speech recognition in pediatric listeners. As an example, Neuman and Hochberg (1983) reported that 5-year-old children with normal hearing obtained less than 80% correct recognition scores for nonsense syllables at an RT of 0.6 seconds. Finitzo-Hieber and Tillman (1978) reported that children aged 8 to 12 years obtained recognition scores of only 76.5% at an RT of 1.2 seconds. Certainly, such diminished perceptual ability, as suggested by the investigations just mentioned, would not be appropriate for maximum learning in the classroom setting.

Recommended Criteria for Reverberation Time

Speech perception in adults with normal hearing is not significantly affected until RTs exceed approximately 1.0 seconds. However, listeners with sensorineural hearing loss need considerably shorter RTs for maximum speech perception. Sources have recommended that listening environments utilized for the hearing impaired should not surpass 0.4 seconds to provide ideal communicative efficiency (ASHA, 1994).

Unfortunately, acoustic criteria for appropriate RTs have not been well established for the diverse populations of children with normal hearing. With these considerations in mind, and until additional research is conducted, a conservative standard for RTs in listening environments for children with normal hearing should follow the same acoustic recommendations utilized for listeners with hearing impairment. That is, RT should not exceed approximately 0.4 seconds. The new American national standard, entitled *Acoustic Performance Criteria, Design Requirements and Guidelines for Schools* (ANSI, 2002), recommends a maximum RT of 0.6 seconds.

Reverberation Times in Classrooms

Available research suggests that classroom environments are often far too reverberant for maximum communication to occur in pe-

diatric listeners. Specifically, the range of reverberation for unoccupied classroom settings is typically reported to be from 0.4 to 1.2 seconds (ASHA, 1994). McCroskey and Devans (1975) reported reverberation levels in classrooms built between 1890 and 1960. Results indicated that the newer classrooms had lower RTs (approximately 0.6 seconds) than older classrooms (approximately 1.0 seconds). Nabelek and Pickett (1974) reported that RTs in medium-sized classrooms ranged from 0.5 to 1.0. Bradley (1986) reported that RTs in medium-sized classrooms ranged from 0.39 to 1.20 seconds (mean 0.72 seconds). In 32 classrooms, Crandell and Smaldino (1994) reported that mean RTs were 0.52 seconds, with a range of 0.35 to 1.20 seconds. The above investigations clearly show that appropriate levels of reverberation (RT = 0.4 to 0.6 seconds) rarely occur in the classroom setting. Indeed, Crandell and Smaldino (1995) reported that only nine of 32 classrooms (28%) exhibited RTs less than 0.4 seconds.

Noise

"Noise" refers to any undesired auditory disturbance that interferes with what a listener wants to hear. Noise can degrade the perception of speech by distorting or eliminating the redundant acoustic and linguistic cues available in the signal. Because it is known that the spectral energy of consonant phonemes is less intense than the energy of vowels, noise primarily affects the perception of consonant phonemes, making them less intelligible to the listener. This reduction of consonant perception can significantly influence speech perception because as much as 90% of a listener's speech perception ability is generated from consonant energy.

The effectiveness of any given noise to reduce or eliminate (mask) speech cues depends upon a number of parameters: (1) the long-term spectrum of the noise, (2) the intensity of the noise relative to the intensity of speech, and (3) the intensity fluctuations of the noise over time (Nabelek & Nabelek, 1985). Generally, low frequency noises in a classroom environment are more effective maskers of speech than high frequency noises because of upward spread of masking (Danaher & Pickett, 1975). The fact that low frequency noises have a greater effect on speech perception than high frequency noises is important because the predominant spectra of noise found in classroom environments are low frequency. It appears that the most effective masking noises are those with a spectrum similar to the speech spectrum because they affect all speech frequencies to the same degree.

Measurement of Classroom Noise

The acoustic characteristics of both the signal (the teacher's voice) and the noise (that sound which is masking the signal) vary considerably in the classroom with time. This variability has made it difficult to measure accurately and reliably classroom noise and its effects in a simple manner. In spite of this, single number descriptions of classroom signal and noise characteristics are widespread. One of the most common single number descriptors is the relative SPL of the signal and the noise at specific points in time. The usual way of doing this is to use a sound-level meter, a device that measures the amplitude of sound. As with reverberation instruments, sound-level meters range from compact inexpensive battery-operated units to computer-based devices that can measure and record numerous properties of a signal. Sound-level meters are classified according to standards set forth in ANSI (1971): type I meters meet the most rigorous standards; type II are general purpose; and type III are for hobby use. Most serious measurement of classroom noise would require at least a type II meter. In addition, many sound-level meters incorporate weighting filter networks. The A-weighting network is designed to simulate the sensitivity of the average human ear under conditions of low sound loudness (40 phons, to be precise). The B-weighting scale simulates loud sounds (70 phons), and the C-weighting network approximates the way the ear would

respond to very loud sounds. Classroom measurement convention uses the A-weighting network. Unfortunately, the single number obtained from a sound pressure measurement performed with the A-weighting can be obtained with a variety of very different sound spectra. The only really accurate and reliable way to measure spectral intensity would be to conduct a spectral analysis of the signal and noise, instead of attempting to use a single descriptor.

Noise criteria (NC) curves can help to determine objectively the suitability of an acoustic spectrum for various human activities (Beranek, 1954). NC curves are a family of frequency and intensity curves based on octave band sound pressure measures across a 20 to 10,000 Hz band and have been related to successful use of an acoustic space for a variety of activities. The value of each NC curve is determined from the highest NC curve the sound pressure intersects. For instance, Figure 12–1 shows an example of an NC curve. NC curves have also been roughly equated to sound pressure measures made using the A-weighting scale. An NC curve of 25 is considered suitable for a classroom.

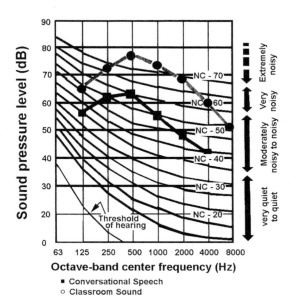

Figure 12–1. An example of noise criteria curves.

The computed equivalent SPL using A-weighting would be approximately 35 dB A. This would then be the target for the long-term average spectrum in the classroom and may be optimal without extensive spectral analysis as a function of time. It is recommended, therefore, that whenever possible, ambient noise levels in classrooms or therapy rooms be measured via NC curve measures because this procedure gives the examiner additional information regarding the spectral characteristics of the noise.

Sources of Noise in Classrooms

Ambient noise in the classroom can originate from a number of possible sources. External noise sources include construction, traffic, and playground areas. Noise can also originate from within the school building but outside the actual classroom (internal noise). Classrooms adjacent to the cafeteria, gymnasium, or busy hallways often exhibit high internal noise levels. Finally, a significant amount of noise is generated within the classroom itself. Classroom noise includes children talking, chairs or tables sliding, hard-soled shoes on noncarpeted floors, and school heating or cooling systems. Classroom noise is typically the most detrimental to a child's perceptual ability because the frequency content of the noise is spectrally similar to the spectrum of the signal (teacher's voice).

Noise Levels in Classroom Settings

Ambient noise levels in the classroom have been reported to be high enough to affect deleteriously even adult communication. For example, Sanders (1965) measured the occupied and unoccupied noise levels of 47 classrooms in 15 different schools. Mean occupied noise levels ranged from an average of 69 dB B in kindergarten classrooms to 52 dB B in classrooms for children with hearing impairment. Unoccupied classroom noise levels were approximately 10 dB lower than the occupied classroom settings, ranging from 58 dB B for kindergarten classrooms to 42 dB B in hearing-impaired classrooms. Nober and Nober (1975) reported that the average intensity of four occupied elementary classrooms was 65 dB A. Bess, Sinclair, and Riggs (1984) measured ambient noise levels in 19 classrooms for children with hearing impairment. Median unoccupied noise levels were 41 dB A, 50 dB B, and 58 dB C. When the classroom was occupied with students, ambient noise levels increased to 56 dB A, 60 dB B, and 63 dB C. Crandell and Smaldino (1995) measured the ambient noise levels of 32 unoccupied classroom settings for children with hearing impairment. Mean unoccupied classroom noise levels were actually higher than previously reported. Specifically, mean unoccupied noise levels were 51 dB A (range: 46 to 59 dB) and 67 dB C (range: 57 to 74 dB).

Criteria for Classroom Noise Levels

The noise levels reported in the investigations just discussed are distressing because acoustic recommendations for children with sensorineural hearing loss suggest that ambient noise levels in unoccupied classrooms should not exceed 30 to 35 dB A or an NC curve of 20 to 25 dB (ASHA, 1994). The new American National Standard (ANSI, 2002) recommends a maximum 1-hour-average A-weighted, steady-state background noise level of 35 dB. Such a recommendation is based on the assumption that appropriate classroom signal-to-noise (S/N) ratios discussed later in this chapter are difficult to achieve if classroom noise exceeds these levels. Unfortunately, a review of the aforementioned investigations indicates that this acoustic recommendation is infrequently achieved. McCroskey and Devens (1975) demonstrated that only one of nine elementary classrooms actually meet the acoustic recommendations. Crandell and Smaldino (1994) reported that none of 32 classrooms met recommended criteria. Overall, it appears that ambient noise levels in the classroom are approximately 10 to 15 dB higher than recommended.

Speech Perception in Noise

The most important consideration for speech perception in the classroom is not the absolute ambient noise level but rather the relationship between the intensity of the signal and the ambient noise at the child's ear. This relationship is referred to as the S/N ratio of the environment. For example, if a speech signal is measured at 65 dB, and a noise is 59 dB, then the S/N ratio is +6 dB. For a given noise and speech material, speech perception scores achieve a plateau for favorable S/N ratios and decline for less favorable S/N ratios. Crum (1974), for example, measured recognition in adult normal hearers at S/N ratios of +12 dB, +6 dB, and 0 dB. Although mean recognition scores were 95% at S/N ratios of +12 dB, percent correct scores declined to 80% and 46% at S/N ratios of +6 dB and 0 dB, respectively.

In general, the perceptual ability of adult listeners with normal hearing is not significantly affected until the S/N ratio decreases below 0 dB (speech and noise are at equal intensities). To obtain adequate communicative efficiency in noise, adult listeners with sensorineural hearing loss require the S/N ratio to be improved by at least 5 to 10 dB and by an additional 3 to 6 dB in rooms with moderate levels of reverberation (Hawkins & Yacullo, 1984). Stated another way, listeners with hearing impairment require considerably better acoustic environments than normal hearers to process and understand speech. As an illustration of the effects of hearing impairment on speech perception, let us examine data from Suter (1978). In this investigation, the author compared speech perception performance in noise for 16 listeners with normal hearing and 32 listeners with various degrees of sensorineural hearing loss. Lists of monosyllables (Modified Rhyme Test) were presented to the two groups at a level of 60 dB SPL. A multitalker babble served as the competing noise and was adjusted to provide S/N ratios of –6, –3, and 0 dB. Results from this investigation revealed that listeners with hearing impairment performed at a significantly poorer level under all listening conditions. At an S/N ratio of –6 dB, for instance, the listeners with sensorineural hearing loss obtained mean perception scores of 27% correct compared with 63% correct for those with normal hearing.

As with reverberation, research has indicated that the group of children with normal hearing discussed previously also requires higher S/N ratios than adult normal hearers to achieve equivalent recognition scores. For example, Elliott (1982) and Nabelek and Robinson (1982) reported that young children require an improvement of approximately 10 dB in S/N ratios to produce perception scores equivalent to those of adults.

Criteria for Classroom Signal-to-Noise Ratios

Acoustic studies and the new standard suggest that S/N ratios in learning environments for children with hearing impairment should exceed +15 dB. These recommendations are based on the finding that the speech perception of children with sensorineural hearing loss tends to remain relatively constant at S/N ratios in excess of +15 dB but deteriorates at less favorable S/N ratios. Moreover, listening effort in children with hearing impairment is minimal at S/N ratios exceeding +10 to +15 dB. At S/N ratios less than approximately +10 dB, children must utilize so much listening effort that they tend to prefer manual communication and speech reading over utilizing auditory input. To date, acoustic standards for S/N ratios are not well defined for "normal hearers." Until such standards are established, the same standards as those advocated for children with hearing impairment should be followed. That is, S/N ratios in learning environments should exceed +15 dB, whereas ambient noise levels should be no more than 30 to 35 dB A or an NC curve of 20 to 25 dB.

Signal-to-Noise Levels in Classroom Settings

Relatively poor S/N ratios have been reported in many educational settings. The range of S/N ratios for classrooms has been reported to be from +5 dB to –7 dB. Sanders (1965) reported that classroom S/N ratios ranged from +5 in elementary classrooms to +1 dB in kindergarten classrooms. Paul (1967) reported an average S/N ratio of +3 dB in classrooms. Blair (1977) measured classroom S/N ratios in a regular classroom at 0 dB and 7 dB in classrooms for children with sensorineural hearing loss. Finitzo-Hieber (1988) reported that classroom S/N ratios ranged from +1 to +4 dB.

In addition to children with hearing impairment, it is reasonable to assume that typical classroom S/N ratios have the capacity of detrimentally affecting speech perception in populations with normal hearing. In the Finitzo-Hieber and Tillman (1978) article previously discussed, the authors also evaluated monosyllabic word perception at different S/N ratios (+12 dB, +6 dB, 0 dB). The most obvious finding from this aspect of the study was that the children with sensorineural hearing loss obtained poorer perception scores under all listening conditions. However, it is also interesting to examine the data obtained from the children with normal hearing. At an S/N ratio of +12 dB (rarely found in a classroom), the children with normal-hearing sensitivity obtained mean perception scores of 89%. At more typical classroom S/N ratios, perceptual abilities were notably poorer. For example, at an S/N ratio of +6 dB, mean perception scores were 80%, and at 0 dB (a common S/N ratio reported in the classroom), mean perception ability decreased to a level of 60%.

In another study of children with normal hearing who exhibit significant perceptual difficulties in noise, Crandell (1993) examined the speech perception of children with minimal degrees of sensorineural hearing loss at commonly reported classroom S/N ratios of +6, +3, 0, –3, and –6 dB. The minimally hearing-impaired children exhibited pure tone averages (0.5 to 2 kHz) from 15 to 25 dB HL. Speech perception was assessed with the Bamford-Koval-Bench Standard Sentence test (Bench, Koval, & Bamford, 1979) presented at a level of 65 dB SPL. Multitalker babble from the Speech Perception in Noise test (Kalikow, Stevens, & Elliott, 1977) was used as the noise competition. Mean sentential recognition scores (in percent correct) as a function of S/N ratio are presented in Figure 12–2. These data suggest that the chil-dren with minimal degrees of hearing impairment had poorer performance across most listening conditions. Moreover, note that the performance decrement between the two groups increased as the listening environment became more adverse. For example, at an S/N ratio of +6 dB, both groups obtained recognition scores in excess of 80%. At an S/N ratio of –6 dB, however, the group that was minimally hearing impaired obtained less than 50% correct recognition compared with approximately 75% recognition ability for those with normal hearing. Interestingly, a similar trend in speech perception was reported by Crandell (1994) for non-native English-speaking (Spanish, Chinese, Japanese) children.

Combined Effects of Classroom Noise and Reverberation

In a real-world classroom environment, noise and reverberation are not independent of each other. In fact, in an actual classroom setting, noise and reverberation combine in a synergistic manner to influence speech perception. That is, the interaction of noise and reverberation adversely affects speech perception to a greater degree than the sum of both effects taken independently. If a child experiences a reduction in speech perception of 10% in a noisy listening environment and a reduction of 10% in a reverberant setting, perceptual deficits may actually equate to 30 to 40% in actual listening environments that contain both noise and reverberation. It is reasonable to assume that these synergistic effects occur because when noise and reverberation are combined, reflections fill in the temporal gaps in the noise, making it more steady state in nature. Recall that the most effective maskers of speech are noises with spectra similar to those of speech. Although noise and reverberation mask speech differently, there are similarities in how these distortions affect overall speech recognition scores and consonant error patterns. As with noise and reverberation in isolation, individuals with hearing impairment experience considerably greater speech perception difficulties in combinations of noise and reverberation than individuals with normal hearing.

Data from several investigations have also suggested that commonly reported levels of classroom noise and reverberation can adversely affect the speech perception of children with normal hearing. For example, Finitzo-Hieber and Tillman (1978) examined the speech recognition of younger children with normal hearing in several conditions of noise and reverberation. Results from this aspect of the investigation are shown in Table 12–2. Note that in typical classroom listening environments, the children with normal hearing generally obtained poor recognition scores. For example, in a relatively good classroom listening environment (S/N ratio = +6 dB; RT = 0.4 seconds), these children were able to recognize only 71% of the stimuli. In a poor but not typical classroom environment (S/N ratio = 0 dB; RT = 1.2 seconds), recognition scores were reduced to approximately 30%.

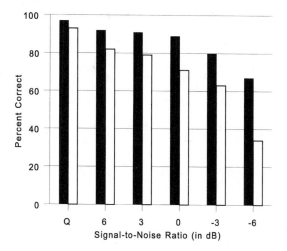

Figure 12–2. Mean sentential recognition scores, in percent correct, as a function of signal-to-noise ratio for children with normal hearing sensitivity (indicated by the closed bars) and children with minimal hearing impairment (indicated by the open bars). (Reprinted with permission from Crandell, 1993.)

Speaker–Listener Distance

In a classroom, the teacher's voice is distributed in several ways (direct sound and indirect sound) that vary as a function of the distance from the source. Figures 12–3 and 12–4 demonstrate several of the paths of direct and indirect sound. At distances relatively near to the speaker, the direct sound field (see Fig. 12–4) governs the listening environment. In the direct sound field, sound waves are transmitted from the teacher to the child with minimal interference from room surfaces. Direct sound pressure decreases 6 dB for every doubling of distance from the sound source, a phenomenon known as the inverse square law. Due to this linear decrease in sound pressure, the direct sound field in a classroom is dominant only at distances close to the teacher. For example, in an average-sized classroom (150 cubic meters) with a typical RT of 0.6 seconds, the critical distance would be slightly greater than 3 meters from the teacher. Thus many

of the children in this classroom will be in the indirect sound field.

At increased distances from the speaker, the indirect or reverberant field (Fig. 12–5) predominates the listening environment. In the indirect sound field (beyond the critical distance), the direct sound from the speaker arrives at the listener first. However, because of the inverse square law, the direct sound is significantly reduced in intensity. In addition to being decreased in intensity, the direct sound is also preceded by numerous reflected sound waves, or reverberation (echoes), which are composed of the original waves that have reflected off hard surfaces within the room (walls, ceiling, and floor). Due to the linear decrease in the intensity of the direct sound, and because the absorptive characteristics of structures in the room affect some frequencies more than others, the reflected sound reaching the listener will contain a different acoustic content in the frequency, intensity, and temporal domains. Acoustic interaction of this modified spectrum with the direct sound can produce reinforcements and diminutions in the direct

Table 12–2.   Mean Speech Recognition Scores*

Testing Condition	Groups	
	Normal Hearing	*Hearing Impaired*
RT = 0.0 seconds		
QUIET	94.5	83.0
+12 dB	89.2	70.0
+ 6 dB	79.7	59.5
0 dB	60.2	39.0
RT = 0.4 seconds		
QUIET	92.5	74.0
+12 dB	82.8	60.2
+ 6 dB	71.3	52.2
0 dB	47.7	27.8
RT = 1.2 seconds		
QUIET	76.5	45.0
+12 dB	68.8	41.2
+ 6 dB	54.2	27.0
0 dB	29.7	11.2

*Percent correct by children with normal hearing ($n = 12$) and children with sensorineural hearing loss ($n = 12$) for monosyllabic words across various signal-to-noise ratios and reverberation times.
Adapted from Finitzo-Hieber and Tillman (1978).

sound. These reinforcements and diminutions of the original signal result in an approximately equal distribution of sound energy beyond the critical distance of the room. A uniform distribution of sound energy, however, may not occur in larger listening environments, particularly if the power of the sound source is restricted. The critical distance refers to that point in a room in which the intensity of the direct sound is equal to the intensity of the reverberant sound (Crandell & Bess, 1986; Puetz, 1971).

Operationally, critical distance can be defined by the following formula:

$$Dc = (0.20)(VQ/nRT)^{-1/2}$$

where V is volume of the room in cubic meters, Q is the directivity factor of the source (the human voice is approximately 2.5), n is the number of sources, and RT is reverberation time of the enclosure at 1400 Hz.

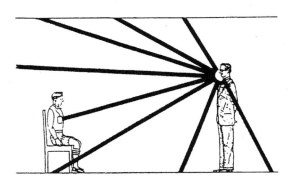

Figure 12–3. Direct sound propagation in a classroom. (Reprinted with permission from Olsen, 1988.)

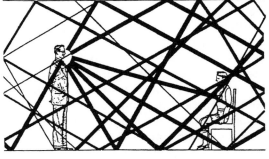

Figure 12–4. Direct and indirect sound propagation in a classroom. The direct sound is indicated by the thickest line, and 1st, 2nd, 3rd, and 4th reflections are denoted by sequentially thinner lines. (Reprinted with permission from Olsen, 1988.)

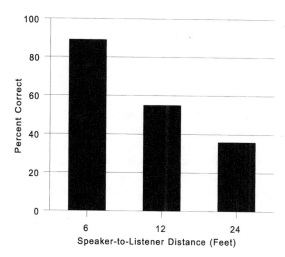

Figure 12–5. Mean sentential recognition scores, in percent correct, as a function of speaker–listener distance for children with normal hearing in a "typical" classroom (signal-to-noise ratio, +6 dB; RT. 0.45 seconds).

Effects of Distance on Speech Perception

The distance from a student to the teacher can significantly affect speech perception in the classroom (Crandell & Bess, 1986). If the student is in the direct field (within the critical distance), reflected sound waves have minimal effects on speech perception. In the indirect field (beyond the critical distance), however, reflections can cause difficulties in perception because there is typically enough of a spectrum or intensity change in the reflected sound to interfere with the perception of the direct sound. Speech perception in a classroom tends to decrease until the critical distance of the room is reached. Beyond the critical distance, perceptual abilities remain essentially constant, particularly in small to moderately sized classrooms. This finding is extremely important because it suggests that speech perception ability can be improved only by decreasing the distance between a speaker and listener within the critical distance of the room. Obviously, increased distance from the teacher more deleteriously affects children with hearing impairment than children with normal hearing sensitivity.

Crandell and Bess (1986) examined the effects of distance on the speech recognition of children with normal hearing in a "typical" classroom environment (S/N ratio = +6 dB; RT = 0.45 seconds). Specifically, PB-K monosyllabic words were recorded through the KEMAR manikin (Knowles Electronics manikin for acoustic research) at speaker–listener distances often encountered in the classroom (6, 12, and 24 feet). Multitalker babble was used as the noise competition. Subjects consisted of children 5 to 7 years of age. Results from this investigation are presented in Figure 12–5. As can be noted, there was a systematic decrease in speech-recognition ability as the speaker–listener distance increased. Overall, these results suggest that children with normal hearing seated in the middle to rear of a typical classroom have greater difficulty understanding speech than has traditionally been suspected. These findings become understandable by examining the findings of a study by Leavitt and Flexer (1991). In this investigation, the authors utilized the Rapid Speech Transmission Index (RASTI) to estimate speech perception in a classroom. RASTI measurements are based on the hypothesis that noise and reverberation in a room will affect a speechlike signal in ways that can be related to speech perception. Results indicated that, in a front row center seat of the classroom, 83% of the speech energy was available to the listener and 55% of the sound energy was available to the listener in the back row center. Clearly, it is reasonable to expect that only a fraction of the speech signal is available to the listener, and poor speech perception will result.

Methods to Improve Classroom Acoustics

The perceptual deficits experienced by children with hearing impairment, and those with normal hearing, emphasize the necessity of providing appropriate acoustic conditions in listening environments utilized by such populations. Unquestionably, stringent acoustic requirements must be used for rooms occupied by such listeners to ensure that noise and reverberation levels are within recommended criteria. Recall that S/N ratios should exceed +15 dB, unoccupied noise levels should not exceed 30 to 35 dB A, and RTs should not surpass 0.4 to 0.6 seconds.

Reduction of Classroom Noise Levels

Ambient noise levels in a classroom can originate from several possible sources (external, internal, or classroom). The most effective procedure for reducing external noise levels in the classroom is through appropriate planning with architects, contractors, school officials, architectural engineers, audiologists, and teachers for the hearing impaired prior to the design and construction of a building. Unfortunately, consultation among such disciplines prior to building construction is rare. In the absence of such consultation, it is critical that rooms intended for learning, therapy, or instruction be located away from high-noise sources, such as traffic, railroads, construction sites, airports, and furnace or air conditioning units. If relocation of the room or the noise source is not feasible, then acoustic modifications of the room must be considered. Acoustic treatments, such as thick or double concrete construction on the exterior wall, will attenuate extraneous noise sources in the classroom considerably more than having doors or windows on the external wall. Of course, to be effective in noise reduction, all walls must be free of cracks or openings that would allow extraneous noises into the classroom. Architects should attempt to achieve a noise reduction, or a Speech Transmission Loss (STL), of at least 45 to 50 dB for external walls.

"STL" refers to the amount of noise that is attenuated as it passes through a particular surface. For instance, if an external noise of 100 dB SPL were reduced to 50 dB SPL in the classroom, the exterior wall of that room would have an STL of 50 dB SPL. A 7-inch concrete wall provides approximately 53 dB attenuation of outside noise, whereas windows and doors provide only 24 dB and 20 dB attenuation, respectively. If windows are located on the external wall, they must be properly installed, heavy-weighted or double-paned, and should remain closed. Unfortunately, during many acoustic analyses of classrooms, the authors have seen exterior windows that remain open the majority of the school day. Landscaping strategies, such as the placement of shrubs, trees (of types that blossom all year long), or earthen banks around the school building can also provide interference and absorption of exterior levels of environmental noise. Moreover, solid concrete barriers between the school building and the noise source can reduce noise radiating into the classroom.

Noise can also originate from internal sources. The most cost-effective procedure for reducing internal noise levels in the room is to relocate the classroom to a quieter area of the building. That is, the classroom must not be located next to the gymnasium, band room, or other high noise source. At least one acoustically dead space, such as a storage area, should separate classrooms from each other or from high-noise sources in the school building. If relocation of the classroom cannot be accomplished, acoustic treatments such as double wall construction of the interior walls, acoustic ceiling tile, carpeting in hallways outside the classroom, and acoustically treated or well-fitting (preferably with a rubber seal) doorways can attenuate internal noise sources. Doors or interior walls should not contain ventilation ducts that lead into the hallways.

Noise also originates from within the classroom itself. Recall that this type of noise may be particularly damaging to speech perception because its spectrum is often similar to the frequency content of the teacher's voice. The simplest procedure for the reduction of classroom noise is the placement of children away from high noise sources, such as fans, air conditioners, or heating ducts. Often, however, these noise sources produce such intense levels that no location in the classroom is appropriate for adequate communication. Classroom noise sources, such as malfunctioning air conditioning units or heating ducts, need to be replaced or acoustically treated. Heating ducts, for example, can be lined with acoustic materials to reduce airborne and vibratory noise. In addition, acoustic modifications such as the installation of thick carpeting or acoustic paneling on the walls and ceiling, placement of rubber tips on the legs of desks and chairs, the use of acoustically treated furniture, and the hanging of thick curtains can also reduce ambient noise generated within the classroom. It is not recommended that children with sensorineural hearing loss, or children with normal hearing, be placed in open plan classrooms because it is well recognized that such classrooms are generally considerably noisier than regular classrooms. In addition, instruction should not take place in areas separated from other teaching areas by thin partitions (particularly those that are not permanently fixed to the floor and ceiling), sliding doors, or temporary walls.

Reduction of Classroom Reverberation Times

Reverberation can be reduced by covering the hard reflective surfaces (bare cement walls and ceilings, glass or mirrored areas, and uncarpeted floors) in a room with absorptive materials. Acoustic paneling on the walls and ceiling, carpeting on the floors, the placement of cork bulletin boards on the walls and curtains on the windows, and the positioning of mobile bulletin boards at angles other than parallel to the walls can decrease reverberation levels in an enclosure. It should be noted that many of the aforementioned acoustic modifications can be achieved at little or no cost to the school system. For example, pieces of carpet strategically placed on a bare cement wall can, at times, dramatically reduce the RT of that learning environment.

Unfortunately, a review of the literature has demonstrated that classrooms often exhibit minimal degrees of acoustic modifications. For example, Bess et al (1984) found that 100% of classrooms had acoustic ceiling tile, but only 68% had carpeting and 13% had draperies. No classroom contained any form of acoustical furniture treatment. Crandell and Smaldino (Crandell & Smaldino, 1994(1)) reported similar findings: all of the

32 classrooms examined had acoustic ceiling tile, but only 19 (59%) contained carpeting. Moreover, only one of the classrooms had drapes (3%), and none of the rooms had acoustic furniture treatments.

Reduction of Speaker-to-Listener Distance

The deleterious effects of noise and reverberation can also be reduced by ensuring that the child receives the teacher's voice at the most advantageous speaker–listener distance possible. Specifically, the child, particularly the child with sensorineural hearing loss, needs to be in a face-to-face situation and in the direct sound field, where the interaction of noise and reverberation are less detrimental to speech-recognition skills. Such a placement would also aid the child in utilizing visual as well as auditory cues. To achieve this recommendation, restructuring of classroom activities must be considered. For example, small group instruction should be considered over more traditional room configuration, where the speaker instructs in front of numerous rows of listeners. Such a recommendation has practical limitations, however, because in typical classrooms the critical distance for maximum speech perception is present only at distances relatively close to the teacher. Hence, the simple recommendation of preferential seating is often not enough to ensure an appropriate listening environment for many children. The utilization of a hearing assistance device, such as a personal frequency modulation (FM) amplification system or sound-field FM amplification system, can also decrease speaker–listener distance and significantly augment speech perception in the classroom. An FM sound field system is essentially a room public address system in which speech is picked up via an FM wireless microphone located near the speaker's mouth, where the effects of noise and reverberation are negligible. The signal is then transmitted to an amplifier and delivered to listeners in the room via several strategically placed loudspeakers. The objectives of such a system are to (1) improve the volume of the teacher's voice approximately 10 dB over the unamplified condition and (2) provide a uniform direct or a speech-reinforcing reflected sound field throughout the classroom. Several investigators have shown that if these objectives are achieved, psychoeducational and psychosocial benefits accrue for children with normal hearing and hearing impairment. For instance, Sarff (1981) utilized a sound-field amplification system in a classroom with children with normal hearing and children with minimal degrees of sensorineural hearing loss. Results indicated that both groups of children, particularly the children with minimal hearing impairment, demonstrated significant improvements in academic achievement when receiving amplified instruction. Moreover, younger children demonstrated greater academic improvements than older children. Crandell (1994) reported that sound-field FM amplification devices can significantly improve the speech perception of nonnative English-speaking children in a classroom setting.

Summary

This chapter has emphasized several of the singular and interactive effects of classroom reverberation, noise, and distance. The acoustic conditions in most classrooms are poorer than what would be recommended for adequate speech perception by children with sensorineural hearing loss and several populations of children with normal hearing. Such findings are alarming because it is well recognized that inappropriate classroom acoustics can deleteriously affect not only speech perception but also psychoeducational achievement. Hence, inadequate classroom acoustics may place many populations of children at risk for language, behavioral, literacy, social, and academic difficulties. To reduce this risk, strategies were suggested to improve classroom S/N ratio and reduce reverberation.

Acknowledgment

Portions of the research cited in this chapter were supported by an Advanced Research Project Grant Texas Higher Education Coordinating Board, and by a Department of Education Research Grant (Listening in Classrooms–Utah State University). Both authors were a part of the ANSI working group responsible for the American National Standard S12.60–2002.

References

American National Standards Institute (ANSI). (1971). Specification for sound-level meters (ANSI S1.4–1971). New York: American National Standards Institute.

American National Standards Institute (ANSI). (1976). Acoustical terminology (ANSI S1.1–1960). New York: American National Standards Institute.

American National Standards Institute (ANSI). (2002). Acoustic performance criteria, design requirements and guidelines for schools (ANSI S12.60–2002). New York: American National Standards Institute.

American Speech-Language-Hearing Association (ASHA). (1994). *Standard on Acoustics in Classrooms.* Rockville Pike: ASHA.

Bench, J., Koval, A., & Bamford, J. (1979). The BKB (Bamford-Koval-Bench) sentence lists for partially hearing children. *Br J Aud, 13,* 108–112.

Beranek, L. (1954). *Acoustics.* New York: McGraw-Hill.

Bess, F., Sinclair, J., Riggs, D. (1984). Group amplification in schools for the hearing-impaired. *Ear Hear, 5,* 138–144.

Blair, J. (1977). Effects of amplification, speechreading, and classroom environment on reception of speech. *Volta Rev, 79,* 443–449.

Bolt. R., & MacDonald, A. (1949). Theory of speech masking by reverberation. *J Acoust Soc Am, 21,* 577–580.

Boney, S., & Bess, F. (1984, November). *Noise and reverberation effects on speech recognition in children with minimal hearing loss.* Paper presented at the American Speech, Language, and Hearing Association, San Francisco.

Bradley, J. (1986). Speech intelligibility studies in classrooms. *J Acoust Soc Am, 80,* 846–854.

Crandell, C. (1993). Noise effects on children with minimal sensorineural hearing loss. *Ear Hear, 14,* 210–217.

Crandell, C. (1994). *Issues in sound field amplification.* Paper presented at the Weekend with the Experts Conference, Improving Classroom Acoustics, Orlando, Florida.

Crandell, C., & Bess, F. (1986). Speech recognition of children in a "typical" classroom setting. *ASHA, 29,* 87.

Crandell, C., & Bess, F. (1987). Sound-field amplification in the classroom setting. *ASHA, 29,* 87.

Crandell, C., & Smaldino, J. (1992). Sound-field amplification in the classroom. *Am J Audiol, 1,* 16–18.

Crandell, C., & Smaldino, J. (1995). The importance of room acoustics. In: R. Tyler, D. Schum (Eds.), *Assistive Listening Devices* (pp. 142–164). Baltimore: William and Wilkins.

Crum, D. (1974). *The effects of noise, reverberation, and speaker-to-listener distance on speech understanding.* Unpublished doctoral dissertation, Northwestern University, Evanston, Illinois.

Crum, D., & Matkin, N. (1976). Room acoustics: The forgotten variable. *Lang Speech Hear Serv Sch, 7,* 106–110.

Danaher, E., & Pickett, J. (1975). Some masking effects produced by low frequency vowel formants in persons with sensorineural hearing loss. *J Speech Hear Res, 18,* 261–271.

Elliott, L. (1982). Effects of noise on perception of speech by children and certain handicapped individuals. *Sound Vibration,* 9–14.

Finitzo-Hieber, T. (1988). Classroom acoustics. In: R. Roeser & M. Downs (Eds.), *Auditory Disorders in School Children* (2nd ed.) (pp. 221–233). New York: Thieme-Stratton.

Finitzo-Hieber, T., & Tillman, T. (1978). Room acoustics effects on monosyllabic word discrimination ability for normal and hearing-impaired children. *J Speech Hear Res, 21,* 440–458.

Gelfand, S., & Silman, S. (1979). Effects of small room reverberation upon the recognition of some consonant features. *J Acoust Soc Am, 66,* 22–29.

Hawkins, D., & Yacullo, W. (1984). Signal-to-noise ratio advantage of binaural hearing aids and directional microphones under different levels of reverberation. *J Speech Hear Disord, 49,* 278–286.

Kalikow, D.N., Stevens, K.N., & Elliott, L.L. (1977). Development of a test of speech intelligibility in noise using sentence materials with controlled word predictability. *J Acoust Soc Am, 61,* 1337–1351.

Knudsen, V., & Harris, C. (1978). *Acoustical Designing in Architecture.* New York: American Institute of Physics for the Acoustical Society of America.

Kurtovic, H. (1975). The influence of reflected sound upon speech intelligibility. *Acoustica, 33,* 32–39.

Leavitt, R., & Flexer, C. (1991). Speech degradation as measured by the Rapid Speech Transmission Index (RASTI). *Ear Hear, 12,* 115–118.

Lochner, J., & Burger, J. (1964). The influence of reflections in auditorium acoustics. *J Sound Vibration, 4,* 426–454.

McCroskey, F., & Devens, J. (1975). Acoustic characteristics of public school classrooms constructed between 1890 and 1960. *NOISEXPO Proc,* 101–103.

Moncur, J., & Dirks, D. (1967). Binaural and monaural speech intelligibility in reverberation. *J Speech Hear Res, 10,* 186–195.

Nabelek, A., & Donahue, A. (1984). Perception of consonants in reverberation by native and non native listeners. *J Acoust Soc Am, 75,* 632–634.

Nabelek, A., & Nabelek, I. (1985). Room acoustics and speech perception. In: J. Katz (Ed.), *Handbook of Clinical Audiology* (3rd ed.) (pp. 834–846). Baltimore: Williams & Wilkins.

Nabelek, A., & Pickett, J. (1974). Monaural and binaural speech perception through hearing aids under noise and reverberation with normal and hearing-impaired listeners. *J Speech Hear Res, 17,* 724–739.

Nabelek, A., & Robinson, P. (1982). Monaural and binaural speech perception in reverberation for listeners of various ages. *J Acoust Soc Am, 71,* 1242–1248.

Neuman, A., & Hochberg, I. (1983). Children's perception of speech in reverberation. *J Acoust Soc Am, 73,* 2145–2149.

Nober, L., & Nober, E. (1975). Auditory discrimination of learning disabled children in quiet and classroom noise. *J Learn Disabil, 8,* 656–677.

Olsen, W. (1988). Classroom acoustics for hearing-impaired children. In: F.H. Bess (Ed.), *Hearing Impairment in Children.* New York: Grune & Stratton.

Paul, R. (1967). *An investigation of the effectiveness of hearing aid amplification in regular and special classrooms under instructional conditions.* Unpublished doctoral dissertation, Wayne State University, Detroit.

Puetz, V. (1971). Articulation loss of consonants as a criterion for speech transmission in a room. *J Audio Eng Soc, 19,* 915–919.

Sabine, W. (1964). *Collected Papers on Acoustics.* New York: Dover.

Sanders, D. (1965). Noise conditions in normal school classrooms. *Except Child, 31,* 344–353.

Sarff, L. (1981). An innovative use of free field amplification in regular classrooms. In: R. Roeser, M. Downs (Eds.). (1981). *Auditory Disorders in School Children* (pp. 263–272). New York: Thieme-Stratton.

Suter, A. (1978). *The ability of mildly hearing impaired individuals to discriminate speech in noise.* (Aerospace Medical Research Laboratory Report No. AMRL-RT-78-4). Wright Patterson Air Force Base, Ohio.

13

Classroom Amplification Systems

CAROL FLEXER

The three great elemental sounds in nature are the sound of rain, the sound of wind, and the sound of the outer ocean on a beach.
—Henry Beston (1888–1968)

We "hear" with the brain. The ears are just a way in. The problem with hearing loss is that it keeps sound from getting to the brain. The purpose of amplification technology is to efficiently and effectively channel sound to the brain.

Recent studies in brain development show that stimulation of the auditory centers of the brain is critical (Boothroyd, 1997; Chermak & Musiek, 1997). Sensory stimulation influences the actual growth and organization of auditory brain pathways. Therefore, anything that can be done to access, grow, and "program" those important and powerful auditory centers of the brain with acoustic detail expands children's opportunities for enhancement of life function. A child's hearing loss can be a roadblock to sufficient sounds getting to the brain unless amplification technologies are used. *Amplification is really about brain stimulation with subsequent brain growth.*

The most common amplification technology is the hearing aid. Unfortunately, hearing aids (and cochlear implants) are not designed to deal with all listening needs. Their biggest limitation is their inability to make the details of spoken communication available to the brain when there is competing noise or when the listener physically cannot be close to the speaker. Because a clear and complete speech signal is essential for the brain growth that leads to the development and expansion of oral expressive language and reading skills, some means for improving the speech-to-noise (S/N) ratio must be provided in every location where a child learns.

One of the most challenging learning locations is the classroom. Children spend a great deal of their time in noisy environments that demand constant, detailed listening to critical instruction that is spoken far from them. Therefore, children with hearing problems require special technologies, in addition to their hearing aids or cochlear implants, that can overcome the barriers of distance and noise. These technologies are personal-worn FM systems and sound-field amplification systems. The secret of their success is the use of a remote microphone that can be placed within 6 inches of the desired sound source, thereby facilitating brain access.

This chapter details the rationale and use of classroom amplification systems.

Definition of Classroom Amplification Systems

Historically, the term "auditory training system" has been applied to any amplification system other than a personal hearing aid. Auditory trainers were introduced into programs for children with hearing impairments about 50 years ago. They were high-power-output amplification units that were used primarily for children with severe to profound hearing impairments who were in self-contained schools or classrooms. The reader is referred to Pimentel (1988), Berg (1993), and Bess and McConnell (1981) for historical descriptions of the following auditory trainers: hard-wired, portable desk auditory trainer, loop (induction), and loop radio frequency (RF) systems. These systems will not be discussed in this chapter.

Because of its history, the term "auditory training system" tends to be associated with a rather restricted population of children (those with severe to profound hearing impairments) in rather restricted settings (self-contained, special education programs) who required high-power-output amplification systems. Please note that the term is not negative; it just might not encompass today's diverse population of children (see Case Study 13–1). It seems that, currently, the term "classroom amplification system" is more appropriate than the term "auditory trainer," and the label "signal-to-noise (S/N) ratio enhancing technology" seems to be even more descriptive of classroom amplification system effectiveness.

Because of the changing demographics and the current mainstream placement of the vast majority of children with hearing problems, this chapter focuses on the two classroom amplification systems most commonly used today: personal and self-contained FM systems, and sound-field amplification systems.

Current Population of Children with Hearing Problems

The use of specific classroom amplification systems is based on the population of children who require the technology. This population has changed over the last few decades (Upfold, 1988). Maternal rubella and Rh incompatibility have been virtually elimi-

nated. Thus there are fewer than half the numbers of children with severe to profound hearing impairments today than there were a few decades ago. Conversely, in the last decade, more than 10 times the number of children with mild to moderate hearing impairments have been identified and fit with amplification.

An additional large population of children who are often not clearly identified are those with hearing problems caused by middle ear dysfunction. Indeed, the incidence of children with persistent minimal to mild hearing impairments caused by otitis media may be much higher than school screenings lead us to believe. Hearing screening environments in schools typically have less than ideal levels of ambient noise, causing hearing to be screened at 20 to 35 dB hearing level (HL). When 15 dB HL is used as the criterion for identifying an educationally significant hearing impairment, the numbers of identified kindergarten and first grade children increase dramatically. A study conducted in Putnam County Ohio found that 43% of their primary-level students failed a 15 dB HL hearing screen on any given day, and about 75% of their primary-level children in classes for children with learning disabilities failed a 15 dB hearing screening (Flexer, 1989). A study by Niskar et al (1998) projected that 14.9% of U.S. school children have hearing loss that can impact their educational progress—that's about 8 million school children!

The point is that the vast majority of children who will require some type of classroom amplification system will be, or certainly ought to be, in mainstream classrooms and not in a self-contained environment. Therefore, audiologists could be even more effective in schools if we expanded our role beyond the special education network into regular education classes.

Rationale for FM Recommendations and Use of a Remote Microphone

School personnel often lack an understanding of the reasons for using classroom ampli-

---

Case Study 13–1   A school-based speech-language pathologist received an audiologist's recommendation for an "FM auditory trainer" for a child who was in a mainstream classroom. The child had a fluctuating hearing loss caused by chronic otitis media. The speech-language pathologist wondered why this child needed the high-power-output unit commonly associated with children with severe hearing impairments in the school's special education program, but he was not familiar with any other kind of "auditory trainer." Because the audiologist's recommendation did not provide a justification for the FM unit, nor did the recommendation state the desired performance characteristics of the FM unit, the speech-language pathologist put an old, high-power output FM unit on the child that had been used in the school's special education program for a child who had a severe to profound sensorineural hearing impairment. That is, this child with a fluctuating, conductive hearing impairment was erroneously fit with a self-contained FM unit (closed earmolds with button receivers, and both environmental microphones on the FM's receiver were activated) that had a 139 dB SPL maximum output.

---

fication systems. Therefore, this section details a compelling rationale for the necessary use of these technologies.

Typical mainstream classrooms are auditory–verbal environments; instruction is presented through the teacher's spoken communication. The underlying assumption is that children can hear clearly and attend to the teacher's speech. Thus children in a mainstream classroom, whether or not they have hearing impairments, must be able to hear the teacher in order for learning to occur. If children cannot consistently and clearly hear the teacher, the major premise of the educational system is undermined.

Levels of Auditory Skill Development

There is a great deal involved in "hearing" the teacher. Erber (1982) was one of the first to identify the levels of auditory skill development associated with "hearing and listening," and Ling (2002) has expanded on them.

- *Detection:* This is the lowest, least sophisticated level of auditory skill development. "Detection" refers to the presence and absence of sound. Obtaining pure tone thresholds is a detection task.
- *Discrimination:* This involves distinguishing between two speech sounds. An example of a discrimination task

would be noting if "pa" and "ba" are the same or different.

- *Recognition:* Selecting a target from a known list of alternatives, recognition is a closed-set task.
- *Identification:* This is an open-set task that involves noting a target from an infinite set of alternatives.
- *Comprehension:* This is the highest level of auditory skill development. Comprehension is achieved when one can answer questions, follow directions, and hold conversations.

It is critical to note that without basic detection, none of the higher levels of auditory processing are available. Therefore, comprehension, the goal of classroom instruction, is completely dependent on the initial detection of individual phonemes that make up the spoken message. Hearing loss, inappropriate amplification and classroom technologies, and challenging acoustic environments all compromise detection. Classroom amplification systems, therefore, function to facilitate detection of the desired auditory signal. Without detection, there can be no comprehension.

Word/Sound Distinctions

Elliott, Hammer, and Scholl (1989) evaluated primary-level children with normal hearing and found that the ability to perform fine-grained auditory discrimination tasks (e.g., to hear "pa" and "ba" as different syllables) correctly classified 80% of the children in their study either as progressing normally or as having language-learning difficulties. The conclusion is that auditory discrimination is associated with the development of basic academic competencies that are critical for success in school. Auditory discrimination cannot occur unless basic detection is first available. A young child who cannot hear (detect) phonemic distinctions is at risk for academic failure.

Audibility versus Intelligibility

The ability to discriminate individual phonemes, to hear word/sound distinctions, is defined as intelligibility. The ability to detect the presence of speech but not identify individual components is called audibility. If, because of poor attending skills, an auditory processing problem, poor classroom acoustics, or a hearing impairment of any degree, a child cannot discriminate "walked" from "walks," for example, he or she will not learn appropriate semantic distinctions unless deliberate intervention occurs.

Invisible Acoustic Filter Effect of Hearing Impairment

The primacy of hearing in the communicative and educational process tends to be underestimated because hearing loss itself is invisible. The effects of hearing loss are often associated with problems or causes other than hearing impairment (Ross, Brackett, & Maxon, 1991). For example, when a child is off-task or cannot keep up with the rapid pace of class discussion, the cause of that child's behavior may be attributed to noncompliant behavior or to attention problems or to slow learning rather than to hearing problems.

One cannot "see" a hearing impairment; therefore, it is easy to confuse the causal hearing loss with the negative consequences of the hearing impairment. To explain, hearing impairment acts like an invisible acoustic filter that interferes with incoming sounds (Ling, 2002). In addition to a reduction in loudness, sounds are often smeared together, or filtered out entirely. Speech, therefore, might be audible but not intelligible. A child with a hearing impairment might be able to hear the presence of speech (audibility), but not be able to hear clearly enough to identify one speech sound as distinct from another. Words like "invitation" and "vacation" might sound the same. It is not difficult to imagine what such word confusions could do to a child's vocabulary and conceptual language development.

This acoustic filter effect is the beginning and the cause of an entire chain of negative events. If speech sounds are not heard clearly, then one cannot speak clearly (one speaks what one hears), unless deliberate intervention occurs. The second step in the chain involves reading ability. If one does not have good spoken language skills, then reading, which is a secondary linguistic function, will also suffer (Robertson, 2000). Said another way, we speak because we hear, and we read because we speak. If reading skills are below average, an individual will have difficulty performing academically. Limited literacy leads to a reduction in professional options and subsequent opportunities for independent function as an adult. The cause of this entire unfortunate chain of events is the ambiguous, invisible, underestimated, and often untreated acoustic filter effect of hearing impairment. Until the primary problem of hearing impairment is identified and managed and the brain has access to detailed sound, intervention at the secondary levels of spoken language, reading, and academics likely will be ineffective.

Computer Analogy

One way to explain the negative effects of any type and degree of hearing impairment on language learning and academic performance is to use a computer analogy. Data input precedes data output. A child must have information or data in order to learn. Information is entered into the brain through the auditory system. If data are entered inac-

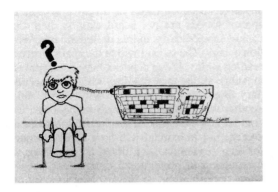

Figure 13–1. Hearing impairment is like having a malfunctioning computer keyboard that enters inaccurate, inconsistent, and incomplete data to the brain. (Illustrated by Josh Klynn.)

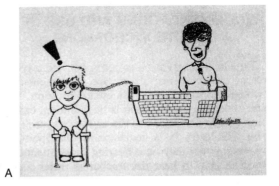

A

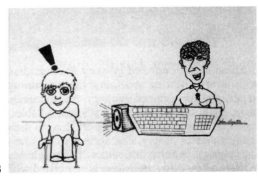

B

Figure 13–2. Classroom amplification systems, such as (A) a personal-worn FM system and (B) a sound-field system, facilitate data entry to the brain by providing a more accessible keyboard. (Illustrated by Josh Klynn.)

curately, like having one's fingers on the wrong keys of a computer keyboard or like having a broken keyboard, then the child will have inaccurate, incomplete, and unreliable data to process (Fig. 13–1). Is it reasonable to expect a child to learn sophisticated spoken communication and to develop academic competencies when the information that reaches the brain is deficient?

Using amplification technology such as a hearing aid, a personal FM system, a sound-field (classroom public address) system, or even a cochlear implant, is analogous to having a better keyboard. The goal in using classroom amplification systems is to provide the best, most consistent and reliable keyboard for instructional data entry (Fig. 13–2A,B). The better a child can detect word/sound distinctions, the better opportunity a child will have for the development of academic competencies.

Once hearing problems are identified and barriers to the clear reception of classroom instruction are removed, analogous to the provision of the best possible keyboard, what happens to all of the previously entered inaccurate and deficient information? Do inaccurate data convert automatically to correct information? Unfortunately, missing data need to be entered and inaccurate data need to be corrected. The longer a child's hearing problem remains unidentified and unmanaged, the more destructive are the negative effects of the acoustic filtering process of that hearing problem.

Managing hearing, beginning with detection, is the crucial first step in the chain of intervention; providing an accurate and reliable keyboard is the prerequisite step to clear data entry. Once hearing has been accessed, a child has an opportunity to learn spoken language as the basis for developing literacy and academic competencies and acquiring knowledge about the world.

Passive Learning/Overhearing/ Distance Hearing

A consequence of hearing impairment and a reason why FM technology needs to be used in a classroom is the concept of distance hearing. Distance hearing is the distance over which speech sounds are *intelligible* and not merely *audible*. Hearing problems of any type and degree reduce the distance over which speech sounds are intelligible, even if one is wearing hearing aids. Typically, the greater the hearing loss, the greater the reduction in distance hearing. Reduction in distance hearing has negative consequences for classroom and life performance because distance hearing is necessary for passive learning (Ross, Brackett, & Maxon, 1991).

A child with a hearing problem, even a minimal one, cannot casually overhear what people are saying. Most children with normal hearing seem to absorb information from their environments; they tend to learn easily information that was not directed to them. Children with hearing problems, however, because of their reduction in distance hearing, need to be directly taught many skills and concepts that other children learn incidentally.

Additional implications of the reduction of distance hearing include lack of redundancy of instructional information and lack of access to social cues. Listening is an active and not a passive process for children with hearing problems. Thus active attention must be directed to appropriate sources at all times. A child's attention will wander often during the school day, causing him or her to miss some of what is being said. Missed information can be offset partially by the use of a remote microphone of a personal FM or sound-field system. The remote microphone can be placed close to the speech or sound source, thereby making information available and alleviating some of the strain and effort of constant disciplined attention.

Level of Effort

Children with hearing problems typically expend a high level of effort as they attempt to learn from classroom instruction. (Case Study 13–2).

As Mark Ross has often stated, the problem with hearing loss is that you do not hear so well. Consequently, you hear what you think you hear, and you do not hear what you do not hear . . . and one does not have a perspective about missed information (Ross, Brackett, & Maxon, 1991).

Speech-to-Noise Ratio

Unfortunately, children are expected to hear meaningful word/sound distinctions in unfavorable acoustic environments. They must listen to a speaker who is not close and who is moving about the room.

S/N ratio is the relationship between a primary signal, such as the teacher's speech, and background noise. Noise is everything that conflicts with the auditory signal of choice and may include other talkers, heating or cooling systems, classroom or hall noise, playground sounds, computer noise, wind, among others. The quieter the room and the more favorable the S/N ratio, the clearer the auditory signal will be for the brain. The farther the listener is from the desired sound source and the noisier the environment, the poorer the S/N ratio and the more garbled the signal will be for the brain. All children—especially those with hearing loss—need a quieter environment and a louder signal than adults do in order to learn.

Persons with normal hearing and intact listening skills require a consistent S/N ratio of approximately +6 dB for the reception of intelligible speech. Because of internal auditory distortion, persons with any type and degree of hearing problem require a more favorable S/N ratio of about +20 dB. Due to noise, reverberation, and variations in teacher position, the S/N ratio in a typical classroom is unstable and averages out to only about +4 dB and may be 0 dB; less than ideal even for children with normal hearing (Crandell & Smaldino, 2002).

Rapid Speech Transmission Index

The negative effects of a typical classroom environment on the integrity of a speech signal probably have been underestimated. Leavitt and Flexer (1991) used the Bruel and Kjaer Rapid Speech Transmission Index (RASTI) to measure the effects of a classroom environment on a speechlike signal. The RASTI signal, an amplitude-modulated broadband noise centered at 500 and 2000 Hz, was transmitted from the RASTI trans-

---

Case Study 13–2 A fifth grade girl with a congenital, mild, sloping to moderately-severe, bilateral, sensorineural hearing impairment and excellent auditory and spoken language skills was earning As and Bs in advanced (mainstreamed) classes. Because she was performing at such a high level, teachers thought that she did not require any support services (such as notetakers, pretutoring of new vocabulary and concepts, captioned instructional materials). She did not use and never had access to FM technology of any kind. Further questioning revealed, however, that she routinely spent 2 to 4 hours per night doing homework, trying to make up for the redundancy of information that she was being denied access to in the classroom. She was expending such a high level of effort that she needed to nap after school; she was also taking antidepressant medication for anxiety. She had no time for extracurricular activities. Children with hearing impairments typically need to exert a higher level of effort than do children with normal hearing to be competitive in school. However, this girl was expending an unnecessary amount of energy trying to gain instructional information on her own that some basic accommodations could have made available to her in the classroom. Interestingly, when initially asked how she was doing in school, she stated, "Everything is fine!" She declined offers of any accommodations such as an FM system. She had no idea that classroom learning could be any easier. She had always worked so hard in school that her perceptions were skewed. This young girl finally agreed to experiment with a personal FM system that provided a favorable acoustic signal and was acceptable socially and visually to her. She also accepted the use of captioned video materials and some preview and review sessions with a tutor. Within one semester, she no longer required naps, homework time dropped to about 1 hour per night, she was taken off the medication, and she joined a soccer team. She was able to maintain her high level of performance with less expenditure of effort and she had time for a life after school.

---

mitter to the RASTI receiver that was placed at 17 different locations around a typical occupied classroom. The RASTI score is a measure of the integrity of signals as they are propagated across the physical space. A perfect reproduction of the RASTI signal at the receiver has a score of 1.0.

Results showed that sound degradation occurred as the RASTI receiver was moved away from the RASTI transmitter as reflected by a decrease in RASTI scores. In the front row center seat, the most preferred seat, the RASTI score dropped to 0.83. In the back row, the RASTI score was only 0.55, reflecting a loss of 45% of equivalent speech intelligibility in a quiet, occupied classroom. Only at the 6-inch reference position could a perfect RASTI score of 1.0 be obtained. Note that the RASTI score represents only the loss of speech fidelity that might be expected at

the student's ear or hearing aid microphone port in a quiet classroom. The RASTI score does not measure the additional negative effects of a child's hearing loss, weak auditory or language base, or attention problems.

Even in a front-row center seat, the loss of critical speech information is noteworthy for a child who needs accurate data entry to learn. The most sophisticated of hearing aids or cochlear implants cannot re-create those components of the speech signal that have been lost in transmission across the physical space of the classroom.

Issue of Acoustic Accessibility

The concept specified by the Rehabilitation Act of 1973, Section 504, that can enable audiologists to recommend classroom amplification systems for children in regular classrooms is called "acoustic accessibility." Audiologists can advocate, proactively, that a child's hearing problem interferes with that child's opportunity to have access to spoken instruction; therefore, that child is being denied an appropriate education. Recognize that schools typically function on a failure-based model. Classroom amplification systems may be provided for children with hearing problems only after they have failed one to three grades or are significantly behind their same-age peers. Because accommodations typically are not allocated to prevent failure, technology is often provided too late to enable the child to catch up to grade level (Flexer, 1999).

Perform Speech-in-Noise Sound-field Testing

By adding only two speech tests to the basic audiometric test battery, an audiologist in a school or clinical setting can provide evidence that a child has a hearing problem that interferes with acoustic accessibility of classroom instruction. *If a child's hearing problem limits acoustic accessibility, then by evoking Section 504 of the Rehabilitation Act of 1973, we can advocate in a proactive fashion for an appropriate classroom amplification system.* That is, we do not have to wait until a child fails and is eligible for special education funding under the Individuals with Disabilities Education Act (IDEA Amendments of 1997), before we can provide services.

To provide functional information about acoustic accessibility, word identification testing should first be performed in the sound field in the unaided condition. If the child wears hearing aids, these same tests can also be performed in an aided condition. Appropriate speech stimuli for the language level of the child should be presented at the average loudness level that a child in a favorable classroom environment (45 dB HL) receives speech. Because the child must also hear soft speech, another list of words should be presented at 35 dB HL. If phonetically balanced (PB) words are presented only at 40 dB sensation level (SL) under ear-

phones, functional information is not provided about accessibility to typical classroom instruction. Words presented at a loud level in perfect quiet always overestimate a child's auditory discrimination ability.

In addition, word identification testing in the sound field ought to be conducted at 45 dB HL using a +5 S/N ratio, a favorable noise level in a primary-level classroom (Berg, 1993). A child might appear to hear very well in the acoustically perfect environment of a sound room but have a great deal of trouble hearing in a typical classroom.

Personnel Involved in Fitting FM Technology

Role of the Audiologist

As specified by the American Speech-Language-Hearing Association (ASHA) Guidelines for Fitting and Monitoring FM Systems (2000), the audiologist is the professional who is uniquely and best qualified to select, evaluate, fit, and dispense FM systems. The necessity of having an audiologist as the "point person" is supported by the American Academy of Audiology, ASHA Codes of Ethics, and federal regulations. There is a great deal of complexity involved in selecting the appropriate FM options and in fitting and evaluating the equipment. An inappropriate FM fit could be worse for a child than not wearing any amplification technology at all. An audiologist can instruct other personnel in performing daily monitoring checks; however, the audiologist must maintain the supervisory position.

Role of the Speech-Language Pathologist

Speech-language pathologists can appropriately perform daily monitoring of classroom amplification systems after they have received instruction from a licensed/certified audiologist. This monitoring role of the speech-language pathologist relative to FM systems is supported by professional organizations. Speech-language pathologists can also (and indeed, should) refer children to an audiologist for an evaluation for FM technology when they encounter children whom they believe would benefit from an improved S/N ratio.

Role of Parents, the Mainstreamed Classroom Teacher, and Other Support Personnel

Parents, mainstreamed classroom teachers, and other personnel who will use the child's FM technology need to receive in-services about the FM equipment. Anyone who is expected to monitor the equipment needs to receive instruction and supervision from an audiologist.

Self-Contained and Personal-Worn FM Systems

Description

An FM unit is an assistive listening device that improves the S/N ratio for a child in a classroom by using a remote microphone that can be placed close to the sound source.

"FM" is a term applied to the radio transmission of signals whereby speech, after being changed into an electrical signal, is frequency modulated onto a carrier wave that is sent from the transmitter to the receiver where it is demodulated and delivered to the listener. A basic FM system consists of two units, a transmitter and a receiver, and is like having an individual private radio station that transmits and receives on a single frequency. The FM receiver worn by the child must be set to the same RF as the microphone/transmitter worn by the teacher, or the child will not receive the desired signal. Because there are no wires connecting the speaker to the listener, both parties have free mobility. The transmission range can vary with different pieces of equipment from about 30 feet to more than 200 feet.

The transmitter microphone is clipped to the speaker's clothing at the midline, no farther than 6 inches from the person's mouth. Think of the FM microphone as the child's third ear and place that third ear within 6 inches of whatever you want the child to hear. The remote microphone of the FM transmitter improves the S/N ratio by being placed close to the primary sound source. The more favorable the S/N ratio, the more intelligible the speech signal received by the brain of the listener. Because sound is degraded as it is propagated across the classroom, the closer the child is to the talker, either physically or technologically, the better acoustic access the child will have. Whenever a child with a hearing problem is in a classroom, technology to enhance the S/N ratio will be necessary to improve intelligibility of the teacher's speech. A hearing aid alone or a cochlear implant alone is never enough in a classroom because the teacher physically cannot be consistently close to the child.

Cautions Regarding Use

FM systems can be of enormous benefit to children who have hearing problems in the classroom. Nevertheless, there are some limitations and cautions that ought to be noted. These issues have been emphasized by Ross (1992), and in ASHA's current Guidelines for Fitting and Monitoring FM Systems (2000).

1. Many FM systems are purchased without consultation with an audiologist because FMs are available commercially. An audiologist should be the professional who is responsible for fitting, evaluating, and dispensing FM systems.

2. Although there is a committee in progress, the American National Standards Institute (ANSI) has not yet issued a standard for performance measurements of FM systems.

3. Currently, there is little regulatory consumer protection for FM fitting and use because most states do not classify these devices as hearing aids. The U.S. Food and Drug Administration may decide differently in the near future.

4. Studies have shown that there are real concerns about specific electroacoustic performance factors. Different FM units and coupling features have shown variability in performance, nonlinearity, lack of stability, and maintenance problems.

5. There are many issues that need to be considered when fitting FM systems on children, including candidacy, a child's many and varied listening/learning domains, effectiveness and flexibility of fit, cost, and psychosocial concerns.

Features of FM Systems

FM systems can be grouped into two general categories, depending on how the signal is delivered to the ear of the listener. A *basic, self-contained FM system* typically delivers the signal via a button receiver/earphone. The FM receiver contains an environmental microphone or microphones, allowing the FM receiver to function also as a hearing aid (usually a body-style hearing aid if the FM receiver is worn on the child's body). A *personal-worn FM system* is similar to a self-contained system except that the child must wear personal hearing aids to deliver the signal.

FM systems can be quite complicated to fit appropriately to a given child because of the many fitting and setting options currently available; there are advantages and disadvantages to each option. The more options available, the better chance we have of providing an appropriate and consumer-acceptable S/N ratio–enhancing device. No single coupling arrangement is automatically superior for all children. The individuality of each child must be considered.

Therefore, not only must an audiologist be the professional to select, evaluate, fit, and dispense FM systems, but that audiologist should also in some way be involved in classroom observations and evaluations of FM settings and function. Ideally, there will be an educational audiologist who can manage the FM technology in school.

Self-Contained FM System

Some FM receivers are designed to function both as hearing aids and as radio receivers. This self-contained system has historically been referred to as an FM auditory trainer. The child who wears hearing aids takes them off when wearing a self-contained unit. The signal is delivered to the child's ears typically through button earphones coupled to custom, snap-ring earmolds. The (hearing aid) environmental microphone or microphones are usually on the FM receiver. Some units have the option of having the environmental microphones and receivers housed in behind-the-ear (BTE) cases for more effective binaural hearing than body-worn microphones can allow.

A bone conduction transducer can be used with some FM receivers. This transducer would be necessary for children who have atresia. A bone conduction transducer could also be a viable option for children who have stenotic earcanals or who experience continually draining ears from chronic otitis media.

Some audiologists fit self-contained FM units as the primary amplification for infants and young children with severe to profound hearing impairments (Madell, 1992). The rationale is that FM units can provide superior auditory access, even in home environments.

An audiologist might fit an FM unit instead of a hearing aid for children with more minimal hearing problems as well. However, in this instance, the FM is not intended to function like a hearing aid but is meant to enhance the S/N ratio in a mainstreamed classroom for children with minimal hearing problems, including unilateral hearing loss, fluctuating hearing impairments, normal peripheral hearing with auditory processing problems, or attending difficulties. This arrangement will be covered under personal-worn FM systems.

Personal-Worn FM Systems—Description

The term "personal-worn FM system" usually refers to an arrangement whereby the FM signal is channeled in some fashion through the child's own hearing aids. For a personal-worn FM system to work, the child's hearing aids must be operating well and efficiently receive the signal from the FM unit. The FM unit cannot work if the hearing aids are not working.

Personal-Worn FM Systems—Recent Advances

There have been several recent advances that have increased ease of use and acceptability of FM technology. All advances involve making the equipment smaller and more flexible. Because of the small size and good sound quality, most students prefer the newer models. However, most of the new technologies are more expensive than the traditional coupling options.

BEHIND-THE-EAR FM RECEIVER/ HEARING AID COMBINATION

Technological developments have provided the option of a hearing aid and FM receiver both housed together in a BTE hearing aid case. There is no body-worn FM receiver. Of course, the talker still needs to wear a microphone transmitter. The child can, by moving a switch, have the unit function as a hearing aid only, an FM receiver only, or as both at the same time. In many school districts, this unit has replaced the traditional body-worn self-contained system.

BEHIND-THE-EAR FM RECEIVER/ NO HEARING AID

Several manufacturers now have FM receivers designed for people with normal or near-normal hearing, built into BTE cases. These devices have low gain and low-power output and may be suitable for children with attention or processing difficulties. There is no hearing aid in the BTE case. Although more expensive than the traditional body-worn FM receiver coupled to Walkman headphones, many children find this unit much more comfortable (fit with an open earmold) and less conspicuous.

FM BOOT

This increasingly popular arrangement is a tiny FM receiver that is built into an audio-input boot (Fig. 13–3). This small boot can be snapped onto certain hearing aids when the FM signal is needed; no body-worn FM receiver is used. Because FM systems also need to be used at home to improve distance hearing and incidental learning, parents find the FM boot user-friendly.

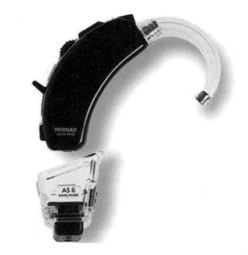

Figure 13–3. Recent technological developments have provided the option of a small FM receiver boot that snaps onto a hearing aid. This small boot replaces a body-worn FM receiver. (Photograph courtesy of Phonak, Chicago, IL.)

FM RECEIVER MODULE FOR A COCHLEAR IMPLANT

An appropriately programmed cochlear implant allows much greater distance hearing than a hearing aid—up to 30 feet, even for voiceless consonants such as "s," "t," "f," and "th." Nevertheless, distance, reverberation, and the movement of sound sources around the room require the use of a remote microphone in order to improve the S/N ratio in a classroom environment.

To date, two companies manufacture small receiver modules specifically designed for cochlear implants. Logicom Ci (AVR Communications, Eden Prairie, MN) is a miniature, synthesized FM receiver, about ½″ × ¾″ × ¾″ that plugs directly into the cochlear implant processor via the auxiliary input. The MicroLink CI and CI+ (Phonak) is a small FM receiver that fits most cochlear implant processors. Both the Logicom Ci and the MicroLink CI and CI+ replace body-worn FM receivers. A caution is that only implant recipients who can report on the quality of the signal they are receiving should use personal FM systems. There is no objective way to determine the quality of sound that is actually being transmitted through the coch-ear implant to the brain of the child. If the child is too young or too inexperienced in listening to provide a reliable report of speech intelligibility, a sound-field system (desktop or whole classroom) can be utilized.

Personal-Worn FM Systems— Traditional Fittings

The traditional coupling options that have been used for years and continue to be used by many school districts include neckloop, silhouette, and direct-input. Each of these coupling arrangements can alter, often in some unpredictable fashion, the output and frequency response characteristics of the hearing aid.

NECKLOOP

With a neckloop coupling, the electrical signal from the FM receiver is sent to a wire or loop that is worn loosely around the child's neck and is attached to the FM receiver. The neckloop generates an electromagnetic field that is picked up by the T attachment on the child's hearing aid or aids and then amplified. Of course, the hearing aids must be equipped with a strong telecoil appropriately positioned in the hearing aid case. To access the many and diverse listening environments that the child must be in, the hearing aids need to have a three-switch setting: M to access the hearing aid's microphone, alone; T to access the hearing aid's telecoil that picks up the signal from the FM microphone, alone; MT together to pick up both the FM signal and environmental sounds and the child's own voice, all at the same time. Each setting has advantages and disadvantages.

A potential problem with neckloop fittings is that a hearing aid's telecoil rarely has the same maximum output and frequency response characteristics as the microphone; the telecoil typically is weaker and tends to roll off the low frequency end of the hearing aid's frequency response. In addition, there can often be an increase in internal noise, and signal strength can change with head

positions. Performance measures need to be obtained.

SILHOUETTE

A T coil in the hearing aid is also needed for a silhouette coupling because this coupling operates on principles similar to the neckloop. The silhouette is actually a wafer-shaped piece of plastic worn between the head and the hearing aid; the silhouette generates an electromagnetic field. A wire connects the silhouette with the FM receiver. A silhouette has the advantage of minimizing signal variation because the position of the silhouette relative to the hearing aid remains constant with changes in head position. A potential wearer-perceived disadvantage is that there is a visible wire.

DIRECT INPUT

For a direct input connection, the electrical signal from the body-worn FM receiver flows through a wire directly into the hearing aid via an audio-shoe or boot. The hearing aid must be equipped with a special feature that will allow it to accommodate a boot. There are many different shapes of boots; some fit snugly on the hearing aid and some fit so loosely that the signal is disrupted easily. The appropriate boot and cords can be obtained from the hearing aid manufacturer. Note that there can be some change in the output signal with FM coupling.

NO HEARING AIDS

Children who do not wear hearing aids and who are fit with FM systems for the single purpose of providing a consistent and favorable S/N ratio are also described as wearing personal FM systems. That is, the FM is not intended to function as a hearing aid, but is fit to enhance acoustic accessibility of intelligible speech and to provide instructional redundancy in a classroom environment. Children who are fit with this intention in mind require a low-power output unit that also has low gain. The gain and output must be specified, known, measured, and controlled by an audiologist. Coupling arrangements used in this instance may include lightweight Walkman earphones, earbuds, stetoclips, and button earphones attached to special custom earmolds.

WALKMAN EARPHONES

Lightweight Walkman-type earphones are commonly used to deliver a monophonic signal (same signal to each ear compared with stereophonic). Because they are lightweight, the child can still hear surrounding sounds. Although suitable for short periods of time, many children find the earphones uncomfortable for 6 hours of daily use. Earbuds and stetoclips, because they are not custom fitted, may also become uncomfortable. For long-term continual use, custom earmolds, or a retention earmold with tubing, may be more acceptable to a child. Keep in mind that any earmold or earpiece potentially changes earcanal resonance.

Children Who Could Benefit from FM Use

Anytime a child with a hearing problem is in a classroom or cannot be close to the speaker, an improved S/N ratio will be necessary to facilitate the reception of an intact, consistent, and clear speech signal. It was thought in the past that preferential seating was enough. However, information about classroom acoustics shows that hearing aids alone, no matter how "good" the hearing aid is, cannot substitute for the remote microphone of an FM unit in a classroom or in any environment in which the speaker cannot consistently be close to the child. FM units can also facilitate communication and incidental learning in the home, car, and grocery store, and at dance lessons, on the soccer field, and other such locales.

FIT AN FM UNIT FIRST ON SOME CHILDREN

There are some instances, such as when a child has a unilateral hearing loss, a fluctuating hearing loss, or a slight permanent hearing impairment, when it might be more ef-fective to fit a mild-gain personal FM unit or a sound-field system instead of, or before, a hearing aid. To explain, a child with the types of hearing problems just mentioned might do fine in a quiet, one-to-one learning situation, but that same child will have difficulty in a typical, noisy, distracting classroom. Thus, it makes sense to address the most pressing concern first: classroom listening.

Audiological Management and Monitoring of FM Equipment

There are many audiological management issues to be considered. A child who has a hearing problem and wears an FM system should hear the teacher much better when the teacher speaks into the FM microphone. If the child does not hear better with the FM system than without it, check the FM. Is the fit appropriate? Is there interference? Any number of problems could occur. Experience has shown that whenever a teacher says a child does not seem to benefit from an FM system, the FM system has been malfunctioning in some way or has not been fitted or used appropriately. Double check the equipment and teacher use first, do not just remove it. Observe, personally, how the equipment is actually set up and used in the classroom (see Case Study 13–3).

Additional management issues to consider involve microphones and both daily and comprehensive monitoring of FM systems.

MICROPHONES

Microphones are critical and often misused elements of classroom amplification systems. There are many microphone options for the talker (Lederman & Hendricks, 2000). There are directional and omnidirectional microphones. In addition, one can choose lapel, collar, or boom microphones for the transmitter. A single directional FM transmitter microphone worn on the head of the talker (boom microphone) would provide the best S/N ratio. However, some teachers resist wearing a head-worn microphone due to comfort or cosmetic reasons.

Case Study 13–3 A mainstreamed kindergarten boy with a moderate, conductive hearing loss due to congenital ossicular malformations told his teacher that he heard much better with his hearing aids than he did with his FM unit; the school system was ready to allocate his FM unit to someone else. The child had been fit with a personal-worn FM using a neckloop coupling. His hearing aids had a good telecoil and M, T, and MT settings. The FM performance features were appropriate for the child, and the teacher had been taught about equipment use. However, a visit to the classroom revealed that the equipment was not being used as intended. The school had substituted a different FM transmitter for the original one. Unfortunately, the new transmitter was set to a different carrier frequency than the child's receiver. In addition, the teacher had put the child's hearing aids on T (they should have been on MT), but the receiver was not picking up the teacher's voice anyway (wrong transmission frequency). That is, the child was hearing only static with the FM. Of course he heard better with his hearing aids. When the personal FM was set, adjusted, and used appropriately, this child heard very well and insisted on wearing his FM unit. This teacher obviously had not been performing listening checks on the equipment or she would have discovered that something was wrong. Moreover, this school system did not have an educational audiologist. The director of special education made the decision to change FM transmitters.

The listener also has several microphone options. Does the listener want to use the FM microphone only? or to use environmental microphone(s) as well? Are the environmental microphones worn at ear level? or are they on the body, in a pocket, on the desk, or in a belt pack? How many microphones are there? What is the relationship between the FM microphone sensitivity and environmental microphone sensitivity? Think of each active microphone as an "ear" and be sure to identify the location of all ears. The more microphones that are activated, the poorer the S/N ratio. Unfortunately, most children object to not hearing their own speech and the speech of their peers. Thus microphone use is not a simple matter, nor is it a fixed variable. That is, sometimes the child needs to hear the teacher only, and sometimes the child needs to monitor the environment, his or her own voice, or the voices of peers.

One solution is to teach the child to control and switch the technology as needed. Another option is to have a teacher (FM) microphone that preempts the child's environmental microphone. Whenever the teacher speaks into the FM microphone, the environmental microphones on the FM receiver are automatically turned off. Some personal FM systems offer this feature.

Another issue about microphone use is that people who are not speaking into the FM microphone will not be heard well, or perhaps not heard at all. So teachers will either have to pass the FM microphone around to classmates or repeat others' comments.

DAILY MONITORING OF FM SYSTEMS

The one certainty about equipment is that it will malfunction at some point in time. FM breakdowns occur even in normal-use situations. Therefore, daily monitoring is essential. A daily visual and listening check should be performed by an audiologist or by someone who has been instructed in the appropriate procedures by an audiologist. Speech-language pathologists, parents, and teachers often fill this role. Someone who has normal hearing should perform the procedure in the environment in which the child will be learning. Spare supplies and equipment should be available to remedy easy-to-fix problems. Examples of supplies include batteries, neckloops, microphones, button receivers, boots, and cords.

COMPREHENSIVE MONITORING OF FM SYSTEMS

Children with hearing impairment who are 3 years and younger should be seen by their audiologist every 3 months for comprehensive evaluation, including FM monitoring. The audiologist should see children over 5 years of age at least yearly. As recommended by ASHA (2000) these assessments may include, but are not limited to: audiological evaluations, assessments of speech recognition, coupler and real ear performance measurements of hearing aids and FM equipment, consultations with school personnel, observation of FM performance in school settings, and subjective scales of performance benefit.

Performance Measures

There are no validated procedures for measuring and fitting FM systems. Several approaches have been proposed and these have been incorporated into the recent updated ASHA guidelines (2000). These 2000 guidelines have been revised from the original 1994 guidelines. They highlight four issues that need to be considered in developing FM measurement strategies:

1. Because the FM microphone is located about 6 inches from the speaker's mouth, the input level of speech to the FM microphone is more intense than to a hearing aid microphone that is located, in a favorable situation, about 1 to 2 m from the speaker. The overall level of speech to the FM microphone is about 80 to 85 dB sound pressure level (SPL), which is about 10 to 20 dB more intense than the typical 60 to 70 dB SPL input to the microphone of a hearing aid. Therefore, if appropriate output measurements are being made to adjust FM systems, then typical input levels should be used. The higher level is particularly important because most FM microphone transmitters use some type of input compression; the gain and output of the FM system could be quite different if lower-level signals are used.

2. Many FM systems have more than one microphone-input possibility. There could be lapel, lavalier, boom, or conference microphones for the FM transmitter. The FM receiver could have one or two environmental microphones and they could be on the body or at ear level. In addition, the microphones could be omnidirectional or directional. Each input channel in the FM system needs to be evaluated and the microphones need to be positioned appropriately. Input levels would be different for environmental microphones and FM microphones.

3. Many FM systems have more than one volume control wheel; some units have one volume control wheel for the FM signal and another one for the environmental microphone or microphones. On personal FM systems, there will be one volume control wheel for the FM system and one for each personal hearing aid. There also might be a volume control on the FM microphone transmitter. Careful thought needs to be given to the setting and measurement of each volume control wheel.

4. FM systems are physically arranged on the user in different ways. Testing procedures need to account for these differences. Please refer to the ASHA (2000) guidelines for the following performance measurements:

   • Outline for FM system gain adjustment using 2 ccc coupler assessment
   • Outline for FM system adjustment using probe-microphone measurements
   • Recommendations for monitored live-voice assessment of speech perception with the FM system

Sound-Field Systems—FM or Infrared

Description

Sound-field technology is an exciting educational tool that allows control of the acoustic environment in a classroom, thereby facilitating acoustic accessibility of teacher instruction for all children in the room (Crandell, Smaldino, & Flexer, 1995). Sound-field systems are like high fidelity, wireless, public address systems. By using this technology, an entire classroom can be amplified through the use of one, two, three, or four wall- or ceiling-mounted loudspeakers. A wireless microphone transmitter worn by the teacher, and just like the one worn for a personal FM unit, sends the teacher's voice via radio waves (FM) or light waves (infrared) to an amplifier that is connected to the loudspeakers. Figure 13–4 shows an example of an infrared sound-field system. There are no wires connecting the teacher with the equipment. The radio or light wave link allows the teacher to move about freely, unrestricted by wires.

Proposed New Term: "Sound-Field Distribution System"

The term "sound-field distribution system" has been proposed as being more descriptive of sound-field function. To explain, some teachers, parents, and acoustical engineers interpret the labels "sound-field amplification" or "classroom amplification" to mean that all sounds in the classroom are made louder. This misunderstanding may give the impression that sound is blasted into a room causing rising noise levels, interfering with instruction in adjacent rooms, and provoking anxiety in pupils. In actuality, when the equipment is installed and used appropriately, the reverse is true. The amplified teacher's voice can sound soothing because it is evenly distributed throughout the room easily reaching every child. The room quiets as students attend to spoken instruction. In fact, the listener is aware of the sound distribution and ease of listening only when the equipment is turned off. The overall purpose of the equipment is to improve detection by having the details of spoken instruction continually reach the brains of all pupils.

Features of Sound-Field Distribution Systems

A sound-field system is one type of assistive listening device. Like a personal FM unit, it improves the S/N ratio by the use of a remote microphone that can be placed close to the desired sound source. Through the loudspeakers, the loudness of the teacher's speech is increased relative to the background noise, allowing all children in the room to benefit from an improved and consistent S/N ratio no matter where they or the teacher are located (Flexer, 1998).

A major difference between a sound-field distribution unit and a personal FM system is that the personal FM, if fit appropriately, can provide the most favorable S/N ratio; +20 to +30 dB. A personal FM unit transfers the speech signal from the microphone transmitter, which is located about 6 inches from the teacher's mouth, directly into the ear of the child who is wearing the FM receiver. A sound-field unit transmits the teacher's speech from the microphone, worn 6 inches from the mouth, to the amplifier/ loudspeakers that are located at some distance from the children. The children can be consistently closer to loudspeakers than they can be to the teacher, but not as close as a child could be to the headphones of the FM unit. Sound-field systems typically improve the classroom S/N ratio by about 10 dB.

Therefore, sound-field units are not replacements for personal FM systems because some children require the more favorable S/N ratio provided by a personal FM unit. Sound-field technology offers audiologists another tool to select from when recommending appropriate classroom amplification systems.

Sound-Field Infrared Technology

A new type of infrared (IR) technology has been developed for the classroom, and it has met with commendable success (Knittel, Myott, & McClain, 2002). IR has the following advantages over the traditional FM tech-

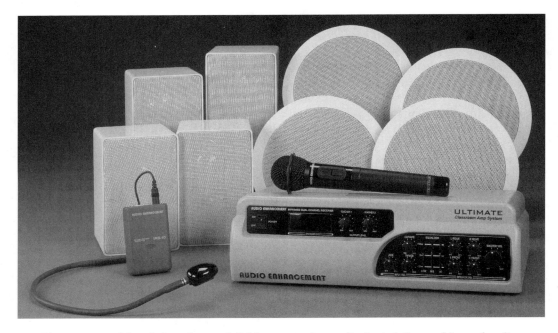

Figure 13–4. New infrared sound-field systems have eliminated the problem of radio-wave interference by using light wave transmission. Also pictured is a handheld, pass-around microphone for use by children in the classroom. (Photograph courtesy of Audio Enhancement, Bluffdale, UT.)

nology: IR systems provide crystal clear, full bandwidth, high fidelity audio; IR signals do not travel through walls, allowing an unlimited number of systems to be used in the same building; importantly, IR is unaffected by any form of RF interference.

Personal/Desktop Sound-Field Amplification

A relatively new type of sound-field FM system is called a personal sound-field unit, or a desktop system (Pillow, 1998). This is a small, lightweight, battery-powered portable loudspeaker that can be carried from class to class and delivers a clear, close-up sound right to the student's desk. Foster, Brackett, and Maxon (1997) found the personal sound-field FM system to be particularly useful for children with cochlear implants due to the proximity of the loudspeaker to the child.

Children Who Might Benefit from Sound-Field Distribution Systems

It could be argued that *virtually all children* could benefit from sound-field distribution systems because the improved S/N ratio creates a more favorable learning environment. If children could hear better, more clearly, and more consistently, they would have an opportunity to learn more efficiently. Some school systems have as a goal the amplification of every classroom in their districts (Knittel, Myott, & McClain, 2002).

No one disputes the necessity of creating a favorable visual field in a classroom. A school building would never be constructed without lights in every classroom. However, because hearing is invisible and ambiguous, the necessity of creating a favorable auditory field may be questioned by school personnel. Nevertheless, studies continue to show that sound-field systems facilitate opportunities for improved academic performance (Arnold & Canning, 1999; Flexer, 2000; Rosenberg et al, 1999).

The populations that seem to be especially in need of S/N ratio–enhancing technology include children with: fluctuating conductive hearing impairments; unilateral hearing impairments; "minimal" permanent hearing impairments; auditory processing problems; cochlear implants; cognitive disorders; learning disabilities; attention problems; articulation disorders; and behavior problems (Crandell, Smaldino, & Flexer, 1995).

Teachers who use sound-field technology report that they also benefit. Many state that they need to use less energy projecting their voices, they have less vocal abuse, and are less tired by the end of the school day. Teachers also report that the unit increases their efficiency as teachers by requiring fewer repetitions, thus allowing for more actual teaching time.

With more and more schools incorporating principles of inclusion where children who would have been in self-contained placements are in the mainstream classroom, sound-field distribution systems offer a way of enhancing the classroom learning environment for the benefit of all children. It is a win–win situation.

The Issue of Literacy and Sound-Field Distribution Systems

Literacy is a national priority, and we still face substantial challenges. In the year 2000, data showed that the percentage of fourth grade students reading at or above "proficient," the level identified by the National Assessment Governing Board (NAGB) as the goal for all students, has increased slightly to 32% from 29% in 1992 (National Center for Education Statistics, 2001). These data mean that only about a third of fourth graders in the United States can read at their grade level. Moreover, although scores for the nation's highest-performing students have improved over the years, scores of the lowest-performing students have declined.

Of critical importance is the fact that there has been no closing of the education gap between students who are white and students who are minorities. Specifically, in the year 2000, 40% of fourth grade students who are white and 46% of students who are Asian/Pacific Islander could read at or above the proficient achievement level (National Center for Education Statistics, 2001). However, only 12% of students who are African American, 16% of students who are Hispanic, and 17% of students who are Native American could read at or above the Proficient achievement level (National Center for Education Statistics, 2001).

There is evidence that sound-field distribution systems can improve literacy development. Numerous studies have been reported (Crandell, Smaldino, & Flexer, 1995). A recent article by Darai (2000) found that sound-field systems, when appropriately used, provided significant improvement in literacy achievement of first grade students. Flexer (2000) reported a study of three first grade classrooms in Utah where 85% of the children were Native American. In the 5 years prior to sound-field use, only 44 to 48% of first grade children scored at the "basic" level and above on the Utah State Core Reading Test. After only 7 months of sound-field use, 74% of the 54 children in the study scored at the basic level and above. Another study found that phonemic awareness skills were most effectively and efficiently taught in preschool and kindergarten classrooms that had sound-field distribution systems. In fact, the fewest at-risk readers came out of the classrooms that routinely used their sound-field distribution systems (Flexer, Biley, Hinkley, Harkema, & Holcomb, 2002).

Audiological Equipment Selection Considerations

There are many issues to consider prior to recommending sound-field distribution technology.

1. Should an audiologist recommend a personal FM system or a sound-field distribution system, or both, for a given child?

Once it is determined that a child has a hearing problem that interferes with acoustic accessibility, the next step involves recommending, fitting, and using some type of S/N ratio–enhancing technology. One thing is certain; one cannot manage hearing by not managing hearing. Children with more severe hearing impairments and with more severe auditory processing and attending problems benefit more from the superior S/N ratio provided by an appropriately fit personal FM system. In addition, children with a permanent hearing impairment will require S/N ratio–enhancing technology throughout their school career, including postsecondary education. It is unlikely that every classroom will be amplified for these children, so a personal FM system would be a more parsimonious recommendation.

The question is often asked if both sound-field distribution systems and personal FM systems can be used in the same room. The answer is yes. In many instances, using both at the same time can create the best listening and learning environment. In fact, this author typically recommends using both because each serves a different purpose. The sound-field distribution system appropriately installed and used in a mainstream classroom improves and equalizes acoustic access for all pupils and creates "listening" in the room. The individual-worn FM system allows the particular child with hearing aids to have the most favorable S/N ratio. The teacher need wear only a single microphone/transmitter if the sound-field unit and the individual FM are on the same RF, or if the personal-worn FM transmitter can be coupled to the sound-field amplifier.

2. Should an audiologist recommend equipment based on a treatment or on a universal design perspective?

Historically, amplification technologies such as hearing aids, personal FM systems, and now cochlear implants have been recommended as treatments for hearing loss. Because there certainly are populations for whom an enhanced S/N ratio can mean the difference between passing and failing in school, sound-field technologies came on the scene as treatments for hearing problems. If viewed as a treatment, sound-field technology is recommended for a particular child and managed through the special education system.

However, with the recognition that all children require an enhanced S/N ratio comes the necessity of moving beyond thinking of sound-field technology as a *treatment.* Sound-field distribution systems need to be integrated into the general education arena. The concept of universal design can be useful in this regard.

The concept of universal design originated in the architectural domain with the common examples of curb cuts, ramps, and automatic doors. After years of use, it was found that the modifications, which were originally believed to be relevant for only a few people, turned out to be useful and beneficial for a large percentage of the population.

In terms of learning, universal design means that the assistive technology is not specially designed for an individual student but rather for a wide range of students. Universally designed approaches are implemented by general education teachers rather than by special education teachers (Research Connections, 1999).

3. Are classroom acoustics a variable in the effective utilization of sound-field distribution systems?

Absolutely! The better the acoustics are in a room, the more effective the sound-field system will be. Other than the children in the room, heating, ventilating, and air conditioning systems (HVAC) are the primary sources of noise (Anderson, 2001).

Reverberation, the noise generated by speech itself that is reflected off of room surfaces, is the most problematic (Boothroyd, 2002). In reverberation, the preceding phonemes blend into the following ones, obscuring the word. Sound-field systems are most effective in overcoming noise and least effective in overcoming reverberation. Therefore, reverberation should be reduced as much as possible before installing sound-field distribution systems.

Classroom acoustics have gained a great deal of attention in the last few years. The American National Standards Institute (ANSI) developed a national standard that was published in June 2002 (ANSI S12.6 2002). The standard calls for noise levels in classrooms to be no higher than 35 dBA. The new standard for reverberation of medium-sized classrooms is 0.6 sec and for large rooms is 0.7 sec (Crandell & Smaldino, 2002). The S/N level is not specified but it is implied to be +15 dB because the noise level should be 35 dBA and the average speech level is 50 dBA. The goal is for the ANSI standard to be adopted into the International Building Code (IBC).

4. What could interfere with the effectiveness of a sound-field distribution system?

Difficulties can result from two primary categories; lack of teacher and administrator information about the rationale and use of the technology, and inappropriate setup and function of the equipment itself.

Initial inservices to teachers and administrators need to emphasize the "brain development" purpose of acoustic accessibility. The relationship of hearing to literacy needs to be targeted, as does the fact that children listen differently than adults. The concept of S/N ratio needs to be explained. Microphone techniques need to be demonstrated to teachers so that they can learn how to use the equipment to teach "incidental listening" strategies. Teachers can use a much softer and more interesting voice because the sound-field distribution system provides the vocal projection. Problems can result when teachers place limitations on their teaching, or when they teach the same way with the technology as without it. A second microphone in the classroom—a pass-around, handheld microphone for the students—can greatly enhance teacher effectiveness (see Fig. 13–4).

Equipment problems can result from improper placement of loudspeakers. In fact, loudspeakers are probably the weakest link. If the primary problem in a classroom is noise, place loudspeakers high for coverage and to reduce feedback (Boothroyd, 2002). If the primary problem in the classroom is reverberation, first acoustically treat the classroom to reduce the reverberation problem as much as possible. Then place the loudspeakers low for proximity (Boothroyd, 2002).

Other equipment problems can include improper microphone placement, lack of sound balance in the room, lack of tuning (not enough high frequencies for consonant enhancement), feedback, interference (if FM transmission is used), and volume that is too soft (Crandell, Smaldino, & Flexer, 1995). Of course, teachers need ongoing support. Someone needs to be designated to troubleshoot the equipment, and replacement parts such as batteries and microphones need to be readily available.

5. Are there efficacy measures that should be used?

Certainly there is a need for a relatively easy measurement tool that teachers can use in a repeated fashion to monitor the effectiveness of the sound-field distribution system. The Screening Instrument for Targeting Educational Risk (SIFTER) is an example of one tool that can be used in this way (Anderson, 1989). The SIFTER relies on the teacher's observations of a child's classroom performance related to listening skills. Areas targeted by the SIFTER include academic performance, attention, communication, class participation, and school behavior. The teacher fills out this brief checklist.

Another tool, the Listening Inventory for Education (LIFE) is a self-report inventory for school-aged children that measures a student's perceptual change (Anderson & Smaldino, 1996). The LIFE consists of pictures of common classroom situations that could provide a listening challenge to the pupil. The child indicates how much difficulty is experienced in each listening situation. The LIFE could be administered before installation of the equipment and then again after about 6 months of use.

Obtaining Funding for Technology

A major issue relative to FM equipment use is money. Who is going to pay for this technology? Some of the newer personal FM technologies can cost up to $2800 for receiver boots and transmitter. For some units, coupling options (earphones, neckloops, direct-input cords, and boots), battery chargers, and patch cords are all extra. Sound-field distribution systems can cost from $850 to $2000—they average $1000 per room.

There are three main options for purchasing the equipment. First, the family could pay and thereby control use of the equipment. Second, community agencies such as local civic groups (like the Lion's club or Quota club), Parent–Teacher Associations, or foundations could be petitioned and fund the technology. Finally, the school could pay and thereby control use of the equipment. There are three primary federal laws that mandate audiological services for children in schools: Education for All Handicapped Children Act of 1975 (Public Law 94–142), the Handicapped Act Amendments of 1986 (Public Law 99–457) that reauthorized and expanded Public Law 94–142), and the Rehabilitation Act of 1973, Section 504. In 1990, Congress amended Public Law 99–457 and changed its name to the Individuals with Disabilities Education Act (IDEA). All of these laws require that children with disabilities have access to a "free appropriate public education (FAPE)."

One point to emphasize when advocating for S/N ratio–enhancing technology for a student is that acoustic accessibility is not a luxury, it is a necessity. Hearing is a first-order event for children in mainstreamed classrooms. If a child cannot clearly and consistently hear classroom instruction, the entire premise of the educational system is undermined. Few families or schools have money for devices that are perceived as frills. However, when hearing takes its proper place at the head of the line relative to academic opportunities, then recommendations for S/N ratio–enhancing technologies are taken seriously.

Summary

This chapter has identified many issues regarding rationale, recommendations, management, and use of classroom amplification systems. Hearing is a first-order event in a mainstream classroom. If a child cannot clearly hear spoken instruction, the entire premise of the educational system is undermined. Due to poor acoustic conditions and a variety of hearing and attending problems, there are millions of children who are being denied an appropriate education due to the lack of acoustic accessibility. Classroom amplification systems can enhance significantly the classroom learning environment by improving the S/N ratio. The better and more consistent the S/N ratio, the more accessible will be the teacher's spoken instruction to the brains of pupils. Audiologists and speech-language pathologists are uniquely positioned to make critical differences for children. We must not underestimate the power of hearing and the necessity of developing the auditory centers of the brain. Our advocacy for a child could mean the difference between success and failure in school.

References

American National Standards Institute (ANSI). (2002, June 26). American National Standard acoustical performance criteria, design requirements and guidelines for schools (ANSI S12.6 2002). New York: American National Standards Insitute.

Anderson, K.L. (1989). Screening Instrument for Targeting Educational Risk (SIFTER). Tampa, FL: Educational Audiology Association.

Anderson, K.L. (2001). Voicing concern about noisy classrooms. *Educational Leadership,* April, 77–79.

Anderson, K.L., & Smaldino, J. (1996). Listening Inventory for Education (LIFE). Tampa, FL: Educational Audiology Association.

American Speech-Language-Hearing Association (ASHA). (2000, Spring). Guidelines for fitting and monitoring FM systems. *ASHA* (Suppl. 20), 20–21.

Arnold, P., & Canning, D. (1999). Does classroom amplification aid comprehension? *Br J Audiol, 33,* 171–178.

Berg, F.S. (1993). *Acoustics and Sound Systems in Schools.* San Diego: Singular.

Bess, F.H., & McConnell, F.E. (1981). *Audiology, Education, and the Hearing-Impaired Child*. St. Louis: C.V. Mosby.

Boothroyd, A. (1997). Auditory development of the hearing child. *Scand Audiol, 26* (Suppl. 46), 9–16.

Boothroyd, A. (2002). *Optimizing FM and sound-field amplification in the classroom*. Paper presented at the American Academy of Audiology National Convention, Philadelphia.

Chermak, G.D., & Musiek, F.E. (1997). *Central Auditory Processing Disorders: New Perspectives*. San Diego: Singular.

Crandell, C., & Smaldino, J. (2002). *Classroom acoustics*. Paper presented at the American Academy of Audiology National Convention, Philadelphia.

Crandell, C., Smaldino, J., & Flexer, C. (1995). *Sound-Field FM Amplification: Theory and Practical Applications*. San Diego: Singular.

Darai, B. (2000). Using sound-field FM systems to improve literacy scores. *ADVANCE for Speech-Language Pathologists & Audiologists, 10*, 5, 13.

Education for the Handicapped Act Amendments of 1986. (Pub.L.No. 99–457, October 8, 1986). *United States Statutes at Large, 100*, 1145–1177.

Education of the Handicapped Act Amendments of 1990. (Pub.L.No. 101–476, October 30, 1990). *United States Statutes at Large, 104*, 1103–1151.

Education for All Handicapped Children Act of 1975. (Pub.L.No. 94–142, November 29, 1975). *United States Statutes at Large, 89*, 773–796.

Elliott, L.L., Hammer, M.A., & Scholl, M.E. (1989). Fine-grained auditory discrimination in normal children and children with language-learning problems. *J Speech Hear Res, 32*, 112–119.

Erber, N. (1982). *Auditory Training*. Washington, DC: Alexander Graham Bell Association for the Deaf and Hard of Hearing.

Flexer, C. (1989). Turn on sound: An odyssey of sound-field amplification. *Educational Audiology Association Newsletter, 5*, 6–7.

Flexer, C. (1998). *Enhancing classrooms for listening, language, and literacy*. (Videotape). Layton, Utah: Info-Link Video Bulletin.

Flexer, C. (1999). *Facilitating Hearing and Listening in Young Children* (2nd ed.). San Diego: Singular.

Flexer, C. (2000). The startling possibility of soundfield. *ADVANCE for Speech-Language Pathologists & Audiologists, 10*, 5, 13.

Flexer, C., Biley, K.K., Hinkley, A., Harkema, C., & Holcomb, J. (2002). Using sound-field systems to teach phonemic awareness to preschoolers. *Hear J, 55*, 38–44.

Foster, S.M., Brackett, D., & Maxon, A.B. (1997). *Cochlear implant users listening in noise: Benefits of sound-field amplification*. Paper presented at the American Academy of Audiology National Convention, Ft. Lauderdale.

Individuals with Disabilities Act Amendments. (1997). 20 (USC §§ 1414).

Knittel, M.A.L., Myott, B., & McClain, H. (2002). Update from Oakland schools sound-field team: IR vs FM. *Educational Audiology Review, 19*, 10–11.

Leavitt, R.J., & Flexer, C. (1991). Speech degradation as measured by the rapid speech transmission index (RASTI). *Ear Hear, 12*, 115–118.

Lederman, N., & Hendricks, P. (2000). A comparison of assistive listening system microphones. *Educational Audiology Review, 17*, 16–17.

Ling, D. (2002). *Speech and the Hearing Impaired Child* (2nd ed.). Washington, DC: Alexander Graham Bell Association for the Deaf and Hard of Hearing.

Madell, J.R. (1992). FM systems for children birth to age five. In: M. Ross (Ed.), *FM Auditory Training Systems: Characteristics, Selection and Use* (Chap. 7). Timonium, MD: York Press.

National Center for Education Statistics, National Assessment of Educational Progress (NAEP). (2001). *1992–2000 Reading Assessments*. Washington, DC: U.S. Department of Education Office of Educational Research Improvement.

Niskar, A.S., Kieszak, S.M., Homles, A., Esteban, E., Rubin, C., & Brody, D.F. (1998). Prevalence of hearing loss among children 6 to 19 years of age: The third national health and nutrition examination survey. *JAMA, 279*, 1071–1075.

Pillow, G. (1998). New personal soundfield from Audio Enhancement: A review. *Educational Audiology Review, 15*, 20.

Pimentel, R.G. (1988). Classroom amplification systems for the partially hearing student. In: R. Roeser, & M. Downs (Eds), *Auditory Disorders in School Children* (Chap. 12) (2nd ed.). New York: Thieme.

Rehabilitation Act of 1973. (Pub.L.No. 93–112, September 26, 1973). *United States Statutes at Large, 87*, 355–394.

Anonymous. (1999). Universal design: Ensuring access to the general education curriculum. *Research Connections in Special Education, 5*, 1–2.

Robertson, L. (2000). *Literacy Learning for Children Who Are Deaf or Hard of Hearing*. Washington, DC: Alexander Graham Bell Association for the Deaf and Hard of Hearing.

Rosenberg, G.G., Blake-Rahter, P., Heavner, J., Allen, L., Redmond, B.M., Phillips, J., & Stigers, K. (1999). Improving classroom acoustics (ICA): A three-year FM sound-field classroom amplification study. *Journal of Educational Audiology, 7*, 8–28.

Ross, M. (1992). *FM Auditory Training Systems: Characteristics, Selection and Use*. Timonium, MD: York Press.

Ross, M., Brackett, D., & Maxon, A. (1991). *Assessment and Management of Mainstreamed Hearing-Impaired Children*. Austin, TX: PRO-ED.

Upfold, L.J. (1988). Children with hearing aids in the 1980s: Etiologies and severity of impairment. *Ear Hear, 9*, 75–80.

14

Assistive Devices

CAROLYN H. MUSKET

"The time has come," the Walrus said, "to talk of many things. . . . "
—Lewis Carroll, *Through the Looking Glass*, 1871

The term "assistive device" is used within the discipline of audiology to refer to any device, other than personal hearing aids or a cochlear implant, designed to improve communication or awareness of auditory signals in the environment for those with hearing loss. The term "hearing assistive technology" is also used in this context. An assistive device may be used alone or may supplement hearing aid or cochlear implant use in specific situations. For example, some assistive devices are used to transmit speech more efficiently or supply text to foster communication between a speaker and a listener with hearing loss. Other devices improve use of the telephone, television, or computer. Finally, there are devices that alert a person to environmental events by transforming an auditory signal into a visual or tactile stimulus. Some assistive devices, such as the frequency modulation (FM) and infrared systems discussed in Chapter 13, greatly improve the classroom learning environment. Others, including many of the devices mentioned in this chapter, are used outside the classroom and improve the functioning of the student with hearing loss in the activities of daily living.

The Individuals with Disabilities Education Act–Reauthorization (IDEA, 1997) includes a broader definition. The term "assis-

tive technology device" refers to "any item, piece of equipment, or product system, whether acquired commercially off the shelf, modified, or customized, that is used to increase, maintain, or improve the functional capabilities of a child with a disability" (34 CFR 300.5). Moreover, IDEA requires that schools consider assistive technology devices when developing a special education student's individualized education plan; they must provide such a device if it is determined that the child requires it in order to receive a free and appropriate education.

There is a need for teachers, clinicians, parents, students, and others to be knowledgeable about the vast assistive device resources available today to help achieve communication access and independent functioning in daily living. This chapter provides an overview of the extensive and versatile array of assistive devices that may benefit students with hearing impairments and acquaints the reader with the various federal laws that mandate and regulate many of them.

Assistive Devices for Telecommunications

It is a necessity to be able to communicate using a phone in our society. The options to make this possible for those with hearing loss are impressive and ever expanding.

Telephones and Hearing Aid Compatibility

Some hearing aids include a telecoil, also known as an induction coil, to help the wearer use the telephone. Telecoils are usually found in behind-the-ear instruments; however, it is also possible to incorporate them effectively into smaller in-the-ear hearing aids. When a conventional hearing aid input switch is on T (telecoil) or the telecoil program of a programmable hearing aid is selected, only the telephone signal will be amplified. For this to occur, the telephone receiver must generate a magnetic field sufficient to induce current flow in the hearing aid telecoil. This is in addition to the acoustic signal of the voice familiar to all. Surrounding noise in the area is not amplified because the hearing aid microphone (M) is not activated.

A series of legislative acts in this country have done much to ensure that all telephone handsets are capable of producing a suitable magnetic field and, therefore, are compatible or usable with hearing aids having a telecoil. The Telecommunications for the Disabled Act of 1982 (PL 97–410) requires that essential telephones, such as pay phones and emergency-use phones, must be compatible with hearing aids and mandates that technical standards be established to guarantee such compatibility. According to PL 97–410, new telephones provided in business and other buildings for use by the public, such as hotel house phones and airport paging phones, must be hearing aid compatible. Moreover, telephone packaging must be labeled to provide information about compatibility with hearing aids. Universal compatibility was furthered when Congress passed the Hearing Aid Compatibility Act of 1988 (PL 100–394), which stated that all corded and cordless telephones manufactured or imported in this country must be hearing aid compatible. After several years of negotiations, in 1996 the Federal Communications Commission issued implementation regulations for PL 100–394 for workplace phones. These rules require that wire-line phones in the workplace, hospitals, nursing homes, hotels, and motels be hearing aid compatible by the year 2000. However, businesses that purchased new phone equipment between 1985 and 1989 have until 2005 to comply. Also, as of 2000, these rules require that new and replacement telephones installed in the workplace have volume controls. This feature is helpful to those who have hearing loss and also to people with normal hearing when there is noise in the background. Companies with fewer than 15 employees are exempt from these requirements.

Amplified Replacement Handset

Telephones with a volume control wheel or touch bar in the handset to increase the intensity of the signal will become more prevalent in the workplace. On other modular phones, it is a simple procedure to install amplified replacement handsets provided the phone does not have the dialing mechanism in the handset. However, replacement handsets are not used very often because of difficulty in matching the style and color of the handset being replaced; other amplification options are available that are easier to obtain.

In-Line Amplifier

In-line amplifiers are convenient to use provided the telephone does not have the dial in the handset. An in-line amplifier may be plugged into the base of a modular telephone after removing the existing handset cord; this cord is then connected to the amplifier. A sliding switch on the amplifier increases the intensity of the telephone signal. An in-line amplifier should have its own power source because the electronic telephones in use today do not provide the necessary power for these add-on devices to operate. Both mild gain and moderate gain in-line amplifiers are available. In-line amplifiers are the option of choice with multiline phones because few of these phones are available with built-in amplification at present.

In-Line Telephone Adapter

This device is similar to the in-line amplifier just discussed because it is also attached to the handset cord jack on the base of the telephone. However, an in-line adapter has an additional component—a cable that may be connected via the input jack to an assistive listening device such as a personal communicator or FM transmitter. This device is especially useful to those with severe hearing impairment because it sends the telephone signal to the listening system they are using and may allow them to hear it binaurally. Telephone adapters are often included as an accessory to an assistive listening device. The Williams Sound TeleLink is an example of this type of device.

Portable Amplifier

A portable amplifier may be carried with the user and placed over the receiver end of a telephone handset when the need arises; the unit is held tightly in place by an elastic strap. A rotary dial or sliding switch controls the intensity; a battery supplies the power. This device offers a mild boost in gain.

Amplified Telephone

Various amounts of gain have been built into a variety of telephones, both corded and cordless (Fig. 14–1). There are mild, moderate, and powerful amplified telephones. These telephones have special features; some, for example, provide greater gain in the high-frequency range, and many offer dual adjustments for both gain and frequency response. In addition, such phones often have an audio output jack so the user may connect the phone to a hearing aid using a direct auditory input cord or inductive coupler (neckloop or silhouette) or to a cochlear implant processor using an adapter cable. Use of a neckloop is an especially helpful option to those with severe hearing loss because it allows binaural hearing if both hearing aids have telecoils. This output

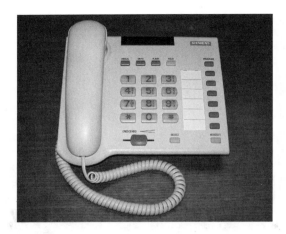

Figure 14–1.   An amplified corded telephone.

jack may also be used to provide binaural hearing through the use of a headset. Usually, these special telephones have large number pads, a visual ring indicator, and controls to adjust the volume and pitch of the ringer. Telephones with more than 18 dB of gain must reset to standard volume when the handset is returned to its base to protect persons with normal hearing who may use the phone (Federal Communications Commission, 2000). Thus the stronger amplified phones have a single button to depress to activate a predetermined amplification level when someone with hearing loss uses the phone.

Speakerphone

A speakerphone allows the child wearing hearing aids to hear the telephone binaurally. This is especially useful for the child who has in-the-ear aids without telecoils. Such an arrangement avoids placing the telephone handset near the hearing aid microphone, which may precipitate acoustic feedback (whistling). It is best if the speakerphone is fully duplex to allow simultaneous two-way conversations without the unnatural clipping of sentences.

Cellular Phone

Digital wireless technology is spreading rapidly and replacing analog cellular phones. When first introduced, digital cell phones often caused interference or a buzzing sound when placed in close proximity to hearing aids in either the microphone or telecoil mode. Manufacturers of current hearing aid models have been successful through design changes and shielding to protect microphones from this interference (Killion, 2001). However, in general, hearing aid wearers who must use a telecoil with a digital cell phone cannot do so in the traditional manner of placing the phone near the hearing aid set on T. The easiest way to confirm this is to try the hearing aid with the particular cell phone (and service provider) in question. More information about susceptibility to such interference should be available to hearing aid users in the future. A new standard has been approved that will provide a rating category for the immunity of a hearing aid (in both microphone and telecoil modes) to electromagnetic interference (American National Standard Institute, 2001). This standard also assigns a rating to the level of the electromagnetic field generated by various digital cell phones. Thus potential cell phone users will be able to match a phone to the capabilities of their hearing aid so that the two devices will function together at an acceptable level of performance. Meanwhile, some manufacturers make an accessory neckloop for cell phones, which counteracts the buzzing interference by separating the phone from the hearing aid telecoil. This arrangement has the added advantage of permitting hands-free use of the phone because the neckloop has a built-in microphone. Finally, there are other types of accessories for a cell phone that are designed to provide amplification to the acoustic speech signal.

Caller ID

It is helpful for the child who reads to have a visual display of the calling party's number and name through Caller ID. Knowing who is calling may enable the child with hearing loss to anticipate certain vocabulary and conversational topics. Also, the phone number for return calls is readily available and

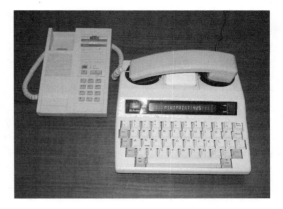

Figure 14–2. A TTY coupled for use with the telephone.

does not have to be understood as part of an auditory message.

Text Telephone

A text telephone (TTY), also known as a telecommunication device for the deaf (TDD), offers visual access via text to telephone communication for those who cannot understand an amplified voice over the telephone or for those who are speech impaired (Fig. 14–2). A TTY typically has a keyboard for touch-typing, an illuminated light emitting diode (LED) screen to display the message, acoustic couplers, and a power supply. Some TTYs provide a hard copy printed record of the conversation. More elaborate models have other options, which may include a voice synthesizer to announce a TTY call, automatic answering, and memory for storing messages. A typical TTY is a little larger than a standard telephone; compact models are available that are small enough to be carried in a purse or briefcase. Versions exist for the pay phone also. When using this device, a telephone handset is placed in the cups of an acoustic coupler on the TTY; some models allow the TTY to be connected directly to an analog telephone line. The user types a message that is converted into tones and conveyed over the telephone line to another TTY, which transforms the message back into visual form. In this arrangement, both the sender and receiver of the message must have a TTY; they communicate by sending a visual, typed message over a telephone connection. It is also possible for a personal computer to be modified to communicate with a TTY.

Telecommunications Relay Service

Telephone calls may occur between TTY users and regular telephone users through a third-party relay service. Title IV of the Americans with Disabilities Act of 1990 (PL 101–336) requires that telephone companies must provide local and long-distance telecommunications relay services (TRS) nationwide. With this service, a TTY user calls a relay operator, known as a communication assistant (CA), who then calls the voice telephone party. When the three-way connection is established, the CA reads aloud what the TTY user types to the person called and transcribes the spoken reply into text for the TTY user. Calls from voice telephones to TTYs follow the same procedure via TRS. Children with intelligible speech and impaired hearing may expedite the process by using the voice carry over (VCO) option. With VCO, once the TRS connection is made, the caller with hearing loss speaks directly to the party called and reads the reply sent by the CA. Because VCO callers only need a screen to view text, and not a keyboard, there are telephones specifically for this purpose (Fig. 14–3). The TRS may also be used to retrieve voice messages on an answering machine or from a voice mail system. TRS is available in Spanish upon request. Several TRS providers offer video relay interpreting (VRI), although it is not required at this time. VRI allows individuals who use sign language to make calls through remote interpreters using desktop computers with videoconferencing capabilities. Other technological innovations, such as higher speed transmission and voice recognition software programs, will increase the speed of TRS calls in the future and help to make them functionally equivalent to voice telephone calls.

Initially, each state had a different phone number to access its TRS. However, in 1997

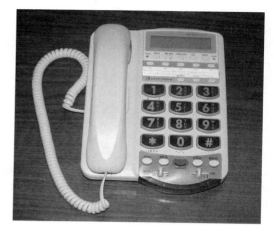

Figure 14–3. A voice carry over (VCO) telephone.

the Federal Communications Commission directed that 711 be reserved nationwide to access relay services. This rule was fully implemented in 2001; now one may dial 711 from any location in the United States and be connected with the area's TRS. Canada also has implemented 711 TRS access in each of its provinces. This abbreviated dialing may not work with certain cellular phones, and some office phone systems may require reprogramming before 711 access is possible.

Internet Protocol Relay Services

Relay calls may be placed via a computer connected to the Internet; it is not necessary to have a TTY. Text to speech calls may be made this way through several Internet relay service providers.

Wireless Messaging Services

Versatile handheld paging devices offer the mobility and convenience of wireless technology to those with hearing loss who rely on text, as opposed to voice, when communicating. The capabilities of modern pagers have been expanded beyond simply receiving messages. These devices now have a small keyboard and a larger screen, yet still remain palm-sized. Special two-way communication services, such as WyndTell, may give the user access to alpha pagers, e-mail, TTY messaging, text-to-voice messaging, and fax machines. Some service plans provide Internet access and target Web sites of interest to those with hearing loss.

E-mail, Fax, and Instant Messaging

Electronic mail (e-mail), facsimile transmission (fax), and instant messaging on the computer are prevalent forms of communication today. They are especially applicable for those with hearing loss because they are text-based systems.

The Telecommunications Act of 1996

Telephone equipment and services are improving for those with hearing loss and other disabilities because of passage of the Telecommunications Act of 1996 and its associated accessibility guidelines. Provisions in section 225 of this law require telecommunication manufacturers and service providers to make their equipment and services accessible to those with disabilities, if readily achievable. If this is not possible, the law directs manufacturers and service providers to make their products and services compatible, where readily achievable, with existing peripheral devices and specialized equipment commonly used by those with disabilities. "Readily achievable" has been interpreted to mean accomplished without much difficulty or expense, relative to the size of the company. For example, a recent innovation allows portable TTYs to be connected to some digital cellular phones; thus TTY users have access to this current wireless telecommunications technology. Section 225 also requires that persons with disabilities must be able to use new products and services; consequently, they must have access to information about them. In the case of hearing loss, this can mean captioned product instructional videos and direct accessibility via TTY to manufacturers' customer service departments. This law and its implementation guidelines will have far-reaching effects in the future because its scope is broad.

Telephone Equipment Distribution Programs

Many states have telephone equipment distribution programs. These programs issue specialized telephone equipment free of charge or at a discount to those with disabilities, which includes hearing loss. Qualifications for participants vary among states. To learn more about a particular state, consult the Web site of the Telephone Equipment Distribution Program Association (www. tedpa.org). This organization coordinates information about existing programs and describes the need for such distribution programs.

Assistive Devices for Television

Assistive devices, using either auditory or visual approaches, are available to improve television viewing for those with hearing impairments; some devices are also suitable for the radio or systems that reproduce music. Those devices involving audition are based on the concept of presenting an amplified audio signal much closer to the ear of the listener with hearing impairment, thereby overcoming the problems associated with distance, room reverberation, and noise. Most personal listening systems, discussed later in this chapter, may also be adapted for use with television.

Hardwire

A simple hardwire arrangement involves plugging a headset into the "phones" jack of a television set; however, this may disconnect the TV speaker for others unless a second jack provides the option of hearing simultaneously via both speaker and earphones. Not all television sets have this output jack. Therefore, it is also possible to position a small microphone by the TV speaker to capture sound; a long cord from this microphone leads to a battery-powered amplifier, which allows the user to select additional volume. Various couplers may be used with this amplifier: monaural or binaural earbuds or button receivers; a headset; and a neckloop or silhouette inductor or a direct auditory input cable to be used with hearing aids. Although many variations of the preceding description are possible, a feature all have in common is that wires connect all components.

Frequency Modulation (FM) Broadcast

The battery-powered transmitter of a personal FM system may be coupled to a television set, either directly through a cable inserted into a phones jack or acoustically with a microphone placed near the speaker. The audio portion of a TV program then becomes an FM radio signal that is broadcast to a battery-powered receiver worn by the viewer. The choice of couplers for the user includes earbuds, a headset, and neckloop or silhouette inductor or direct auditory input to a hearing aid. Instead of a personal receiver, some manufacturers offer a small, remote loudspeaker that may be located next to the listener with hearing impairment. FM systems are wireless between the TV and the viewer.

Infrared Light

An infrared (IR) system is also wireless from the TV set to the viewer (Fig. 14–4). An AC powered IR transmitter is situated near the TV and connected to either a microphone to pick up sound from the speaker or to a cable

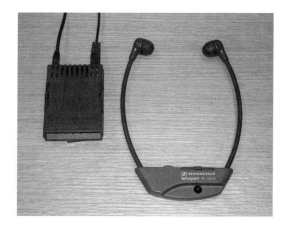

Figure 14–4. An infrared assistive listening device for TV has a transmitter (left) and stethophone receiver (right).

leading to the television's audio output jack. This transmitter contains several LEDs that send invisible beams of infrared light to a receiver used by the viewer. The type of receiver varies; it may be worn suspended under the chin (stethophone), as a headset, or lavalier-style around the neck. All receivers contain a small diode that must be exposed to the infrared beams from the transmitter to operate. Some receivers may interface with a hearing aid having a telecoil or direct auditory input capability (see Case Study 14–1).

Induction Loop

An area induction loop may be used during television viewing. Again, a microphone placed near the TV speaker serves as input to an AC-powered amplifier; the electrical signal from this amplifier is sent throughout a closed wire loop antenna that encircles the listening area. The loop may extend around the room or enclose only the chair of the viewer. To benefit from the electromagnetic signal emanating from the loop, the listener needs either a hearing aid or a personal body-worn receiver containing a telecoil.

Television-Band Radio

A simple, yet effective, way to amplify TV sound for those with impaired hearing is with a portable or tabletop radio that has very high frequency channels 2 to 13 for the audio portion of TV programs. TV sound is transmitted in FM bands outside the range of most FM radios, but special radios with this feature are available. The radio may be located beside the viewer, tuned to the station also selected for the TV, and adjusted to a comfortable volume. An earphone, headset, or inductive coupler may be plugged into an output jack. A limitation of this device is that it cannot be tuned to UHF or cable channels and must be readjusted every time the TV channel is changed.

Closed-Captioned Television, Videos, and DVDs

"Closed captions" refers to a text display of spoken words presented on the television

Case Study 14–1 A.T., age 9 years, had a moderately severe, bilateral, sensorineural hearing loss above 500 Hz and wore binaural behind-the-ear hearing aids most of the time. She was enrolled and mainstreamed in a third grade classroom. A.T. enjoyed watching TV, but sat very close to the TV set at home and did not wear her hearing aids. Mrs. T brought A.T. to our Assistive Devices Center to investigate help for A.T.'s TV viewing. The use of closed captions was recommended and a captioned version of the previous day's *Sesame Street* program, which had been recorded in anticipation of their appointment, was shown. In addition, A.T. was fitted with an infrared receiver coupled via a silhouette inductor to her hearing aid set on T (telecoil). A wireless system was chosen because of other small children in the family. Amy watched and listened from across the room. "Gee, Mom," she volunteered, "I never knew that fellow's name before!" A.T.'s parents purchased an infrared system for TV. Moreover, Mrs. T moved the infrared system to another room in the evenings to use as a personal communicator, with a microphone as the input, when she tutored Amy in her lessons. Next, A.T. started taking the infrared system to school whenever use of a TV, VCR, or other audio source was scheduled for the class. Her teacher used the system when announcing the weekly spelling test words. In fact, A.T.'s use of an infrared system with her personal hearing aids demonstrated to both family and teachers that improved performance was possible in certain situations. At the last meeting of her school's Admission, Review, and Dismissal Committee, the decision was made to provide a personal FM system for her to use daily in the classroom. Surely, A.T.'s use of assistive devices is a success story.

screen. The Television Decoder Circuitry Act of 1990 (PL 101–431) requires that TV sets with screens 13 inches or larger and manufactured or imported into this country after July 1993 contain built-in decoders for displaying captions. A closed-caption decoder may be purchased separately and connected to older television sets. With a decoder, the audio portion of a TV program appears as captions on the screen, much like subtitles for a foreign film. Thus a viewer with impaired hearing may read dialogue and narration to supplement what is heard; for the deaf, captions replace the sound track. Closed captions are transmitted on line 21, field 1 and field 2, of the TV broadcast signal, which has been reserved by the Federal Communications Commission (FCC) for this purpose. Multilingual captioning is possible; for example, *Plaza Sesamo,* the Spanish language version of *Sesame Street,* may be seen with Spanish captions. Internal circuitry to decode closed captions may also be found in videocassette and DVD players.

The United States Congress established the National Captioning Institute (NCI) in 1979 to provide closed-captioning services for TV broadcasts. NCI, along with some other companies, continues to caption all types of TV programs. Prerecorded shows are captioned in advance of the broadcast. News programs and live events, such as sports, are captioned as they occur through realtime captioning; these captions are created on a computerized stenotype machine. The Telecommunications Act of 1996 promotes the use of closed-captioned programming; implementation guidelines from the FCC became effective in January 1998. For programming that first aired prior to the effective date, a 10-year transition period is allowed; by the end of this time, 75% of the old programming must be closed captioned. Programs initially broadcast after the FCC ruling became effective have an 8-year transition period to achieve captioning for 100% of these new programs. Spanish-language programs have similar FCC guidelines. Prerule Spanish-language programs have a 14-year time frame to implement closed captioning for 75% of these programs. All new post-rule Spanish-language programs must be closed captioned within 12 years of January 1998 (National Association for the Deaf, 2000). Notable exemptions to this mandate are programs in languages other than English or Spanish and nonvocal musical programming. Program listings in the newspapers and magazine guides identify a closed-captioned program through use of the initials "CC."

A large number of movies are closed captioned in their videocassette and DVD versions and are identified as such on the packages. In addition, most DVDs offer subtitles in multiple languages. However, closed captions and subtitles have different formats; closed captions include information about sound effects (phone ringing, car horn) because they are intended for those with hearing loss.

Studies have shown that students with hearing impairments who read at or above the third grade level significantly increase their comprehension of televised programs when closed captions are added (Braverman, 1981; National Captioning Institute, 1983). Captioned TV has the potential not only to increase comprehension of a program but also to improve reading and language skills when used over a period of time. Children with hearing losses, like all children, find televised material highly interesting and the addition of closed-captions gives them greater access to spoken language and a means of enriching vocabulary. It is an effective tool, also, for non-English-speaking students learning English.

Alerting Devices

As a part of daily activities, one must respond appropriately to a variety of non-speech auditory signals. The ring of the telephone, the chime of a doorbell, and the buzz of an alarm clock are essential cues for independent living (see Case Study 14–2). Moreover, one's actual safety depends on being able to hear the sound of a smoke detector or security alarm. Those with impaired hearing may not hear these auditory signals. Consequently, there is a wide array of devices and systems that offer help in this area. Primarily, these assistive devices must detect and announce the occurrence of a specific sound by converting it into a stimulus that will be perceived in various places. The number of options and possible combinations makes this a complex topic. First, sounds may be detected via (1) a monitoring microphone, (2) a direct electrical connection, or (3) inductive coupling. Then the occurrence of a sound may be converted into (1) a more suitable auditory signal that is louder or lower in pitch, (2) a visual signal, such as a flashing light or strobe, or (3) a vibrotactile signal, such as a pager or bed shaker. Finally, these devices may signal the existence of a sound (1) near the original sound or (2) in a remote location. To add further possibilities, there are single-purpose devices as well as systems designed for total facility monitoring. The following sections describe common solutions for certain situations and should help acquaint the reader with the type of help available to improve the detection of alerting and warning sounds.

Telephone Ring

Portable telephone ring amplifiers may be plugged into any modular telephone jack. These amplifiers have controls to increase the volume and to change the actual ring into a warble tone or low-pitched sound more likely to be heard by those with hearing loss. Other units are available that feature a strobe light or make it possible for an incandescent lamp to become a flashing signaler in any room. A vibrotactile receiver worn on the body can be activated by the ring of the telephone through use of a remote transmitter connected to the telephone jack. A slightly different problem occurs when it is desirable to distinguish incoming TTY calls from conventional voice calls once the phone rings. A telephone service, usually known as "Distinctive Ring," will provide two numbers on one phone line. This feature

Case Study 14–2 Mrs. H. telephoned the Assistive Devices Center on behalf of her son to inquire about alarm clocks modified for use by those with impaired hearing. She was told such clocks were available with either a flashing visual or a vibrotactile signal; in standard or travel size; and as a single-function clock or combined with an alert for the ring of the telephone. She was amazed—and so were we. Her son was 23 years old! Why did this mother wait until now to learn about this option? Why did she, rather than her son, contact us? How can our educational system help those with impaired hearing learn about assistive devices to enable them to make telephone calls and to awaken at the proper time each morning—to enable them to have communication access and independence?

may be used to differentiate incoming TTY phone calls from other calls.

Doorbell

Doorbell chimes may be replaced with an extra-volume bell or buzzer and extended by use of remote receivers in other rooms. Visual signaling systems, which use flashing lamps or strobes, may be installed with or without an existing doorbell. A doorbell transmitter may also trigger a wearable vibrotactile receiver.

Door Knock

A device containing a strobe may be attached to a dormitory room, bedroom, or bathroom door and will flash in response to a knock at the door. It may also be obtained in a model that works in conjunction with a body-worn vibrotactile receiver.

Wake-up Alarm

Modified alarm clocks have outlets for connection to a lamp or bed vibrator to act as an alternative signal (Fig. 14–5). In some systems, this clock may serve as a remote receiver for the telephone, doorbell, or baby cry transmitters. A smaller, travel-size clock clipped to a pillow contains a battery-powered vibrator. Still another electrical device, a universal sound signaler, is sensitive to any nearby sound and may be used with a regular alarm clock. It will activate a lamp or bed vibrator plugged into it when the alarm sounds.

Smoke Detector

One type of device activates a strobe light or bed shaker when its microphone senses the occurrence of the sustained, intense sound of a smoke alarm. In other systems, the smoke detector and transmitter are combined in one unit that activates a visual or vibrotactile alert.

Computer Accessibility

A flashing screen or blinking words may replace the audible prompt on a computer to relay an attention-getting visual warning signal. These visual alerts are available as customized options on computer operating systems such as Windows and Mac. It is noteworthy that the computer speaker volume may also be increased. Other options

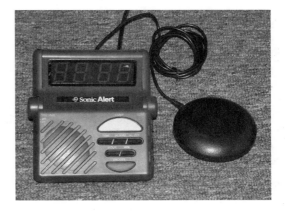

Figure 14–5. An alarm clock with a vibrotactile bed shaker (right).

display captions for speech and sounds on software with these features.

Multipurpose System

Monitoring several different auditory signals in a residence may be accomplished through a single multipurpose system. Access to remote alerting signals may be accomplished several ways. There may be a radio transmission link between different locations, such as between telephone and doorbell transmitters and a body-worn vibrotactile receiver. Also, the existing electrical wiring in a home may be used to carry the signal from a transmitter to a remote receiver. Thus a transmitter plugged into both an electrical outlet and a phone jack will send a signal when the phone rings to receivers connected to both a lamp and an electrical outlet in other rooms. A central controlling unit will recognize input from various sensing transmitters and give a response unique to each. In a visually based system, a light may flash a distinctive coded pattern to differentiate the doorbell from the telephone. For a vibrotactile system, each remote sensor transmitter may be identified by a specific light and symbol on a body-worn receiver.

Hardwire Assistive Listening Devices

Personal assistive listening devices (ALDs) improve interpersonal communication in difficult listening situations. In most instances, they offer the user a way to overcome problems due to noise. To some extent, they may reduce the effects of speaker distance depending upon the length of the cords used. Hardwire devices are for stationary, one-on-one communication situations and are less mobile and less expensive than the personal FM systems described in Chapter 13. A hardwire ALD has the basic components of an amplification system: a built-in or removable microphone, an amplifier, and a receiver, which is usually a single mini-earphone or headset (Fig. 14–6). In the most flexible configuration, an extension cord may be used to allow some distance be-

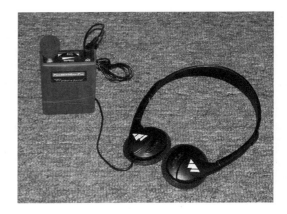

Figure 14–6. A hardwire personal communicator.

tween the speaker's microphone and the user's amplifier/receiver. Then it is possible for the person speaking to hold this remote microphone 6 to 8 inches from the mouth, or clip it to a lapel, making the message spoken much more intense than any surrounding noise. The listener, a comfortable conversational distance away, is tethered to the talker with cords, but profits from the enhanced speech-to-noise ratio that this system allows. Such a listening arrangement may be helpful in restaurants and automobiles, for example, to an aided listener who can connect the ALD to a hearing aid through direct auditory input or by induction. An unaided listener may require less amplification and wear a mini-earphone or headset. Several manufacturers produce hardwire ALDs. It is also possible to assemble a simple system from components readily available at electronics stores. One needs a lapel-clip or handheld microphone, a low-gain mini-amplifier-speaker, and a monaural headset. A speech-language pathologist, counselor, or diagnostician might use a hardwire ALD when working one-on-one with some children. It is helpful with a child whose hearing aids are not functioning. When the device is used with a child who has a very mild hearing loss or normal peripheral hearing and an auditory processing disorder, it should provide only minimal amplification. In the latter case, a program of supervision and monitoring has been recommended (ASHA,

1991). A hardwire ALD is not appropriate in the regular classroom; instead, a wireless personal or desktop FM system for the teacher and student will provide both flexibility and the desired speech-to-noise ratio (see Chapter 13).

Large Area Assistive Listening Systems

Assistive listening systems (ALS) for the benefit of those with impaired hearing may be found in large assembly areas, such as auditoriums, convention center meeting rooms, concert halls, stadiums, cinemas, and theaters due to federal law. Houses of worship may offer this assistance voluntarily. These listening systems are classified according to the transmission technology they use: FM broadcast, infrared light, or induction loop.

Frequency Modulation Broadcast

In addition to classroom use (see Chapter 13), FM assistive listening systems may be installed in large assembly areas. A base station transmitter is connected to a facility's existing public address system. Low gain FM receivers compatible with the transmitting frequency of the base station are available on site for use by those with hearing loss. Provision may be made for these receivers to interface with hearing aids having a telecoil or direct auditory input or with a cochlear implant. If more powerful or nearby transmitters share the same frequency, radio wave interference could potentially occur. However, FM systems are economical for large areas and free of electrical interference, and they allow mobility among users. These advantages have promoted the use of FM assistive listening systems in assembly areas such as cinemas and houses of worship.

Infrared Light

Infrared assistive listening systems are confined to large indoor areas because bright sunlight is a source of interference. Panels containing large LED arrays are connected to a public address system or a movie's soundtrack, for example, and positioned strategically above the assembly area; they transmit information by radiating invisible infrared light waves over the entire audience. Infrared receivers, described in a previous section of this chapter, are available for use by those with impaired hearing in attendance. Infrared light cannot penetrate walls; consequently, this technology is often chosen for adjoining rooms or settings where security of the information transmitted is of prime importance. Infrared systems operate on different subcarrier frequencies. Persons who use IR receivers at home when viewing TV may take these same receivers to use at facilities equipped with an IR assistive listening system only if both systems operate on the same transmitting carrier frequency. Infrared systems have been installed in many live performance theaters throughout the country and also in courtrooms.

Induction Loop

Because an induction loop (IL) is simply a loop of wire, it may encircle a listening area of any size; the two ends of the wire are attached to a loop amplifier whose input is a microphone or other signal source. The current passing through the wire creates an electromagnetic field that reflects the strength and frequency of the input signal. This electromagnetic field generates voltage proportional to the current in the loop in another coil of wire (such as a telecoil) within its range. Thus, to benefit from an IL arrangement, those with hearing loss need either a hearing aid with a telecoil or a special receiver equipped with a telecoil. The latter may be pocket-sized with earphones attached or a wand held to the ear like a telephone handset.

High-powered amplifiers are needed for a large area loop. If only a smaller assembly area is looped, then listeners using the IL system must sit in a designated place, and some view this as a disadvantage and discriminatory. Induction loop systems are susceptible to electromagnetic interference from electrical wiring, fluorescent lighting, transformers, electric motors, and similar sources.

Moreover, the strength of the signal varies according to location within the loop; a signal is stronger near the perimeter and weaker in the center. An electromagnetic field will pass through walls; thus spillover to receivers in adjacent rooms is possible. Oval Window Audio has developed a three dimensional (3-D) induction loop embedded in a special mat designed to be placed beneath a classroom's carpet (Hendricks & Lederman, 1991). Major advantages of the 3-D system are reported to be greater uniformity of the signal and minimal spillover. Induction loops are used widely as assistive listening systems in Europe, where telecoils in hearing aids are common. However, IL assistive listening systems are not prevalent in the United States at this time (Ross, 2002).

Architectural Barriers Act of 1968

The Architectural Barriers Act (ABA) of 1968 prohibits architectural barriers in federally funded buildings and facilities to ensure accessibility to people with disabilities. Regulations known as the Uniform Federal Accessibility Standards (UFAS) apply. Assembly areas with audio amplification systems are required to have a listening system to assist persons with hearing loss. Induction loops and radio frequency systems, which include light wave systems, are listed as acceptable. For assembly areas without amplification systems, a permanently installed or portable listening system is mandated (Architectural and Transportation Barriers Compliance Board, 1982).

Americans with Disabilities Act of 1990

The Americans with Disabilities Act (ADA) of 1990 extended communication access for those with disabilities to the public sector (state and local governments) and the private sector (public accommodations). The term "public accommodation" refers to 12 categories of privately operated entities, including places of exhibition (museums); entertainment (theaters, stadiums, concert halls); and public gathering (auditoriums, convention centers). Private membership clubs and religious organizations are exempt. According to present ADA accessibility guidelines (ADAAG, 1994), a public accommodation must provide auxiliary aids to remove communication barriers for those with hearing loss unless doing so would result in an undue burden or a fundamental alteration in the nature of the goods or services being provided. Among the auxiliary aids listed by the ADA are assistive listening systems. Permanently installed assistive listening systems are required for existing or new assembly areas that (1) accommodate at least 50 persons or have audio amplification systems and (2) have fixed seating. The minimum number of receivers to be provided is based on the total number of seats. In other assembly areas either a permanent or portable ALS shall be provided.

The Architectural and Transportation Barriers Compliance Board

The Architechtural and Transportation Barriers Compliance Board (ATBCB), usually referred to as the Access Board, is the federal agency that enforces the ABA. The Access Board is also responsible for determining the standards for the ADA accessibility guidelines (ADAAG). The accessibility guidelines for both the ABA and the ADA are being revised and updated. Moreover, the Access Board has proposed incorporating these revisions into one ruling. As a result, future accessibility standards for facilities in the federal, public, and private sectors may be more uniform and consistent.

Portable Assistive Listening Systems

Portable desktop sound-field assistive listening systems are available. The teacher or speaker has a choice of microphones—head-worn, neck, or lapel—that may be connected to a body-worn FM transmitter. Some manufacturers offer a handheld transmitter/microphone that interacts with the desktop unit. The unique feature of this type of ALS is that the amplifier and FM receiver/speaker are combined into one unit to be placed on a child's desktop. It is actually a small, portable radio receiver tuned to the teacher. A carrying case is included for transporting the system from classroom to classroom, if needed. This arrangement may be useful for children with cochlear implants, fluctuating or mild hearing loss, unilateral hearing loss, or auditory processing disorders. Other portable FM systems have larger amplifier/speakers and may be used as an assistive listening system in small classrooms. At least one manufacturer makes this latter product using infrared technology.

Visual Displays in the Classroom

Some students benefit from the addition of visual information along with an assistive listening system in the classroom. Others must rely largely on visual assistance because of the severity of their hearing problem. Technology may provide visual information in the classroom for those with hearing loss in several ways.

Audiovisual-FM System

Visual cues of speech are available by speechreading the lip movements and facial expressions of the speaker. This information supplements and enhances the auditory message, especially in the presence of competing noise. AudiSee is an audiovisual-FM system designed to provide the student with both auditory and visual speech signals (Gagne, 2001; Ross & Levitt, 2001). The teacher wears a headset that has both a miniature camera and a microphone positioned in front of the face by a support arm. A transmitter worn at the waist broadcasts both the voice and facial image to the student. There are three types of receivers: (1) a desktop monitor-receiver, which has a 5½-inch screen and a built-in speaker; (2) a computer monitor; and (3) a television screen. It is also possible to broadcast the audio portion to a child's personal FM receiver. Thus speech perception may be maximized with this system because the student receives combined auditory and visual cues regardless of the distance or orientation of the teacher in the classroom. Also, more detailed visual information for speechreading may be available to the child via the projected image of the face.

Text Supplements

Several methods exist for providing the student with an ongoing text or printed presentation of spoken language in the classroom. They enable the student with hearing loss to fully participate in a class because both the words of the teacher and the comments or questions of the students appear as text. In addition, text-based systems offer the potential to improve and enhance a student's reading skills. The most extensive text supplement is obtained using realtime captioning through a method referred to as either communication access realtime translation or computer-assisted realtime transcription (CART). CART provides a complete and almost instantaneous written account of what is said in the classroom. It requires the services of a court reporter skilled in using a stenotype machine, which transcribes speech phonetically. These stenotype codes are sent to a computer with realtime software to convert this information into English text. A student may view the transcription on a computer or television monitor or it may be projected via a liquid crystal display (LCD) panel and overhead projector to a larger screen for all to view. Later, it is possible for the student to review the lecture and class discussion in either a printed or an electronic format. In educational settings, CART has been used primarily in secondary and postsecondary programs (Steinfeld, 2001). The potential exists for a classroom with a conference telephone to be linked with a stenographer in a remote location using two telephone lines for the connections (Preminger & Levitt, 1997). The National Court Reporters Association has a Web site, www.CARTinfo.org, that provides information about CART and assistance in locating CART providers.

Other transcription or notetaking systems exist that do not require the use of a stenotype machine. They are similar in that each requires a computer for the operator that is linked to a computer for the student. Type-Well® uses a standard computer keyboard and special word abbreviation software and condensing strategies; typists complete a 5-day training program and learn to produce notes or summaries of a class rather than verbatim text. Details are available at the Web site, www.typewell.com. Another approach is C-Print™, which is a system developed at the National Technical Institute for the Deaf for students in a mainstream classroom environment (Stinson, Elliot, McKee, & Francis, 2001). Operators undergo 6 weeks of training to become proficient. In its most recent version, C-Print Pro, the operator uses a computer with specialized software that combines IBM's ViaVoice automatic speech recognition software and a keyboard-based word abbreviation system (Francis & Stinson, 2003). Thus the operator may dictate continuously into a microphone connected to a computer or type on a keyboard to produce an ongoing text summary. Finally, the term "computer-assisted note-taking" (CAN) refers to having a good typist take notes or provide a summary of a class as it progresses using a computer word processing program (Compton, 1992; Youdelman, 2001). The student with hearing impairment reads this text on a monitor.

Methods have been developed that use only automatic speech recognition (ASR) technology to produce text in the classroom. An example of this approach is the iCommunicator™ software program, V 4.0 (Interactive Solutions, Inc., 2003). With this system, it is not necessary to have a special typist or speaker in the classroom. Instead, the teacher talks directly into the headset microphone of a body-borne FM transmitter. A wireless remote FM receiver is connected to a student's computer, which has ASR software (Dragon NaturallySpeaking Professional, Version 7.0) to convert continuous speech into electronic text (and/or video sign language) in realtime on the computer monitor. This speech may also be converted in realtime to a computer-generated voice and delivered directly via a cable to hearing aids, an FM receiver, or a cochlear implant

processor. Of course, instructors must undergo prior speech and voice recognition training with the software so that their individual speech and voice patterns will be transcribed as accurately as possible. Moreover, text typed on the student's keyboard may be converted in realtime to a computer-generated voice (or video sign language) for participation in class. A student user must be trained in the operation of this program and possess the computer skills necessary for working in a Windows environment. iCommunicator was initially developed to meet the needs of those who are deaf or hard of hearing, but it is also helpful to many others with special communication needs. Consult the Web site, www.myicommunicator.com.

Captioned Educational Media

The Captioned Media Program (CMP), formerly the Captioned Films/Videos (CFV) program, provides the free loan of over 4,000 open-captioned titles on video, CD-ROM, and DVD to students with hearing loss, their parents, and teachers (see Appendix). Open captions are always present and do not require a caption decoder. This program was established in 1958 and is funded by the U.S. Department of Education and administered by the National Association for the Deaf. In addition, the CMP serves as a clearinghouse for information and materials on captioning by providing descriptions and sources of open- and closed-captioned educational media available for purchase.

The Challenge

Certainly, there have been many technological advances and innovations with regard to assistive devices for those with hearing impairments. Such progress continues. In addition, important federal laws mandate and regulate the use of some devices, systems, and services. The challenge now is to introduce more students with hearing loss, their families, and school personnel to all the help possible with assistive devices. The need for this information is great and largely unmet.

There are many factors to consider in selecting appropriate assistive technology. The process begins, however, with an awareness and understanding of the various options. A school library, for example, might add assistive device catalogs and videotapes that demonstrate assistive devices to its collection (see the Appendix). A program about assistive devices might be scheduled periodically in connection with parent meetings. A school-based assistive device fair, similar to a health fair or book fair, where area vendors display and demonstrate their products is another possibility. The overall goals should be to incorporate assistive devices whenever possible into classroom learning and to help students identify which assistive devices will best meet their daily needs. Only then will communication access and independent functioning become a reality for those with hearing loss.

Summary

This chapter acquaints the reader with the outstanding breadth of assistive devices available today for the child with hearing loss. There are numerous options. Consideration is given to telecommunication devices and television, alerting devices, assistive listening devices and systems, and visual displays for the classroom. In addition, federal laws that mandate and regulate the use of these assistive devices are mentioned.

Appendix: Resources

Videotapes

League for the Hard of Hearing, 71 W. 23rd St., New York, NY 10010–4162. Phone: 917–305–6600. www.lhh.org. *Come Hear with Me* (1998).

Johns Hopkins Center for Hearing and Balance and Self Help for Hard of Hearing People. Available from SHHH, 7910 Woodmont Ave., Suite 1200, Bethesda, MD 20814. Phone: 301–657–2248. www.shhh.org. *The Telecoil: Plugging Into Sound* (1996).

Captioned Media

Captioned Media Program, National Association for the Deaf, 1447 E. Main Street, Spartanburg, SC 29307. Phone: 800–237–6213. www.cfv.org.

Assistive Devices Catalog Vendors

ADCO Hearing Products, Inc., 359 North First Avenue, Littleton, CO 80210. Phone: 800–726–0851. www.ADCO-hearing.com.

Harris Communications, 15159 Technology Drive, Eden Prairie, MN 55344. Phone: 800–825–6758. www.hariscomm.com.

HITEC Group Intn'l., 8160 Madison, Burr Ridge, IL 60527. Phone: 800–288–8303. www.hitec.com.

LS&S Group, Inc., P.O. Box 673, Northbrook, IL 60065. Phone: 800–468–4789. www.LSSGroup.com.

Sound Clarity, 359 North First Avenue, Iowa City, IA 52245. Phone: 888–477–2995. www.soundclarity.com.

WCI, 2716 Ocean Park Blvd.. Santa Monica, CA 90405. Phone: 800–233–9130. www.weibrichtcom.com.

References

Americans with Disabilities Act of 1990. (Pub.L.No. 101–336, 104 Stat. 327).

Americans with Disabilities Act Accessibility Guidelines (ADAAG). (1994). 36 CFR Part 1191, Accessibility Guidelines for Buildings and Facilities.

American National Standards Institute (ANSI). (2001). *American National Standard for Methods of Measurement of Compatibility between Wireless Communications Devices and Hearing Aids*. (ANSI/IEEE C63.19–2001). New York: American National Standards Institute.

American Speech-Language-Hearing Association (ASHA). (1991). Amplification as a remediation technique for children with normal peripheral hearing. *ASHA, 33* (Suppl. 3), 22–24.

Architectural Barriers Act of 1968. (Pub.L.No. 90–480, as amended, 42 USC § 4151–4157).

Architectural and Transportation Barriers Compliance Board (ATBCB). (1982). 36 CFR Part 1190, Minimum Guidelines and Requirements for Accessible Design: Final Rule.

Braverman, B. (1981). Television captioning strategies: A systematic research and development approach. *Am Ann Deaf, 126*, 1031–1036.

Compton, C. L. (1992). Assistive listening devices: Videotext displays. *Am J Audiol, 1*, 19–20.

Federal Communications Commission (FCC). (1996). *In the Matter of Access to Telecommunications Equipment and Services by Persons with Disabilities*, Report and Order, CC Dkt. No. 87–124, June 27.

Federal Communications Commission (FCC). (1997). *In the Matter of Using 711 Codes and Other Abbreviated Dialing Arrangements*, First Report and Order and Further Notice of Proposed Rulemaking, CC Dkt. No. 92–105, FCC 97–51, February 19.

Federal Communications Commission (FCC). (2000). 47 CFR 68.317 (f).

Francis, P., & Stinson, M. (2003). The C-Print speech-to-text system for communication access and learning. *Technology and Persons with Disabilities 2003 Conference Proceedings*. Available online: http://www.csun.edu./cod/conf/2003/proceedings/157.htm (accessed February 18, 2003).

Gagne, J.P. (2001). Audiovisual-FM system is found more beneficial in classroom than auditory-only. *Hear J, 54,* 48–51.

Hearing Aid Compatibility Act of 1988. (Pub.L.No. 100–394, 102 Stat. 976).

Hendricks, P., & Lederman, N. (1991). Development of a three-dimensional induction assistive listening system. *Hear Instruments, 42,* 37–38.

Individuals with Disabilities Education Act–Reauthorization (IDEA). (1997). 20 USC §§ 1400 et seq.

Interactive Solutions, Inc. (2003). i*Communicator Version 4.0 Training Manual.* Sarasota, FL: Interactive Solutions.

Killion, M.C. (2001). Digital cell phones and hearing aids: The problem is mostly solved. *Hear J, 54,* 10–19.

National Association for the Deaf (2000). Television. In: *Legal Rights: The Guide for Deaf and Hard of Hearing* (pp. 192–196) (5th ed.). Washington, DC: Gallaudet University Press.

National Captioning Institute (1983). *Hearing Impaired Children's Comprehension of Closed Captioned Television Programs.* Research Report 83–5. Falls Church, VA: National Captioning Institute.

Preminger, J.E., & Levitt, H. (1997). Computer-assisted remote transcription (CART): A tool to aid people who are deaf or hard of hearing in the workplace. *Volta Review, 99,* 219–230.

Ross, M., & Levitt, H. (2001). Developments in research and technology: An FM system for speechreading. *Volta Voices, 8,* 30–31.

Ross, M. (2002). Telecoils: The powerful assistive listening device. *Hear Rev, 9,* 22–26, 57.

Steinfeld, A. (2001). The case for realtime captioning in the classroom. *Volta Voices, 8,* 6–8.

Stinson, M.S., Elliot, L.B., McKee, B.G., & Francis, P.G. (2001). Accessibility in the classroom: The pros and cons of C-Print. *Volta Voices, 8,* 16–19.

Telecommunications Act of 1996. (Pub.L.No. 104–104, 110 Stat. 56).

Telecommunications for the Disabled Act of 1982. (Pub.L.No. 97–410, 96 Stat. 2043).

Television Decoder Circuitry Act of 1990. (Pub.L.No. 101–431, 104 Stat. 960).

Youdelman, K.S. (2001). Computer-assisted notetaking in the mainstream classroom. *Volta Voices, 8,* 8–10.

15

Cochlear Implants

ROSS J. ROESER AND PAUL BAUER

Security is mostly a superstition. It does not exist in nature. . . . Life is either a daring adventure or nothing.

—Helen Keller

The U.S. Food and Drug Administration (FDA) approved cochlear implants for adults with profound hearing loss in 1985 and for children with severe-to-profound hearing loss in June 1990. When cochlear implants were approved for children there was considerable controversy. On the one hand, it is well recognized that there are major consequences for severe-to-profound deafness, especially for infants and children with congenital losses. Without cochlear implants, children with profound deafness will rely on total communication or sign language as their means for providing language skills. Language learning and speaking will be significantly impaired, with marked delays in vocabulary development and reading skills. For example, compared to a vocabulary of 5000 to 26,000 words for the normal 5-year-old child, a child who is deaf will have a speaking vocabulary of about 200 words. Moreover, studies have shown that 50% of children having hearing losses greater than 85 dB HL had no reading comprehension at all (Berliner & Eisenberg, 1985). Severe-to-profound deafness impacts all aspects of educational and psychosocial development and subsequently will greatly influence socioeconomic factors.

On the other hand, during the research and development stages of cochlear implants there were uncertainties about the po-tential benefits that could be derived from this new technology. Then, and even now, it is not possible to predict those who will benefit and the amount of benefit a child will obtain from a cochlear implant. Degree of neural survival in the impaired ear is probably the single most significant physiological factor to predict success of cochlear implant use. However, there are no preoperative procedures available to measure neural survival in the cochlea (Fryauf-Bertschy, 1993). In addition, costs (monetary, psychological, time, effort, etc.) are high. These are critical factors to be considered as part of the decision to implant a child.

Since FDA approval in 1990, through December 2002 over 8000 infants and children have received cochlear implants in the United States. Moreover, the number of implants is increasing significantly; in the United States alone in 1999 over 3000 people received cochlear implants (Garber, Ridgely, Bradley, & Chin, 2002). It has been estimated that since 1978 over 60,000 patients worldwide have received cochlear implants (Josefson, 2002). Although there remain some who do not derive significant benefits, performance with cochlear implants has been no less than remarkable for many users (see Case Study 15–1). Even though considerable variability is seen in oral communication

Case Study 15–1   K.S. had no significant medical history, except for a series of ear infections beginning at about 2 years of age. At 2 years, 7 months, K.S. contracted meningitis. Following hospital discharge, her parents noted a lack of awareness to sound and had K.S. evaluated by an audiologist. Despite her visual attentiveness, behavioral testing over two sessions revealed a lack of behavioral responses to auditory stimuli, except for low frequencies presented at the limits of the audiometer. Immittance testing revealed no apparent middle ear disease and otoacoustic emissions were absent bilaterally. Auditory brainstem response testing indicated no responses at audiometric limits in either ear, confirming a severe-to-profound bilateral sensorineural hearing loss.

At 2 years, 11 months, K.S. was fit with high-gain binaural hearing aids, and she and her family were placed in a parent education program for children with hearing impairment. Aided testing showed improved awareness to pure tones and awareness to speech in the 55 to 60 dB range. No improvement in speech recognition could be documented. Both parents noted increased response to environmental sounds and speech when K.S. was wearing her hearing aids, and felt that she was receiving benefit.

At 3 years, 4 months, K.S. was placed in a preschool program for children with hearing impairments, which she attended daily. Her teachers felt that K.S. had excellent learning potential, but her limited speech was unintelligible, and she was significantly delayed in her language skills on formal tests. None of her teachers felt that she was benefiting from hearing aid use, as was evident from her performance on listening tasks. She was consistently unable to perform auditory tasks whether aided or unaided. On occasion, routine daily checks of her hearing aids would reveal that one or both instruments were not functioning, and she did not indicate that she knew the difference.

At 3 years, 9 months, K.S. underwent cochlear implant surgery and 5 weeks later her processor was fitted and mapped. Within a few weeks her parents reported she was aware of speech and environmental sounds at normal levels. In addition to her educational placement she was enrolled in private speech-language therapy, and within 6 months her speech intelligibility had improved significantly and language testing showed a 2-year increase from baseline measures. At 6 years, 6 months of age K.S. entered first grade with her normal-hearing peers with the use of resource support and continued speech therapy.

outcomes among children who have been implanted (Kirk, 2000), cochlear implant technology is improving and expected user benefits in recognizing sounds and understanding speech are increasing. With these improvements it is highly probable that the numbers of patients eligible for implants will increase dramatically and that school services programs for children with hearing loss will be impacted significantly by this new technology.

This chapter covers the topic of cochlear implants with a particular focus on topics of interest to school-based professionals, including how implants work, the devices that are currently available, candidacy, risks, benefits, cochlear implants in the schools, and cochlear implants and the deaf culture. For children with profound hearing loss who cannot benefit from cochlear implants, tactile hearing aids are available and they are described here as well.

What Are Cochlear Implants?

Cochlear implants are like hearing aids in that they attempt to process acoustic signals so they are audible and have meaning. However, cochlear implants differ from hearing aids because they use more sophisticated electronic technology and deliver an electrical signal, rather than an acoustic signal, to the ear through a surgically implanted multiple electrode array having several channels. Because surgery is required, the technique requires the expertise of a specially trained otolaryngologist (otologist) for implanting the electrode, and it is expensive. First-year costs, including the hardware, hospitalization, surgery, and rehabilitation, range between $45,000 and $50,000, which includes about $20,000 to $25,000 for the device. In the United States, third-party coverage is available for the cochlear implant device, hospitalization, and surgery. Medicaid covers these costs in some states. However, coverage for the critically important postoperative rehabilitation and device adjustment can be difficult to secure; some insurance policies specifically exclude any type of therapy, education, or rehabilitation. As a result, there are many school children in the United States using cochlear implants in the classroom without insurance support for special services.

Unfortunately, the high cost of cochlear implants, as well as the need for comprehensive rehabilitation programs, limits their availability to some children and adults with profound deafness in developed countries. However, many factors make them virtually unavailable in developing countries. Berruecos (2000) surveyed 11 countries in Latin America and Spain and found that there were over 90,000 eligible candidates, but fewer than 1400 cochlear implants had been provided. Factors contributing to the lack of implant programs in developing countries include the large number of possible candidates, the relationship between the cost of programs and socioeconomic considerations, low per capita annual income, the limited participation of official institutions, and very limited resources. Developing countries must employ rigorous candidate selection criteria to maximize the benefits that cochlear implants provide.

How Do Cochlear Implants Work?

Figure 15–1 is a diagram showing one type of body-worn cochlear implant system. Most systems use the basic components shown here, but smaller ear-level processors are now available. The device consists of an

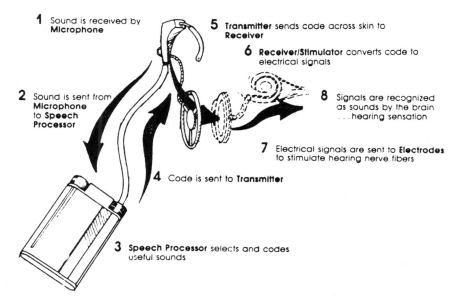

1 Sound is received by **Microphone**

2 Sound is sent from **Microphone** to **Speech Processor**

3 **Speech Processor** selects and codes useful sounds

4 Code is sent to **Transmitter**

5 **Transmitter** sends code across skin to **Receiver**

6 **Receiver/Stimulator** converts code to electrical signals

7 Electrical signals are sent to **Electrodes** to stimulate hearing nerve fibers

8 Signals are recognized as sounds by the brain . . . hearing sensation

Figure 15–1. Illustration of how cochlear implants produce sound sensations (see text for detailed explanation). (Courtesy of Cochlear Americas.)

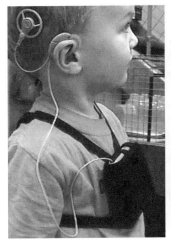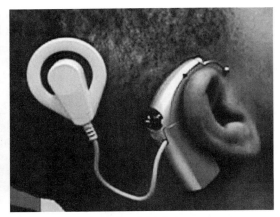

Figure 15–2.   Comparison of a body-worn (left) and ear level (right) processor.

external system (a microphone, speech processor, and externally worn transmitter) and an internal system (implant receiver and electrode). During surgery, an electrode array is placed through an opening near the round window of the cochlea into the scala tympani, and the implant receiver is secured in the temporal bone above and behind the ear. As sound is delivered to the microphone (1) it is converted into an electrical signal and delivered to a speech processor, which can be either a body-worn or an ear-level instrument (Fig. 15–2) (3), where selected acoustic characteristics are coded. The primary function of either type of processor is to prepare and code the incoming acoustic information for delivery to the electrode array. The electric code from the speech processor is delivered to a transmitter coil (5) and is electromagnetically induced across the skin to an internal receiver/stimulator (6). The internal receiver/stimulator converts the code to electric signals that are delivered to the electrode or electrodes placed in the cochlea (7). As the electric signals stimulate the structures in the inner ear and cranial nerve VIII they are recognized as sounds, and a sensation of hearing occurs.

Some manufacturers are developing preformed electrode arrays from elastic materials that are designed to conform to the coiled shape of the cochlea and inner (modialar) wall of the cochlea (Fig. 15–3). The purpose of the design is to elicit better contact between the electrodes and the neural tissue so that less electrical voltage is required to stimulate the tissue and elicit a sound percept. The reduction in required voltage may improve performance and has the added advantage of increasing battery life.

It should be noted that not all channels can be or always are activated. Instead, only the channels found to be functional through testing (or mapping) are turned on. In fact, recent studies have shown that using only seven or eight channels provides enough spectral information to allow cochlear implant wearers to perform like normal-hearing listeners (Friesen, Shannon, Baskent, & Wang, 2001). Moreover, some implants have been placed in cochleas obliterated by bony growth (ossification). In these cases, less than a full array of electrodes is placed in the cochlea. Interestingly, many patients with partially inserted electrodes do very well with their implants, and data from adults indicate that less than a full array of electrodes does not always affect speech perception performance.

Currently Available Cochlear Implant Devices

Dr. William F. House was the first surgeon in the United States to implant a wearable

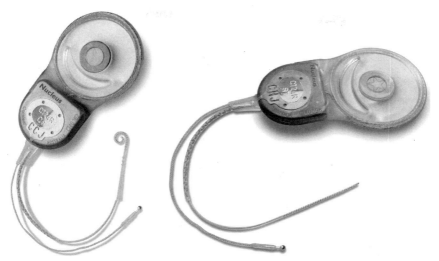

Figure 15–3. A multichannel electrode is surgically implanted into the inner ear. On the right is a nonconforming electrode, whereas an electrode designed to form around the snail-shaped cochlea is shown on the left. (Courtesy of Cochlear Americas.)

cochlear implant. His efforts led to the development of the single-channel 3M/House cochlear implant system. Although this instrument represented a major breakthrough at the time, clinical studies began showing that as a group, patients performed better with multiple-channel instruments, and single-channel instruments are no longer implanted in the United States.

An important clinical observation is that some patients implanted with single-channel analog devices were explanted and successfully reimplanted with a multiple-channel digital device in the same (homolateral) ear (Hamzavi, Baumgartner, & Pok, 2002). Moreover, homolateral explantation/reimplantation is needed in other cases due to electrode dislocation, local infection, technical failure, or damage from manipulation. Typically, the process does not impair auditory perceptions and performance; in fact, better speech perception has been reported after reimplantation for some children (Chute, Hellman, Parisier, Tartter, & Economou, 1992). In a report on seven adult patients who were reimplantated with the same multichannel, digital device in the same ear, Hamzavi et al (2002) found that five regained their speech recognition performance within 3 months, one showed a slight decline, and one showed a significant decline. The significant performance decline in the one patient was related to central auditory system involvement. These data indicate that reimplantation is a possibility without performance decrements, but that before reimplantation surgery, patients should be carefully counseled regarding expectations of subsequent performance.

Currently, three manufacturers have cochlear implants approved by the FDA for use with children in the United States: Advanced Bionic Corporation, Cochlear Americas, and Med El Corporation. The FDA process requires manufacturers of all new regulated medical devices to undergo in-depth premarket approval (PMA) trials to show safety and effectiveness prior to release. PMA trials have been conducted on cochlear implants first on adults and then on children in the United States over the past 25 years. It is important to know the status of a device, whether it is in the PMA or approved category, because during the PMA process some insurance companies will not provide funding for a device that has not yet received FDA approval.

Table 15–1 provides basic features of the three cochlear implant systems with FDA approval for children and adults in the

Table 15–1.   Basic Features of Cochlear Implant Systems*

Manufacturer	Name of Device	Speech Processor(s) Names	No. Electrodes	No. Channels	Electric Waveform	Coupling to Internal Transmitter/ Electrode
Advanced Bionics Corp 12740 San Fernando Rd. Sylmar, CA 91342 1–800–678–2575 (V) 1–818–362–7588 (V) 1–800–678–3575 (TDD) www.bionicear.com	Clarion S-Series Clarion Hi-Focus Clarion CII Bionic Ear	S-Series (Body), and Platinum (BTE) Platinum Series (Body), and Platinum (BTE) Platium Series and CII (BTE)	8 Intra-cochlear	16	Analog or pulsatile	Transcutaneous
Cochlear Americas 4100 Inverness Drive South #400 Englewood, CO 80112 1–800–523–5798 www.cochlear.com	Nucleus CI-22 Nucleus CI-24	Spectra (Body), and ESPrit 22 (BTE) Sprint (Body), ESPrit 24 and 3GB (BTE)	22 24 (22 intra-cochlear & 2 extra-cochlear)	22 22	Pulsatile	Transcutaneous
Medical Electronics Med-El 2222 East Highway 54 #180 Beta Building Durham, NC 27713 1–888–633–3524 www.medel.com	Med-El Combi 40+	CIS Pro+ (Body) Tempo+ (BTE)	24	12	Pulsatile	Transcutaneous

*Approved by the U.S. Food and Drug Administration for use with children in the United States.

United States. A comprehensive review of current cochlear implant technology with an in-depth description of additional hardware features and a description of the fitting process has been published by Moore and Teagle (2002). However, the rapid technological development of cochlear implants makes it impossible for any printed materials to be current for more than just a few months. As a result, information from manufacturers is the only way to stay current with available technology; contact information for each of the current manufacturers is included in Table 15–1.

Advanced Bionics Corporation manufactures the Clarion Multi-Strategy implant system, including the S-Series, Hi-Focus,

and CII Bionic Ear. The Clarion device was developed through collaborative efforts at the University of California at San Francisco, the Research Triangle Institute (in North Carolina), and MiniMed Technologies (Sylmar, California). In March 1996 the Clarion device was approved for use in postlingually deafened adults and in 1997 for use in children. The Clarion device permits more than one type of speech coding; that is, the user can select between analog or pulsatile electric waveforms. This versatility allows patients to choose the electric code that offers the most advantageous sound reception in different environments.

Cochlear Americas manufactures the Nucleus CI-22 and 24 M, CI 24K, and CI-24

Contour devices. The initial work that led to the development of CI-22 was performed at the University of Melbourne in Australia. The initiation of clinical trials in the United States began in 1986. The Nucleus CI-22 was the first device approved for children in 1990 and, as a result, more patients (both children and adults) have been implanted with this device than any other cochlear implant.

Medical Electronics (Med-El) Corporation was founded in 1975 and developed the first hybrid multichannel cochlear implant in Vienna. The first implant in the United States was in 1995, and FDA approval was granted for adults and children in 2001. Med-El Corporation manufactures the Combi 40+, 40+ S, and Combi 40+ G systems.

Because of the success of cochlear implants and the potential for expanded use for hearing loss and other auditory disorders, such as reducing or eliminating tinnitus, it will not be surprising if additional manufacturers come into the market place. Those interested in current technology should also contact the Web sites listed in the Appendix of this chapter.

Which Implant Is Best?

There is a wide variety of instrumentation with different speech processing strategies, and it appears that there is no one optimal strategy best for all users (Arndt, Staller, Arcaroli, Hines, & Ebinger, 1999; Moore & Teagle, 2002). Some perform better with processors that emphasize frequency components of speech, others are designed to represent timing characteristics, and the newer "hybrid" strategies attempt to give the patient a combination of both frequency and temporal characteristics. Parents of children (as well as adults) who are candidates for cochlear implants will need to select among the available devices. In addressing this important issue they should be advised to seek current information about available systems from audiologists and otologists who are on implant teams. In addition to the technical capabilities of the system, factors to be considered in selecting a cochlear implant include the following:

- Availability of service and the number of centers that will provide support for the system
- Time required for repair
- Availability of a loaner external signal processor in the event that the unit malfunctions
- Ability of the device to interface with external components, such as FM systems (see Chapter 13)
- Manufacturer's research and development capabilities including readily available resources and a commitment from the manufacturer to continue supporting the device

Who Are Candidates?

For children, cochlear implantation involves a series of steps through which the child and parents must proceed. The stages include candidacy, surgery, device activation, and rehabilitation. The initial step, candidacy, is one of the most important in the implant process, especially for children, and should be performed by a multidisciplinary team of professionals with knowledge and clinical experience in deafness and childhood development. Minimally, the decision regarding candidacy should involve an audiologist, otologist, and speech-language pathologist; ideally input from a teacher of deaf children and psychologist should also be included.

Candidacy requirements have changed significantly from when cochlear implants were first introduced in 1985 to the present. Table 15–2 shows the evolutions that have occurred. Initially, only adults were eligible and they were required to have postlinguistic, profound deafness and no recognition ability for open-set sentences. However, as the available benefits from cochlear implants have been documented through clinical trials, candidacy criteria have changed dramatically. Since the time that children were approved for cochlear implants in 1990, the degree of hearing loss was modified to include severe-to-profound deafness for adults in 1998 and children in 2000. Candidacy now includes those with speech

Table 15–2.   Expanding Cochlear Implant Candidacy Criteria

Factor	1985	1990	1998	2000
Age for implantation	Adults	Adults Children (2 yrs)	Adults Children (18 mo)	Adults Children (12 mo)
Age of onset of hearing loss	Postlinguistic	Postlinguistic adults Pre- and postlinguistic children	Adults and children pre- and postlinguistic	Adults and children pre- and postlinguistic
Degree of sensorineural hearing loss	Profound	Profound	Adults: severe-to-profound Children: profound	Adults and children > 2 yrs: severe-to-profound Children < 2 yrs: profound
Adult (open-set sentences)	0%	0%	40% or less (CID Sentences)	≤ 50% (HINT) in implanted ear < 60% in nonimplanted ear
Pediatric (speech scores)	Not candidates	0% open-set	Lack of auditory progress ≤ 20% (MLNT/LNT)	Lack of auditory progress ≤ 30% (MLNT/LNT)

From Cochlear Americas.
HINT, Hearing In Noise Text; MLNT, Multisyllabic Lexical Neighborhood Test (Iler-Kirk, Pisoni, & Osbergr, 1995); LNT, Lexical Neighborhood Test (Iler-Kirk et al, 1995).

recognition performance on word/sentence tests in the 30 to 50% range.

In all cases, candidacy will be based on results from audiological evaluation, and medical tests that must include an x-ray [computed tomographic (CT) scan or magentic resonance imaging (MRI)], to verify the status of the cochlea. Candidacy requirements differ by country. In the United States, FDA requirements determine whether a device is approved for safety and effectiveness, as well as third-party reimbursement. The Nucleus 24 Contour device is approved for children 12 months of age and older, the Med-El COMBI 40+ for 18 months and older, and the Clarion Hi-Focus for 24 months and older. FDA approval is just a guideline. It does not mean that implanting a child younger than 12 months old is not allowed or that it is not effective. It is important to note that the FDA does not regulate clinical activity.

Currently, candidacy requirements for cochlear implants differ for infants 12 months to 2 years, toddlers through adolescents 2 through 17 years, and adults 18 years and over as follows:

Infants ages 12 months to 2 years
- Profound bilateral deafness
- Little or no benefit from hearing aids, preferably fit for at least 3 months
- Lack of progress in development of auditory skills
- Realistic expectations of results
- Family or caregiver is proactive with rehabilitation exercises

Toddlers and adolescents (ages 2 through 17 years)
- Severe to profound bilateral sensorineural hearing loss
- Little or no benefit from hearing aids, preferably fit for at least 6 months
- Lack of progress in the development of auditory skills

Ages 18 years and over
- Severe to profound bilateral sensorineural hearing loss [greater than or equal to 70 dB hearing level (HL)]

- Pre- or postlinguistic onset of hearing loss
- Receive little or no useful benefit from hearing aids, defined as score of 50% or less on sentence recognition tests in the ear to be implanted and 60% or less in the nonimplanted ear or bilaterally

It should be noted that the minimum duration of hearing aid use is waived for infants and toddlers if x-rays indicate ossification of the cochlea.

Contraindications for both children and adults include:

1. Deafness due to lesions of the acoustic nerve or central auditory pathway
2. Active middle ear infections
3. Absence of cochlear development as determined through preoperative high-resolution CT scan
4. Tympanic membrane perforations
5. The presence of contraindications for surgery (i.e., significant heart disease)

At one time, postlinguistic deafness was considered an important candidacy requirement. However, it is now becoming clear that children and adults who are prelinguistically deaf also derive benefits from implants. After implantation, some adults with prelinguistic deafness will use sign language in conjunction with listening, others rely exclusively on spoken language. In fact, after implantation some prelinguistically deaf adults are able to achieve open-set speech intelligibility and use the telephone (Sorkin, 2002).

All of the above criteria have value in determining candidacy, but results from the audiological evaluation and past experience with hearing aids weigh more than any other single presurgical consideration. The audiological data and results from the hearing aid trial are the primary considerations used to determine candidacy for infants and children. Patients who receive cochlear implants must have severe-to-profound deafness and not be able to receive significant benefit from conventional amplification.

A trial period with appropriately fit amplification is an important step prior to cochlear implantation. The trial period should be used to determine if hearing aid(s) will provide enough benefit for language and speech development as determined through standardized language tests and auditory speech perception and speechreading with a suitable hearing aid when possible. However, as the benefits derived from cochlear implants in young children are being documented, it is becoming more acceptable to shorten the hearing aid trial to 1 to 2 months when profound deafness is firmly established.

The earliest age at which cochlear implants should be provided has been debated by many. The requirement that children be at least 2 years of age does not arise from technical surgical considerations, but rather from the need to establish firmly the presence of deafness and the lack of benefit from traditional amplification. Such a time period is required when deafness is established at birth. Even though the age of 2 years has been set as a minimum criterion for cochlear implant candidacy, there are those who believe that this is too young. They argue that audiometric testing on children age 2 years and younger is much too variable to ensure with 100% accuracy that profound bilateral deafness is present. Although auditory brainstem evoked response (ABR) audiometry is available, the maximum stimulation levels are limited and low frequency hearing can be present when ABR responses are absent.

Behavioral audiometry using observation techniques can be used, but responses are influenced by the attention and maturational level of the child and the observers' experience and response criteria (see Chapter 3). In addition, especially for the child with acquired deafness, at 2 years of age the benefits of hearing aid use cannot always be firmly established. Sufficient time is needed with appropriately fit amplification before the decision is made to implant a young child. Based on these concerns many believe that specifying a minimum age for a cochlear implant is not appropriate. Unfortunately, this minimum age becomes the accepted standard for all children to receive an implant. Instead, each child must be considered individually, and candidacy must be determined only when deafness and the inability to benefit from appropriately fit amplification are firmly established.

Risks

The risks involved with cochlear implants are low, but their existence must be recognized. With any surgical procedure, consideration must be given to the low-incidence risks associated with general anesthesia and possible infection. Besides these general considerations, there are several others that are specific to the cochlear implant. Initially, concern was raised about the possibility of bone growth in the cochlea because animal studies have shown that electric stimulation of the cochlea will cause this condition to occur, which results in disruption of hair cell function (Northern, Black, & Brimacombe, 1986). However, clinical experience has demonstrated that many patients have used cochlear implants for years without significant changes in electric threshold sensitivity. This finding would suggest that there are no obvious adverse affects of cochlear implant use for these time periods, but it does not address the important question of lifetime use for periods of 70 to 80 years for the infant wearing a cochlear implant. However, the question remains as to the possible effects on the discrimination ability or recognition of more complex sounds over extended use.

A particular concern with children is head growth. At birth, the cochlea has reached adult size. However, the temporal bone that houses the components of the cochlear implant continues to grow and enlarge as the infant develops. As a result, allowances need to be made with infants so that the intracochlear electrode will not be extracted from the cochlea. One study found that maximum head growth occurs in the first 2 years of life and recommended prolonging surgery until after this age (O'Donoghue, Jackler, Jenkins, & Schindler, 1986). These investigators recommended that a stretching allowance of 1 to 3 cm be made for the intracochlear electrode array in young children to account for head growth. Surgeries are now being performed outside the United States on infants as young as 8 months without apparent complications.

Device malfunctions have occurred in some patients. In fact, several years ago one manufacturer voluntarily called a moratorium on implanting a device due to a failure of the internal coil in several patients. When device malfunctions occur, reimplantation is necessary, and reports have indicated auditory sensations are possible from the reimplanted electrode array (Luxford & House, 1985).

Recently, concern has been raised that children may be more at risk of developing meningitis after cochlear implantation (FDA, 2003; Wooltorton, 2002). In the United States, 52 cases of postimplant meningitis have been reported: Clarion (29), Nucleus (22), and Med-El (1). According to the manufactures, the Nucleus and Med-El cases had predisposing factors for meningitis unrelated to the implant (Mondini inner ear deformity, preimplantation history of meningitis, etc.). Culture results were available for 23 of these cases: *Streptococcus pneumoniae* (16), *Haemophilus influenzae* (4), *Streptococcus viridans* (2), and *Escherichia coli* (1) (FDA, 2003).

To prevent or decrease the risk of meningitis in children after cochlear implantation the FDA has made the following recommendations (FDA, 2003).

1. Diagnose and treat otitis media promptly. The cochlear implant, because it is a foreign body, may act as a conduit for infection from otitis media to reach the cerebral spinal fluid or brain.

2. Use the pneumococcal vaccinations Prevnar and Pneumovax. This vaccination will build immunity to the most common strains of *Streptococcus pneumoniae*.

3. Use the Hib vaccination. This vaccination will build immunity to *Haemophilus influenzae*–type B.

Other possible complications include tinnitus, dizziness, and facial muscle twitching (the latter is most likely with extracochlear devices). Although these potential complications exist, their occurrence is reportedly rare because they have been found in only a few patients (Tyler, Davis, & Lansing, 1987).

Benefits

Once the FDA approves a device, manufacturers can then label the device and advertise the benefits that can be expected from using the device. However, the claims made must be based on the data that were collected during the FDA approval process. Quite obviously, the expected benefits from cochlear implants are different for children and adults, and separate claims are available for the two populations.

For children who receive cochlear implants the expected benefits are as follows:

1. Implant patients are able to detect medium to loud environmental sounds, including speech, at comfortable loudness levels.
2. Some (34 to 52%) children can identify environmental sounds chosen from a closed set of alternatives, at comfortable loudness levels.
3. Many (more than 52%) children can identify the timing and rhythm of speech as well as identify words from a closed set of alternatives without lipreading.
4. Some (34 to 52%) children demonstrate enhancement of their lipreading abilities.
5. For many (more than 52%) children, speech production is improved after training and experience with the device.
6. A few (5 to 34%) children demonstrate the ability to recognize speech without lipreading.
7. Children who are born deaf or become deaf shortly thereafter may derive less benefit than children who acquire deafness later in life.

Despite careful screening of implant recipients, significant variability exists in speech perception performance. Some recipients perform remarkably well, being able to discriminate open-set sentences and talk over the telephone, whereas others do not. Neural survival in the cochlea, correct fitting of the device, and speech processor coding strategy are possible factors. In children, personality, cognitive ability, and the availability and quality of rehabilitation and educational support are also variables. Studies have shown that educational setting and mode of communication are additional factors influencing cochlear implant use (Fryauf-Bertschy, 1993; Somers, 1991).

Predicting Outcomes

Common questions heard during any preimplant evaluation include, How well will my child do with their implant? How much will a cochlear implant help my child? Will a cochlear implant help my child learn to talk? Unfortunately, the answer to these questions, for any given child, is unique to each child, and nobody knows. In reality the performance level that any one child will achieve after implantation will not be realized until months or years after the implant is in and turned on.

When parents ask about outcomes, the factors known to influence performance after implantation can be discussed. Geers et al (2002) found that children who receive cochlear implants before 5 years of age are presented with auditory information at a crucial time for speech and language development. In addition, they found the extent to which a child will use this information to achieve speech and language competence is affected by a variety of factors, including:

What the child brings to the learning environment
What the implant contributes
What the rehabilitation program provides

The most important factor that a child brings is a good nonverbal intelligence. In fact, if this variable is held constant, earlier age at implant and later age at onset of deafness do not contribute significantly to speech perception and production skill.

It is important to note that the actual device selected by the family has not been shown to significantly influence outcome (the device selected should be determined by the parents). The only variable contributed by the implant that affected the outcome was duration of use of the updated SPEAK coding strategy. The duration of use of the SPEAK coding strategy had a substantial impact in all outcome areas examined. Better outcomes were also associated with a larger number of active electrodes in the cochlear implant map (Geers et al, 2002).

The primary rehabilitative factor associated with desirable performance outcomes was educational emphasis on oral–aural communication. Communication mode was more important to auditory and spoken language development than any other rehabilitative factor examined. Communication mode was more important than classroom placement, amount of therapy, experience of therapist, or parental participation in therapy. Children in programs that emphasized oral–aural communication were better able to use information from their implant to: hear, speak, and read (Geers et al, 2002). To answer the question, How well will my child do with the implant? it is important for parents to understand that from the predictive factors already outlined here, those that appear to be most influential are communication mode and the educational setting in which their child is enrolled for postimplant rehabilitation.

Strong family support is another critical ingredient for successful cochlear implant usage and outcomes for children. The obligations and responsibilities associated with cochlear implants are considerable and critical to the child's overall success. The family must be aware of the requirements through preimplant counseling, and then be in agreement to meet the increasing needs following

Table 15–3. Evidence of Strong Family Support

Accepts and is knowledgeable about child's hearing loss

Shows interest by asking questions and seeking outside information

Has appropriate and realistic expectations for child

Is prompt to appointments and participates in treatment when asked

Is knowledgeable about instrumentation

Communicates well with child

Displays high interest and motivation levels

Spends ample time with child and participates in treatment/educational activities

Uses same language at home and school

Has concern for child's educational and physical development

surgery. Table 15–3 provides examples of how family support can be documented objectively.

Children with Developmental Disabilities

Advances in technology, improved performance, and expanded criteria to include very young and older children with more residual hearing have raised questions about implanting children with significant cognitive, developmental, and physical comorbidities. Traditionally these exceptional children have not been considered appropriate candidates because of questionable benefit from implantation. At one time it was even strongly suggested that children with autism and significant learning disabilities be eliminated from candidacy (ASHA, 1985).

Some centers choose not to implant deaf children with multiple co-morbidity because of potentially poor results. Others will implant these children in anticipation of some benefit from long-term acoustic input. Recent work has shown that children with significant comorbid conditions, such as seen in CHARGE syndrome, do receive benefit from cochlear implantation (Bauer, Wippold, Goldin, & Lusk, 2002).

Part of the difficulty in deciding to implant these exceptional children is in objectively quantifying "benefit" after implantation. "Benefit" can mean something that promotes well-being (a useful aid). However, it is important to point out that as the age of implantation has been reduced to 12 months and sometimes below in special cases, it is inevitable that some children with developmental disabilities, especially children with cognitive impairment, will be implanted because most are not identified until after 12 months of age.

The current battery of audiological and perceptual testing provides the basis to demonstrate objective benefit after a cochlear implant. However, in children with significant cognitive, developmental, and physical disability the current limitations with the standard test battery limit the ability to demonstrate objective benefit in these children. Often it is more subjective measures, reports by parents and other caregivers, that serve as early indicators of benefit.

Research has shown that children with motor or cognitive delays develop improved speech perception more slowly than other implanted children; however, they do progress in their speech and auditory skills over time (Pyman, Blamey, Lacy, Clark, & Dowell, 2000; Waltzman, Scalchunes, & Cohen, 2000). In a study of 10 children with developmental delays who received cochlear implants, Hamzavi et al (2000) report that eight showed either subjective or objective benefit from their implants. These results emphasize that, even though children with multi-handicaps are not considered to be good candidates, many of them become good implant users. The important point is in the preimplant education of the parents. Due to the variations in the amount of benefit these children may achieve after implantation, it is important to ensure that parents have been counseled thoroughly and have appropriate, realistic expectations of what their children will be able to accomplish before proceeding with cochlear implantation.

Children with Auditory Neuropathy/Dys-synchrony

Auditory neuropathy (AN), also referred to as auditory dys-synchrony, involves a dysfunction of timing in the auditory system that results in poor auditory neural function and a significant impairment in speech recognition ability (see Chapter 3). Hearing sensitivity for patients with AN can range from normal to severe-to-profound, making some eligible candidates for cochlear implants. Because AN is potentially a confounding issue for cochlear implants, a number of recent studies have focused on this intriguing topic. Initial reports on individual patients suggested that children with AN derived significant benefits from cochlear implants (Miyamoto, Kirk, Renshaw, & Hussain, 1999; Trautwein, Sininger, & Nelson, 2000). Shallop, Arndt, & Turnacliff (1992) were among the first to report data from multiple patients. They studied five children diagnosed with AN who had received cochlear implants. Results showed that all children improved in their listening skills, enabling them to take advantage of different communication options. Reporting on retrospective data from a data pool of 18 patients, Madden, Hilbert, Rutter, Greinwald, & Choo (2002) found that all children showed varying amounts of improvement in auditory and verbal development. Similar findings are now available from a number of additional studies (Buss et al, 2002; Mason, De Michele, Stevenson, Ruth, & Hashisaki, 2003). Overall, it appears that cochlear implants are able to overcome the desynchronization hypothesized to underlie AN, at least to the point that speech becomes more intelligible.

Cochlear Implants in the Schools

The introduction of cochlear implants into the educational environment has had a major impact on the educational process for children who are deaf. Successful cochlear implant (re)habilitation, especially for young infants, requires the combined and coordinated efforts of each member of the child's "team," which includes family members, caretakers, teachers, and other school personnel. The process must have the necessary daily quantity and quality for it to be successful. Meaningful auditory input from all daily living experiences becomes crucial for the child to be able to associate environmental and speech sounds with meaning and build them into relevant language constructs. Parents and other caregivers must be taught that everyday experiences are opportunities to learn language and speaking skills: meal times become therapy sessions, a trip to the store an opportunity to experience new environmental sounds, and bedtime stories an opportunity to learn new vocabulary words.

When young children who are deaf and use cochlear implants present themselves to the school for the first time, school personnel must enlist team support. Parents should be given specific assignments to carry out at home. Weekend activities should be designed to reinforce activities from the classroom and speech therapy programs. As part of the regular curriculum, lessons that include activities to be carried out at home in the morning and evening hours, as well as on weekends and during vacations, should be provided to caregivers. Such team cooperation will ensure continuous exposure to meaningful experiences to reinforce sound association and language development.

Educators have long known that children perform to the level that their teachers expect. As a result, teacher expectations should be significantly different for the child wearing a cochlear implant. Prior to cochlear implant technology, the probability for a child with severe/profound deafness to have intelligible speech was not high; the thought that a child with severe/profound deafness would have open-set speech recognition was nonexistent. However, today with a cochlear implant it is possible that a child will have open-set speech recognition. Assuming the implant is functioning properly, all children with implants will perceive speech at normal conversational levels, and many children will be able to understand speech at normal conversational levels with lipreading. When children are enrolled in an effective (re)habilitation program, many will have open-set speech recognition.

School personnel must realize that infants and children with cochlear implants have the potential to perform at extraordinarily high levels. The expected performance for children with implants must be raised to a level that will promote the highest level of performance for each child. School personnel must create the expectation that children with implants will be able to learn at normal rates. Visual cues can be used, but should be gradually reduced to increase the dependence on acoustic information.

Teachers and speech-language pathologists who are first confronted with a child wearing a cochlear implant must realize that there are some basic procedures that need to be followed. Every sound a child hears through the implant system is new. Children who had hearing prior to their deafness or who wore hearing aids prior to using their cochlear implant may not readily respond because they hear sound very differently. Each sound and each word must be heard many times before it will be recognized. This basic principle must be incorporated into each lesson developed for the child's daily team efforts. Continuous repetition of sounds and words for the young cochlear implant user is a critical technique for successful listening; it requires patience and persistence.

Cochlear implants are electronic devices, with the likelihood that they may have failures. Once children become adept at using implants they will signal when it is not functioning. However for young children, checking the device several times each day is important. Spare batteries and simple spare parts should be available for nonfunctional units.

Background noise in the environment can mask and distort sounds heard by implant users (see Chapter 13). Such interference should be avoided in the teaching/listening environment by reducing reflective surfaces (floor tile and hard walls) and treating the environment with acoustic tile and using carpeting on the floors (see Chapter 12). Other ways to improve the listening are: to point the implant microphone toward the primary speaker, avoid moving while speaking, and point to the speaker when multiple speakers are presenting so the implant user can orient to the speaker.

All team members should also assume that children with cochlear implants hear sounds at normal conversational levels. That is, when it is fit, the audiologist adjusts the processor to a level that normal conversational speech sounds are heard at a comfortable listening level. Speaking at higher intensities can overload the implant processor and distort sounds.

Parents must become advocates for their children and work together with school personnel as a team to provide the child with the necessary learning experiences and acoustic stimulation to maximize the benefits that can be derived with the use of the cochlear implant. For all children with handicaps parents must act as advocates; with cochlear implants it is even more critical that the parent assume the advocacy responsibility. Cochlear implants are relatively new to school systems, and many educators and educational systems have limited experience with them. When this is the case, parents should become the resource for educators and familiarize them with the necessary conditions needed for success with cochlear implants. Parent advocacy and parent/school cooperation constitute the ideal formula to maximize the benefits from cochlear implants in school children.

Cochlear Implants and the Deaf Culture

Cochlear implants do not restore normal hearing, but they can restore a level of hearing where virtually all implant patients are able to perceive sounds at intensity levels where normal hearers respond. In addition, with appropriate postimplant (re)habilitation, many recipients are able to recognize environmental sounds and understand speech at high levels of comprehension. However, even with the documented benefits that cochlear implants provide, this topic is a sensitive issue for the deaf community. The deaf community does not view deafness as a disability; rather it is considered a "culturally defining characteristic." This philosophy views deaf individuals as being different due to the use of an alternate mode of communication—sign language. As such, the deaf community feels that the use of cochlear implants has the potential to eliminate their culture.

However, by all definitions deafness is a disability. For example, the Americans with Disability Act of 1990 defines "disability," including loss of hearing, as an impairment that substantially limits major life activities. Individuals who are deaf have a significant impairment or disadvantage in competing in many areas, such as employment. A person who is deaf operates from a deficit position in the part of the world that includes spoken language, the sounds of nature, or the sounds of a musical instrument. An important fact when considering this issue is that deaf people participate in disability programs and benefits.

The concern by the deaf community that cochlear implants have the possibility of eliminating their culture is a reality. The fact is that if the technological advances continue as they have been, and the costs associated with cochlear implants are reduced significantly, making them more available to a larger population, there is a high possibility of eliminating deafness—worldwide. Today, with cochlear implants it is possible to provide a child who is deaf, or a deafened adult, the means to enter into the world of sound. It is possible to eliminate the disability of deafness.

Although there was initially major concern about cochlear implants among the deaf community, there has been gradual understanding and acceptance. An important development in this area is that Gallaudet University in Washington, D.C., the only university in the world for deaf students, has established a cochlear implant program, providing some validation that the deaf community has started to accept and realize the importance and value of cochlear implants.

Tactile Hearing Aids

With tactile hearing aids, acoustic signals are changed into vibratory (or possibly electri-

Table 15–4. Commercially Available Tactile Hearing Aids

Name of Device	Type of Stimulation	Channels	List Price (US $)
Tactilator (LTD)	Vibrotactile	2	$975
Tactaid 7	Vibrotactile	7	$2400
Tactaid 2000	Vibrotactile	6	$2400

Available from Audiological Engineering, 9 Preston Road, Somerville, NMA 20143. Phone: 800 283–4601. E-mail address: www.tac-taid.com.

cal) patterns, which are delivered to the skin. The goal of a tactile communication system is to extract relevant information from the acoustic signal and to present it to the individual in a tactile mode as a means of supplementing or replacing the auditory reception of the acoustic signal—with the successful reception of speech as the ultimate goal. Surgery is not required for tactile stimulation, and the typical cost of a tactile aid ranges from about $950 to $2600.

There is a vast literature on the development and assessment of tactile hearing aids (Roeser, 1985). Based on the positive laboratory and clinical reports, a number of manufacturers developed both vibrotactile and electrotactile instruments having from single to multiple channels; one study evaluated the effectiveness of a 256-channel electrotactile instrument stimulating the thorax, although the device was never made available

for clinical use. Currently, only one manufacturer has commercially available instruments (Table 15–4). As shown, three vibrotactile instruments (2-channel, 6-channel, and 7-channel) are available.

Surprisingly, the use of tactile hearing aids provides benefits similar to cochlear implants. Table 15–5 provides a comparison between expected performance on nine different auditory functions for the two devices. As shown by this comparison, it is possible to perform seven of the nine auditory functions successfully with either cochlear implants or tactile hearing aids. In fact, sound awareness can be obtained at virtually the same hearing levels for both devices. However, for two functions, the ability to discriminate between environmental sounds and to discriminate open-set speech, cochlear implants are clearly superior, indicating that those eligible for cochlear implants will

Table 15–5. Comparison of Cochlear Implant and Tactile Hearing Aid Expected Performance

Task	Cochlear Implant	Tactile Hearing Aid
Discriminate loud and soft sounds	Yes	Yes
Discriminate continuous and interrupted sounds	Yes	Yes
Discriminate long and short sounds	Yes	Yes
Differentiate number of sounds	Yes	Yes
Differentiate number of sounds in words	Yes	Yes
Differentiate number of syllables in sentences	Yes	Yes
Differentiate different types of sounds in the environment (e.g., door knock versus speech)	Yes	No
Recognition of closed-set speech (Assist in lipreading)	Yes	Yes
Recognition of open-set speech	Some/Most Of The Time	No

derive significantly more benefit than they would from tactile hearing aids.

Despite being less available commercially, vibrotactile hearing aids continue to be a viable option for use with children and adults with profound deafness. Because they are noninvasive, totally safe, and fit easily to the skin of the hand, forearm, abdomen, or chest, they can be used with infants when their deafness is first identified. Tactile hearing aids are valuable tools during the time when cochlear implant candidacy is being pursued, and following surgery until initial mapping takes place. Tactile hearing aids are also a consideration for patients who are unable to benefit from hearing aids and are not candidates for cochlear implants, such as patients having bilateral eighth nerve involvement (neurofibromatosis).

The Future

Alessandro Volta (1880) is credited with the first observation that electrical current applied to metal rods placed in the earcanals at a voltage approximating 50 V created a sensation of "une recousse dans la tete" (a boom within the head) followed by a sound similar to that of boiling, thick soup. Current understanding of how electrical stimulation of the auditory system creates sound that can be interpreted by the brain has certainly advanced since 1880. Advancements have been made to the point where it is realistic to expect that most implanted children will achieve open-set speech recognition.

There are multiple avenues that can still be explored, including improved implant design, implant drug delivery to stimulate neural growth, perimodiolar positioning, depth of insertion, and speech processor programming strategies to name just a few. One of the most exciting new areas of future research is bilateral cochlear implantation. One goal of bilateral implantation is to achieve the "binaural effect."

It is known from studies on hearing-impaired patients who utilize hearing aids in both ears that they can understand speech better, especially in noise, compared with wearing a hearing aid in one ear (Bronkhorst & Plomp, 1989). In fact, little doubt exists regarding the advantages of bilateral amplification for hearing aid users, and bilateral fitting is now the rule rather than the exception for hearing-impaired children aided by hearing aids.

What is the "binaural effect"? When speech and noise come from different directions, the signal-to-noise ratio will be more favorable at one ear than at the other because of the size of the head. Listeners who are aided in both ears can selectively attend to the ear that presents a better signal. This is called "head diffraction." The auditory system and the brain can combine information from both ears to produce a central representation of the signal that is more salient than that resulting from information extracted by one ear alone. Localization of sound in the horizontal plane is strongly dependent on perception of interaural differences in time, phase, and intensity. The advantages gained from wearing bilateral hearing aids is better speech intelligibility, better sound localization, and better performance in noise.

Combine this knowledge with earlier statements that the audiometric selection criteria for cochlear implant candidates are changing and there is a growing number of children with cochlear implants who also have useable residual hearing in the contralateral ear.

Studies have looked at postlingual adults that use a cochlear implant in one ear and a conventional hearing aid in the other (Armstrong, Pegg, James, & Blamey, 1997; Dooley, Blamey, & Seligman, 1993). These studies have shown that the binaural condition was consistently the best condition for vowel and consonant identification and for reception of sentences when compared to the monaural condition. In addition, binaural amplification in comparison to monaural consistently showed an advantage in noise for word and sentence scores.

A major concern in implementing this technology in adults as well as children is the potential problem arising from the "incompatibility" between sensations elicited by electrical stimulation via an implant and by acoustic stimulation via a hearing aid (Blamey, Dooley, Parisi, & Clark, 1996). Ching, Psarros, Hill, Dillon, and Incerti (2001) investigated sensation "incompatibility" with 16 children having unilateral cochlear implants. The mean hearing threshold levels of this group of children would be described as profound bilateral hearing loss; this was not a group of children with reasonably good hearing on one side. They asked three questions: Do hearing aids need to be adjusted differently for use with cochlear implants? Is there any binaural interference or negative effect? And do children benefit from wearing hearing aids with cochlear implants in the contralateral ear? They found that hearing aid gain needs to be adjusted to amplify speech to an overall loudness that is similar to that perceived in the implanted ear. Binaural interference did not occur for any of the individual children in their study. In addition, there were significant benefits in speech perception, localization, and aural–oral function in everyday life when the children used cochlear implants with adjusted hearing aids compared with when they used cochlear implants alone (Ching et al, 2001).

The natural assumption leads to the conclusion that if bilateral hearing aids are better than unilateral hearing aids, and hearing aids combined with an implant are better than an implant alone, then shouldn't bilateral implants be even better? This is not an easy question to answer.

Stepping back from performance outcome measures, the financial cost of cochlear implantation has to be considered. There are no research reports addressing the cost of bilateral implantation. What is known is that the costs associated with profound deafness are substantial. The expected lifetime cost to society for a child with prelingual onset of profound deafness exceeds US $1 million, largely because of special education and reduced work productivity (Mohr, Feldman, & Dunbar, 2000). Cost utility studies have established that pediatric cochlear implants are highly cost effective, with a net expected savings of $53,198 over a child's lifetime

(Cheng et al, 2000). In the United States alone over 4000 children will be born each year with profound hearing loss. Assuming that these children are implanted as a result of newborn hearing screening, a net savings to society of over $212,792,000 will be realized in 1 year alone.

The difficulty in justifying a second implant financially is that current data are only for unilaterally implanted children. It is hard to imagine that the savings from a second implant, if there are any, will be justified based on improved performance. Without question, there is a large, significant monetary cost associated with achieving the binaural effect.

It has been shown that unilateral pediatric cochlear implantation has a positive effect on quality of life at reasonable direct costs and results in a net savings to society (Cheng et al, 2000). However, with bilateral implants, extra cost of the device, extra rehabilitation time, extra time in the operating room, and increased risk to the patient's facial nerve and sense of taste are significant factors. Is it worth it? Is the child going to gain any appreciable benefit from having bilateral implants? Do the data concerning bilateral hearing aid use or combined hearing aid/implant use transfer or improve with bilateral implant use?

What is known can be taken from several sources. There are a few case reports of bilateral 3M/House single-channel implants (Green, Mills, Bell, Luxford, & Tonokawa, 1992a). A few case reports of bilateral, one side 3M/House single-channel and the other side Nucleus 22M are available (Balkany, Boggess, & Dinner, 1988; Green, Mills, Bell, Luxford, & Tonokawa, 1992b). Several reports are also available on bilateral Nucleus 22M implants (van Hoesel & Clark, 1997; van Hoesel, Tong, Hollow, & Clark, 1993). And now there is one case series of 10 patients implanted with bilateral Med-El Combi-40+ devices (Muller, Schoen, & Helms, 2000).

Balkany et al (1988) reported on one postlingually deafened female patient with a 3M/House device on one side and a Nucleus 22M on the other side. The good news from their report was that open-set testing using both devices simultaneously demonstrated improved function over either device alone, which provided evidence of combined central representation, and that binaural integration and enhancement can take place with bilateral implants. The bad news was that both the visual enhancement scores and the speech tracking results caused a slight, but consistent, decrement when using both devices compared to using the Nucleus 22 device alone.

The advantage of the report by Muller et al (2000) is that all patients were implanted with the same device using the same speech processing strategy. They report some very impressive results with a few of their patients having very impressive performance in speech understanding in noise. However, their small population of patients includes patients with pre- and postlingual hearing loss, a variety of etiologies of their hearing loss, and a variety of intervals of deafness prior to implantation. In general, the population was too heterogeneous to draw any conclusions and the data are incomplete for every patient.

There are studies under way investigating bilateral cochlear implantation using the Nucleus 24 Contour device and the Med-El Combi 40+ device in postlingually deafened adults. These studies are complete, although the data are not yet published. A recent industry-sponsored protocol has been approved for bilateral Nucleus 24 Contour devices in prelingually deafened children. Bilateral cochlear implantation is specifically not regulated by the FDA. Therefore, patients who desire a second cochlear implant can be implanted with a second device if the funding is available.

It is important to note that the benefit gained from the binaural effect is not the only rationale for considering bilateral cochlear implantation. It is known that speech recognition ability gets worse in the unaided ear for individuals who have bilateral hearing loss but unilateral hearing aid amplification. This deterioration is often attributed to a lack of auditory stimulation or "auditory deprivation" in the unaided ear, and its effects can be observed as soon as 3 months after monaural

fitting (Gelfand & Silman, 1993; Gelfand, Silman, & Ross, 1987). This led to the theory that implanting the second ear may preserve and actually promote the peripheral and central neural development of the auditory system.

What is known about prelingual deafness, neural development, and cochlear implantation has been gleaned from animal studies. Several groups of examiners have studied auditory neural development in mammalian models, most often cats or guinea pigs. Beitel, Snyder, Schreiner, Raggio, and Leake (2000) have extensively studied auditory nerve survival with and without electrical stimulation in congenitally deafened cats. They have shown that spiral ganglion cell survival (the beginning of the auditory nerve in the cochlea) and the central nervous system tonotopic organization are dependent upon and preserved by early stimulation. In addition, not only does electrical stimulation promote survival of the auditory nerves, but placing the electrode closer to the spiral ganglion (the auditory nerve) further minimizes the loss of nerves. This supports the concept of perimodiolar positioning (having the electrode as close as possible to the nerve).

Some argue to "save the nerve." What if hair cells can be regenerated some day? What if a better device comes along some day? Devices and their programming strategies are always improving. If the ear is implanted now it might be "ruined" so that the child may not be a candidate for advances in the future.

What the future holds for cochlear implants is impossible to know. In addition to the current work on bilateral cochlear implants, work is always ongoing to create better processing strategies and the age of implantation continues to decrease. Perhaps some day totally implantable devices will be a reality (Huttenbrink, Zahnert, Bornitz, & Hofmann, 2001; Maniglia et al, 1999).

Summary

This is an exciting era for professionals who provide services to infants and children with hearing loss. As a result of the development of cochlear implants, the potential of improving educational performance is impacted for those with severe-to-profound hearing losses. Current cochlear implant technology, when accompanied by effective (re)habilitative programs, gives those who are appropriate candidates the means to achieve high levels of speech perception and production performance. And, there is good reason to believe that additional technological advances will continue to improve the benefits derived from cochlear implants. Perhaps one day those with moderate levels of hearing loss will be candidates for cochlear implants. With this as a possibility, all who provide services and educational programs to infants and children with hearing loss must continue to keep up with advances in all (re)habilitative technology, with cochlear implants being among the most promising area of future development. Although many of those with severe-to-profound hearing losses are candidates for cochlear implants, there remains a small minority who cannot benefit, and clinicians should be aware of alternate rehabilitative techniques, including tactile hearing aids.

Appendix: Web Sites on Cochlear Implants

Facts about Cochlear Implants

http://www.deafblind.com/cochlear.html
http://deafness.about.com/cs/cochlear implants/
http://members.aol.com/DrDaveLink/ci.htm
http://www.nidcd.nih.gov/health/hearing/coch.asp
http://www.utdallas.edu/~loizou/cimplants/tutorial/
http://www.zak.co.il/deaf-info/old/ci-faq.html

Computer Simulation of Cochlear Implants

http://www.utdallas.edu/~loizou/cimplants/

Cochlear Implant Manufacturers (see Table 15–1)

Advanced Bionics—Clarion: http://www.cochlearimplant.com
Cochlear Corporation—Nucleus: http://www.cochlear.com
MED-EL—Combi 40+: http://www.medel.com

References

Armstrong, M., Pegg, P., James, C., & Blamey, P.J. (1997). Speech perception in noise with implant and hearing aid. *Am J Otol, 18* (Suppl. 6), S140–S141.

Arndt, P., Staller, S., Arcaroli, J., Hines, A., & Ebinger, K. (1999). *Within-Subject Comparison of Advanced Coding Strategies in the Nucleus 24 Cochlear Implant.* Englewood, CO: Cochlear Corporation.

American Speech-Language-Hearing Association (ASHA). (1985). Ad Hoc Committee on Cochlear Implants. *ASHA, 28,* 29–52.

Balkany, T., Boggess, W., & Dinner, B. (1988). Binaural cochlear implantation: Comparison of 3M/House and Nucleus devices with evidence of sensory integration. *Laryngoscope, 98,* 1040–1043.

Bauer, P., Wippold, F., Goldin, J., & Lusk, R. (2002). Cochlear implantation in children with CHARGE association. *Arch Otolaryngol Head Neck Surg, 128,* 1013–1017.

Beitel, R.E., Snyder, R.L., Schreiner, C.E., Raggio, M.W., & Leake, P.A. (2000). Electrical cochlear stimulation in the deaf cat: comparisons between psychophysical and central auditory neuronal thresholds. *J Neurophysiol, 83,* 2145–2162.

Berliner, K., & Eisenberg, L. (1985). Methods and issues in the cochlear implantation of children: An overview. *Ear Hear, 6,* 6S–13S.

Berruecos, P. (2000). Cochlear implants: An international perspective—Latin American countries and Spain. *Audiology, 39,* 221–225.

Blamey, P.J., Dooley, G., Parisi, E., & Clark, G.M. (1996). Pitch comparisons of acoustically and electrically evoked auditory sensations. *Hear Res, 99,* 139–150.

Bronkhorst, A., & Plomp, R. (1989). Binaural speech intelligibility in noise for hearing-impaired listeners. *J Acoust Soc Am, 86,* 1374–1383.

Buss, E., Labadie, R.F., Brown, C.J., Gross, A.J., Grose, J.H., & Pillsbury, H.C. (2002). Outcome of cochlear implantation in pediatric auditory neuropathy. *Otol Neurotol, 23,* 328–332.

Cheng, A., Rubin, H.R., Powe, N.R., Mellon, N.K., Francis, H.W., & Niparko, J.K. (2000). Cost-utility analysis of the cochlear implant in children. *JAMA, 284,* 850–856.

Ching, T., Psarros, C., Hill, M., Dillon, H., & Incerti, P. (2001). Should children who use cochlear implants wear hearing aids in the opposite ear? *Ear Hear, 22,* 365–380.

Chute, P., Hellman, S., Parisier, S., Tartter, V., & Economou, M. (1992). Auditory perception changes after reimplantation in a child cochlear implant user. *Ear Hear, 13,* 195–199.

Dooley, G., Blamey, P.J., & Seligman, P. (1993). Combined electrical and acoustical stimulation using a bimodal prosthesis. *Arch Otolaryngol Head Neck Surg, 119*, 55–60.

Friesen, L.M., Shannon, R.V., Baskent, D., & Wang, X. (2001). Speech recognition in noise as a function of the number of spectral channels: Comparison of acoustic hearing and cochlear implants. *J Am Acad Audiol, 110*, 1150–1163.

Fryauf-Bertschy, H. (1993). Pediatric cochlear implantation: An update. *ASHA, 35*, 13–16.

Garber, S., Ridgely, M.S., Bradley, M., & Chin, K.W. (2002). Payment under public and private insurance and access to cochlear implants. *Arch Otolaryngol Head Neck Surg, 128*, 1145–1152.

Geers, A.E., Brenner, C., Nicholas, J., Uchanski, R.M., Tye-Murray, N., & Tobey, E.A. (2002). Rehabilitation factors contributing to implant benefit in children. *Ann Otol Rhinol Laryngol Suppl, 189*, 127–130.

Gelfand, S., & Silman, S. (1993). Apparent auditory deprivation in children: Implications of monauralversus binaural amplification. *J Am Acad Audiol, 4*, 313–318.

Gelfand, S., Silman, S., & Ross, L. (1987). Long-term effects of monaural, binaural and no amplification in subjects with bilateral hearing loss. *Scand Audiol, 16*, 201–207.

Green, J.D., Mills, D.M., Bell, B.A., Luxford, W.M., & Tonokawa, L. (1992a). Binaural cochlear implants. *Am J Otol, 6*, 502–506.

Green, J.D., Mills, D.M., Bell, B.A., Luxford, W.M., & Tonokawa, L. (1992b). Binaural cochlear implants. *Am J Otolaryngol, 13*, 502–506.

Hamzavi, J., Baumgartner, W.D., Egelirer, B., Franz, P., Schenk, B., & Gstoettner, W. (2000). Follow up of cochlear implanted handicapped children. *Int J Pediatr Otorhinolaryngol, 56*, 169–174.

Hamzavi, J., Baumgartner, W.D., & Pok, S.M. (2002). Does cochlear reimplantation affect speech recognition? *Int J Audiol, 41*, 151–156.

Huttenbrink, K., Zahnert, T., Bornitz, M., & Hofmann, G. (2001). Biomechanical aspects in implantable microphones and hearing aids and development of a concept with a hydroacoustical transmission. *Acta Oto-Laryngologica, 121*, 185–189.

Iler-Kirk, K., Pisoni, D.B., & Osbergr, M.J. (1995). Lexical effects on spoken word recognition by pediatric cochlear implant users. *Ear Hear, 16*, 470–481.

Josefson, D. (2002). Cochlear implants carry risk of meningitis agencies warn. *BMJ, 325*, 298–299.

Kirk, K.I. (2000). Challenges in the clinical investigation of cochlear implant outcomes. In: J.K. Niparko, A.M. Mellon, D. Robbins, D. Tucci, & B.S. Wilson (Eds.), *Cochlear Implants: Principles and Practices* (pp. 225–258). Baltimore: Lippincott, Williams & Wilkins.

Luxford, W., & House, W. (1985). Cochlear implants in children: Medical and surgical considerations. *Ear Hear, 6*, 20S–24S.

Madden, C., Hilbert, L., Rutter, H., Greinwald, J., & Choo, D. (2002). Pediatric cochlear implanation in auditory neuropathy. *Otol Neurotol, 23*, 163–168.

Maniglia, A., Abbass, H., Azar, T., Kane, M., Amantia, P., Garverick, S., Ko, W.H., Frenz, W., & Falk T. (1999). The middle ear bioelectronic microphone for a totally implantable cochlear hearing device for profound and total hearing loss. *Am J Otol, 20*, 602–611.

Mason, C., De Michele, A., Stevenson, C., Ruth, R., & Hashisaki, G.T. (2003). Cochlear implantation in patients with auditory neuropathy of varied etiologies. *Laryngoscope, 113*, 45–49.

Miyamoto, R.T., Kirk, K., Renshaw, J., & Hussain, D. (1999). Cochlear implantation in auditory neuropathy. *Laryngoscope, 109*, 181–185.

Mohr, P.E., Feldman, J.J., & Dunbar, J.L. (2000). The societal costs of severe to profound hearing loss in the United States. *Int J Assess Health Care, 16*, 1120–1135.

Moore, J.A., & Teagle, H.F.B. (2002). An introduction to cochlear implant technology, activation and programming. *Lang Speech Hear Serv Sch, 33*, 153–161.

Muller, J., Schoen, F., & Helms, J. (2000). Bilateral cochlear implant: New aspects for the future? *Adv Otorhinolaryngol, 57*, 22–27.

Northern, J., Black, F., & Brimacombe, J. (1986). Selection of children for cochlear implantation. *Seminars in Hearing, 7*, 341–446.

O'Donoghue, G., Jackler, R., Jenkins, W., & Schindler, R. (1986). The problem of head growth. *Otolaryngol Head Neck Surg, 94*, 78–81.

Pyman, B., Blamey, P.J., Lacy, P., Clark, G.M., & Dowell, R. (2000). The development of speech perception in children using cochlear implants: Effects of etiologic factors and delayed milestones. *Am J Otol, 21*, 57–61.

Roeser, R.J. (1985). Tactile aids for the profoundly deaf. *Seminars in Hearing, 6*, 279–298.

Shallop, J.K., Arndt, P., & Turnacliff, K.A. (1992). Expanded indications for cochlear implantation: Perception results in seven adults with residual hearing. *Speech Language Pathology Association, 16*, 141–148.

Somers, M. (1991). Speech perception abilities in children with cochlear implants or hearing aids. *Am J Otol, 12*, 174S–182S.

Sorkin, D.L. (2002). Cochlear implant candidacy and outcomes: 2002 update. *Hear J, July/August*, 12–17.

Trautwein, P.G., Sininger, Y.S., & Nelson, R. (2000). Cochlear implantation of auditory neuropathy. *J Am Acad Audiol, 11*, 309–315.

Tyler, R., Davis, J., & Lansing, C. (1987). Cochlear implants in young children. *ASHA, 29*, 41–49.

U.S. Food and Drug Administration (FDA). (2003). Cochlear implant recipients may be at greater risk for meningitis. Available online: www.fda.gov/cdrh/safety/cochlear.html (accessed July 24, 2003).

van Hoesel, R.J.M., & Clark, G.M. (1997). Psychophysical studies with two binaural cochlear implant subjects. *J Acoust Soc Am, 102*, 495–507.

van Hoesel, R.J.M., Tong, Y., Hollow, R., & Clark, G.M. (1993). Psychophysical and speech perception studies: A case report on a binaural cochlear implant subject. *J Acoust Soc Am, 94*, 3178–3189.

Waltzman, S.B., Scalchunes, V., & Cohen, N.L. (2000). Performance of multiply handicapped children using cochlear implants. *Am J Otol, 21*, 329–335.

Wooltorton, E. (2002). Cochlear implant recipients at risk for meningitis. *CMAJ, 167*, 670.

16

Techniques and Concepts in Auditory Learning and Speechreading Enhancement

Helen McCaffrey Morrison

That music always round me, unceasing, unbeginning—yet long untaught I did not hear; But now the chorus I hear, and am elated; I hear not the volumes of sound merely—I am moved by the exquisite meanings
—Walt Whitman, 1819–1892

Auditory learning is the process by which a child develops the skills necessary to extract meaning from the acoustics of spoken language. For the overwhelming majority of human cultures, audition is the preeminent route for language comprehension. The phonological systems in spoken languages have evolved to take advantage of the processing capacities of the human auditory system (Gopnik, Meltzoff, & Kuhl, 2000; Lindblom, MacNeilage, & Studdert-Kennedy, 1983; Sussman, McCaffrey, & Matthews, 1992; Syrdal, 1985). Furthermore, acoustic speech information is more accessible to the perceiver than visual information. Auditory information travels over distance, across obstacles, and around corners; visual information does not. In localizing sound one need not direct the ear to the source. With vision, however, one must see the source and time is lost in reception when movement for visual access is required. Nevertheless visual cues do serve an important function in the reception of spoken language, predominantly to enhance or disambiguate auditory perception.

The person who has a hearing impairment must overcome the challenge of perceiving spoken language through a degraded auditory signal that may be enhanced by visual information contributed by speechreading. When the person with a hearing loss is a child, the perceptual challenge impacts spoken language acquisition and academic performance. Intervention targets skill and strategy development as well as perception, as shown in Case Study 16–1. The ultimate goal in intervention is the child's successful use of primary acoustic and secondary visual cues to acquire spoken language, to gain academic skills, and to communicate successfully throughout the life span. This chapter outlines some fundamental concepts associated with auditory learning and the enhancement provided by speechreading. A description of typical auditory development, followed by discussion of the essential elements and the interactive nature of auditory learning is covered first. The related issues of speechreading, beginning auditory learning later in life, and speech production will be addressed. The chapter closes with suggestions for implementing an auditory learning program.

Auditory Development

Typical Development

Humans are innately predisposed to decode spoken language. Many auditory behaviors

Case Study 16–1   S.W. was a 6-year-old boy with a severe-to-profound bilateral sensorineural hearing loss. S.W. was first fit with hearing aids at age 18 months and enrolled in a parent–infant program. At the time of therapy, S.W. was mainstreamed in a first grade classroom. His support services included the use of a frequency modulation (FM) system, individual speech/language therapy, tutoring with an itinerant teacher of the hearing impaired, and private therapy. S.W. uses auditory–verbal communication. Among his language and speech goals were comprehension and expressive use of complex sentences, including passives and relative and subordinate clauses, comprehension and use of new vocabulary from the classroom, expressive use of negative contractions and the /s/-/z/ morphemes, reduced stopping of fricatives, and reduced neutralization of the vowels /1/, and /e/. Auditory skills assessed revealed that he had difficulty remembering more than three critical elements and the details of a short story. In addition, S.W.'s teacher and parents observed that he did not consistently cue the teacher when he did not understand what was being said in the classroom.

S.W.'s auditory goals were shaped by his speech and language goals as well as the results of auditory skills testing. His auditory memory improved with practice listening to and identifying lists of words with increasing numbers of elements. Nevertheless, greater effort was directed toward improving comprehension of sentences made more complex by added phrase structures. Elaboration of the phrase structure served to increase critical elements within the sentence.

Simple stories were presented during the therapy sessions. S.W. answered questions about these stories and retold them. Questions were directed toward exposing S.W. to story grammars (Who is in the story? Where was the boy? Was there a problem?) in preparation for his second grade language arts curriculum. In the classroom he had showed some difficulty reading "short vowels" during phonics lessons. These were essentially the same vowels that were neutralized in his speech productions. S.W. and the clinician read stories to each other from primers that were loaded with words containing short vowels.

Most auditory work proceeded at the comprehension level with connected discourse, with some exceptions appearing for the purpose of highlighting a target. For example, S.W. demonstrated auditory awareness and discrimination of fricatives, all vowels, and negative contractions when these were presented in syllables or single words. However, these elements were difficult for him to perceive in running speech and as a consequence he did not establish rules for the use of these speech sounds or morphemes in receptive or expressive language. S.W. practiced auditory identification and production of these targets in syllables, words, and phrases, and rules for their use were explicitly presented (Is there more than one boy? What do you add at the end of the word?). Because these elements tend to be less audible in running speech, he also practiced identification via speechreading as well.

S.W.'s reticence to cue the teacher when he did not understand came from two sources. First, S.W. did not always know when he did not understand. Second, he needed skills to notify the teacher. The clinician embedded vocabulary that S.W. did not know throughout her conversations with him, and he practiced finding these words and asking for an explanation. The clinician and S.W. talked about different ways to clue the speaker if the person were a teacher talking to a class, an adult talking to him individually, or a teammate on the soccer field.

are "hardwired" into the perceptual system from birth (Kuhl, 1992, 1993, 2000). From the first moments of life, audition provides a bridge between infants and their environment. Newborns demonstrate an awareness to sound (Schneider & Trehub, 1992); they show a listening preference for speech in general and for their own mother's voice in particular (Fernald, 1985). During the first year of life, auditory behavior is increasingly selective, constraining recognition to cues that are linguistically important in the parent language. As early as 1 month of age infants discriminate among speech sounds, including sounds not present in their "mother" tongue (Aslin, Pisoni, & Jusczyk, 1982). This ability declines at around 8 to 12 months of age when most infants discriminate only those speech sounds that are native to their language (Werker & Tees, 1984). The infant has learned what to pay attention to and what to ignore. This perceptual process develops in step with cognitive skill in categorization (Gopnik, Meltzoff, & Kuhl, 2000). Using innate learning strategies, infants exploit the statistical properties of language input to detect recurrent patterns that form the bases of phonetic categories (Kuhl, 2000).

Notwithstanding the typically hearing infant's demonstrated ability to discriminate individual speech sound contrasts presented in the experimental context, the acquisition of receptive language appears to be generally a top-down process, founded on developing skill in segmenting spoken language into meaningful units (Nittrouer, 2002). Prosodic perception supercedes phonetic perception in the acquisition of meaning (Jusczyk, 1998). Peters (1983) proposed four strategies that the child applies in breaking down language input into meaningful units: (1) pay attention to perceptually salient stimuli, (2) discriminate stimuli along salient dimensions, (3) remember stimuli, and (4) classify stimuli according to the result of the discrimination. Peters's algorithm requires sufficient repetitiveness and predictability of the input so that many opportunities are present for attention and discrimination. There should be a consequence to the child's response that will provide feedback as to the correctness of the child's behavior, allowing classification and storage into memory.

The child first applies these strategies to chunks of speech that can be as large as the daily routines of dressing or feeding. Daily routines occur with regularity and tend not to vary in linguistic content, providing predictability. Routines also provide communication turns for the child's participation, requiring appropriate, discriminated response (Ninio & Bruner, 1978). Caregivers give saliency to spoken language by using "motherese": simplifying the lexical content, reducing utterance length, paraphrasing, repeating, and providing contextual support (Newport, Gleitman, & Gleitman, 1977). Motherese is characterized by a communicative style that serves to acoustically highlight meaningful units in the input. Clause boundaries are marked by more consistent use of change in fundamental frequency (F_0), more frequent pauses, and increased syllable durations. Content words have greater duration than function words. Nouns tend to have more syllables than verbs (hence the diminutives "doggie" and "kitty"). Motherese scaffolds prosodic processing by being easier to segment and process for discrimination and comprehension.

Among the first words comprehended by young children with normal hearing are simple labels and action nouns (Benedict, 1979). At this point, the observation of auditory development in children with typical hearing is essentially an observation of the acquisition of receptive language and linguistic comprehension skills. Linguistic comprehension appears to be strategy based, at least in the early stages of language development (Milosky, 1992). Children apply comprehension strategies to figure out meaning on the basis of situational cues and past experience. The evidence that children use strategies suggests that comprehension is a cognitive process as well as linguistic, and subject to general notions about learners and skill development.

Ultimately children with normal hearing comprehend spoken language automatically, with little reliance on context or personal experience. This ability appears with the onset of school age. The school-age child is expected to acquire knowledge and academic skills through comprehension of instructional language that is presented with increasing abstraction and departure from direct experience as each year ensues. A child in the fourth grade is expected to function independently in the use of receptive language (listening and reading) and expressive language (speaking and writing) to acquire knowledge and think critically.

Implications for Children with Hearing Loss

Intervention that targets auditory learning by children with peripheral hearing loss is shaped by principles gained from observing auditory development by children with normal hearing. The foundation of an auditory learning program is the provision of an audible, learnable signal through amplification or cochlear implantation. Once an audible, learnable signal breaches the peripheral hearing loss, innate universal auditory abilities can be manifested. A child with a peripheral hearing loss possesses an intact auditory system beyond the periphery that is waiting to be nourished with spoken language.

Subsequent to hearing aid fitting or cochlear implantation, children with hearing loss have similar potential as their normally hearing peers to apply learning strategies to segment the ongoing speech stream into meaningful units, categorize the speech sounds of the language, and gain information from listening. Audibility provided by amplification must be supported by input and experience that provide guided practice in using the learning strategies that children ordinarily apply to the process of learning to comprehend language. Caregivers and therapists provide guided practice in the form of the daily language routines experienced by the child, acoustic qualities of the input, and skill demands of conversational interaction.

The input that assists normally hearing children segment speech into meaningful units is particularly beneficial for children with hearing loss. Clause markers that incorporate F_0 variation and syllable duration, or lexical cues that incorporate duration or syllable number, are available auditorially to most children with hearing loss, including many children with profound hearing loss wearing conventional amplification. Hence, an auditory learning program that at the outset targets recognition at the simple phrase level within the context of repetitive language routines is not only developmentally appropriate but is also well suited to the child with hearing loss.

Finally, an auditory learning program is ultimately a program that targets the acquisition of receptive language and linguistic comprehension. Initial teaching guides children with hearing loss to decode spoken language using situational cues and their own experience. As the receptive language base grows, these children are guided to use their language knowledge to achieve comprehension of new information.

Aspects of an Auditory Learning Program

Table 16–1 displays the elements that constitute an auditory learning program. The language used, or the input stimulus, in an auditory learning program will be selected with regard to the audibility of the signal, the linguistic level, and the predictability of the subject matter. The auditory skill that the child will use in decoding the auditory stimulus must also be considered. Auditory learning programs take various forms, ranging from guided opportunities for the child to learn from conversational interaction to more structured task-oriented approaches. Finally, ideal listening settings are ones in which the signal is presented within 3 feet of the listener in quiet, nonreverberant environments. Once an auditory skill is mastered in the ideal listening environment, skill development in less than ideal acoustic environments is targeted.

Stimulus Features

CHARACTERISTICS OF THE SPEECH SIGNAL

The sounds of spoken language can be described along three acoustic dimensions: in-

Table 16–1. Aspects of an Auditory Learning Program

	Stimulus Features					
Acoustic	Phonologic/ Linguistic	Predictability	Skill	Structure	Stimulus Distortion
Basic: Intensity Frequency Time	Prosodic feature	"Closed" to "open" set:	Basic skills: Detection Discrimination Identification Comprehension	Conversational Informal Adaptive Play based	Distance Direction Noise
	Speech segment: Consonant	Response visible Topic known			
Specific to the speech signal: F_0 F_1 F_2 Steady state and transient qualities	Vowel Syllable Morpheme Word Phrase Clause Sentence Paragraph Conversational turn	Unknown topic	Supporting skills for comprehension Classroom listening	Discrete skill Task oriented Stimulus-response Traditional	

tensity, frequency, and time. The average conversational speech intensity measured from a distance of about 1 m is 65 dB sound pressure level (SPL), ranging from faint speech at 45 dB SPL to a shout at 85 dB SPL (Fletcher, 1953). Vowels have the greatest intensity among English speech sounds, and the fricative consonant /θ/ has the weakest. The frequency spectrum of speech ranges from 50 to 10,000 Hz, with greatest energy appearing from 100 to 600 Hz, or the region where suprasegmentals and vowels lie. F_0 carries suprasegmental information including rhythm, intonation, and stress.

Vowels are differentiated by the location of peaks in the frequency spectrum known as formants. Formant peaks differentiate the extent of jaw movement (vowel height) and location where the tongue is raised for production (vowel place). Vowel height is signaled primarily by the first formant peak (F_1); vowel place is signaled primarily by the second formant peak (F_2). The predominant energy of consonants is weaker in intensity than vowels and appears at higher frequency ranges. The primary cues of consonant manner of production appear at and below 1000 Hz; consonant place of produc-

tion is cued in the region between 2000 and 4000 Hz. Temporal characteristics of a speech segment may be described as (1) the duration of a segmental aspect or (2) the transition, or change over time, from one aspect to another. For example, the voice/voiceless distinction among consonants can be characterized by a difference in the time of onset of voicing (duration of silence) in the case of an initial plosive or in the duration of the preceding vowel in the case of a final stop. Semivowels contrast with diphthongs by differences in the speed of formant transitions within the segments.

A simple description of the acoustic characteristics of speech does not fail to specify those aspects that best cue speech recognition. Some characteristics have greater importance than others. For example, despite the predominance of speech energy from 100 to 600 Hz, the sounds most important for English speech recognition do not lie in this frequency region. The more crucial segments are the consonants, which lie in higher frequency regions of lower intensity (Dubno & Ahlstrom, 1995).

Furthermore, each speech sound possesses a variety of acoustic cues that can lead to its identification. Trading relationships exist among perceptual cues such that when an acoustic cue is not available to the listener, others will take prominence, both in the case of experimental manipulation of the speech signal (Diehl & Walsh, 1989) and in the case of hearing impairment (Fry, 1978). Finally, the acoustic characteristics of a speech sound vary from one context to another. Speech sounds influence the acoustic characteristics of adjacent sounds by way of coarticulation. It benefits the child to practice speech sound recognition in a variety of phonetic contexts to take advantage of facilitative context effects.

Sensorineural hearing loss affects the audibility of suprasegmentals and speech segments by reducing the sensation level of the conversational speech spectrum and filtering frequency components of speech. The majority of cases of sensorineural hearing loss tend to have greater effect on high frequency speech components than on low frequency speech. The result is greater ease of perception of speech features that are of the strongest intensity, lowest frequency, or coded temporally. These include number of syllables, suprasegmentals, vowel height, consonant manner, and for some listeners, consonant voicing. Table 16–2, adapted from Boothroyd (1984), lists unaided hearing threshold levels at which the probability of identification of various speech features drops to 50%.

The information in Table 16–2 can contribute to the selection of speech features for listening practice, but cannot be the sole source. Stimuli are selected from analyses of (1) the aided or implant audiogram, (2) the speech processing algorithm of the hearing aid or cochlear implant, and (3) auditory confusions on discrimination tasks. Analysis of speech information that is furnished by the cochlear implant or hearing aids should not eliminate cues for training but should instead guide the clinician in organizing stimuli from the easiest perceptions to the most difficult.

In summary, intensity, frequency, and temporal features may describe speech sounds. As a rule, the high frequency characteristics of speech sounds are lower in intensity than mid or low frequencies, and are less likely to be audible to the listener with hearing impairment. Each speech sound possesses a variety of acoustic characteristics that may serve as cues to the identification of a sound. A listener need not utilize all cues to identify a segment. The listener with hearing impairment may perceive cues differently than someone with normal hearing.

Table 16–2. Hearing Levels at Which Identification of Speech Characteristics Drop to 50% Probability*

Speech Feature/ Characteristic	Hearing Level
Consonant place	75 dB HL
Initial consonant continuance	85 dB HL
Initial consonant voicing	90 dB HL
Vowel place	100 dB HL
Speaker gender	105 dB HL
Syllabic pattern	115 dB HL
Vowel height	In excess of 115 dB HL

*Adapted from Boothroyd (1984).

PHONOLOGIC/LINGUISTIC LEVEL OF THE STIMULUS

Children attend to a variety of phonologic and linguistic units in the process of developing comprehension skills. The items in listed in Table 16–1 under this category appear in a continuum of informativeness. Movement along this continuum can be bidirectional. Although larger linguistic units (sentences, conversational discourse) possess more available information for comprehension, the amount of information that a child can use is constrained by developmental language level, attention, memory, and the ability to segment meaningful units from speech. The clinician may restrict the length and complexity of the stimulus to accommodate these constraints or to highlight or isolate a linguistic unit for processing. For example, the child who exhibits confusion among speech sounds may benefit from syllable-level drill with sound contrasts.

PREDICTABILITY

A number of constraints function to limit the range of possible responses to auditory input, and thus provide predictability. The set of possible responses may be limited by restricting the number of items or pictures from which a child might choose in an auditory task. Keying the child in to the topic of conversation can also limit the range of responses. Closed sets are those responses that are constrained in the auditory learning session. Open sets are those responses that have no constraints, or have constraints that are not applied by the child. Some children will benefit from experiences geared toward learning to recognize response constraints, such as identifying the topic of conversation from hearing sets of related words or phrases, or considering a picture of a communicative setting and talking about what is typically said (see Case Study 16–2).

Auditory Skill

Auditory skills range from the simple awareness that sound has occurred, to full comprehension of the spoken message. The majority of auditory learning curricula tend to be organized according to Erber's (1982) hierarchy of auditory skills, listed in Table 16–1 under "Basic Skills" and described below:

1. Detection: awareness of the presence or absence of sound. Detection responses include indication that sound is "on" or "off"; "I heard that!"
2. Discrimination: perception of differences between sounds. Responses indicate that sound is "same" or "different."
3. Identification: association of sound with meaning. Identification responses include pointing to, naming, or writing the label associated with the auditory input.

4. Comprehension: understanding the meaning of an auditory message. Responses at the comprehension level include answering questions, following directions, paraphrasing, and maintaining a conversation.

When the auditory learner is a child who is also acquiring language, some adaptation of the hierarchy is necessary. For example, young children cannot engage the metacognitive process required at the discrimination level to establish whether words or syllables are the same or different auditorially. Therapists working with young children frequently cite imitative speech approximation of the auditory input as evidence of discrimination—the child indicates hearing one particular stimulus and not another (Estabrooks, 1994, 1998; Pollack, Goldberg, & Caleffe-Schenck, 1997).

Clinicians and educators also combine practice at the discrimination and identification levels by asking the listener to identify objects or pictures from closed sets of choices that vary in selected speech sound contrasts, thus requiring that specific discriminations be made as part of the process of identification. Table 16–3 lists a hierarchy of speech sound discriminations found in various curricula and training materials. The hierarchy is ordered by two converging principles, likely audibility to persons with hearing loss, and multiplicity of acoustic features that differ.

The leap from association of sound with meaning at the identification level to comprehension of a message requires substantial linguistic development and the establishment of supporting auditory skills. Targeting developmentally appropriate receptive language goals frames the structure of the basic skills hierarchy to enable a child to bridge the gap between single-word auditory identification and message comprehension. Four supporting auditory skills are also essential: auditory attention and tracking, auditory memory, sequencing, and closure. Auditory attention and tracking enable the listener to follow a message. Unlike the written word, which remains on the page

Case Study 16–2 A.P. was an 8-year-old boy with a profound bilateral sensorineural hearing loss. He was first fit with hearing aids at age 31 months and was enrolled in an auditory–oral preschool. When A.P. entered therapy, he had received a cochlear implant and had been wearing the device for 3 months. He was mainstreamed in a second grade classroom. His support services included individual speech/language therapy, tutoring with an itinerant teacher of the hearing impaired, and private therapy.

Prior to implantation, A.P. received intensive auditory therapy and had developed a number of auditory skills. Nevertheless, A.P.'s aided hearing levels barely reached the conversational speech spectrum, and he relied heavily on speechreading for ordinary communication. When A.P. entered therapy, he demonstrated the following auditory capabilities in a closed set: word identification by syllable number, sentence identification by length, and vowel discrimination on the basis of the second formant. A.P. also demonstrated emerging recognition of common sentences or expressions (How old are you? It's time for PE.). He also expressed a desire to use the telephone with his implant.

Auditory goals incorporated language and speech goals in the same manner as seen with S.W. in Case Study 16–1. Specifically, auditory goals included:

1. Recognition and comprehension of open-set speech material
   a. Common sentences or expressions
   b. Sentences within a given topic
   c. Unrelated sentences with clue words
   d. Unrelated sentences without clue words
2. Participation in interactive telephone practice following the goals listed
3. Process three and four critical elements with known vocabulary, two to three critical elements with less familiar vocabulary

Therapy was directed toward bridging open- and closed-set identification skills. A.P. easily identified what he heard when the choices were explicitly available, either in picture or in written form. A.P. practiced identifying sentences or answering questions after listening to an auditory message and looking at pictures that were related to what was said, but did not contain all the information. He listened to sentences describing events while looking at pictures that illustrated these events and then sequenced the pictures. Later, foils were included among the pictures that could logically be sequenced, but were not contained in the message. Still later, the simultaneous presentations of pictures and message were changed to presentation of the message first, followed by pictures.

A.P. progressed to message identification with the message topic first announced by the speaker. Conversations were practiced at this stage. A.P. and the clinician would select a topic ("Let's talk about the Horned Frogs football game.") and the conversation would continue in an auditory-only mode. In the beginning, there would be some discussion about what might be said to give A.P. an opportunity to practice anticipatory strategies. A.P. made a list of anticipatory and repair strategies that he could refer to during the session, and these were modified as he determined what was most effective for him. A.P. needed to be able to determine the topic of a conversation on his own in order to develop open-set auditory skill. He practiced listening to groups of related words, short descriptions, and definitions and identifying what the speaker was talking about.

Case Study 16–2   *(continued)*

Telephone practice proceeded at a slow and careful pace. When A.P. was successful with an auditory task during the therapy session, he completed the same kind of task with the message delivered over the telephone. A.P. also explored the components of a telephone conversation, including how to recognize that a speaker was ready to change a topic or to end a conversation. He wrote conversations and rehearsed them on the telephone with his clinician.

Six months after A.P. was first stimulated with the cochlear implant, he achieved a word discrimination score of 68% to monosyllables presented in a closed set at 50 dB HL. A.P.'s error responses were analyzed to catalog his auditory confusions. These formed the basis of syllable-level drill to give A.P. practice in identifying these speech sounds. He created variations to make the drill more interesting, moving to different locations in the therapy room and introducing different kinds of background noise

---

once inscribed, a spoken message disappears as it is delivered. Auditory memory permits the spoken message to be retrieved and analyzed subsequent to delivery. Auditory sequencing works hand in hand with auditory memory, and is an important skill in decoding an order-based syntax such as English. Lastly, auditory closure is an especially important skill for comprehension by listeners with hearing loss. Hearing loss renders aspects of the signal inaudible; additional features are obliterated by distance and noise. The listener who is able to take advantage of context and fill in these gaps is

Table 16–3.   Hierarchy of Speech Contrasts for Discrimination and Identification Practice

Suprasegmentals

Syllable number

Varied consonant and vowels

Vowel height

Vowel place

Initial consonant manner

Final consonant manner

Final consonant voicing

Initial consonant voicing

Initial consonant place

Final consonant place

From Sindrey (1997, Appendix A).

better equipped to achieve auditory comprehension.

Classroom listening necessitates advanced comprehension skills. The language of instruction increases in complexity and abstraction as a child's education progresses. The skills already described that support auditory comprehension play an important role in the classroom. In addition, the child must acquire the ability to process material with reduced contextual predictability. Table 16–4 lists additional auditory comprehension goals pertinent to classroom listening collected from three auditory learning curricula.

The child with hearing loss operates from several dimensions of skill development, and each influences the clinician's plan as well as the child's response. These include (1) the skill level of the perceptual task to be trained; (2) the level of expertise with language form, content, or use in which the perceptual task is embedded; and (3) the child's competency with the response required. The language levels of school children with hearing loss are often notably lower than those of their peers with normal hearing, even among those children who participate in mainstream classes (Davis, 1974; Osberger, 1986; Rhoades & Chisolm, 2001). Consequently the child with hearing loss may utilize comprehension strategies more typical of younger children. The clinician thus has two tasks with regard to intervention. First, when planning

Table 16–4. Advanced Skills with Connected Speech: The Bridge to Classroom Listening

Speech Perception Instructional Curriculum and Evaluation (SPICE) (Moog, Biedenstein, & Davidson, 1995)

Comprehends key words in sentence contexts

Identifies and repeats practice sentences

Converses using picture context
    Responds to questions, directions, statements
    Repeats questions, directions, statements

Engages in discussion about a familiar topic
    Answers questions
    Converses

Engages in connected discourse tracking
    Repeats sentences
    Answers questions

Auditory Skills Instructional Program (ASIPS) (Thies, 1979)

Demonstrates auditory/cognitive skills within a structured listening set
    Multielement directions
    Identifications based on several related descriptors
    Listens to passage and
        Sequences three events
        Recalls five details
        Sequences five events
        Understands main idea

Demonstrates auditory–cognitive skills in conversation
    Answers questions
    Paraphrases remarks of other speakers
    Offers spontaneous relevant remarks

The Developmental Approach to Successful Listening II (DASL II) (Stout & Windle, 1992)

Using an open set, without discussion beforehand, learns new vocabulary through audition alone

Using an open set, without discussion beforehand, listens to a story and answers questions

Using an open set, without discussion beforehand, listens to a story and then retells story

Carries out a conversation through audition alone, clueing in to topic changes auditorially

---

auditory learning tasks, accommodate the level of comprehension strategies used by a particular child. The second is to foster more sophisticated strategies that will give the child greater access to the instructional language in the classroom.

The acquisition of auditory skills does not necessarily follow a linear hierarchical path. Multiple skills develop simultaneously. Progress can plateau. Auditory learning may even appear to regress. For example, as children attempt to process more complex language and less predictable input they may need to return to lower skill levels. Paying attention to the dimensions along which au-

ditory skills are attained permit an understanding of the varied routes that children may take within an auditory skills hierarchy.

Structure

Auditory learning programs for children fall into two general categories: discrete skill or language based (Paterson, 1986). Erber's (1982) skill objectives are fundamental to both discrete skill and language based auditory learning curricula. Discrete skill programs tend to train specific auditory skills in a context separate from learning experiences that target the development of other communicative behaviors. Clinicians applying a discrete skill program will select stimuli based on audibility and the perceptual task. Examples of discrete skills programs include the Auditory Skills Instructional Program (Foreworks, 1979), SPICE: Speech Perception Instructional Curriculum and Evaluation (Moog, Biedenstein, & Davidson, 1995) and DASL: The Developmental Approach to Successful Listening (Stout & Windle, 1992).

The stimuli in a language-based approach are encased within an interactive language development program. Clinicians employ audibility and skill criteria similarly to a discrete skill approach while also selecting stimuli that teach specific linguistic principles (Estabrooks, 1993, 1994; Nevins & Chute, 1996; Pollack, Goldberg, & Caleffe-Schenck, 1997; Rhoades & Chisholm, 2001). Auditory skills are positioned within the more pervasive context of targeting objectives according to what would be expected according to normal language development. Ling (1986) first applied the term "auditory learning" to describe the language based process. He observed that real-life experiences develop listening skills more effectively than isolated tasks. Learning to listen occurs when children extract meaning from everyday acoustic events. Language based approaches integrate auditory learning experiences into activities that target language and communication. Examples of language based curricula and materials are found in Estabrooks (1994, 1998), Pollack et al (1997), and Sindrey (1997, 1998).

The most efficacious approach to developing auditory skills judiciously applies the best of discrete skill and auditory learning methods. There are times that a child will benefit from separating auditory tasks from other language or communication tasks to introduce a skill or to allow for practice of a skill toward developing automaticity. Discrete skill training also permits easier observation of auditory performance in isolation from other language behaviors and can be introduced throughout the auditory learning program as a check on progress. One must also keep in mind that integrating au-

ditory learning into the more general language intervention program requires careful planning in order to avoid burdening the child with too many new skills targeted in a single experience.

Discrete skill training sessions tend to be more structured than language based auditory learning experiences. Simser (1993) describes an effective auditory training program as one that moves in and out of structured tasks, to the extent that structure does not overpower conversational interaction. Patterson (1986) points out that auditory training programs tend to vary in the amount of structured adult-directed activities so that in the real clinical setting there may be no clear dividing line between discrete skill training or language based approaches, but rather a continuum of sorts. Erber (1982) describes a continuum of structure among auditory learning programs:

1. Structured practice on specific tasks
2. A moderately structured approach that first elicits identification within a closed set and follows with a related comprehension task
3. Natural conversational approach

Tye-Murray (1993a) utilizes short, intense sessions of formal training, 10 to 15 minutes per day, similar in practice to Ling's (1989, 2002) recommendations for phonetic-level speech production drills. Formal objectives are then pursued informally throughout the day in the natural context.

Speechreading

Speechreading incorporates information appearing on the lips, in a speaker's facial expressions and body language, and in the situational and linguistic context. Visual speech cues enhance or disambiguate the auditory signal. Features that are potentially the least audible, such as consonant place of articulation, tend to be visible. Other speech features, however, are characterized by low visibility or ambiguous visual cues. Suprasegmental aspects are not cued visually. Vowels and diphthongs may be differentiated visually by lip shape and jaw height, but tongue position is generally not visible. Adjacent vowels are easily confused visually. Among consonants, few acoustic manner features are available visually. Some manner features such as frication and plosion can be contrasted visually by duration of position, but these are difficult to resolve in connected speech. Voicing contrasts cannot be visually differentiated within the spoken signal. As a consequence, some 60% of the spoken message is visually uninterpretable. Approximately 50% of English phonemes and words are so reduced in contrastiveness that they are identical (Berg, 1972).

Acoustic and visual cues in speech combine to provide an intelligible message. For the listener with normal hearing, the acoustic signal is ordinarily sufficient for speech recognition, provided that there is little interference from noise, distance, or reverberation. The listener with hearing loss will miss crucial auditory information and rely on information from other sources to supplement audition, including visual cues in spoken language. Ambiguity and low visibility of visual cues, however, render sole reliance on vision to be a difficult route to comprehension.

Interactive Auditory Learning

The comprehension of spoken language is interactive, necessitating attention to strategies used by both the listener and the talker. The child who succeeds in comprehending spoken language is likely to have internalized communication strategies for preventing or repairing breakdowns that occur in everyday communication. A perceptual training program that is designed with communicative interaction in mind will facilitate the development of these strategies. Kaplan, Bally, and Garretson (1985) describe communication strategies as two types: anticipatory and repair. Anticipatory strategies are applied before a message occurs and minimize potential problems. Anticipatory strategies include anticipation of the vocabulary, topic, and dialogue that may take place in a particular situation, and preparation for the auditory environment with plans for modifications. Repair strategies address a breakdown after it has occurred. Repair strategies include requests for repetitions, paraphrasing, saying or spelling key words, gestures or writing, or asking questions about the message.

While a child is developing communicative strategies, clinicians and educators adapt auditory input in order to provide a facilitative context or to respond to communicative breakdowns. Adaptive strategies influence the input presented by the clinician based on the child's response to a perceptual task. If the child is successful, the clinician maintains the task, introduces new semantic content or more complex linguistic form, or moves to a higher level of perceptual demand. If the child is not successful, a task analysis reveals the nature of the unsuccessful response and the clinician applies strategies to facilitate success. Breakdowns may be behavioral, linguistic, perceptual, or based on the child's knowledge about the topic.

Tye-Murray (1994) points out three challenges to incorporating communication strategies training in a program designed for children: (1) presenting strategies that children can understand; (2) choosing strategies appropriate for children's conversation; and (3) developing interesting materials and procedures. Skits and role-playing provide an avenue for illustrating the need for and use of conversational strategies (Elfenbein, 1992; Trychin, & Bonvillian, 1992). Furthermore, children with hearing impairment may require training to use the structure of conversation. Practice of conversational routines, or scenarios, is one way to establish conversational function and makes use of routinized language from which linguistic rules may be derived.

Starting "Late"

The age at which auditory learning begins influences progress. The ideal is to provide amplification or a cochlear implant and intervention during the optimal language-learning period (Brackett, 1991; Yoshinaga-Itano, 1998). One can apply the notion of "hearing age" to establish expectations for performance based on the length of time that a child has been fit with amplification or has been stimulated by an implant (Northcott, 1972; Pollack, 1970). The application of hearing age to predictions of auditory behavior is most straightforward when the child is fit with amplification or receives a cochlear implant in infancy and the discrepancy between chronological and hearing age is minimal.

As the gap between chronological and hearing age widens, intervention may be initiated at ages beyond the optimal period for acquiring auditory language. Nevertheless, motoric, cognitive, and experiential levels that are present in the older child must be taken into account, as well as the potential for auditory neural plasticity (Tallal, Merzenich, Miller, & Jenkins, 1998). The effect of starting intervention beyond the optimal period may slow progress, but maturity in other skill areas may actually positively influence performance.

Although the ideal age for implementation of an auditory learning program is during infancy or early childhood, some children with hearing loss do not begin auditory learning until school age. This can happen when a child receives a cochlear implant during the school years. The child is likely to have a language base of some sort, probably highly visually organized, using speechreading, a sign system, cuing, or attending to a combination of visual information sources. For this child, the fundamental task is one of transitioning from attending to language visually to becoming a listener. The long-term goals for new listeners of this sort are to:

1. Self-identify as a listener
2. Develop auditory skills
3. Integrate auditory skills into the existing communication system
4. Decrease dependence on visual cues in receptive and in expressive communication

If the child is to integrate hearing into his or her personality, the older child who has new auditory potential via the cochlear implant must discover that potential and be an active participant in the learning process. Without self-motivated involvement, the development of auditory skills is likely to remain a discrete ability, not integrated into the communication system. Orienting the child to the acoustic landscape by providing guidance and identifying the sources and meaning of sounds in the daily environment begins this process. Another approach is journaling. Wayner and Abrahamson (1998) provide a template for newly implanted listeners to keep a journal about their discoveries and personal responses to changes subsequent to implantation. The approach can be adapted to accommodate the student's skills and preferences; journals need not take written form nor must all entries be shared with educators. The journal, whatever form it takes, is a tool to engage the student's insight and encourage self-directed learning. Some journaling topics suggested by Wayner and Abrahamson include:

What new sounds/pleasant/nice/terrible/irritating?
What are your reactions/feelings?
What have you noticed about your interactions with others?
Have you tried anything you have avoided before?
How does music sound?
What has surprised you?
What advice would you give?

Many school-aged children who are newly implanted have minimal knowledge about spoken language. This may be particularly true for a student who is dependent on a sign system and may not have been encouraged to develop speechreading skills in conjunction with sign acquisition. Auditory learning must include discovery of the phonological system. Systematic, discrete skill training at the discrimination level is useful in this case, providing the student with information describing how sounds contrast acoustically as well as multiple examples with a variety of consonant–vowel contexts. The training materials authored by Nancy Tye-Murray (1993b, 1997) provide practice of this nature.

Friendships and social activities are vital to school children, and the telephone is an important device. Telephone conversations may be considered the ultimate open-set, auditory task. Speechreading cues are unavailable, and conversational topics can change quickly with minimal cuing by the speaker. Fully independent telephone use may be a long way off for new implant users who are visually dependent in communication and have minimal English proficiency. Nevertheless, the telephone can be a useful tool in an auditory learning program. Skills that are practiced in live voice can be practiced on the telephone. The child is able to see progress toward the ultimate goal, and is motivated to attend to skill training at levels below open-set comprehension.

Speech Production

A final word must be said about a related area of learning that appears within many auditory skills hierarchies, the establishment of the productive phonology, or the speech sound system, in the child's native language. Residual hearing and auditory skill acquisition fundamentally influence speech abilities in children with hearing loss, establishing auditory feedforward and auditory feedback (Ling, 2002; McCaffrey, Davis, MacNeilage, & von Hapsburg, 2000; Tye-Murray, 1992). Auditory feedforward enables the child to set an acoustic target for the production of a speech sound. This is not easily achieved without the auditory experience and practice that establish the phonology both motorically and auditorially. Auditory feedback enables continual monitoring of speech production and ongoing adjustments as needed to maintain accuracy. The child who has not established an auditory-based phonology will utilize other less effective sources for feedback, such as proprioception or tactile information (Higgins, Carney, McCleary, & Rogers, 1996; Higgins, McCleary, & Ide-Helvie, 2002). The inclusion of speech production tasks within the auditory learning program facilitates both speech production and auditory skills development

more effectively than auditory training alone (Novelli-Olmsted & Ling, 1984).

Implementing Auditory Learning

The following suggestions are not intended to be a cookbook for developing an auditory learning program from start to finish. A cookbook approach would fail to meet the varied needs of school children with hearing loss, as is shown in Case Study 16–3. Instead, a scaffold is provided to facilitate the reader's own design.

1. *Assess auditory learning.* An auditory learning program begins with assessment. Assessment of auditory learning provides information regarding a student's current level, determines teaching objectives, and documents progress if assessment is conducted over time. Table 16–5 organizes several of these according to the aspects laid out in Table 16–1. Selection of an assessment instrument will be dictated by the skill level targeted, the acoustic features of the linguistic aspect that one wishes to probe, and the level of predictability that the student is expected to be able to accommodate. Assessment is incomplete without a determination of the child's receptive and expressive language level. The reader is referred to the Cottage Acquisition Scales (Wilkes, 1999) for an example of a checklist that is useful for documenting language ability and selecting comprehension goals within an auditory learning framework.

   Assessment may also compare a child's receptive language abilities across auditory and visual modalities. This is particularly important in planning for a child who is transitioning from a visual language approach to the acquisition of auditory skills, such as in the case of a newly implanted student. Table 16–6 profiles data from assessments conducted across domains. The child who transitions from dependence on a visual sign system to establishment of listening skills will likely have

Table 16–5. Features of Auditory Skill Assessments

Test	Ages	*Scoring	Stimuli/ Features Assessed	Skills Assessed	Response Set	Comments
Early Speech Perception Test (ESP) (Moog & Geers, 1990)	2 through teens	CR	Syllable number Spondees differing in consonant and vowel content Vowels	Discrimination Identification	Closed	Toys available for use by young children
Test of Auditory Comprehension (TAC) (Trammel, 1976)	4–12 yrs	STD-HI	Environmental sounds Nonverbal human sounds Words, phrases, sentences, short stories	Discrimination Identification Memory for two and four critical elements Sequencing Recalling details Listening in noise	Closed	Out of print, but widely used in programs for children with hearing loss; normative data from children with cochlear implants not available
Auditory Perception Test for the Hearing Impaired (APT-HI) (Allen & Serwatka, 1994)	5 through teens	CR	Syllables Pitch Vowels Consonant difference in words Sentences	Auditory awareness Discrimination Identification Comprehension of questions	Closed Open set for compre-hension	
Test of the Auditory Percepual Skills–Revised (TAPS-R) (Gardner, 1996)	4–13 yrs	STD-NL	Words and numbers Words differing in vowel or consonant content Sentences	Memory Discrimination Comprehension	Open	
The Listening Test (Barrett, Huisingh, Zachman, Bladgen, & Orman, 1992)	6–12 yrs	STD-NL	Paragraphs	Getting the main idea Remembering details Applying conceptual vocabulary Inferring answers Story comprehension	Open Concepts section supplies pictures for topic	
Speech Perception Instructional Curriculum and Evaluation (SPICE)— Rating form (Moog, Biedenstein, & Davidson, 1995)	3–12 yrs	CR	Syllables Words Sentences Questions	Detecton Suprasegmental discrimination Vowel and consonant discrimination Identification of words and sentences Comprehension	Ranging from closed to open set	This is a rating form for placement on the DASL curriculum and for documenting progress

Table 16–5. Features of Auditory Skill Assessments (continued)

Test	Ages	*Scoring	Stimuli/ Features Assessed	Skills Assessed	Response Set	Comments
Developmental Approach to Successful Listening II (DASL-II)— Placement test (Stout & Windle, 1992)	3–18 yrs	CR	Syllables Words Sentences	Detecton Suprasegmental discrimination Vowel and consonant discrimination Identification of words and sentences Comprehension	Ranging from closed to open set	This is a rating form for placement on the DASL curriculum and for documenting progress

*Scoring categories: CR, criterion referenced; STD-NL, standardized with children with normal hearing; STD-HI, standardized with children with hearing impairment.

different levels of function across the two modalities. The profile identifies a place to begin auditory learning as well as to establish level of comprehension in the visual modality.

2. *Specify the learning objectives.* Consider perceptual skill to be the learning objective with language form and content as stimuli for the intervention. Academic content also influences the stimuli for school children. The educator or clinician may move back to an earlier-developing auditory skill if new language or academic content are being acquired.

3. *Plan for exposure.* The development of listening skills demands enormous amounts of input before similar output from the child is observed. An exposure, or stimulation, period is often necessary even for higher levels of listening skills. The inclusion of an exposure phase in training requires simultaneous

---

Implanted thresholds for Case Studies 16–2 and 16–3:

    250 Hz: 25 dB HL
    500 Hz: 20 dB HL
    1000 Hz: 25 dB HL
    2000 Hz: 30 dB HL
    4000 Hz: 25 dB HL
    6000 Hz: 25 dB HL

---

targeting of future and current objectives so that exposure and stimulation are provided on an ongoing basis.

4. *Consider the guidelines found in milieu language teaching (Kaiser, Yoder, & Keetz, 1992).*
   a. Follow the child's interest.
   b. Provide multiple, naturally occurring examples.
   c. Explicitly prompt the child's production or response.
   d. Embed the teaching episode in ongoing interactions.
   e. Program for generalization by using multiple encounters in multiple conversational contexts.

5. *Employ linguistic prefacing.* Before an activity is presented, describe it to the child so that the child first attends to spoken language. Repeat this language throughout the activity.

6. *For each learning objective, provide a variety of response alternatives and learning experiences.* These will accommodate the various comprehension strategies that might be applied by the novice learner. If necessary, target the development of mature comprehension strategies.

7. *Provide negative examples.* Disequilibrium precedes the formation of new knowledge structures. Activities that do not produce expected results allow for disequilibrium. The child develops the expectation that there will be a cer-

Table 16–6. Communication Modality Profile

Closed set			
Perceptual Skill/Stimulus	*Auditory*	*Speechreading*	*Sign + Speech*
Suprasegmentals			
Single word: feature identification			
Stereotypic phrases			
Phrases/sentences			

Memory:
  Two elements
  Four elements
  More			

Passage comprehension:
  Sequences
  Recalls details
  Answers questions
  Main idea
  Learns new information/vocabulary			

Open Set			
Perceptual Skill/Stimulus	*Auditory*	*Speechreading*	*Sign + Speech*
Suprasegmentals			
Single word: feature identification			
Stereotypic phrases			
Phrases/sentences			

Memory:
  Two elements
  Four elements
  More			

Passage comprehension:
  Sequences
  Recalls details
  Answers questions
  Main idea
  Learns new information/vocabulary			

Scale: 0 Never observed
    1 Rarely: Approximately 25% correct, or observed in 25% of opportunities
    2 Occasionally: Approximately 50% correct, or observed in 50% of opportunities, restricted to only a few contexts
    3 Frequently: Approximately 75% correct, or observed in 75% of opportunities
    4 Always: Generalized to all contexts

tain amount of unpredictability in what is heard.

8. *Learning is active and interactive.* The child should do something with what is heard.

9. *Integrate content and process.* Integrate the process of listening while teaching content of academic subject areas.

10. *Plan auditory learning experiences along the dimensions of linguistic level, linguistic unit, and response constraint.* Target auditory skill development according to the child's performance within these levels. Add on, rather than check off, skills.

Case Study 16–3 T.S. was an 11-year-old girl who was seen for a consultation at the request of her parents and school. She had a congenital bilateral profound sensorineural hearing loss of unknown etiology. She was first fit with hearing aids at age 20 months and was enrolled in a total communication preschool. T.S. received a cochlear implant at age 9 years. At the time of consultation, T.S. had been wearing her implant for 18 months. T.S. is partially mainstreamed in a third grade classroom with an educational interpreter. She receives instruction in language arts and reading in a self-contained classroom with other children with hearing loss. T.S. also received individual therapy with a speech-language pathologist at her school in two 15-minute sessions per week. Her school program used a manually coded English sign system.

The school and parents expressed disappointment at T.S.'s progress in the production and comprehension of spoken language since the cochlear implantation. They asked for suggestions for improving T.S.'s skills. In addition, her parents wanted to know if signs should be removed from her daily communication to facilitate the establishment of oral skills.

Formal language measures, observation of T.S. in school and in the clinic, and school and parent interviews showed T.S. to be functioning within 2 years of her chronological age in the form, content, and use of English-based sign language. Speech use was greatly reduced relative to language. T.S. rarely used her voice when she signed. Nevertheless, T.S.'s speech-language pathologist reported an increase in her phonetic inventory in the therapy setting since receiving the cochlear implant. Generalization to the phonological level was limited.

Observation of T.S. in the classroom revealed that most of the language input she received was signed and generally unaccompanied by spoken language. When T.S. was in the mainstream setting, she made good use of her educational interpreter to follow classroom instruction, but the signal she was attending to was primarily signed with few speechreading cues accompanying the signal. In T.S.'s class with other children with hearing loss, instruction presented by the teacher occurred without voice some 40 to 60% of the time that was observed. In all settings, T.S. was rarely encouraged to accompany her signed communications with spoken language.

Assessment of auditory skills showed that T.S. had an awareness of sound, recognized some environmental sounds, and differentiated human from environmental sounds. Speechreading assessment revealed that she had little recognition of common words through the combined modalities of speechreading and listening, despite the fact that she understood the words when they were signed. The observation of the clinician was that T.S. was not aware of information available through speechreading and listening.

T.S. received her implant relatively late in life. The timing of the implantation suggested that auditory learning would be slow and her skills may not progress to the same level as a child with similar capacities who receives an implant during the optimal language-learning years. In addition, T.S. had established a visual language system that was English based but did not have the underlying auditory phonology that exists in spoken English. The presence of an already established visual language system and the absence of functional use of audition or speechreading suggested that auditory language learning should be mapped onto existing signed structures, and removal from a signing environment was not recommended.

Case Study 16–3 *(continued)*

The recommendation that signs remain as part of T.S.'s communication system did not mean, however, that the learning environment did not require modification. Despite the fact T.S. possessed a higher level of auditory potential following implantation, the expectations and interactions in the school program had not changed to accommodate this new potential. Without opportunities throughout the day to listen to, speechread, and produce spoken language, prognosis for improvement beyond the level of rudimentary auditory awareness seen at the time of assessment was considered to be poor.

The program for this child did not follow a model of consultation with the family and school to modify the learning environment and assist personnel in developing techniques that had not previously been incorporated into the curriculum. In addition, the school program increased T.S.'s time with the speech-language pathologist for auditory skill practice. The school also provided for increased participation of the speech-language pathologist in T.S.'s self-contained and mainstream classrooms to assist in the incorporation of added techniques.

T.S.'s auditory skills improved to the level of closed set identification of familiar phrases and there was an increase in her vocalizations. In addition, other children in the program showed improvements in auditory skills as a result of the incorporation of auditory techniques in the instructional program.

---

11. *Once mastery of a skill has occurred, provide opportunities for reinforcement and generalization.*

12. *Proceed at an appropriate pace.* Goals and activities should be distributed among a variety of levels of skill mastery.

13. *Listening is an internal process that cannot be measured directly.* Include some tasks in a stimulus-response framework, so that training will elicit a specific response to each activity and performance can be monitored (Pollack, 1993). This should not be confused with testing. It may be necessary to teach the response and give the child experience with the correct response before performance is observed.

14. *Prepare the child to take responsibility for successful communication.* Allow for breakdowns in the therapy session, and guide the child in the repair and prevention of these.

15. *Identify influences on performance and account for these in expectations of performance.*

Child characteristics such as degree of hearing loss or age at identification that might slow the attainment of learning objectives should not rule out the application of an auditory training program. Instead, realistic expectations for the rate of learning and final level should be considered as training ensues.

References

Allen, S.G., & Serwatka, T.S. (1994). Auditory Perception Test for the Hearing Impaired (APT/HI). Burlingame, CA: Psychological and Educational Publications.

Aslin, R.N., Pisoni, D.B., & Jusczyk, P.W. (1982). *Auditory Development and Speech Perception in Infancy.* Research on Speech Perception, Technical Report No. 4. Bloomington: Indiana University Infant Perception Laboratory, 132–143.

Barrett, M., Huisingh, R., Zachman, L., Bladgen, C., & Orman, J. (1992). The Listening Test. East Moline, IL: LinguiSystems.

Benedict, H. (1979). Early lexical development: Comprehension and production. *J Child Lang, 6,* 619–635.

Berg, K.W. (1972). Visemes and homophenous words. *Tch Deaf, 70,* 396–399.

Boothroyd, A. (1984). Auditory perception of speech contrasts by subjects with sensorineural hearing loss. *J Speech Hear Res, 27,* 134–144.

Brackett, D. (1991). *Rehabilitation/Education Strategies for Children with Cochlear Implants.* Clinical Bulletin. Englewood, CO: Cochlear Corporation.

Davis, J.M. (1974). Performance of young hearing impaired children on a test of basic concepts. *J Speech Hear Res, 17,* 342–351.

Diehl, R.L., & Walsh, M.A. (1989). An auditory basis for the stimulus-length effect in the perception of stops and glides. *J Acoust Soc Am, 85,* 2154–2164.

Dubno, J.R., & Ahlstrom, H.B. (1995). Masked thresholds and consonant recognition in low-pass maskers for hearing-impaired and normal-hearing listeners. *J Acoust Soc Am, 97,* 2430–2441.

Elfenbein, J. (1992). Coping with communication breakdown: a program of strategy development for children who have hearing losses. *Am J Audiol, 1,* 25–29.

Erber, N.P. (1982). *Auditory Training.* Washington, DC: Alexander Graham Bell Association for the Deaf and Hard of Hearing.

Estabrooks W. (1993). Still listening . . . auditory–verbal therapy for "older" children. *Volta Rev, 95,* 231–252.

Estabrooks, W. (Ed.). (1994). *Auditory–Verbal Therapy for Parents and Professionals.* Washington, DC: Alexander Graham Bell Association for the Deaf.

Estabrooks, W. (Ed.). (1998). *Cochlear Implants for Kids.* Washington, DC: Alexander Graham Bell Association for the Deaf.

Fernald A. (1985). The perceptual and affective salience of mothers' speech to infants. In: L. Feagans, C. Garvey, & R. Golinkoff (Eds.), *The Origins and Growth of Communication* (pp. 285–306). New Brunswick, NJ: Alkex Press.

Fletcher H. (1953) *Speech and Hearing in Communication.* New York: D. Van Nostrand.

Fry, D.B. (1978). The role and primacy of the auditory channel in speech and language development. In: M. Ross & T.G. Giolas (Eds.), *Auditory Management of Hearing-Impaired Children* (pp. 15–43). Baltimore: University Park Press.

Gardner, M. (1996). Test of Auditory Perceptual Skills–Revised (TAPS-R). Los Angeles: Psychological & Educational Publications.

Gopnik, A., Meltzoff, A.N., & Kuhl, P.K. (2000) *The Scientist in the Crib: What Early Learning Tells Us about the Mind.* New York: Quill.

Higgins, M.B., Carney, A.E., McCleary, E., & Rogers, S. (1996). Negative intraoral air pressures of deaf children with cochlear implants: Physiology, phonology, and treatment. *J Speech Hear Res, 39,* 957–967.

Higgins, M.B., McCleary, E., & Ide-Helvie, D. (2002). *Speech and voice physiology of children who are hard of hearing.* Paper presented at the annual meeting of the American Speech-Language-Hearing Association, Atlanta, GA.

Jusczyk, P.W. (1998). *The Discovery of Spoken Language.* Cambridge: MIT Press.

Kaiser, A.P., Yoder, P.J., & Keetz, A. (1992). Evaluating milieu teaching. In: S.F. Warren & J. Reichle (Eds.), *Causes and Effects in Communication and Language Intervention* (pp. 9–47). Baltimore: Brookes.

Kaplan, H.F., Bally, S., & Garretson, C. (1985). *Speechreading: A Way to Improve Understanding.* Washington, DC: Gallaudet.

Kuhl, P.K. (1992). Psychoacoustics and speech perception: internal standards, perceptual anchors, and prototypes, In L.A. Werner & E.W. Rubel (Eds.), *Developmental Psychoacoustics.* (pp. 293–332).Washington, DC: American Psychological Association.

Kuhl, P.K. (1993). Innate predispositions and the effects of experience in speech perception: The native language magnet theory. In: B. deBoysson-Bardies, S. de Schonen, P. Jusczyk, P. McNeilage, & J. Morton (Eds.), *Developmental Neurocognition: Speech and Face Processing in the First Year of Life* (pp. 259–274). Dordrecht, Netherlands: Kluwer Academic Publishers.

Kuhl, P.K. (2000). A new view of language acquisition. *Proc Natl Acad Sci, 97,* 11850–11857.

Lindblom, B., MacNeilage, P., & Studdert-Kennedy, M. (1983). Self-organizing processes and the explanation of phonological universals. In: B. Butterworth, B. Comrie, & O. Dahl (Eds.), *Explanations of Linguistic Universals* (pp. 181–203). Mouton: The Hague.

Ling, D. (1986). Devices and procedures for auditory learning. *Volta Rev Monog, 88,* 19–28.

Ling, D. (1989). *Foundations of Spoken Language for Hearing-Impaired Children.* Washington, DC: Alexander Graham Bell Association for the Deaf and Hard of Hearing.

Ling, D. (2002). *Speech and the Hearing-Impaired Child: Theory and Practice* (2nd ed.). Washington, DC: Alexander Graham Bell Association for the Deaf and Hard of Hearing.

McCaffrey, H.A., Davis, B.L., MacNeilage, P.F., & von Hapsburg, D. (2000). Multichannel cochlear implantation and the organization of early speech. *Volta Rev, 101,* 5–29.

Milosky, L.M. (1992). Children listening: The role of world knowledge in language comprehension. In: R.S. Chapman (Ed.), *Processes in Language Acquisition and Disorders* (pp. 20–44). Baltimore: Mosby Year Book.

Moog, J.S., & Geers, A.E. (1990). Early Speech Perception Test. St. Louis: Central Institute for the Deaf.

Moog, J.S., Biedenstein, J.J., & Davidson, L.S. (1995). SPICE: Speech Perception Instructional Curriculum and Evaluation. St. Louis: Central Institute for the Deaf.

Nevins, M.E., & Chute, P.M. (1996). *Children with Cochlear Implants in Educational Settings.* San Diego: Singular.

Newport, E.L., Gleitman, L.R., & Gleitman, H. (1977). Mother, I'd rather do it myself: Some effects and non-effects of maternal speech style. In: C.E. Snow & C.A. Ferguson (Eds.), *Talking to Children: Language Input and Acquisition.* New York: Cambridge University Press.

Ninio, A., & Bruner, J. (1978). The achievement and antecedents of labelling. *J Child Lang, 5,* 1–15.

Nittrouer, S. (2002). From ear to cortex: A perspective on what clinicians need to understand about speech perception and language processing. *Lang Speech Hear Serv Sch, 33,* 237–252.

Northcott, W. (1972). *Curriculum Guide: Hearing Impaired Children—Birth to Three Years.* Washington, DC: Alexander Graham Bell Association for the Deaf and Hard of Hearing.

Novelli-Olmsted, T., & Ling, D. (1984). Speech production and speech discrimination by hearing-impaired children. *Volta Rev, 86,* 72–80.

Osberger, M.J. (1986). *Language and Learning Skills of Hearing-Impaired Students.* ASHA Monogr, 80.

Paterson, M. (1986). Maximizing the use of residual hearing with school-aged hearing-impaired students-a perspective. *Volta Rev Monog, 88,* 93–106.

Peters, A.M. (1983). *The Units of Language Acquisition.* London: Cambridge University Press.

Pollack, D. (1970). *Educational Audiology for the Limited Hearing Infant and Preschooler* (1st ed.) Springfield, IL: Charles C. Thomas.

Pollack, D. (1993). Reflections of a pioneer. *Volta Rev, 95,* 197–204.

Pollack, D., Goldberg, D., & Caleffe-Schenck, N. (1997). *Educational Audiology for the Limited Hearing Infant.* (3rd ed.). Springfield, IL: Charles C. Thomas.

Rhoades, E.A., & Chisolm, T.H. (2001). Global language progress with an auditory–verbal approach for children who are deaf or hard of hearing. *Volta Rev, 102,* 5–24.

Schneider, B.A., & Trehub, S.E. (1992). Sources of developmental change in auditory sensitivity. In: L.A. Werner & E.W. Rubel (Eds.), *Developmental Psychoacoustics* (pp. 3–46). Washington, DC: American Psychological Association.

Simser, J. (1993). Auditory verbal intervention: Infants and toddlers. *Volta Rev, 95,* 217–230.

Sindrey, D. (1997). *Listening Games for Littles.* Washington, DC: Alexander Graham Bell Association for the Deaf and Hard of Hearing.

Sindrey, D. (1998). *Cochlear Implant Auditory Training Guidebook.* Washington, DC: Alexander Graham Bell Association for the Deaf and Hard of Hearing.

Stout, G., & Windle, J. (1992). The Developmental Approach to Successful Listening II (DASL). Denver: Cochlear Corporation.

Sussman, H.M., McCaffrey, H.A., & Matthews, S.A. (1991). An investigation of locus equations as a source of relational invariance for stop place categorization. *J Acoust Soc Am, 90,* 1309–1325.

Syrdal, A.K. (1985). Aspects of a model of the auditory representation of American English vowels. *Speech Communication, 4,* 121–135.

Tallal, P., Merzenich, M.M., Miller, S., & Jenkins, W. (1998). Language learning impairments: Integrating basic science, technology, and remediation. *Exp Brain Res, 123,* 210–219.

Thies, T.L. (1979). *Auditory Skills Instructional Program (ASIPS).* Portland, OR: Foreworks.

Trammel, J.L. (1976). Test of Auditory Comprehension. Portland, OR: Foreworks.

Trychin S., & Bonvillian, B. (1992). *Actions Speak Louder: Tips for Putting on Skits Related to Hearing Loss.* Bethesda, MD: Self Help for Hard of Hearing Press.

Tye-Murray, N. (1992). Articulatory organizational strategies and the roles of audition. *Volta Rev, 94,* 243–259.

Tye-Murray, N. (1993a). Aural rehabilitation and patient management. In: R. Tyler (Ed.), *Cochlear Implants: Audiological Foundations* (pp. 87–144). San Diego: Singular.

Tye-Murray, N. (1993b). *Communication Training for Hearing-Impaired Children and Teenagers: Speechreading, Listening, and Using Repair Strategies.* Austin: PRO-ED.

Tye-Murray, N. (1994). Communication strategies training. *J Acad Rehabil Audiol Monogr, 27,* 193–207.

Tye-Murray, N. (1997). *Communication Training for Older Teenagers and Adults: Listening, Speechreading, and Using Repair Strategies.* Austin: PRO-ED.

Wayner, D.S., & Abrahamson, J.E. (1998). *Learning to Hear Again with a Cochlear Implant.* Washington, DC: Alexander Graham Bell Association for the Deaf and Hard of Hearing.

Werker, J.F., & Tees, R.C. (1984). Cross-language speech reception: Evidence for perceptual reorganization during the first year of life. *Infant Behav Devel, 7,* 49–63.

Wilkes, E.M. (1999). *Cottage Acquisition Scales for Listening, Language and Speech.* Washinton, DC: Alexander Graham Bell Association for the Deaf and Hard of Hearing.

Yoshinaga-Itano, C. (1998). Language of early and later-identified children with hearing loss. *Pediatrics, 102,* 1161–1171.

17

Remediation of Auditory Processing Disorders in Children: An Overview

CAROL G. COKELY AND PHILLIP L. WILSON

The future belongs to those who believe in the beauty of their dreams.
—Eleanor Roosevelt, 1884–1962

Children evaluated for auditory processing disorders (APD) almost always have deficits in a myriad of areas, resulting in poor performance in educational settings and sometimes very obvious poor pragmatic communication skills. Parents of these children often come to clinics when the children are preschoolers with speech and language difficulties, or when the children are school-aged and having academic or behavioral problems. The diagnostic challenge is to assess pertinent auditory, language, and cognitive capabilities adequately and to determine whether language problems, academic difficulties, and questionable communication skills result or partially result from auditory processing deficits. After diagnosis, the management challenge is to discern the best way to improve the children's listening and communication abilities and to resolve any academic difficulties. Simply remediating auditory deficits (though seldom simple) will not erase language, reading, learning, and other impairments that may be longstanding and entrenched.

The development of treatment programs is very much a team effort. Members of a team might include an audiologist, a speech-language pathologist, a psychologist, a reading specialist, an occupational therapist, a physician, and an educational diagnostician,

among others. The nature of the processing problems will define the roles members play in the intervention plans. In some cases speech-language pathologists lead the management teams, working on improving language competence and pragmatic communication skills or implementing computerized training. In other cases audiologists are case managers developing plans to enhance the children's listening environments with FM systems and implementing specific auditory training exercises to improve auditory processing skills. Rarely, however, does any one person serve as the only professional contact.

In recent years, there has been an increased interest and debate about the existence, nature, and consequences of APD. Professionals and parents alike have a plethora of information available, which often creates uncertainty as to the best courses of action. As a result, speech and hearing professionals are conducting much needed efficacy research, essential for the development of valid and effective treatment programs. Outcomes of robust, large-scale studies should add precision to the evaluation and management of problems now attributed to APD. As a discipline, it is important to be ready to provide clinicians access to the best practices in diagnosis and management of children who often present complex language, educational, and social needs.

ASHA Task Force

In 1995, the American Speech-Language-Hearing Association (ASHA) Task Force on Central Auditory Processing Consensus Development prepared the technical report, *Central Auditory Processing: Current Status of Research and Implications for Clinical Practice,* which ASHA later approved (ASHA, 1996). The working group defined central APDs as both a dysfunction of the auditory system specifically, as well as dysfunction of the auditory system as part of a multimodal deficit. The task force also reached consensus regarding what it considered four critical issues related to APD:

1. What does basic science tell about the nature of central auditory processing and its role in audition?
2. What constitutes an assessment of central auditory processing and its disorders?
3. What are the developmental and acquired communication problems associated with central APDs?
4. What is the clinical utility of a diagnosis of central APDs?

Of particular interest to the management of APD are the task force's opinions on issues 3 and 4. With regard to communication problems associated with APD, the task force noted that although language learning ability and language use are very likely to be deficient in children with APD, clinicians should not infer the presence of APD simply because of the existence of language learning or language comprehension deficits. Instead, careful audiological assessment is necessary to determine whether language impairments of children are the result of APD or the consequences of other factors. With regard to the clinical utility of an APD diagnosis, the task force was not clear whether a differential diagnosis offered a treatment advantage.

Auditory Processing Deficit Profiles

According to current philosophy, successful management of APD hinges on identifying specific auditory, language, and learning deficits. The 2000 Consensus Conference on the Diagnosis of APD in School-Aged Children and stressed that appropriate intervention stems from precise diagnosis (Jerger & Musiek, 2000). Diagnosis of impairments involves in-depth appraisals of fundamental auditory processes using any number of tests that evaluate auditory discrimination, auditory temporal pattern recognition, degraded speech understanding, and dichotic listening. Assessment must also address language, educational, emotional, and cognitive skills, as well as impulsivity and attention deficits, the latter of which can be evaluated using measures such as the Auditory Continuous Performance Test (ACPT) developed by Keith (1994). Further, primary caregivers and teachers should complete questionnaires or listening profiles [e.g., Screening Instrument for Treating Educational Risk (SIFTER) (Anderson & Matkin, 1996), Fisher's Auditory Problem Checklist (Fisher, 1985), and the Children's Auditory Performance Scale (CHAPS) (Smoski, Brunt, & Tanahill, 1998), all available from the Educational Audiology Association]. Although the information obtained from the various disciplines and diagnostic measures might prove redundant, most professionals agree that skills should be assessed from multiple perspectives. Moreover, clinicians recognize that most assessments will likely yield a complex pattern of children's abilities and deficits.

To help organize the multitude of symptoms that children might exhibit, some researchers have created matrices, or deficit profiles, that group impairments presumed to stem from a common underlying factor (Bellis, 1996; Bellis & Ferre, 1999; Katz, 1992; Masters, Stecker, & Katz, 1998). Others have identified specific listening and learning processes without categorizing them into profile patterns (Chermak & Musiek, 1992, 1997, 2002). The Katz, or Buffalo Model, and the Bellis/Ferre and Chermak/Musiek plans

Table 17–1. Processing Deficit: Auditory Decoding/Auditory Closure

(+) Test Findings:
  Monaural degraded speech tests:
    Filtered words
    Time compressed
    Speech in noise
  Phonemic analysis/synthesis
  Temporal tasks
  Dichotic tasks

Academic/Language/Learning Deficits:
  Receptive language
  Expressive language
  Slow responder
  Reading
  Spelling
  Writing

Table 17–2. Processing Deficit: Temporal Processes

(+) Test Findings:
  Temporal pattern recognition—bilateral
    (verbal and hummed response modes):
    Pitch patterns
    Duration patterns
  Gap detection
  Multitask items

Academic/Language/Learning Deficits:
  Pragmatics, humor
  Prosody
  Nonverbal speech, affect
  Memory
  Reading
  Music

are three popular comprehensive approaches that pair identification of specific deficits with specific remediation techniques. Defining processing difficulties specific to the auditory system, along with language, and learning problems points to appropriate courses of therapy.

Tables 17–1 through 17–6 provide the characteristics representative of APD profiles compiled from the three models. The first six tables describe what are presumed to be distinctive performance patterns. For each profile specified, common auditory test findings and related academic/learning difficulties are provided.

Table 17–1 reflects an auditory decoding/auditory closure deficit. Children with a decoding profile reveal a combination of auditory closure and speech sound discrimination problems. They have difficulty discriminating the fine intensity, frequency, or durational components of speech and are hampered by background noise or any condition that degrades the acoustic signal. Poor vocabulary and contextual skills typically impede learning. This class of deficits is typically revealed by degraded speech tasks, speech-in-noise tasks, or tasks that require analysis and synthesis of phonemes. Dichotic tests may be poorly performed bilaterally.

Table 17–2 cites temporal processing deficits, another common APD profile. Children who cannot process auditory temporal patterns will have difficulty perceiving and interpreting running discourse. Temporal deficits, in fact, are often considered the root of auditory processing deficits. Children have difficulty perceiving intonation patterns and display poor pragmatics or socially inappropriate communication behaviors. Tasks requiring recognition and repetition of pitch or duration pattern sequences are difficult for children with a temporal processing deficit for both hummed and verbal response formats. Gap detection tests may also implicate temporal-based inadequacies.

Table 17–3 summarizes deficits in binaural listening. Tasks that require the coordination of information presented to both ears necessitate interhemispheric communication. Impaired communication between the right and left hemispheres of the brain presumably implicates immature development of the corpus callosum. Children with integration deficits have difficulty combining information from both ears (binaural integration) or attending to a message addressed to the one side while suppressing information from the other (binaural separation). Multimodal tasks (e.g., verbal–motor or auditory–visual) require interhemispheric trans-

Table 17–3. Processing Deficit: Binaural Listening

(+) Test Findings:
 Dichotic tests—left ear deficit:
  digits, words, sentences, Staggered Spondaic Word
 Masking level difference (MLD)
 Temporal patterns (verbal response)
 Speech-in-noise
 Phonemic synthesis

Academic/Language/Learning Deficits:
 Reading
 Spelling
 Writing
 Multimodality tasks
 Music
 Prosody

Table 17–5. Processing Deficit: Auditory Language

(+) Test Findings:
 Degraded speech—bilateral
 Dichotic speech—bilateral

Academic/Language/Learning Deficits:
 Receptive language
 Expressive language
 Pragmatics
 Auditory memory
 Reading
 Writing
 Distractible
 Impulsive

fer of information and may be poorly performed in the face of integration deficits. Auditory and visual information provided in tandem, for example, may be difficult to process. Further, children might not reconcile information carried via rhythm and patterns with the rest of the auditory message. The dominant finding in the binaural listening profile is poor ability for dichotic listening tasks, most notably left-ear deficits. Dichotic test paradigms include digits, words, or sentences. Also, performance is poor when children are asked to label the components of a pitch or duration pattern, but the task is executed well when they are asked to hum the same pattern.

Table 17–4 illustrates tolerance fading memory (TFM), a profile specific to the Buf-

falo Model. TFM highlights short-term memory deficits and is diagnosed following administration of the Staggered Spondaic Word (SSW) Test, Phonemic Synthesis Test, and a speech-in-noise test. It is characterized by speech understanding difficulties in noise, abnormal phonemic synthesis (omitting the first sound of a target word), and several SSW errors illustrating dichotic difficulties and temporal effects. Following directions is difficult, and children with TFM often resemble those with attention deficits. Children may exhibit both expressive and receptive language problems.

An auditory language profile (Table 17–5) illustrates children who display significant language deficits across a wide range of skills, including semantics, syntax, and pragmatics. Note that auditory language deficits are not always depicted as a distinct APD category but rather as a subprofile (Bellis/Ferre) or as a typical by-product of APD (Chermak/Musiek) because they are present for almost all children with APD. In fact, language-related problems in the absence of any of the auditory processing deficits described in Tables 17–1 through 17–3 would not be classified as APD. Children may perform poorly on degraded speech and dichotic tests bilaterally.

Table 17–6 describes the executive control profile. As with language-related problems, metacognitive abilities, or executive functions, often are compromised in children with APD. These deficits are mediated by higher

Table 17–4. Processing Deficit: Tolerance Fading Memory

(+) Test Findings:
 Speech-in-noise
 Phonemic synthesis
 Spondaic Staggered Word (SSW)—Left Competing Condition
 SSW—order/ear effects
 Hyperacusis

Academic/Language/Learning Deficits:
 Auditory memory
 Receptive language
 Expressive language

Table 17–6. Processing Deficit: Executive Control/Planning

(+) Test Findings:
  Tasks with multi-item responses
  Reversals

Academic/Language/Learning Deficits:
  Organization, planning
  Expressive language
  Memory
  Motor skills
  Writing

order, cognitive functions. Children are unorganized and have trouble completing tasks or completing them effectively and efficiently. They may exhibit numerous reversals or perseverative responses for tests that require sequencing or implementing listener strategies as needed for dichotic tests, for example. These shortfalls are addressed by comprehensive management plans, whether as a primary profile (Buffalo Model), as a secondary profile (Bellis/Ferre), or as a universal manifestation of APD (Chermak/Musiek).

Table 17–7 identifies the six profiles previously discussed as they relate to the Buffalo, Bellis/Ferre, and Chermak/Musiek management approaches in an effort to illustrate their similarities. Whereas the majority of deficits are common to the three programs,

TFM is not readily interchanged with other designs. Its features, although clustered in a unique way, are seen in the other profiles. Furthermore, although memory deficiencies constitute a primary profile only in the Buffalo Model, Bellis/Ferre implicate weak memory trace and recall as part of a receptive-language based subprofile of APD. Musiek also links poor performance across multiple processes to auditory memory deficits.

Although profiles provide a means to organize or relate many pieces of a diagnostic puzzle, the outcomes of APD evaluations often illustrate mixed findings. Typically weaknesses point to more than one processing category. Clinicians may be able to indicate which profiles are primary and which are secondary, but this is not always the case. Furthermore, although interdisciplinary evaluations are desired, their outcomes do not always converge.

Multidimensional Management

Following comprehensive and multidimensional assessment, each program specifies a management plan that suits specific needs gleaned from the evaluation process. Although the terms "remediation," "management," and "treatment" are often used inter-

Table 17–7. Identification of Auditory Processing Disorders According to Comprehensive Approach

Deficit Profile	Buffalo Model	Bellis/Ferre	Chermak/Musiek
Decoding	Decoding deficit	Decoding deficit	Auditory discrimination Auditory closure
Temporal processing		Prosodic deficit	Temporal analysis Temporal synthesis
Binaural listening	Integration deficit	Integration deficit	Binaural separation Binaural summation Binaural integration Interhemispheric transfer
Tolerance fading memory	Tolerance fading memory		
Auditory language		Auditory association	Metalinguistics
Executive control	Organization deficit	Organization/output deficit	Metacognition

changeably, some distinctions are worth noting. "Management" refers to coping and compensatory tactics whereas "treatment" implies reducing or eliminating a deficit. "Remediation" addresses both management and treatment and is often presented as a three-step method. This approach to intervention includes (1) direct therapeutic techniques that habilitate auditory processing deficiencies via auditory training, (2) compensatory strategies that circumvent listening and learning hindrances, and (3) modifications of the listening environment to optimize access to communication. The Buffalo Model parcels remediation into audiologic, speech/language, and academic components that clearly summarize the same goals. Likewise the ASHA Task Force (1996) identifies two general approaches for intervention: enhancing language resources and improving signal quality.

The multitier system, in fact, takes advantage of time-honored combined bottom-up and top-down approaches for remediation of auditory disorders. Top-down processes reflect context-driven knowledge that requires receptive language, memory, and attention proficiencies. Bottom-up initiatives focus on the processing of the incoming auditory signal via auditory training techniques. Comprehensive plans are redundant, offering multiple avenues to offset any deficit. In addition to other resources cited throughout the chapter, Bellis (2002), Kelly (1995), and Mokhemar (1999) offer a wide variety of activities and suggestions regarding auditory training, compensatory strategies, and environmental modifications.

Direct Therapy/Auditory Training

Auditory training (AT), or intensive teaching of sound distinction or attributes, is a decades-old approach to improving auditory perception for individuals with hearing loss. AT has been extended to the population of children (and adults) with APD. Several authors have outlined AT programs for APD with the knowledge that animal and human research suggests that the brain undergoes structural and functional changes following intensive auditory training (Chermak & Musiek, 1997, 2002; Sloan, 1986). Brain and concomitant behavioral change is referred to as neural plasticity. The brain may change in neurochemical, physiological, and structural capacities, and it is anticipated that listening abilities, receptive language, and academic achievement likewise improve. The belief that immature or underdeveloped auditory neural systems are treated—not merely compensated for—underlies the use of intensive, systematic, and varied AT techniques.

Training addresses the requisite auditory processes for speech perception: detection, discrimination (phonemic training), temporal processing, memory, auditory closure, vigilance, auditory memory, and binaural listening (Musiek & Berge, 1998; Musiek, Shinn, & Hare, 2002). Regardless of the auditory training techniques used, it is imperative that the child is motivated to bring about change, is committed to the therapy process, and expends the effort necessary for a successful outcome.

Auditory Vigilance Training

Auditory vigilance involves maintaining a high level of attention prior to the presentation of a target. Teachers and parents often complain that students with suspected APD have a difficult time maintaining attention for a substantial period of time. Tasks that strengthen auditory vigilance require children to attend to a target embedded within a stream of nontarget stimuli. Children are asked to respond quickly each time the target is presented. Although the ACPT is an evaluation tool to assess inattention and impulsivity, it may serve as a training tool as well. The word "dog" is the target, presented amid scores of repetitions of the 10 other words in an unpredictable sequence. A target can be a designated word in a story, a sound in a specified position (e.g., initial /s/ or medial /m/) or a prosodic target like rising intonation. Auditory vigilance training may be ineffective if the underlying condition is not specific to audition but related to attention deficits across modalities.

Temporal Training

Training techniques have been developed in response to a body of work that implicates temporal processing capabilities as the foundation of auditory speech perception. In addition to computer-based programs like Fast ForWord or Earobics, discussed in a following section, training methods include traditional methods for strengthening temporal analysis. The discrimination and identification of pitch or duration patterns is suggested. The Pitch Pattern Sequence (PPS) or Duration Pattern Sequence (DPS) tests may be used as training tools. These come in a standard version as well as a pediatric version, with longer stimuli and interstimulus interval durations. Likewise, the detection of gaps, or interruptions, placed within a continuous signal is another temporal training task. The Random Gap Detection Test or Auditory Fusion Test may be used as temporal training tasks. These tests are available from Auditec of St. Louis in CD or audiotape formats. As well, Auditec customizes CDs to offer various stimulus frequency, intensity, and duration characteristics.

In addition, rapid intensity and frequency changes provide the intonation and rhythmic patterns in our speech that manifest acoustically by the stress placed on word segments, words, or parts of sentences. Interpreting the prosody, or the melody, of speech requires the recognition of temporal aspects of speech. Activities designed to improve timing, sequencing, and discrimination skills should be targeted.

Auditory Discrimination/ Phonemic Training

Children with APD often have difficulty processing at the phoneme level with both the speed and the accuracy necessary to comprehend speech. Fortifying auditory discrimination abilities is a first step in training. In phoneme discrimination training, children practice same/different determinations for vowels, consonants, consonant blends, and words. In particular, children with APD may have inordinate trouble with the discrimination and identification of short vowels. First, children must be able to distinguish long and short vowels and learn to identify the corresponding sound to the orthographic symbol for the vowel. Vowel discrimination should be completed with vowels in isolation, then consonant–vowel (CV) format, followed by short vowels in consonant–vowel–consonant (CVC) or word contexts. A confusion matrix that maps a child's particular consonant or vowel confusions will help determine appropriate discrimination tasks. Consider the following CVC pairs that may be used in a same/different task for discrimination of short vowels at the word level.

Short-Vowel Discrimination
cast–cast slip–slap bad–bod chip–chop
bill–ball rest–rust hip–hop bit–bat

Task difficulty increases by introducing consonant pairs whose acoustic characteristics are progressively similar.

Only after children demonstrate the ability to discriminate speech sounds, phonemic synthesis and analysis therapy training should be implemented to strengthen encoding and decoding capabilities. Phonemic synthesis is the ability to combine single-unit sounds into a word. The sounds of a word are provided in isolation and the child must put them together in the modeled sequence. For example, /b . . . o . . . l/ is given and the child must repeat the three sounds in rapid succession to form the word "bowl." The opposite of phonemic synthesis is phonemic analysis, the division of a word into its component sounds. Phonemic analysis is more difficult than synthesis and directly addresses speech-decoding skills. The word "bowl" is recited and separated into its individual sounds, /b . . . o . . . l/. Katz (1983) and Sloan (1986) provide programs that facilitate phonologic awareness and speech sound discrimination.

Computerized Auditory Training Programs

As previously stated, treatment of APD using AT techniques is based upon theories of neural plasticity, which suggest that changes in neural function follow intensive adaptive listening exercises. To create changes in neural function of the central auditory nervous system the participant must be fully engaged over a considerable length of treatment (Musiek, 2003). Thus sustaining a child's motivation and effort is of paramount importance.

The use of computer software producing high quality, appropriate listening activities using a game format has the potential to increase the motivation of children participating in auditory training activities. Computerized auditory training software is currently available from a number of sources. The product that has received the most attention is Fast ForWord™ (FFW) produced by Scientific Learning Corporation. FFW, developed after many years of research by Paula Tallal and her colleagues, is based on the hypothesis that disordered language development in children results from their inability to process rapidly changing acoustic inputs (Tallal & Piercy, 1974).

Tallal and colleagues compared children with language impairment and children with normally developing language with regard to their ability to process short vowels and consonants when presented with brief interstimulus intervals. They found a consistent and significant correlation between language impairment and poor performance on tests requiring perception of frequency transitions on the order of 40 msec or less. Inability to perceive transitions of this short duration has implications for an individual's ability to distinguish, for example, /ba/ from /da/. Failure to make these distinctions is deemed primarily as a temporal processing deficit and is a proposed etiology for

language processing impairment (Tallal, Miller, & Fitch, 1993).

The FFW program is designed to treat these temporal processing deficits. It is composed of seven exercises presented in a game format. Three of the exercises focus on children's ability to process information at the phonemic level, whereas the remaining four exercises focus on words and sentences. Initially, children hear stimuli in which speech segments are selectively lengthened and amplified. When the child performs at the specified criteria, the stimuli are gradually modified to more closely approximate normal frequency transitions, making the proper identification of stimuli more difficult. Children then must master each new stimulus. This adaptive process continues until children are able to perceive stimuli delivered with normal frequency transitions (Friel-Patti, Loeb, & Gillam, 2001).

Studies by Tallal, Merzenich, and colleagues report significant improvement in scores on standardized language tests as well as improved performance on an auditory perception task for children who have participated in FFW (Merzenich et al, 1996; Tallal et al, 1996). More recent and small independent studies of FFW efficacy have been undertaken. Attempts to replicate results in Tallal's studies were mixed. That is, some gains were seen in certain language areas but not others, and many were not statistically significant. Gillam and colleagues looked at the efficacy of FFW as a treatment program for language impairment and concluded that a large-scale, randomized clinical trial is needed to evaluate the effectiveness of FFW. They reported that all of the children in this series of studies had improved language after treatment, but that more information is needed to (1) validate FFW's effectiveness to improve language and literacy, (2) determine what mechanisms might underlie the effectiveness, and (3) determine whether the particular therapy setting influences outcome (Gillam, Crofford, Gale, & Hoffman, 2001; Gillam, Loeb, & Friel-Patti, 2001). At least one large-scale clinical trial as described by Gillam is currently under way. This study's goal is to determine (1) if a computer program specifically designed to treat auditory temporal processing (Fast ForWord–Language™) demonstrates measurable changes in language performance; (2) if computer-assisted language intervention programs that do not specifically address auditory temporal processing demonstrate measurable changes in language; (3) if individual language therapy delivered by traditional clinical methods, but over the same time course as the computerized intervention, demonstrate measurable changes in language; and (4) if general academic enhancement activities demonstrate measurable changes in language.

Computerized auditory training activities designed to improve language skills and literacy are currently available from other vendors. Most prominent in this group of other programs is the Earobics™ software from Cognitive Concepts. Earobics™ offers a family of software products designed to offer adaptive auditory training activities that impact phonological awareness, vocabulary, fluency, phonics, and comprehension. The Cognitive ConceptsWeb site presents outcome data collected independently from a number of different school sites that have purchased and used the product. Although these outcome data seem to indicate that children have made significant gains on a variety of measures, as of yet no controlled research has been published in peer reviewed journals validating these gains.

Other computerized auditory training software exists, but clinicians and parents should carefully review the needs of the child and the claims of the manufacturers before deciding that a particular product is appropriate for the problems the child exhibits. Even for more extensively studied computer-assisted therapy programs, it is not yet clear which diagnostic profiles of children are more likely to benefit from these treatment methods. More research looking at the effectiveness of all such therapeutic techniques may clarify which children are most likely to benefit from these programs, the processes affected, and the benefits associated with each of these auditory training products. Case Study 17–1 illustrates dramatic improvements in language following implementation of FFW, whereas significant changes are not as clear in Case Study 17–2 with this intervention strategy.

Binaural Listening Activities

The transfer of information between the two cerebral hemispheres, via the corpus callosum, facilitates binaural listening abilities. Binaural integration, binaural separation, and interhemispheric transfer exercises are recommended when dichotic listening ability is poor. To improve binaural listening, Musiek (2003) recommends using dichotic stimuli where a more intense signal is delivered to the deficit ear while the better ear receives a weaker signal. This type of training, called Dichotic Interaural Intensity Difference (DIID) Training, initially lowers strong ear intensity levels until weak ear performance increases to a satisfactory level. Then the intensity level to the strong ear is gradually increased so that high performance is maintained in the weak ear. With training, the intensity to the strong ear is increased to match weak ear levels. Training sessions may take place in a sound field or with earphones. Musiek maintains that such training should be given four to five times per week for up to 30 minutes per session. Preliminary studies indicate that improvements in weak ear performance of 10 to 15% can be achieved in as little as 1 month of training when a child is motivated and an active participant. Stimuli are varied and include sounds, words, phrases, and sentences. This task can be modified to strengthen binaural separation skills (attend to one ear only) or binaural integration skills (attend to both ears). The use of a variety of different dichotic paradigms trains a variety of subtle processing difficulties and serves to maintain the child's interest (Musiek, 2003; Musiek et al, 2002).

Case Study 17–1   S.P. is 5 years, 7 months old, and was referred for Fast ForWord™ (FFW) home-based treatment for a severe receptive/expressive language delay. His preschool teacher noticed his language difficulties when he was 3 years old.

Prenatal history includes gestational diabetes. He was born at 41 weeks gestation by cesarean section with mild hyperbilirubinemia. He has a history of an allergy to iodine, frequent colds and sore throats, tonsillitis, pneumonia, and bronchitis. He had nearly continuous episodes of otitis media between 2 and 3½ years of age. At the time of his assessment for entrance into FFW, his mother reported that he communicated mostly with single words and short sentences. Other children teased him at school because of inappropriate responses or comments in social situations, and his mother felt he suffered from low self-esteem.

Prior to enrollment in the FFW program the Clinical Evaluation of Language Function–Revised (CELF-R) indicated expressive and receptive language significantly below age level. The Test of Auditory-Perceptual Skills–Revised (TAPS-R) revealed poor auditory memory and word discrimination. The Test of Auditory Processing Disorders in Children–Revised (SCAN-C) illustrated at-risk performance for competing words and sentences. Based upon the results of this and previous assessments, S.P. was enrolled in a home program of FFW. His mother supervised the 10-week program and progress was monitored by a speech-language pathologist through Internet report. Posttreatment results indicated a dramatic improvement in all test measures to within the normal range. Pre- and posttreatment scores are provided:

Test	Pretreatment	Posttreatment
CELF-R		
Receptive	72	122
Expressive	80	108
TAPS-R		
Auditory Number Memory		
Forward	70	92
Reversed	86	109
Auditory Sentence Memory	74	107
Auditory Word Memory	76	96
Auditory Interpretation of Directions	84	117
Auditory Word Discrimination	70	117
Auditory Processing	106	114
SCAN-C		
Filtered Words	9	11
Auditory Figure-Ground	10	11
Competing Words	7	9
Competing Sentences	7	10

In addition to substantial gains in test scores, S.P.'s parents and teacher report that he engages in social conversation and is more confident when communicating. His speech is characterized by more complex words and sentences. S.P. has begun to use

---

Case Study 17–1 *(continued)*

the irregular verb tense. Furthermore, he is able to follow multilevel instructions and has gained understanding of the concepts "same" and "different."

S.P. exhibited a wide array of speech and language and auditory-related deficits with substantial objective and subjective gains following FFW. However, it is still uncertain which diagnostic findings from his language and auditory processing profile were the best predictors for success with FFW. Continued research and collection of treatment efficacy data are needed to answer this question.

Interhemispheric transfer is necessary for tasks that require processing across multiple modalities; for example, verbal labeling of an unseen object manipulated by the left hand. When children must find a verbally specified object with their left hand, without being able to see the object, interhemispheric transfer of information is again required. Other activities to stimulate information exchange across the corpus callosum include telling a story while simultaneously illustrating it, music activities, and auditory directives. Auditory directives, or the ability to follow auditory directions, require integration of speech understanding and a motor response. Activities include drawing directives that progressively increase in difficulty:

Draw a dot.
Draw a dot connected by a line to another dot.
Draw a dot connected by a line to another dot and draw another line underneath.

Interhemispheric transfer may be facilitated by asking children to respond to verbal commands that require action from the left side of the body: "Simon Says hop on your left foot; raise your left hand; touch your left pointer finger to your nose. . . . " Interhemispheric transfer tasks tend to be fun and are easily implemented at home.

Speech-in-Noise Training

Several intervention approaches specifically address speech perception ability in the presence of noise. Katz (2002) proposes a word identification task in the presence of noise that systematically increases in intensity. Performance should be maintained at 70 to 80%, but when performance falls below criteria, the noise level is reduced to below audibility for relief and relaxation before it is again increased. Relaxation training may be a useful component of therapy to help children approach difficult listening situations without excessive tension. The aim of the training as described by Katz is to acclimate children to listening in noise and increase performance to their maximum capability.

Ferre (1998) adapted an auditory–visual program originally designed for individuals with hearing loss for use with children with APD. Noise tolerance training requires recognition of everyday sentences or single-syllable words in the sound field in the presence of noise presented ipsilaterally. The signal-to-noise (S/N) ratio, linguistic redundancy of the message, type of background noise, availability of visual cues, and number of allowable repetitions are manipulated. Parameters are changed so that conditions get harder but success remains high. Good performance for sentences at a –10 dB S/N ratio and for words at –5 dB S/N ratio in auditory-only conditions is expected by completion of training. Skilled performance for combined auditory–visual modes should be maintained to –20 dB S/N ratio for sentences and –10 dB S/N ratio for single-syllable words. Children are required to repeat targets verbatim so that sufficient attention is afforded to reception of the speech signal.

Case Study 17–2 K.S. is 11 years, 5 months old, and is currently in a regular education classroom in the fifth grade. She qualifies for special education services in the areas of listening comprehension and mathematical calculation. Over the past several years K.S. has had several comprehensive language evaluations, APD assessments, educational assessments, and a neuropsychological evaluation. Noteworthy is K.S.'s motivation and that of her parents and educators.

Language evaluations consistently revealed weaknesses in word-finding abilities, vocabulary, following auditory directions, sentence memory, and reasoning skills. A neuropsychological evaluation completed in the third grade revealed deficient memory and learning ability, particularly with information presented in a cross-modal manner. Behavioral/emotional assessment suggested slightly lower than expected self-esteem, some lack of self-control, and apprehension. Although the neuropsychological battery indicated average auditory discrimination and auditory processing abilities, an APD evaluation also completed when K.S. was in the third grade showed a combination of language-related deficits and abnormal binaural listening skills distinguished by a greater than expected left ear advantage for both dichotic digits (binaural integration) and sentences (binaural separation), and poor pitch pattern sequencing in a verbal-response mode in the presence of good performance in a hummed-response mode. When K.S. was in the fourth grade, deficiency in interhemispheric transfer of information was observed following a comprehensive electrophysiological test battery. Details of this evaluation are reported elsewhere (Jerger et al, 2002).

Academically, K.S. has remained at or near grade level, except in mathematical problem solving. Intervention has consisted of auditory training, speech and language therapy, and significant instructional and environmental modifications. She has received expressive and receptive language intervention since age 5, with concomitant focus on auditory memory. Intervention also included FFW during the summer after the second grade. Following training, receptive language scores for the Clinical Evaluation of Language Fundamentals (CELF-3), particularly in sentence structure, word classes, and word structure, significantly improved. Auditory memory and auditory processing subtests of the Test of Auditory Perceptual Skills (TAPS) revealed depressed scores. Her parents did not observe significant advances in communication, academic, or language skills following FFW.

Instruction style and curriculum alterations have included homework reduction, test adaptations, use of paraphrase, reinstruction and repetition, an inclusion teacher in the classroom, and note takers. Environmental modifications include preferential seating, with the left ear toward the teacher. K.S. began consistently wearing a MicroEar FM system in the fifth grade. The system includes a teacher microphone and a behind-the-ear FM receiver coupled to her ear via an open earmold. She has alternated the receiver across ears but prefers to wear it on her right. Her parents and teacher report that the personal FM system has made a "tremendous and profound" difference in her classroom performance and listening abilities. K.S. is more attentive, absorbs more information, and has significantly reduced her reliance upon tutors, the inclusion teacher, and note takers. K.S.'s confidence has grown significantly and she has become a consistent participant in class discussions, which represents a significant change in behavior from previous grades.

Educational placement evaluation in the fifth grade showed gains of 1 to 2½ grade levels for word recognition, reading comprehension, and listening comprehension between the fourth and fifth grades, with the greatest improvement seen for listening

---

Case Study 17–2   *(continued)*

comprehension. Similarly, Children's Auditory Performance Scale (CHAPS), completed by her teachers, highlighted normal to near normal listening skills with use of her MicroEar. Note that between the third and fourth grades, improvement was less than one grade level for the content areas previously noted, and teacher ratings for the CHAPS indicated at-risk listening behaviors for all environments.

Despite steady academic improvement, reading comprehension and auditory memory remain areas of concern. Additionally, K.S. has trouble understanding jokes and riddles and enjoying age-appropriate movies. Her parents are considering enrolling her in a small, private middle school next year when she leaves elementary school. To facilitate continued progress, intervention might focus on additional memory enhancement training, pragmatics, and metatcognitive strategies.

Auditory Memory Training

Poor auditory memory is common in children with APD. Attention, feature extraction, and auditory pattern recognition may be compromised secondary to auditory memory deficits. Memory deficits are typically evaluated via comprehensive receptive language assessment or psychological evaluation. Poor performance across a wide range of tests that employ multiple items such as the dichotic paradigms or pattern recognition tests may implicate poor auditory memory as well.

Auditory memory enhancement (AME) is a technique used to improve recall (Musiek, 1999). AME procedures include imagery, spatial elaboration, generative processes, multimodality representation, and organizational perspectives. Comprehension exercises that focus on main idea extraction may be a necessary precursor to AME. In AME therapy, children are asked to read or listen to a story, broken into segments containing at least one identifiable main idea. After the segment is read, the child has a time window of 1 minute or less to sketch the main idea of the passage. The 1-minute time limit forces the child to reduce a bulk of information to its basic components. This process is repeated for all segments of the story. After all segments have been sketched, children use their pictures to retell the story.

Segment:

Mr. and Mrs. Jones and their two children were at a cabin by a lake for their summer vacation. One afternoon, the Jones family packed a picnic lunch and their fishing poles and set out on the lake in their rowboat. After some time, Mrs. Jones felt a tug on her fishing pole. She pulled and pulled but couldn't reel in the fish. Mr. Jones grabbed onto the pole and together they pulled and pulled. They couldn't reel in the fish. The two children grabbed the pole, and together they all pulled and pulled but couldn't reel in the fish. Then, with one last tug they all fell back and their catch of the day landed in the boat. To their surprise, they had caught a car tire!

The final sketch should contain a boat on a lake, a family of four with fishing poles, and a tire.

AME training forces a multidimensional representation of auditory or verbal information. The combination of visual, auditory, and motor components enhances internal representation and coding of the concepts, and ultimately recall. As a result, the depiction by drawing reflects a more holistic or gestalt representation. The transfer from verbal to gestalt representation requires mental imagery, another successful recall enhancement procedure. Presumably, the recall of well-represented general concepts requires less memory obligation than does the recall of large amounts of detail. Although known to improve memory, efficacy data on the use of AME specifically for management of APD are not available.

Compensatory Strategies

Intensive auditory training that addresses the impaired auditory system is important, but it is not the only component of the remediation process. Comprehensive intervention should also include compensatory strategies and environmental modifications. Children with APD must learn strategies that improve their access to spoken language. These strategies are often referred to as metalinguistic skills. As well, children must learn problem-solving skills, develop internal motivation, and maintain self-direction toward successful communication. These compensatory strategies are referred to as metacognitive abilities and are intended to provide access to underutilized resources to develop new skills. Modifications to the environment cover an array of management techniques that make the acoustic message clearer and easier to understand.

Metacognitive Strategies

Metagcognitive knowledge, often referred to as executive control, reflects understanding task requirements, allocating sufficient attention to a task, and using appropriate self-monitoring and self-correcting mechanisms. These abilities are crucial to the development of problem-solving skills and learning in general. Children with APD must be taught what adept listeners learn naturally. First, children with APD must understand their listening and learning difficulties so they face their environment with appropriate expectations. Incorporating metacognitive training into a comprehensive plan facilitates children as active participants in intervention. The reader is referred to Chermak and Musiek (1992) and Chermak (1998) for detail regarding metacognitive training.

Some of the major components are described following here.

Attribution Training

Children must learn to identify when to attribute task failure to lack of effort. Conversely, they also must realize that success follows hard work. This type of feedback serves to increase motivation and improve performance. The clinician and child, together, determine whether sufficient effort has been sustained. Clinicians provide consistent statements relating effort to outcome. Tasks must pose a problem, but one that the child is capable of solving. Attribution training does not disregard that listening abilities are impaired or that children will sometimes be unsuccessful; however, it illustrates that consistent effort and implementation of appropriate strategies can yield success over the long term.

Behavior Modification

Behavior modification techniques foster self-control and responsibility. Training emphasizes clients as decision makers. Do children identify when background noise interferes with listening? Do they recognize a noise source and know how to circumvent it? Do successful strategies bring internal reward? Children are taught to focus on the pertinent components of a task, to implement a viable strategy, and to evaluate its success. Assertiveness, another goal of behavior modification training, emphasizes self-expression and self-confidence. Assertive clients tend to make more progress in therapy and implement new skills in novel environments.

Cognitive behavior modification is divided into four non–mutually exclusive categories: self-instruction, problem-solving training, self-control, and cognitive strategies. Self-instruction is a means by which clients are taught to verbalize task requirements before, during, and after their completion. Cognitive problem solving emphasizes the communication breakdown as a problem to be solved and is particularly useful in addressing anxiety and stress. Difficult situations are divided into their component parts, multiple solution sets are devised, and the most adaptive solutions are recognized. Self-control or self-regulation procedures promote self-centered assessment, monitoring, and reinforcement. Internal feedback systems and response to failure are prominent components of self-regulation. Improving cognitive strategies provides tools for successful task performance. Specific strategies include reciprocal teaching, whereby the child monitors the clinician's performance. Implementing appropriate cognitive style or reasoning techniques is another cognitive strategy. Children with APD often do not recognize which approach works best or do not routinely differentiate their problem-solving approach according to the class of problem. For example, when faced with difficulty understanding speech, a child might universally employ a phoneme synthesis approach (bottom-up) to improve understanding even when the use of context or inference (top-down) might be the better choice.

Metalinguistic Strategies

Metalinguistics is the recognition and use of the implicit rules of language and aids in the understanding of spoken discourse. The acquisition of language-based skills comes incidentally to most children with normal auditory processing capabilities. Expansion of the number and breadth of vocabulary, construction of cohesive discourse, utilization of contextual and nonverbal cues all develop naturally with inclusion in normal home, school, and social environments. These skills, however, must be taught to children with APD.

Auditory Closure/Vocabulary Building Activities

Vocabulary deficiencies are common to most children with APD. Exercises that foster contextual relations, understanding of multiple meanings, and inference will enhance expressive and receptive vocabulary and aid in the development of auditory closure. Musiek (1999) describes a 1-week vocabulary-building program that emphasizes context derivation, review, and classroom usage of target words. Teachers can provide a list of words pertinent to upcoming science, social studies, spelling, or reading lessons. Parents or clinicians can look ahead in children's textbooks. In this way, the child will be better prepared to learn new material.

The use of context to deduce an unknown or missing word is pivotal to building vocabulary and closure skills:

> The apple was a beautiful *crimson* color.

Pointing out that apples are typically red will aid in the addition of "crimson" to vocabulary.

> The woman read the *p*_____ she bought from the newsstand.

The missing word is "periodical" but knowing that "newspaper," "paper," or "magazine" satisfy the content of the message improves the likelihood of adding the word "periodical" to an existing semantic category.

Using words that rhyme is another technique to increase predictability for missing words:

> I love you, you love me. We're a happy _____ (family).

Know which songs, books, television or video programs children enjoy as some of our old favorites do not provide a familiar context. Nonsense words also may be used in activities that strengthen closure capabilities:

> On Planet X, you can see the flubbawug swinging from tree to tree in the jungle. What do we call a flubbawug on the planet Earth?

Riddles or "Get a Clue" games offer a wonderful venue to strengthen the development of semantic relations among words. Clues are provided until the riddle is solved:

> It has four legs. (no not a dog)
> It's flat. (??)
> You eat on it. (Yes, a table)

Children are encouraged to create riddles as well. Also, it may be beneficial to promote the use of visual imagery to strengthen semantic relationships by having a child verbalize a mental picture.

Addressing multiple meanings of words will expand the child's semantic network as well. In addition, learning how to apply multiple uses and meanings for words is a cornerstone in the development of humor.

> Have you ever seen an ocean *wave*?
> Knock knock. . . . *Orange* you glad I didn't say banana?
> Why did the coach go in to the bank? He wanted to get his *quarterback*.

These jokes may not be understood by children with restricted vocabularies and limited implicit knowledge about the rules and sound system of language. When a child "doesn't get the joke," he faces exclusion from a socially important area of growth for elementary school-aged children. (Ask any third grade teacher!) For many reasons, therapists should be armed with age-appropriate joke and riddle books. Refer to Miller and Gildea (1987) for greater detail.

Prosody and Segmentation Skills

The normal variations in rhythm, timing, and intensity of speech that provide lexical, semantic, and syntactic cues are often undetected by children with APD. Prosodic and segmentation skills are closely related to temporal aspects of speech addressed in the previous section, Auditory Training. Only after a child demonstrates recognition of stress-pattern differences should work emphasize stress and intonation changes that alter the meaning of an utterance. Consider the sentence pair:

> Do *YOU* see that dog?
> Do you see *THAT* dog?

Word emphasis in the first sentence signals that the speaker is drawing attention to a communication partner, whereas for the latter sentence, the speaker's focus is on a particular dog. Understanding the subtle differences between the two sentences, implied by the stress pattern, allows the listener to respond appropriately and to meet the expectations of the speaker.

Children should be asked not only to identify which words in a phrase or sentence carry stress but also to imitate a speaker's intonation pattern. Also, exercises should have children match emotions to statements.

> I won a new bike!!! (Am I scared, excited, or bored?)
> You had two weeks to finish your report. (Am I annoyed, scared, or happy?)

Once children are able to interpret and mimic intonation patterns, they should create statements reflecting target emotions. (Though parents may not appreciate it later, include the recognition and use of sarcasm with older children.)

Discourse Cohesion and Schema Utilization

Discourse cohesion tools are strategies used to connect simple ideas to make complex messages. Although cohesion training often resembles a grammar lesson, it is imperative that children with APD are explicitly taught how pronouns are used as referents, for example, or that the connectives "because," "instead," "however," and "but" are not interchangeable but carry specific meanings. Utilizing successful discourse cohesion tools results in more efficient message relay and reception. Children who know that the words "but" or "however" in a spoken or written message signal a contradiction or conditional circumstance will interpret the meaning more readily.

> She wanted to go to the State Fair, however she had to study.

Children who are unable to effectively utilize discourse cohesion devices might not realize that the girl, unfortunately, did not go to the State Fair.

As children become more sophisticated communicators, they incorporate shortcuts to comprehension when they recognize patterns from their experiences that allow them to predict outcomes. These shortcuts, available via learned linguistic and contextual knowledge, are referred to as schema or scripts. For example, understanding connectives provides a linguistic aid in the construction of schema or scripts that facilitate message comprehension. Also, scripts are used when outcomes of typical events are anticipated—ordering food at a restaurant, speaking to a customer service representative, or checking out at the grocery store. Children's schema for daily sequences might include typical classroom rules and behavior: First you raise your hand, then the teacher calls your name, and last you respond. Without a repertoire of scripts or schema, greater resources than necessary would be continually required when one is facing repetitive situations. Children with APD must learn to draw appropriate conclusions that support the development of schema. Encouraging mental imagery, discussing target concepts in reference to children's experiences, using visual aids for concept reinforcement, and asking questions that will elicit appropriate responses are techniques that aid development of internal schema. See Chermak (1998) and Chermak and Musiek (1992, 1997) for additional discussion.

Pragmatic Skills

Poor social use of language is a common finding for children with APD. Children who have not learned the implicit rules governing language style or choice of words may have difficulty communicating with both their peers and adults. Improper language behavior may be recognized via role-playing exercises. Children can be taught which choices are interpreted as "bossy" or "rude" or out of sync with communication partners.

> Which statement is made by Bossy Bess?
> Give me that pen.
> I need a pen.
> May I please have a pen?

Children with APD may need explicit instruction to recognize important characteristics of the speaker (age, status, familiarity) or the communication situations that dictate style differences.

Auditory Memory Strategies and Aids

Understanding spoken discourse necessitates effective attention, encoding, pattern recognition, and comprehension skills. These abilities rely, in part, upon various aspects of memory. Children with APD may exhibit auditory memory weaknesses and benefit from strategies that foster improvement of auditory memory. Auditory memory enhancement may be approached from multiple perspectives. A training or direct therapy perspective aims to improve recall ability. These techniques were reviewed in the previous section on AT. A compensatory-based perspective to improving performance provides organization techniques that foster retrieval of information. Strategies may reflect internal or external resources.

Mnemonic tools are internal strategies used to remember unfamiliar or large amounts of information. Mnemonics are often language based and include elaboration, transformation, chunking, and coding. Elaboration techniques are often used to remember the 12 cranial nerves. Transformation requires that difficult material is translated into something simpler so that it is remembered more easily. Chunking involves organizing a large amount of information into categories because smaller pieces are easier to remember. The original 13 colonies were made up of _____ southern states, _____ mid-Atlantic states, and _____ northeastern states. Coding occurs when mental images are created to recall detail or pair difficult information with a specific experience. Picturing two desserts instead of one provides a code to remember that "dessert" contains not one "s" but two.

Rehearsal is an effective strategy for helping poor auditory memory. It is quite natural to repeat a locker combination or phone number to yourself until you have successfully opened the lock or dialed the number. Children with APD employ this technique ineffectively, if at all. Children should be instructed to repeat aloud directions to themselves. At first, they may have to learn to extract the key elements. Then they must be taught to reduce the volume of the voice until rehearsal is subvocal, or lips move without voice. Following subvocalization, a child may be taught silent rehearsal, or to repeat directions without vocalization or lip movement. Rehearsal processes are also referred to as reauditorization. Subvocalization or reauditorization strategies should be monitored until they are used routinely, without prompting.

External-based approaches to facilitate memory emphasize the use of compensatory devices such as calendars, palm pilots, or cue cards. Children should carry an agenda or semester planner so that all assignments and important events are properly noted. Teachers or classroom buddies should check the agenda until it is clear that the child correctly records all pertinent information.

Environmental Modifications

Modification of the environment is a universal component to intervention. Alterations of the physical environment, adaptations to an academic curriculum, and use of assistive listening technology have long been advocated by audiologists and speech pathologists to ensure proper quality of the acoustic environment.

Changes to the Physical Environment

Although all school children face a hostile listening environment, children with APD confront exacerbated difficulties. External barriers combine with internal degradations to impede the processing of auditory information. The "typical" classroom provides a less than ideal, if not poor, listening environment secondary to a combination of noise levels, reverberant surfaces, and distance between the student and teacher. Placement of rubber tips on the bottom of chairs and desks, creation of small listening spaces with placement of room-dividing structures like bookshelves or movable bulletin boards, introduction of corkboards, curtains, and carpet to sound-reflective surfaces are but a partial list of room modifications that may reduce noise and improve auditory access to instruction (see Chapter 12).

Curriculum/Instructional Modifications

Adjustments in both the presentation of information and the task requirements are typically necessary for children with APD to succeed academically with minimal frustration. Preferential seating close to the teacher and away from extraneous noise is a first consideration. In addition, teachers should be instructed to use "clear speech." Naturally produced clear speech occurs when a speaker consciously produces each word carefully. Without training, a plea to "speak clearly" prompts speakers to slow their speaking rate, increase number and length of pauses, employ a higher pitch and greater variation, raise the intensity of consonants relative to vowels, and articulate vowels more precisely. A recent study revealed that speech understanding in noise improved significantly for children with learning disabilities when speakers used naturally produced clear speech (Bradlow, Krauss, & Hayes, 2003). As well, teachers should be reminded to repeat new information offered by fellow students as the level and clarity of other children's speech is often less than optimal. Although the use of naturally produced clear speech is not a substitute for direct therapy or other compensatory strategies, it is an effective means to improve speech understanding in difficult listening environments for children who have difficulty processing speech.

Although repetition may be needed for a child with APD to understand the spoken message, it will be most beneficial if repetition is accompanied by increased clarity. If difficulty arises from understanding the linguistic components of a message, restating the material, despite clarity, may not be appropriate. Active statements should replace passive statements, complex sentences should be reduced to their simpler components, and specific information should substitute for general statements. Whereas children who have significant language-based sequelae might find rephrasing more helpful than repetition, children who have difficulty integrating multiple inputs might find that rephrasing adds yet another component to reconcile, thus making repetition a better strategy for emphasis.

Animated teachers offer a style conducive to message reception, particularly for children who have a difficult time understanding facial expressions and interpreting prosodic and segmental cues. No matter the teaching style, teachers need to recognize and reward the small successes.

Often, by using an outline or vocabulary list in advance, parents and therapists can preteach new words and concepts so as to enhance the contextual cues available to children. Note that the same concept can be extended to books, movies, and television shows. Preteaching or previewing the plots often results in greater understanding and enjoyment for some children with APD.

Use of tape recorders, note takers, or teacher-provided outlines reduces the demand on the child, allowing greater attention for the information presented by the teacher. Although note taking is an arduous task for children with APD, increased independence should be encouraged for children in middle school and beyond. Parents might reread the complete set of notes using slow and clear speech while the child underlines key words. Children should rewrite notes from outline form into paragraphs or be asked to recite them. Students should likewise proofread their own notes to make sure they understand them. A well-picked classroom buddy may be appropriate, wherein one child can help to keep the other on the right page or to make sure the correct homework assignment is copied.

Test and assignment modifications may include shortened or closed-set examinations rather than open-ended essays, less writing requirements, nonrestrictive time limits, and a quiet room or use of earplugs to limit extraneous noise. Of course, curriculum and instructional modifications will not be successfully implemented without the parent, teacher, child, and case manager working in concert to establish and work toward common goals. See Ferre (2002) for additional detail regarding modifications for home and school.

Assistive Listening Devices

The deleterious effects of noise, distance, and reverberation for any student in a typical classroom are well documented (see Chapters 12 and 13). It is expected that these detractors are substantially more problematic for children with APD. The use of assistive listening devices (ALDs) is the best means to improve the S/N ratio in the classroom (see Chapter 14). Careful consideration of FM system options is important in providing the system best suited to the child, family, and school.

As described in Chapter 14, personal FM systems may be body worn or self-contained, ear-level devices. Placement of a microphone transmitter close to the teacher's mouth offers a 15 to 20 dB S/N ratio advantage for the child wearing a personal FM system. Receiver options include a headset, monaural or binaural earbuds, or custom earmolds.

As described in Chapter 13, sound-field FM systems are another receiver option that provides enhanced auditory access to the teacher in the presence of background noise. The teacher wears a transmitter microphone, and a small speaker may be placed on the child's desk or several speakers may be mounted strategically around the classroom. The S/N ratio advantage is approximately 5 to 10 dB, significantly less than that of a personal FM system but improved relative to a normal classroom environment.

Regardless of the receiver choice, there are several microphone/transmitter options. Microphones may be directional, have noise-cancellation options, or have team-teaching capabilities. Teachers should be acquainted with receiver and microphone alternatives and be involved in the decision making so that they are more invested in the child's management.

Improved attentiveness and listening behaviors, auditory comprehension, speech recognition scores, on-task behavior, and spelling have all been reported in association with FM use. Several populations have benefited from FM systems, including children with language delays (Flexer & Savage, 1993), children with mild hearing loss (Ross & Giolas, 1971), and those with normal hearing in standard academic placements (Rosenberg et al, 1999). One case study illustrated that a child with APD demonstrated significant improvement in both speech perception and academic performance with the use of an FM system (Stach, Loiselle, Jerger, Mintz, & Taylor, 1987).

An FM evaluation should include a pre-use observation report such as the SIFTER, the Fisher's Auditory Problems Checklist, or the Children's Auditory CHAPS, and an assessment of the listening and learning barriers in the classroom. Objective measurements of FM benefit should incorporate speech recognition measures that will provide insight as to whether children are able to meet the listening demands of a classroom. Administer word or sentence recognition tests at a soft level as well as in the presence of substantial noise (S/N ratio of 0 or 5 dB). Children with normal auditory function perform very well under these listening conditions. Furthermore, an S/N function may provide useful information when considering sound-field options. If children do not reach maximum speech recognition until a 15 dB S/N ratio is provided, for example, the sound-field system will not meet the children's needs. Also, consider that an audiologist must fit a personal FM system, and medical clearance is required. Furthermore, children, teachers, and parents must be adequately educated regarding its use, maintenance, and expected advantages and limitations. Teachers and parents should complete a follow-up observation report after several weeks of FM trial use to monitor its effectiveness.

Multidimensional Treatment and Profile Specificity

The pervasive impact of APD on language throughout the lifespan, academic perfor-mance, social and vocational engagement, and self-concept emphasizes the need for joint effort in both assessment and management. In such a collaborative model of patient management, the child, family, educators, and health and communication professionals share information and expertise and formulate a remediation plan. When applying this treatise to management, one first assumes children with APD represent a heterogeneous group. Second it is assumed there are recognizable auditory and other behaviors that signal abnormal development, and third that test findings offer insight to unique patterns of auditory processing and learning shortfalls. Finally, it is presupposed that intervention should be multidimensional but narrowly focused toward specific deficits. Current practice does not favor handouts for parents and teachers that outline generic "dos and don'ts" meant for all children with APD.

Tables 17–8 to 17–11 illustrate remediation techniques for four of the profiles: auditory decoding, temporal processing, binaural listening, and tolerance fading memory. For each, current trends are provided in direct therapy, compensatory strategies, environmental modifications, and home-based activities.

Management and treatment options for both auditory language and executive control deficiencies are not offered separately but are addressed in the remediation plans of the other auditory-based deficit profiles. The ASHA Task Force (ASHA, 1996, p. 42) states, "regardless of the nature of the processing deficit, most persons who have difficulty with the comprehension of spoken language will profit both from procedures that enhance the acoustic signal and from procedures that increase the scope and control of central resources, particularly language resources." Additionally, metacognitive approaches should be investigated for all children with APD. However, particular strategies are not matched to specific auditory deficits or profiles because there is no indication that a given deficit or profile requires a unique metacognitive tactic. All children with APD are at risk for inadequate motiva-

Table 17–8. Management Components for Auditory Decoding/Closure Deficits

Direct Therapy/Auditory Training
   Auditory vigilance training
   Auditory discrimination of frequency, intensity, and duration
   Phonemic analysis and synthesis training/phoneme discrimination activities
   Speech-in-noise training
   Fast ForWord™/Earobics™

Compensatory Strategies
   Metalinguistic Strategies: vocabulary building, auditory closure activities, discourse cohesion,
      schema and scripts
   Speech/language therapy
   Metacognitive Strategies

Modifications to Environment
   Preferential seating
   Supplement with visual cues (notes, outlines)
   Repeat/rephrase
   Preteach new words, concepts
   Naturally clear speech
   Assistive listening devices to improve signal-to-noise ratio
   Bilateral earplugs to minimize noise
   Tape lectures
   Changes to physical environment to reduce noise and reverberation

At Home
   Listening games: Telephone, Simon Says, and alphabet games
   Games to enhance vocabulary/relationship among words: Catch Phrase™, Scattergories™,
      Taboo™, Wheel of Fortune™, word puzzles/searches
   Phonemic analysis: MadGab™
   Read "popular" magazines to help provide social context
   Read age-appropriate joke and riddle books together
   Review/discuss upcoming movies to aid in comprehension of plots
   Select several "words of the week" from school material and use them daily
   Prepare/rehearse for new situations
   Avoid important communication from a different room or in background noise

tion, self-monitoring, or problem-solving skills and would benefit from learning cognitive behavior modifications to increase goal oriented and on-task behaviors.

Profile or deficit-specific management is an attractive concept because it connects a defined problem to an organized plan. However, because children often demonstrate combinations of profiles, remediation may be broad in scope, and specificity in management may be an ideal rather than a reality. For example, outcomes may implicate combined TFM and integration deficits or decoding deficits in conjunction with abnormal temporal and integration profiles. The blurring of profile distinctions may pose a predicament if the plan becomes too cumbersome. Children who demonstrate combined TFM, binaural listening, or decoding

deficits would face quite a daunting list of direct therapy goals that perhaps incorporates memory enhancement, listening in noise, phonemic training, vocabulary building, interhemispheric transfer exercises, and appropriate metacognitive and metalinguistic strategies. Furthermore, in the presence of multiple deficits, divergent recommendations may apply to the same child. Consider, for example, that rephrasing and repetition are not interchangeable message modifications. Repetition is often recommended in lieu of rephrasing for children with binaural listening or temporal processing deficits. Conversely, rephrasing is often suggested for children with language-based processing deficits. The dilemma is obvious because binaural listening or temporal deficiencies do not typically occur without language-

Table 17–9.   Management Components for Temporal Processing Deficits

Direct Therapy/Auditory Training
    Gap detection
    Pattern recognition training: pitch, duration, intensity
    Prosody/segmentation training
    Fast ForWord™/Earobics™
    Auditory memory enhancement

Compensatory Strategies
    Vocabulary building: key word extraction; language and humor, discourse cohesion
    Schema/scripts
    Counseling if social/emotional concerns
    Speech-language therapy
    Reading program
    Music activities
    Metacognitive strategies

Environmental Modifications
    Animated teacher
    Naturally clear speech
    Repetitions with key word emphasis
    Preteach material
    Visual aids as supplements
    Untimed tests
    Examinations with closed-set questions

At Home:
    Games that require sequencing, synthesis, pattern recognition: Simon™, SuperSimon™, Bop-It™, Bop-It Extreme™, Taboo™, Gestures™ (charades), Pictionary™
    Games/activities that require following auditory directions: Simon Says, Say After Me (child as leader and participant)
    Read aloud together
    Recite poems, limericks, and rhymes
    Review jokes and riddles together
    Avoid plays on words and sarcasm
    Keep instructions short and simple
    Check for understanding
    Prepare/rehearse for new social situations

based manifestations. Always keep in mind that it is essential to follow a plan of action with assessment of its success.

Also at issue is whether FM systems are beneficial to all children with APD. Rosenberg (2002) advocates personal FM systems for children who demonstrate speech-in-noise deficits as part of decoding, TFM, or organization output profiles. For these children, noise degrades speech cues in an already ineffective speech-decoding system, and S/N ratio enhancement is necessary to counterbalance these problems. Conversely, it has been suggested that children with deficits in binaural listening or temporal processing, for example, may not benefit from enhancing the S/N ratio as long as signal clarity is preserved. Consider Case Study 17–2, a child with both interhemispheric transfer deficiencies and language deficits for whom a MicroEar personal FM system afforded substantial listening advantages. Regardless of the presenting profile or profile combinations, providing unimpeded access to the teacher eases the listening requirements for children with APD, and FM use should be evaluated.

Auditory Neuropathy (Dys-synchrony) as a Special Case of APD

Processing failures, unrelated to sensitivity loss, may occur below the level of the brainstem and cortex and result in significant

Table 17–10. Management Components for Binaural Listening—Integration Deficit

Direct Therapy/Auditory Training
  Auditory vigilance training
  Interhemispheric transfer exercises
  Phoneme training
  Prosody training
  Speech-in-noise training
  Auditory memory enhancement

Compensatory Strategies
  Linguistic: vocabulary building
  Speech/language intervention
  Reading program
  Content mastery/tutoring for academic weaknesses
  Memory aids: mnemonics, rote memory, drills, chunking, rehearsal
  Metacognitive strategies

Environmental Modifications
  Preferential seating
  Evaluate use of assistive listening devices
  Unilateral earplug to minimize weak-ear effect
  Untimed tests
  Examinations with closed-set questions
  Quiet environment for test taking
  Content mastery/tutoring for specific academic weaknesses
  Reduce need to listen *and* write: Note-taking assistance, provide outlines
  Repetition might be preferable to rephrasing
  Avoid visual cues as concurrent supplement

At Home
  Activities to strengthen verbal and motor coordination: Name That Tune, Bag of Surprises (child
    must identify unseen/unnamed objects or search for target item); have child talk about a picture
    while drawing it
  Activities to strengthen multimodality processing: Bop-It™, Bop-It Extreme™, Simon™, Super
    Simon™, Charades, Pictionary™
  Listen to imbalanced stereo to detect loudness differences
  Reduce to single modality in face of comprehension difficulty: listen—then look

---

roadblocks to speech perception and development of oral language. Auditory neuropathy (AN), also termed auditory dyssynchrony, is a disorder wherein cochlear outer-hair cell function is preserved in the face of impaired auditory neural function (see Chapter 3). Clinically, it is characterized by robust otoacoustic emissions (OAEs), asynchronous or absent auditory brainstem response (ABR), absent acoustic reflexes (ARs), audiograms that range from normal to severe-to-profound, and arrested speech and language development in young children. The presence of other sensory neuropathies is not unusual. The premise, "What we do with what we hear" (Lasky & Katz, 1983), often applied to the treatment of

APD, may be extended to management of children with AN.

Children with AN typically have inordinately poor speech perception abilities despite appropriate amplification. In fact, the presence of AN may account for some of our most difficult cases whereby children exhibited poor auditory capabilities and oral language progress in the face of substantial residual hearing and "doing all the right things." The prevalence of AN in individuals with severe to profound hearing impairment may be 12 to 14% (Berlin et al, 1998; Krauss, Ozdamar, Stein, & Reed, 1984).

Intervention options for children with AN are controversial, and systematic evaluation of treatment options is in progress but cur-

Table 17–11. Management Components for Tolerance Fading Memory

Direct Therapy/Auditory Training
    Noise desensitization training
    Auditory memory training

Compensatory strategies
    Memory strategies
    Schema/scripts

Environmental Modifications
    Outlines/note-takers/tape recorder
    Assistive listening devices
    Preferential seating
    Earplugs
    Test taking in quiet

At Home
    Memory games: Simon™, SuperSimon™, alphabet sequencing games (I went to the store, and I bought . . .)
    Organizational/memory strategies: use of calendar; daily planner; dry-erase board for messages; review classwork and create mnemonics where appropriate
    Listening games in noise: maintain high success
    Prepare/rehearse for new situations

rently limited. As for all children with hearing loss, early intervention is a key factor in the development of communication and language skills for children with AN. Children with AN may require combined auditory and visual/manual communication systems to learn language. Thus hearing aids, cochlear implants, sign language, and cued speech are all viable options facing parents.

Cochlear implants have become a more common habilitation option for children with severe sensory hearing loss, and many advocate their use for children with AN once it has been demonstrated that hearing aids are not beneficial (see Chapter 15). Although intuition might argue against a cochlear implant for an auditory system without synchronous neural discharge, the efficacy of direct stimulation of the auditory nerve has been demonstrated. Many case studies have highlighted significant gains in speech and oral language capabilities for some, but not all, children with AN who have received a cochlear implant and intensive auditory training and speech-language

therapy (Miamoto, Kirk, Svirsky, & Seghal, 1999; Trautwein, Shallop, Fabry, & Friedman, 2001). The need for total communication rather than oral-only methods may increase for children with AN and coexisting disabilities such as developmental and cognitive delays.

Despite evidence supporting cochlear implants for young children and infants with AN, their use should not be considered the universal treatment option. First, several cases of spontaneous reversal of AN in children 1 to 2 years of age have been reported (Madden, Rutler, Hilbert, Greinwald, & Choo, 2002; Neault & Kenna, 2003). Second, some children with AN who use hearing aids also show significant development of speech perception skills. Children fit with wide dynamic range (WDRC) hearing aids appropriate for their degree of loss, in concert with habilitation emphasizing a combined auditory and visual approach, showed significant improvement in auditory awareness and speech perception. Approximately 50% of a study group of children with AN who wore hearing aids demonstrated open-set speech perception ability comparable to that of children with sensorineural hearing loss of similar degree but without AN. Of course, an equal number of children with AN failed to demonstrate benefit from their hearing aids (Cone-Wesson, Rance, & Sininger, 2001; Rance, Cone-Wesson, Wunderlich, & Dowell, 2002). The use of unilateral, low-gain amplification for children with AN is a more conservative approach advocated to prevent deterioration of outer hair cells (OHC) as might happen with use of high-gain aids (Hood, 1998). However, it is unclear whether preserving OHCs for these hearing systems is functionally significant or that low-gain amplification serves their amplification needs.

Event-related potentials (ERPs) may be a useful tool in monitoring habilitation for children with AN. The P1, an auditory-evoked response generated by auditory thalamic and cortical regions, has been used to assess the neuromaturational status of the central auditory pathways for children with sensorineural hearing loss following cochlear implantation (Sharma, Dorman, & Spahr, 2002). In general, children implanted prior to the age of 3½ years of age demonstrated normal P1 latencies whereas those implanted after the age of 7 had delayed P1 latencies. In addition, a rapid time course in the development of the P1 response was noted for early-implanted children, with the P1 response apparent 1 week following implantation and age-appropriate latencies by 8 months postimplantation (Sharma, Dorman, Spahr, & Todd, 2002). Data describing the development or time course of the N1 response following implantation for children with AN are not yet available.

The P1 response may be a good predictor for the development of auditory speech perception capabilities because it appears to be highly correlated with speech perception scores. Strong correlations have been observed between P1 response and open-set word recognition for groups of children using cochlear implants (Sharma, Dorman, Todd, Fainberg, & Martin, 2003) as well as for children with AN who use hearing aids (Rance et al, 2002). The use of age-appropriate and sensitive speech perception measures and parent inventories of auditory development in the assessment of speech perception capabilities of young children cannot be overstated. Case Study 17–3 describes a child with AN and developmental delays who received a cochlear implant at 18 months of age.

Treatment Efficacy

Numerous case studies highlight successful intervention plans consisting of auditory training techniques, language and cognitive-based compensatory strategies, and environmental modifications in treatment for children with APD. Although numeric change in the positive direction for any measurement is encouraging, its interpretation needs further clarification as factors like test–retest reliability, learning effects for test measures, and real-world validity need to be evaluated.

On a patient by patient basis, status of identified auditory deficits, academic performance, receptive and expressive lan-

guage proficiencies, and emotional adjustment should be revisited but with care. Reassessment might overestimate improvement if training techniques mirrored test paradigms. Pitch-pattern or duration pattern sequence tests become limited in their usefulness as diagnostic tools if they are used during therapy, for example. Post intervention questionnaires (SIFTER, CHAPS, Fisher Auditory Checklist) for teachers and parents are important efficacy tools as they have high face validity.

Determining the benefit of APD remediation plans is essential from an intervention-approach perspective as well. Although deficit-specific management plans (whether the deficit is considered a single auditory skill or bundled into a profile) are currently popular and appeal to common sense, they are still limited to controlled clinical trials that evaluate their efficacy in contrast to generic treatment approaches. Currently, there is some question whether specificity is the key to successful remediation. Gillam and colleagues revealed similar outcomes for treatment regimens that targeted different language processes (Gillam, Crofford et al, 2001; Marler, Champlin, & Gillam, 2001). Likewise, children who received temporal-based auditory training made gains on temporal-based psychoacoustic tests similar to children who did not receive specific training using temporally altered speech. Thus, it remains to be seen whether each deficit identified in these recommended test batteries warrants intervention or even represents a unique process. Perhaps it is the intensity and frequency of intervention, together with motivational factors, that are more important than is targeting specific auditory or learning processes. Furthermore, "intense" and "frequent" remain to be defined.

In addition to subjective and objective behavioral indices of treatment efficacy, electrophysiological measures may be used to objectively monitor the maturation of the auditory central nervous system as part of a comprehensive evaluation and management plan. The middle latency response (MLR); mismatch negativity (MMN); long-latency N1, P1, and P2 components; and P300 event-

Case Study 17–3   D.S. is a 3-year-old male born 8 weeks prematurely. He was jaundiced and required mechanical ventilation for 12 days. He remained in the neonatal intensive care unit (NICU) for 5½ weeks and was diagnosed with chronic lung disease. D.S. failed a hearing screening at birth, and by 2 months of age, auditory neuropathy was confirmed by ABR and OAE measurements. Hearing, ABR, and OAE status were closely monitored. Hearing evaluations indicated sporadic responses to speech stimuli at 60 to 75 dB hearing level (HL) but consistently no response to tonal stimuli. A trial with binaural low-gain amplification failed to illustrate any benefit from hearing aids, and D.S. often pulled the hearing aids out. His parents feel that many audiologists are not up-to-date regarding current evaluation and treatment options for AN. They added that, whereas the term "synchronicity" was used often during the diagnostic process, the concept remained foreign until they realized that lack of synchronicity translated into lack of "clarity."

A multidisciplinary cochlear implant evaluation at 15 months of age indicated significantly delayed receptive and expressive oral language skills with gestures, facial expressions, and a few signs as the primary means of communication. In addition, neuropsychological evaluation revealed mild to moderate delays in motor and cognitive development. At 18 months of age, D.S. was implanted in the right ear with a cochlear Nucleus 24. His initial reaction to auditory stimulation was unfavorable and it took several days to adjust but he never pulled off the external receiver. His parents noted increased but inconsistent awareness to environmental sounds like the telephone or the vacuum within the first few days of device hookup. Audiometrically, D.S. responded to tonal and speech stimuli at approximately 35 to 40 dB HL. He has worked with an auditory–verbal therapist and an occupational therapist on a weekly basis. Auditory–verbal therapy is intended to provide children with hearing aids or cochlear implants maximum accessibility to audition in order to understand speech and learn to speak. Typically, auditory–verbal therapy is not accompanied by visual communication methods, but this varies on a case-by-case basis. D.S.'s mother is a deaf educator and has been teaching him sign language at home.

At 14 to 15 months postimplant, or "auditory age," (33 months chronologic age), D.S. responded to auditory stimuli in his environment and vocalized more consistently, sometimes accompanied by gestures or signs. He became interested in music. The Infant Toddler Meaningful Auditory Integration Scale (IT-MAIS) (Zimmerman-Phillip, Osberger, & Robbins, 1997), a parent survey that provides useful information for monitoring auditory development, yielded a 30% score—consistent with performance of normal-hearing children at approximately 3 to 6 months of age. Late-evoked potentials were attempted but no clear response was recorded. At 18 months auditory age (36 months chronologic age), D.S.'s implant was reprogrammed with the benefit of neural response telemetry (NRT), a technique that allows audiologists to program the CI by monitoring electrically evoked action potentials (ECAPs). The new program represented a vast change in threshold and comfort levels. D.S. responded to tonal and speech stimuli at 25 dB HL, and his parents noted increased auditory awareness and vocalization. An IT-MAIS of 60% suggested auditory development comparable to a child 9 to 12 months of age. Late-evoked potentials yielded a repeatable response but one difficult to interpret. Continued evaluation using late-evoked potentials is planned. His mother describes an overall "developmental burst." D.S. has recently begun to use eating utensils. Communicatively, he understands simple commands and uses approximately 40 to 50 words, divided about equally between spoken and sign language.

Case Study 17–3 *(continued)*

Speech consists primarily of vowel productions, but he is beginning to demonstrate repetitive babbling. Both his mother and auditory–verbal therapist note an increase in the functional use of language through the auditory channel. According to D.S.'s mother, the use of sign language facilitates the mapping of concepts to labels, fosters expressive language, and minimizes his frustration. Receptive capabilities continue to exceed expressive, but both are delayed. A neuropsychological evaluation is scheduled for the near future. D.S. will attend a total communication classroom in a Regional Day School for the deaf. His parents are encouraged by continued progress and cannot overemphasize the value of resources such as the AN Listserv, www.auditoryneuropathy.tripod.com, and other parents of children with AN.

---

related potentials (ERPs) have been used to document neurophysiological changes following treatment on a case-by-case basis [see Jirsa (2002) for a review]. In addition, functional magnetic resonance imaging (fMRI) techniques have documented increased brain activity in multiple brain areas following computerized auditory training and oral language therapy. The magnitude of physiological change was positively correlated with improved oral language scores (Temple et al, 2003). Moreover, Jerger et al (2002) use an array of 32 electrodes to obtain topographic maps to reflect brain activation patterns over both hemispheres during completion of various auditory or visual tasks. This technique might offer insight into posttreatment brain changes. Research in this area is progressing at a rapid pace and conclusive outcomes are anticipated from large numbers of children with APD to determine whether various electrophysiolgical and neuroimaging techniques document progress in treatment.

Summary

The evaluation and remediation of APD in children remains an exciting and complex science. Audiologists, speech-language pathologists, educators, psychologists, and parents have at their disposal a large, growing, and sometimes conflicting body of work devoted to APD. Current trends favor deficit-specific evaluation of APD together with a multidimensional remediation plan. Treatment of APD is addressed via intensive auditory skills training. Management of language, academic, and communication problems associated with the disorder is accomplished via compensatory techniques and environmental modifications. Large-scale and careful research regarding the efficacy of remediation techniques is essential for the delivery of efficient and successful intervention for APD.

References

Anderson, K., & Matkin, N.H. (1996). Screening Instrument for Targeting Educational Risk (SIFTER). Tampa: Educational Audiology Association.

American Speech-Language-Hearing Association (ASHA). (1996). Central auditory processing: Current status of research and implications for clinical practice. *Am J Audiol, 5*, 41–54.

Bellis, T.J. (1996). *Assessment and Management of Central Auditory Processing Disorders in the Educational Setting.* San Diego: Singular.

Bellis, T.J. (2002). *When the Brain Can't Hear: Unraveling the Mystery of Auditory Processing Disorder: Treating APD.* New York: Pocket Books.

Bellis, T.J., & Ferre, J.M. (1999). Multidemensional approach to the differential diagnosis of central auditory processing disorders in children. *J Am Acad Audiol, 10*, 319–328.

Berlin, C., Borderlon, J., St. John, P., Wilensky, M., Hurley, A., Kluka, E., & Hood, L. (1998). Reversing click polarity may uncover auditory neuropathy in infants. *Ear Hear, 19*, 37–47.

Bradlow, A.R., Krauss, N., & Hayes, E. (2003). Speaking clearly for children with learning disabilities: Sentence perception in noise. *J Speech Lang Hear Res, 46*, 80–97.

Chermak, G.D. (1998). Managing central auditory processing disorders: Metalinguistic and metacognitive approaches. *Seminars in Hearing, 19*, 379–392.

Chermak, G.D., & Musiek, F.E. (1992). Managing central auditory processing in children and youth. *Am J Audiol, 1,* 61–65.

Chermak, G.D., & Musiek, F.E. (1997). *Central Auditory Processing Disorders: New Perspectives.* San Diego: Singular.

Chermak, G.D., & Musiek, F.E. (2002). Auditory training: Principles and approaches for remediating and managing auditory processing disorders. *Seminars in Hearing, 23,* 297–308.

Cone-Wesson, B., Rance, G., & Sininger, Y. (2001). Amplification and rehabilitation strategies for patients with auditory neuropathy. In: Y. Sininger & A. Starr (Eds.), *Auditory Neuropathy: A New Perspective on Hearing Disorders* (pp. 233–249). Canada: Singular, Thompson Learning.

Ferre, J.M. (1998). The M³ model for treating central auditory processing disorders. In: M.A. Masters, N. Stecker, & J. Katz (Eds.), *Central Auditory Processing Disorders: Mostly Management* (pp. 103–115). Boston: Allyn and Bacon.

Ferre, J.M. (2002). Managing children's auditory processing deficits in the real world: What teachers and parents want to know. *Seminars in Hearing, 23,* 319–326.

Fisher, L.I. (1985). *Learning Disabilities and Auditory Processing Addministration of Speech-Language Services in the Schools.* San Diego: College Hill Press.

Flexer, C., & Savage, H. (1993). Use of mild gain amplifier with preschoolers with language delay. *Lang Speech Hear Serv Sch, 24,* 151–155.

Friel-Patti, S., Loeb, D.F., & Gillam, R.B. (2001). Looking ahead: An introduction to five exploratory studies of Fast ForWord. *Am J Speech Lang Pathol, 10,* 195–202.

Gillam, R.B., Crofford, J.A., Gale, M.A., & Hoffman, L.M. (2001). Language change following computer-assisted language instruction with Fast ForWord or Laureate Learning Systems software. *Am J Speech Lang Pathol, 10,* 231–247.

Gillam, R.B., Loeb, D.F., & Friel-Patti, S. (2001). Looking back: A summary of five exploratory studies of Fast ForWord. *Am J Speech Lang Pathol, 10,* 269–273.

Hood, L.J. (1998). Auditory neuropathy: What is it and what can we do about it? *Hear J, 51,* 10–18.

Jerger, J., & Musiek, F.E. (2000). Report of consensus conference on the diagnosis of auditory processing disorders in school-aged children. *J Am Acad Audiol, 11,* 467–474.

Jerger, J., Thibodeau, L., Martin, J., Mehta, J., Tillman, G., Greenwald, R., Britt, L., Scott, J., & Overson, G. (2002). Behavioral and electrophysiologic evidence of auditory processing disorder: A twin study. *J Am Acad Audiol, 13,* 438–460.

Jirsa, R.E. (2002). Clinical efficacy of electrophysiologic measures in auditory processing disorders management programs. *Seminars in Hearing, 23,* 349–355.

Katz, J. (1983). Phonemic synthesis. In: E. Lasky & J. Katz (Eds.), *Central Auditory Processing Disorders: Problems of Speech, Language and Learning* (pp. 269–295). Baltimore: University Park Press.

Katz, J. (1992). Classification of auditory processing disorders. In: J. Katz, N. Stecker, & D. Henderson (Eds.), *Cental Auditory Processing: A Transdisciplinary View* (pp. 81–91). St. Louis: Mosby Year Book.

Katz, J. (2002). *Evaluation and remediation of CAPD: Part II.* Paper presented at the 14th Annual Convention and Expo of the American Academy of Audiology, Philadelphia, PA.

Keith, R. (1994). ACPT: Auditory Continuous Performance Test. San Antonio: Psychological Corporation.

Kelly, D. (1995). *Central Auditory Processing Disorder: Strategies for Use with Children and Adolescents.* San Antonio: Communication Shell Builders.

Krauss, N.A., Ozdamar, O., Stein, L., & Reed, N.C. (1984). Absent auditory brainstem response: Peripheral hearing loss or brainstem dysfunction? *Laryngoscope, 94,* 400–406.

Lasky, E.Z., & Katz, J. (1983). *Central Auditory Processing Disorders: Problems of Speech, Language and Learning.* Baltimore: University Park Press.

Madden, C., Rutler, M., Hilbert, L., Greinwald, J., & Choo, D. (2002). Pediatric cochlear implantation in auditory neuropathy. *Otol Neurotol, 23,* 163–168.

Marler, J.A., Champlin, C.A., & Gillam, R.B. (2001). Backward and simultaneous masking measured in children with language-learning impairments who received intervention with Fast ForWord or Laureate Learning Systems software. *Am J Speech Lang Pathol, 10,* 258–268.

Masters, M.G., Stecker, N.A., & Katz, J. (1998). *Central Auditory Processing Disorders: Mostly Management.* Boston: Allyn and Bacon.

Merzenich, M.M., Jenkins, W.M., Johnston, P., Schreiner, C., Miller, S.L., & Tallal, P. (1996). Temporal processing deficits of language-learning impaired children ameliorated by training. *Science, 271,* 77–80.

Miamoto, R.T., Kirk, K.I., Svirsky, M.A., & Seghal, S.T. (1999). Communication skills in pediatric cochlear implant recipients. *Acta Otolaryngolica (Stockholm), 119,* 219–224.

Miller, G.A., & Gildea, P.M. (1987). How children learn words. *Scientific American, 257,* 94–99.

Mokhemar, M.A. (1999). *The Central Auditory Processing Kits.* East Moline, IL: Linguisystems, Inc.

Musiek, F.E. (1999). Habilitation and management of auditory processing disorders: Overview of selected procedures. *J Am Acad Audiol, 10,* 329–342.

Musiek, F.E. (2003). *Auditory processing disorders: New trends.* Paper presented at the 15th Annual Convention and Expo of the American Academy of Audiology, San Antonio, TX.

Musiek, F.E., & Berge, B. (1998). A neuroscience view of auditory training/stimulation and central auditory processing disorders. In: M. Masters, N. Stecker, & J. Katz (Eds.), *Central Auditory Processing Disorders: Mostly Management* (pp. 15–32). Boston: Allyn and Bacon.

Musiek, F.E., Shinn, J., & Hare, C. (2002). Plasticity, auditory training and auditory processing disorders. *Seminars in Hearing, 23,* 263–275.

Neault, M., & Kenna, M. (2003). *Auditory dys-synchrony of infancy: Implications for implantation.* Paper presented at the 9th Symposium on Cochlear Implants in Children, Washington D.C.

Rance, G., Cone-Wesson, B., Wunderlich, J., & Dowell, R. (2002). Speech perception and cortical event-related potentials in children with auditory neuropathy. *Ear Hear, 23,* 239–253.

Rosenberg, G.G. (2002). Classroom acoustics and personal FM technology in management of auditory processing disorder. *Seminars in Hearing, 23,* 309–317.

Rosenberg, G.G., Blake-Rahter, P., Heavner, J., Allen, L., Redmond, B.M., Phillips, J., & Stigers, K. (1999). Improving classroom acoustics: A three-year FM sound field classroom amplification study. *J Ed Audiol, 7,* 8–21.

Ross, M., & Giolas, T.G. (1971). Effect of three classroom listening conditions on speech intelligibility. *Am Ann Deaf, 116,* 580–584.

Sharma, A., Dorman, M., & Spahr, A. (2002). A sensitive period for the development of the central auditory system in children with cochlear implants: Implications for age of implantation. *Ear Hear, 23,* 532–539.

Sharma, A., Dorman, M., Spahr, A., & Todd, N.W. (2002). Early cochlear implantation in children allows normal development of central auditroy pathways. *Ann Otol Rhinol Laryngol, 11,* 38–41.

Sharma, A., Dorman, M., Todd, N.W., Fainberg, J., & Martin, K. (2003). *Relationship between central auditory development and speech perception abilitiy in children with cochlear implants.* Paper presented at the IXth Symposium on Cochlear Implants in Children, Washington, D.C.

Sloan, C. (1986). *Treating Auditory Processing Difficulties in Children.* San Diego: College Hill.

Smoski, W.J., Brunt, O.M., Tanahill, J.C. (1998). Children's Auditory Performance Scale. Tampa: Educational Audiology Association.

Stach, B., Loiselle, L., Jerger, J., Mintz, S., & Taylor, C. (1987). Clinical experiences with personal FM assiting listening devices. *Hear J, 5,* 1–6.

Tallal, P., Miller, S., & Fitch, R.H. (1993). Neurobiological basis of speech: A case for the preeminence of temporal processing. *Ann N Y Acad Sci, 682,* 27–47.

Tallal, P., & Piercy, M. (1974). Developmental aphasia: Rate of auditory processing and selective impairment of consonant perception. *Neuropsychologica, 12,* 83–93.

Tallal, P., Miller, S.L., Bedl, G., Byman, G., Wang, X., Nagarajan, S.S., Schreiner, C., Jenkins, W.M., & Merzenich, M.M. (1996). Language comprehension in language-learning impaired children improved with acoustically modified speech. *Science, 271,* 81–84.

Temple, E., Deutsch, G.K., Poldrack, R.A., Miller, S.L., Tallal, P., Merzenich, M.M., & Gabrieli, D.E. (2003). Neural deficits in children with dyslexia ameliorated by behavioral remediation: Evidence from functional MRI. *Proc Natl Acad Sci USA, 100,* 2860–2865.

Trautwein, P., Shallop, J., Fabry, L., & Friedman, R. (2001). Cochlear implantation of patients with auditory neuropathy. In: Y. Sininger & A. Starr (Eds.), *Auditory Neuropathy: A New Perspective on Hearing Disorders* (pp. 203–231). Canada: Singular, Thompson Learning.

Zimmerman-Phillip, S., Osberger, M.J., & Robbins, A.M. (1997). *Assessment of auditory skills in children two years of age or younger.* Paper presented at the Vth International Cochlear Implant Conference, New York, New York.

18

Classroom Intervention Strategies and Resource Materials for Children with Hearing Impairment

Virginia Berry

The eye is the mirror to the soul; The ear is its gates.
—Helen Keller, 1880–1968

The child with hearing impairment in the mainstream or an inclusion setting is often manipulated by the well-meaning educator falling prey to the self-fulfilling prophecy. The Individuals with Disabilities Education Act (IDEA) and other laws regulating services for children with disabilities are often a double-edged sword. Certainly, one of the most positive outcomes has been an increased sensitivity to identifying children with handicaps and improved awareness of the importance of meeting their educational needs. The result has been the rapid development of services within the local education agency, the home school district.

In turn, an outgrowth of these positive trends has been the surfacing of increased labeling of children. Granted, a necessary evil, categorizing a child is a prerequisite to providing service. However, it is, in fact, this process that is the catalyst for the educator's submission to the self-fulfilling prophecy.

Teachers react, although often indirectly, to labels assigned to children. When they are told a child is "gifted," expectations are set. This child is often given increased attention and special privileges. If creativity is expected, a child frequently responds accordingly. After reading a previous teacher's notes on the discipline difficulties associated with a child there is often a tendency to mis-

judge those small misbehaviors, frequently overlooked or excused in other children, as outrageous disruptive acts.

Teachers who have had a child with hearing impairment in their class, particularly if the child comes with the label of "deaf," may also create some inappropriate assumptions. Well-trained and experienced educators are outstanding professionals in many areas. However, with limited exposure to children with hearing impairments, they are likely to be holding on to many misconceptions. Thus the self-fulfilling prophecy begins.

This chapter provides the tools an educator needs to successfully manage the child with hearing impairment in the classroom. Also, it is hoped, this chapter will illustrate that the strategies needed for the child with hearing impairment are no more overwhelming than those basic strategies that make for a good educational setting in general.

Certainly, if an educator is modifying or redirecting all teaching to serve the child with hearing loss, then placement staff should ask the question, "Was mainstreaming or inclusion premature?" Successful inclusion should include only a few overt classroom changes, with most techniques being subtle differences in style. One of the most important keys to the process will be a teacher with a positive attitude and confidence, who is not being transformed into an educator of the deaf. This chapter will discuss the skills necessary to eliminate forever the fear of deafness and, therefore, bury for good the self-fulfilling prophecy.

Who Are the Kids?

So often, professionals are plagued with the attitude that the only children who have special needs are those with the most obvious, most visible, and, therefore, the most severe problems. It is ironic to think that the child who is hearing impaired and who often has the least difficulty "making it" in the regular classroom is the child with the more severe hearing loss.

The reason for this is likely attributed to the direct relationship between severity of handicap and level of intensity of staff involvement. The child who is mainstreamed with a severe hearing impairment is often older than the child with a mild hearing impairment, has received years of previous direct intervention, utilizes interpreters/tutors, has use of special assistive devices, and so forth. In addition, teachers selected to serve these children are chosen after careful consideration of knowledge and experience (Brackett, 1990b).

On the other hand, children with lesser degrees of hearing loss of varying natures are often not afforded such advantages. Are their special needs any less important? In fact, these children are often more difficult to serve in the regular classroom. Children with mild hearing losses, fluctuating losses, unilateral deficits, or high-frequency disorders are often overlooked when needs are outlined or programs are planned. Chapter 10 in this book clearly points out that learning for these children is impacted by their hearing losses. Table 18–1 provides helpful tips for identifying these children.

Certain techniques specific to all populations of students with hearing impairment are essential to incorporate in the classroom. Professionals must recognize the unique differences among children with hearing loss. In many states, for a number of years the

Table 18–1. Helpful Tips for Identifying a Child with Hearing Impairment

Inattention

Frequently requests to have a statement or word repeated

Frowns or strains forward when addressed

Fatigues easily

Fails to participate in class discussions

Unable to localize sound

Gives inappropriate answers to simple questions

Chooses isolation or is isolated by peers

Is overly dependent on visual clues

Becomes easily frustrated

Often speaks too loudly

Has poor reading skills

Tends to do better in mathematics than in reading

Uses poor spoken or written language

Distorts or omits sounds from words

Has a voice that is harsh, breathy, nasal, or monotone

Uses inappropriate pitch, rhythm, stress, and inflection

Has a history of frequent earaches or ear discharge

Uses mouth breathing or shows other nasal symptoms

Complains of ringing, buzzing, or other noises in the ears

guidelines that qualify and quantify special education funding have considered hearing impairment a low incidence handicap. Such a distinction often translates into less funding applied to public education needs and services for students with hearing impairment. In considerations of only severe-to-profound, bilateral hearing losses, perhaps such an equation is justified. However, if other types and degrees of hearing loss are factored into the formula, a drastic increase in numbers occurs (Ross, Brackett & Maxon, 1991). Examining those figures and including fluctuating, conductive, and numerous acquired losses, some studies have noted in excess of 3 million school children who reveal educationally significant hearing disorders (Schow & Nerbonne, 2002). These figures should certainly reinforce the critical need to reexamine how education of the hearing impaired is prioritized and funded.

Where Are the Kids?

In addition to overlooking certain populations of children who are hearing impaired, educators and other professionals often neglect the issue of what placement is chosen for the child. Currently, only 46% of children with hearing impairment are served in some form of special placement or itinerant service (Schow & Nerbonne, 2002). However, "mainstreaming" can be a fairly generic term, sometimes simply meaning a child attends lunch or recess with regular classes. For the remainder of the day, the child's educational needs may best be met in a noncategorical, self-contained special education classroom. In many districts there are not enough children with hearing impairment to justify a teacher for children who are deaf. Children with hearing loss are often served successfully by special education teachers holding certification in another area and in classrooms housing a variety of children with disabilities and with differing needs. The intent of this chapter is not to debate the validity or appropriateness of such placement.

Rather, the point to be made is that professionals serving children with hearing impairment often assume that information on hearing loss and intervention goals do not need to be provided to any special educator (Ross, 1991). In fact, the goal should be to direct the teaching strategies of the regular classroom teacher who has no experience with children having special needs. After all, special educators received all the training they needed in every exceptionality, including deafness. Experience has proven that, with the exception of certified teachers of the deaf, special education classroom teachers need suggested techniques and guidance in working with the hearing impaired and are eagerly receptive to such information.

The environment in which the child is placed cannot be neglected. Regardless of whether the child with hearing impairment is in a full-time regular classroom, or a resource room for a portion of the day for isolated tutoring in selected areas, or in a self-contained room for the entire day, neither the child's special needs nor the intervention plan to meet these needs changes. Equal time and energy should be placed on informing all varieties of educators of these needs.

Getting Ready

Teacher Motivation

Successful implementation of any educational program is only as strong as the professional responsible for it. All the training and experience do not guarantee the will to succeed. Success hinges on the motivational level and attitude of those involved with the program.

Many hearing professionals assume that simply supplying school staff with pertinent case history information on the child, a previous services summary, and tips for teaching will provide the basis for a trouble-free classroom. Although these materials are important, other support is needed.

One all-important variable, motivation, should not be forgotten. Regardless of what role particular school staff plays in the program for a child with hearing impairment, that person must have a receptive attitude toward serving the child. The responsibility of working with this child means extra work for everyone, including the child (Sexton, 1991).

The first important step in establishing the necessary receptive climate is to ensure the classroom teacher feels a part of the child's total program. Too often, hearing professionals enter a school situation bringing in their "better mouse trap." It is important to keep in mind that educators do have some critical insight to add about good teaching practices. Their suggestions or concerns are often ignored (Sexton, 1991).

In addition, hearing professionals typically have one goal when approaching school staff: meeting the needs of the child with hearing impairment. Although commendable, the needs of the educator must be included in developing the educational program.

In many situations, individuals are significantly more receptive to hard work or change if asked for input into the direction of the change. Therefore, enthusiasm for a better mouse trap should be tempered and school staff should be asked for input and take an active part in the planning of any special training. Specific teaching strategies are much more likely to be incorporated in the classroom if the manager of the classroom has assisted in the design.

Administrative Preparation

An individual who is often overlooked as a critical element in the success of a mainstreamed child who is hearing impaired is the school administrator. Familiarization of administrative staff to the design of the program will have lasting effects on the outcome.

Administrators can assist in the commitment to the child and supply confidence to the teaching and support staff. They can foster the positive attitude of, "We can make a difference for this child." They can arrange for the redistribution of duties for teachers serving children who have special needs. Administrators can support the funding of equipment and materials essential to school staff implementing teaching strategies necessary for success (Ross, 1991).

Therefore, professionals working with schools must include administrators in all activities, particularly during the initial stages of program development. They have needs that should be addressed just as classroom staff do. Information should be provided that is relevant to their role; utilize strategies directed to meeting their needs; provide answers geared to eliminating their fears. The end result will be a cohesive program with a long-term emotional, professional, and financial commitment.

Team Management

If a child with hearing impairment is truly expected to succeed in a mainstreamed educational environment, it is naive to consider this a "one man show." It is certainly a team effort. Members of the team are all individuals concerned with this child's progress. Each member has specific responsibilities and goals and, therefore, requires specific intervention practices and strategies (Conway, 1990).

The recognition of the importance of team management is a prerequisite to getting ready for any program. Identifying the team members and providing useful and relevant management information are essential. One individual should be designated team manager. Too often, hearing professionals who are not school staff and are brought in only on a random consultant basis feel they are this designee. However, the role of the team manager is to provide consistency and continuity among members in the implementation of classroom strategies. Is it possible for an individual who visits a school only a few times to serve in this capacity?

Granted, although the hearing consultant is likely the individual with extensive knowledge and expertise in the area of the needs of the hearing impaired, this is not the individual who can guarantee daily application of good educational principles. For example, the primary teacher might be the more appropriate choice for team manager. This individual can assist the school counselor, the speech-language pathologist, the music teacher, the school secretary, and others in carrying over successful management strategies from the classroom.

However, the underlying assumption here is that this primary teacher has been given the necessary tools for effective management to continue. Enter the hearing professional. Although these consultants cannot guarantee continuity of daily programming, they can take responsibility for intensive training and education of school staff, particularly the team manager. If adequate staff preparation occurs, the team manager and, subsequently, each team member can take charge of consistent implementation.

Team professionals often ignore the parents. So often, parents are considered a nuisance, a threat, or intimidating. Certainly, there are parents who make it difficult to enjoy working with the child because of their demanding, "You work for me" attitude. However, if this aggression was traced back through the child's special service career, one may find that it stems from parent needs that were ignored, questions that were unanswered, or concerns that were pushed aside and not addressed.

Most parents want to have an active role in their child's programming, but not to the point of domination, as many professionals often think. Parents can be important assistants in the process of identifying strategies that work. Who better to explain some techniques in successful communication practices than the individual who uses them 24 hours a day?

Professionals need to listen carefully and attentively to parents. Information they supply will give insight into the child that educators often miss. Communicate to parents that their input is important and that their suggestions will be incorporated into the child's program.

Finally, one essential member of the team is the child. For those children who are old enough to provide meaningful input, use it. The child is the only true expert on what facilitates learning. Allow him or her to set the example for strategies that are useful. If the child is too young to describe these strategies specifically, then observation and manipulation of various procedures will provide the answer.

In-Service Training

No matter what specific information is included as part of the in-service training sessions or what style or form these sessions take, the intent should be to develop a knowledgeable and accepting attitude toward hearing loss and students with hearing loss. The outcome of such training should be the establishment of a realistic educational environment in which children with hearing impairment can function and progress (Ross, 1991).

Hearing professionals who are likely to be responsible for conducting in-service training must not be dogmatic. Remembering the principles of teacher motivation and team management, it is critical that participants do just that—participate (Maxon & Brackett, 1992). They must feel that the information presented gives them options for intervention (Hall, Oyer, & Hass, 2001). Preparing staff for working with children with hearing impairment should not take away from their flexibility or creativity.

When establishing an in-service training program for a school, it is helpful if the information presented can be specific to the child with hearing loss in the school. It is the responsibility of the professional conducting the in-service to know the child in question. Rather than general information on hearing loss, hearing aids, or teaching practices, present the topics chosen for discussion as they relate to the specific child with hearing impairment. Discuss the child's loss and its educational implications. Discuss classroom activities as they are understood. It is helpful to observe in some sort of teaching environment so that specific examples can be given. Know the specific curriculum and textbooks used in the child's class so you can explain modifications necessary to them in terms of vocabulary, content, and so forth (Ross et al, 1991). Many sources are available that can provide specific information to be gathered during the observation. There are several observation protocols that are commercially available or professionals can create their own. Data should be collected that describes the participation of the child in classroom activities, such as interactions among child, teacher, and classmates; communication style, level, and modality; physical environment; teaching style, and curriculum structure. If possible, it is certainly meaningful to have the child attend a portion of the in-service so that demonstrations of certain teaching strategies can be given.

Table 18–2 provides topics for in-service training for teachers, other school staff, and classmates of children with hearing loss. As shown, there is a wealth of information that

Table 18–2. In-Service Training Topics: Teacher, Other School Staff, Classmates, and Children with Hearing Loss

Definition of hearing loss and nature of the problem

Specific assessment information as it relates to each child who is hearing impaired (audiological data, previous academic history, speech/ language abilities, etc.)

Orientation to hearing aids and FM systems, including operation, placement, and maintenance

Auditory training

Speech and language activities

Behavior management

Individual educational planning and implementation

Teaching strategies

Materials and resources

Use of an interpreter, tutor, note taker, or other supportive staff

Acceptance in the classroom

Communication needs

Sign language classes

---

hearing professionals can convey to school staff during in-service preparation. The goal of such training is to instill an attitude that students with hearing impairments are a challenge not a burden and they can be an asset to the school. Often hearing professionals are overambitious and attempt too much during the preparation stage of programming. Certainly ambition is well meaning in recognizing several areas of need that warrant discussion. Staff preparation should include information on language, communication, reading, behavior management, peer orientation, speech, hearing aids, and classroom techniques.

The timing and scheduling of in-service training can be the variables that dictate the success of the program in general. School staff are already burdened with many extracurricular assignments. Care must be taken to guard against lengthy, after-school

meetings. Also, brief, frequent meetings are often better received than 2- to 3-hour workshops. Each session could focus on one particular issue.

Although some initial in-service preparation is certainly necessary prior to a teacher assuming responsibility for a child with hearing impairment, educators will have a much better understanding of this child's needs following time in direct classroom contact. Therefore, it is critical that in-service training be an ongoing, continuous process. Staff preparation sessions preceding direct child contact do just that—prepare staff. It certainly is not possible to acquaint staff with all situations that may arise. Individuals responsible for staff education should be willing to schedule several meetings throughout the school year (Ross, 1991).

In addition, professionals should keep in mind that in-service training cannot meet its goals if it does not keep the interest of its audience. Therefore, a straight lecture format is typically not effective. Demonstrations, visual aids, and open discussion forums are generally excellent techniques to maintain interest level. Also, although there are, as previously mentioned, many areas that need discussion, some areas are more relevant to certain school staff than others. It is helpful, therefore, to conduct in-service training on specific topics with specific types of staff. Specialized sessions can be scheduled for speech-language pathologists, school nurses, and others.

Intervention Strategies

General Considerations

Previous educational structures met the needs of children with exceptional needs by removing them from the mainstream of regular classrooms, serving them in self-contained classes or separate schools. With the shift in emphasis toward the least restrictive environment of the regular classroom, all teachers are now expected to meet the needs of the exceptional child, with little preparation (Sexton, 1991). During a school day, children are expected to listen and respond, integrate information, and generalize. They must interact with spoken language, written language, peers, and adults. They must apply thinking skills to learning and problem solving.

When a regular teacher is asked to enroll a child with a hearing impairment in a school program, it is likely that teacher's first contact with such a youngster. For this reason, it is critical that some basic elements of the mainstreamed program be analyzed before specific educational strategies can be addressed. These elements are child, family, class, and teacher centered. Each of these partners in the program represents varying priorities, needs, personal characteristics, demographics, and expectations. As much as possible, these differences should find the best balance to optimize the child's learning potential. For example, placing children with hearing impairment in classrooms in which their classmates are similar in age and academic level, the teacher uses a teaching style that is hands on, the physical arrangement is conducive to improved comprehension, and parents have appropriate expectations.

Classroom Arrangement and Environment

As described in several other chapters in this book, classroom acoustics are important for children with hearing loss. Noise levels in every classroom should be kept as low as is practical. There is certainly no elementary school class where no noise is present. As normal hearers, it is easy to take for granted sources of classroom noises, such as papers rustling, pages turning, hallway traffic, pencil sharpeners, playground activity, student chatter, and classroom animals. With normal hearers, adequate comprehension of orally presented information is found to occur in the presence of a +30 dB signal-to-noise ratio (English, 1995). Considering an average vocal volume of 60 dB, combined with often present classroom noise of 60 to 70 dB, the chances of such a listening condition occurring are obvious (Berg, 1993). For the child with hearing impairment, even with the utilization of personal amplification, the effects

of these conditions are even more devastating. It is important to remember the limitations of personal hearing aids. All sounds are amplified, thus prohibiting the child with hearing impairment from sorting out the important from the unimportant. Teachers should be aware that hearing aids do not correct a hearing loss but only assist in improving awareness or discrimination. The presence of excessive noise often counteracts the benefits of these improvements. As discussed in Chapter 13, the use of frequency modulation (FM) systems can eliminate many of the adverse effects of classroom noise.

In addition, the teacher should be aware of classroom acoustics. Although there is usually little a teacher can do to alter the construction of the room, controlling some of the adverse effects is possible. Hard surfaces, such as glass, wood floors, and blackboards reflect sound and can add to extraneous noise. Reverberation results as speech is repeatedly reflected back and forth from each surface with a time differential. This will cause the child with a hearing impairment to pick up echoes of several different words at the same time (Flexer, 1994).

There are some materials in the room that can absorb sounds and, therefore, assist in decreasing noise. Soft porous materials such as fabrics, paper, carpet, window shades, and cork can be used strategically throughout the room. The rear wall of the classroom is often the starting point for reverberation. Posters or cork bulletin boards arranged in this area as well as on the blackboard and shades or curtains on windows are certainly helpful. Carpet squares can be placed under each desk to help with sound absorption. The human body also provides effective dampening of sound. If the teacher can stagger the students' desks instead of arranging them in straight rows, less sound will travel to hard surfaces. The physical size of the classroom and the number of students will also be contributing variables to room acoustics.

Teachers should take care not to schedule a verbal presentation or lecture during periods of high activity or noise, either in other parts of the classroom or directly outside. Lighting is a variable that can also significantly affect the comprehension of a child with a hearing impairment. There is an obvious correlation between lighting and speech-reading ability, which will be discussed in more detail in another section. The best situation is the use of overhead lights and natural lighting, which can supply sufficient light but not be so bright as to cause shadows or a glare. If lighting comes primarily from one wall, the teacher should arrange so that it is the back wall of the class. It is best if the light comes from behind the child and falls on the teacher's face. This illuminates the teacher's face and the child is not blinded by the glare. The teacher should be careful not to stand near a window in bright sunlight because it often casts a shadow on the face. The teacher should also be aware of the effects of changes in lighting throughout the day and make appropriate adjustments (Brackett, 1990a).

The importance of preferential seating cannot be underestimated. The seating placement of a child with a hearing impairment certainly depends in part on the type of hearing loss, but it also is important to look at classroom format and activity.

If a bilateral loss is present, placement should be in a central location approximately 3 to 5 feet from the teacher, which allows for optimum use of the hearing aids. The teacher needs to take care not to be too close so that voice is not directed above the child with a hearing loss. Therefore, second row seating near the center is typically most effective. This can also help eliminate back and neck strain from the child's looking up at the teacher. If a significant asymmetry exists between the ears or a unilateral loss is present, a similar placement in the second row is recommended but with the child seated off-center so that the better ear is angled toward the teacher.

Special seating should not necessarily isolate, separate, or further identify the student with a hearing loss as "special." The front row is not only a disadvaantage for optimum hearing aid use, but also, at times, puts the child on the periphery of the class and causes the child to "stand out."

Preferential seating by itself is not the complete answer to the problems of a child with a hearing loss. The teacher does not perform all the talking or teaching in a classroom. Much information comes from class participation. Incidental or third-party learning is critical to each child's progress. A child should be allowed some flexibility in seating or orientation. This might mean different seats for different class activities. Or, if such movement is too attention-getting, the student should be placed where turning the body will assist in monitoring other students' questions or discussions, thus improving overall comprehension. The teacher may need to cue those students with hearing impairment who are unaware of other classmates' participation. Whenever possible, a circular class arrangement could be utilized that allows for better peer monitoring (Northern & Downs, 2002). Case Study 18–1 provides an example of improvements that can be made in the classroom to improve acoustical characteristics and placement.

Communication

Speechreading is a skill on which all children with hearing impairment exhibit heavy reliance. The success of speechreading is based on the principle of redundancy (the ability to predict the total message after receiving only a part of that message). Speechreading is not absolute. There are many more speech movements per second than the eye is capable of perceiving. In addition, many speech movements are not visible and many sounds and words look identical. Such homophenous elements can confuse a child and certainly affect the accuracy of comprehension. Imagine the frustration of thinking the teacher said to "sit by Pat," when the actual instruction was to "sit on your mat." The following are some guidelines to assist in optimum speechreading abilities and to guarantee improved comprehension.

1. It is critical to make sure the child with hearing loss is attending, not just listening. However, it is unrealistic to expect continuous attention of a child with hearing impairment. After all, such a level of attention from children with

Case Study 18–1   A.K., age 11, exhibits a moderately severe sensorineural hearing loss in his right ear and a profound, fragmentary loss in his left. A.K. utilizes an ear-level hearing aid on his right ear and no amplification on his left due to its minimal hearing. He receives excellent benefit from his monaural aid, responding within normal limits.

A.K. entered the fifth grade this school year. He has consistently been placed in regular classrooms throughout his school experience, receiving resource room instruction and speech/ language services. A.K. functions near grade level in all academic areas and has good communication skills.

A.K.'s fifth grade teacher has complained that he often has difficulty following directions and understanding orally presented class material. She finds him a bright student who is capable of all work, with minimal resource assistance. However, she is concerned about A.K.'s auditory comprehension skills and questioned his ability to maintain adequate progress because of this deficit.

Examination of the class by the area's consultant for the hearing impaired found a large room with wooden floors. One wall had all windows with no shades. Two walls were long blackboards. The back wall of the class was plaster. In addition, the class often divided into groups to complete different activities or projects. Significant background noise is often present caused by the hum of the heating or cooling unit in the rear of the class, pupils' conversations during small group work, and street noise from the unshaded windows.

Several recommendations were made to improve the class signal-to-noise ratio. Window shades were added. Also, corkboard was placed on the rear plaster wall, which was also used as a class bulletin board. Inexpensive room dividers were used to section off small group work. Also, such a divider was placed around the heating and cooling unit. Portions of each long blackboard were used to display class projects, assisting with decreasing the amount of hard surface. Student desks were staggered so as to create a body-baffle effect for noise and reverberation.

Further examination also revealed inappropriate seating for A.K. He was seated in the front desk on the far right-hand side of the class. Such a seat places A.K.'s unaided, poorer left ear nearer the teacher. It was recommended that he be moved to the second row, off-center to the left. Such placement would provide A.K. improved auditory clues, placing his better, aided right ear toward the teacher. Also, such seating would provide A.K. better visual access to both blackboards. The teacher was also encouraged to allow A.K. flexible seating so as to be better able to follow orally presented materials from all points in the room.

To monitor A.K.'s comprehension, his teacher had been asking questions such as, "Did you understand what to do?" A.K.'s response was typically a head nod for yes. It was recommended that the teacher begin asking open-ended questions such as "Which pages in your science book are you to read?"

These simple recommendations were well implemented. A 9-week review conference was held to examine A.K.'s progress. His teacher was surprised at the changes in A.K.'s abilities. She particularly commented on the effectiveness of flexible seating and the use of open-ended questions. In addition, some of her other children with normal hearing had mentioned how much easier it was to concentrate with the decreased noise.

normal hearing is not expected. Some inattention should be tolerated if the child is not to be worn out. Speechreading can be exhausting. Therefore, presenting as many important lessons in the morning hours can help avoid fatigue (Conway, 1990).

2. Teachers should speak clearly with moderate speed. The voice should be pleasant and unstrained. Lip movements should be natural and not exaggerated. Raising the voice or overarticulating will make understanding more difficult for the child (Brackett, 1990a).

3. Teachers should try to speak to the class from a position in the room that allows adequate light to fall on the face. It is nearly impossible to speechread in a glare; therefore, abundant light should be avoided. Also, teachers should not stand with their back to the window for this places their face in a shadow.

4. Teachers should avoid excess movements during critical speechreading times. They should try to stand as still as practical for their teaching style.

5. Teachers should try to face the class as much as possible. Writing on the blackboard and talking at the same time should be avoided. In addition, teachers should keep books and papers down from their faces when speaking.

6. Teachers should expect adequate speechreading behaviors from other students as well. They should be instructed to speak normally. The child with hearing impairment should be encouraged to turn and face other children while they are speaking.

7. Teachers should be aware that many words look alike on the lips. They should, therefore, always put single words into a sentence so that the child with a hearing impairment can take advantage of the principle of redundancy. More contextual clues result in better comprehension. Also, teachers should be patient and understanding with any confusions that occur in comprehension.

8. Teachers should be aware that it is difficult for the student with a hearing impairment to speechread a new person who might come into the classroom. Also, although lipstick often assists speechreading abilities, fancy hairstyles, certain clothes, moustaches, and beards will detract from speechreading.

9. It can be helpful to have one location in the classroom that is routinely used for oral presentations by both the teacher and other classmates.

Although part of the communication success that takes place in a classroom is dependent on visual clues, many students with hearing impairment can also rely on audition. Therefore, the teacher must use strategies that ensure adequate comprehension through listening. Auditory and visual clues should be used together to ensure that the child is obtaining as much information as possible. However, as with speechreading for many students with hearing impairments, auditory clues will not be absolute. As normal hearers, it is possible to forget the subtle language/meaning changes that occur simply with inflectional or intonational differences. Emphasizing one word over another in a sentence can change its meaning. A statement can be turned into a question simply by altering our inflection. Also, the phonemes of /s/ and /z/ are responsible for a significant amount of linguistic information (Flexer, 1994). Plurals, possessives, or some verb tenses are conveyed by these speech sounds. These high frequency sibilants are difficult to discriminate through audition alone. Even with the ambiguity of much of the auditory information received, children with a hearing loss should be encouraged to use their listening skills to the fullest extent possible. From responding correctly to roll call to following a story read aloud, any traditional auditory activity successfully completed will allow the child with a hearing impairment to feel like a part of the class.

As mentioned previously, it is important that the teacher makes sure the child is attending. Asking an open-ended question requiring a specific response can often determine if the child is alert to the content. Teachers cannot assume that the child with a hearing impairment understands information presented one time. These children are "famous" for the neutral response technique, and teachers should learn never to trust a nod (Johnson, Bensen, & Seaton, 1997). However, it must be emphasized that simply repeating what was said a second time does not guarantee comprehension. Rephrasing information is helpful, using different vocabulary, less complex sentence structure, and shorter sentences. Such practices are even more important when dealing with new or complex information or when listening conditions are poor. Here again, asking a question can check the child's ability to use or apply what was presented. Children with hearing impairments hear in a distorted manner and encounter unfamiliar vocabulary and language structures daily (Flexer, 1994).Teachers will find it necessary to go over any verbal instructions or directions given to the child.

In addition, classmates' presentations will require similar strategies. It is difficult for the child to follow discussion when speech is coming from several different directions. Teachers will often need to repeat or rephrase the main points stated by other students during such discussion. The consistent use of repetition with rephrasing provides the child with a hearing impairment increased input and the advantage of redundancy, thereby aiding comprehension (Johnson et al, 1997).

Hearing professionals often place so much emphasis on the communication skills of teachers that they forget there are strategies the child should practice as well. Teachers must remember that children with hearing impairments have special vocabulary limits. Many words that children with normal hearing use may not be common to the student with a hearing impairment. Teachers should encourage activities that strengthen vocabulary and enrich communication. Dictionary assignments are helpful. In addition, professionals should promote an interest in read-

ing. Teachers should reinforce and reward attempts to learn or use new vocabulary, and professionals must remember that the use of slang is important to communication (Ross et al, 1991). Children with hearing impairments should have the benefit of this exposure as well.

Teachers need to make the child with a hearing loss speech conscious (Johnson et al, 1997). Goals should be developed that address communication skills, posture, attitude, and fluency. Classroom staff can work closely with speech-language pathologists so they can be aware of specific speech goals and targets. Encourage the children to "practice" their speech goals in class and modify speech as appropriate. Naturally, this is not to mean the use of constant interruption or speech nagging. Sometimes rather than correcting poor speech the teacher should simply model appropriate production.

Teachers should compliment correct speech, as well. Reinforcement and reward are important keys to carry over. Often, children with hearing impairment cannot hear improvements but must depend on the listener to judge their accuracy. Educators should not protect children with hearing impairments from speaking assignments. They should be provided the same opportunities as other children (Northern & Downs, 2002). Depending on the degree of the hearing loss, the speech of the child with a hearing impairment may be difficult to understand at times. As the teacher becomes more familiar with the child's pattern of speech production, intelligibility will improve. Teachers who are unsure should not hesitate to ask the child to repeat what was said. When requesting information or a response, it is helpful to give the child time to "attack" and organize the communication attempts. Also, providing the child with a limited number of choices to use in selecting responses will assist the teacher in interpreting the answer.

Many children with hearing impairments may exhibit inappropriate volume by talking either too loudly or too softly. Teachers should assist children to work out their own "measuring stick" for monitoring the loudness of their voice (Hall et al, 2001). Teachers can help the child recognize the loudness level to maintain. Also, at times, children with hearing impairments vocalize to themselves or make unnecessary noises. This can be disturbing to the class so the child should be taught to identify these times through cuing or other means.

It is important that educators instill feelings of speech competency in children with hearing impairments. Also, they must learn not to be ashamed or embarrassed if they do not understand. Children should express their confusion immediately. Teachers should watch for signs of poor understanding and not be impatient if the child with a hearing impairment asks for clarifications. The art of asking questions is a critical skill for all children to master.

Teaching Methodology Hints and Recommendations

No amount of in-service training or chapters in books can prepare classroom teachers for all situations they will encounter with children with hearing impairments or develop in them all skills necessary for successful management of these children. Each class-room is different, as is each teacher and each child. However, there are many areas of common ground and, therefore, many universal methods that should be incorporated in classrooms housing children with hearing impairments.

Teachers must be realistic. No teacher is expected to be all things to all students, particularly those with disabilities. Textbooks often emphasize how professionals should not frustrate children with hearing impairments, but they forget to stress the frustration of the teacher and its negative effects. Educators cannot reinvent the wheel with every lesson. Rather, they should be expected to simply be aware of this population's special needs, to be eager to meet them, and to do their best. A failure to grasp the concept of multiplication in a student with hearing impairment is not necessarily a reflection of poor teaching or an absence of teacher enthusiasm. Table 18–3 outlines some strategies for impacting learning in children with hearing loss.

Teachers of students with hearing impairments must be aware that the active listening and concentration required of these children will cause them to fatigue more easily than others. Greater effort is necessary of these students, and as a result, they will tire (Maxon & Brackett, 1992). At the end of a

Table 18–3. Tips for Impacting Learning in Students Who Are Hearing Impaired

Be careful about the assumptions made about the child

Be word and vocabulary conscious. The child encounters new words daily that other children may already know

Be conscious of students' questioning abilities

Be aware of opportunities to develop word attack abilities, including both phonetic and contextual analysis

Keep up with all available resources and materials useful to the hearing impaired

Be aware of the importance of figurative language, syntax, memory, sequencing, inferencing, and comprehension, not only to reading but to all learning areas

Be alert to students' attitude and motivational level

Develop test-taking abilities of students

Recognize importance of expanding students' general world knowledge

Expose students to a variety of printed materials

Read to children daily and provide time daily for children to read silently school day, they may appear not to be paying attention or to be daydreaming. In actuality, they may be exhausted. It is helpful to alternate class activities that require close attention or precise comprehension. Listening breaks are useful. Give the class seatwork to complete (Ross et al, 1991). This is not to mean, however, that teachers should not expect the student with a hearing loss to pay as close attention as others.

Teachers should organize their schedule so that children with hearing impairments can anticipate subjects and thereby predict vocabulary, and so forth. It is helpful to provide for the student with a hearing impairment a preview of topics or subjects to come. They could be given assignments to read ahead to become familiar with new concepts and vocabulary. Vocabulary lists could be sent home. Early exposure to subjects to come can prepare children for the visual properties of the new vocabulary and acquaint them with contextual clues.

Teachers should reduce as much to writing as practical to their classroom style. New vocabulary words should be written on the board, as well as said. Blackboard outlines of topics being discussed assist in orienting students to the subject matter and allow them to keep up with the sequence. Homework assignments should also be written on the board as they are given. It is helpful if the same portion of the blackboard is consistently used to note assignments.

Teachers should use natural gestures just as they would during informal conversation. Gestures and cuing assist children with hearing impairments with comprehension. When talking about a specific child or object, point to, walk over to, or touch the child or the object (Schow & Nerbonne, 2002).

Visual aids are very helpful to comprehension. Diagrams, graphs, pictures, maps, and the like are excellent supplements to lecture materials. They assist in reinforcing verbally presented material and increase visual input. Such aids give context and clarify the message. Overhead projectors are particularly helpful. Information may be written on a transparency as the lecture progresses,

cuing students with hearing impairments to new vocabulary, subject changes, and so forth. Visual aids increase the number of sensory associations.

The use of slides, movies, and tapes is often not as helpful, however. Their sound tracks are frequently poor and the pictures are too small and far away for adequate speechreading. If these are used, it is often beneficial to provide to the student with a hearing impairment a script or summary before the noncaptioned film or slides are shown (Hall et al, 2001).

Instituting a buddy system for the child with a hearing impairment can be of great benefit to both the teacher and the child. One or two students in the class can be named as the assistant to the child with a hearing loss. Such "buddies," if chosen appropriately, can take some of the demands off the teacher. Buddies can alert the child with a hearing impairment to critical listening times. The buddy can repeat directions or instructions to ensure comprehension. In addition, note takers can be assigned to help the student with a hearing impairment. Not that the child with a hearing loss should be excused from note taking, but teachers must remember that it is difficult to write and speechread at the same time. Notes supplied by another student can supplement any information missed. Carbonless paper copies are excellent tools for note takers. When choosing a buddy for the child with a hearing impairment, it should be a classmate who is reliable, willing, and an above average student (Northern & Downs, 2002).

With the implementation of cooperative learning centers in many classrooms, the child with a hearing loss will face some new, yet needed, challenges in education. The purpose of cooperative learning is to provide students the opportunity to work together in small groups and to target a specific task, such as reviewing for a test, solving mathematical problems, or writing a book report. The advantages to this practice are obvious. Students learn how to share ideas, encourage participation from others, become responsible for their own learning, and increase their attention to tasks (Sexton, 1991). For the child with a hearing impairment, these are also important outcomes of cooperative learning. In addition, however, the child will develop improved social skills and acquire necessary exposure to pragmatic skills, such as turn-taking and interactive communication. It will also provide increased opportunity to utilize targeted auditory, speechreading, and speech production skills. It is critical that teachers not eliminate children with hearing impairments from cooperative learning experiences (Northern & Downs, 2002).

Teachers should recognize that subjects that involve manipulative activity or experimentation such as home economics, mathematics, or science are more readily understood than those subjects with high language content, such as reading or creative writing (Brackett, 1990a). Experimental activities assist in comprehension, as well. After discussing farm animals, a trip to a farm will reinforce learning. Pictures can be taken by the students to bring back to class, which helps with carryover and provides consistent exposure to new concepts. Also, the use of role-playing or dramatic play assists concept development. All children learn best by doing. Table 18–4 provides some suggestions for the teacher to maintain school and learning as a positive experience.

Teachers should avoid "yes" or "no" questions. This type of response provides no guarantee that the child with hearing impairment grasped the material. Teachers can have the child repeat or summarize what was said. This reveals if the student with

Table 18–4. School and Learning Can Be Fun

IF YOU . . .
  Provide for individual differences
  Avoid overarousal
  Work on strong areas
  Allow time for response

AND . . .
  Work sequentially
  Watch vocabulary
  Increase redundancy

hearing impairment did understand the message.

Teachers should avoid introducing new topics without preparing or cuing the child with a hearing impairment. Verbal and visual connectives and transitions should be used between subjects. Situational clues can be provided, which can clue children to what is to come (Hall et al, 2001). In lower grades where vocabulary enrichment is a daily event, teachers can label items in the room so that the child is exposed to the vocabulary in printed form.

Obviously, poor auditory memory is associated with impaired hearing. Teachers should break verbal directions down into a step by step explanation so that the child is not required to process multiple components. For complex written directions, it might be helpful for either the teacher or the student to highlight each stage or component with a different-color marker. Again, although it is critical for children with hearing impairments to be held accountable for similar levels of responsibility as other students, at times it may be necessary to provide them additional time to complete some assignments. Based on the complexity of the language used or reading requirement, some extra time will allow the child to sort through the information presented, process the task, and provide a more accurate picture of the child's true abilities on that activity. Also, there may be times due to difficulties in timely task completion that some assignments need to be decreased in length to safeguard self-esteem. Perhaps the child with hearing loss could complete 15 of the 25 mathematical problems. It is also helpful to increase the spacing between questions or problems on a page, decrease the number on a page, enlarge the print, and put all information on one page to avoid page turning because the child with a hearing impairment is often distracted by too much material. Also, teachers must remember that word order is not always the same as meaning order. The direction "Before you do your spelling assignment, complete your math worksheet," can be confusing to a child with a hearing impairment. Again, when possible, teachers should be concrete and specific in their language, rephrase the information if confusion appears, or check the level of comprehension by asking the child to repeat what was said.

Oral tests place the child with a hearing impairment at an obvious disadvantage. Although written tests are recommended, they cannot always be used. When oral testing is used, an overhead projector could be utilized to reveal one question at a time after it is presented orally. This does preserve some of the elements of oral testing. Teachers should be confident that they are testing the knowledge, rather than the listening or language skills, of the student who is hearing impaired (Hall et al, 2001). Also, children with hearing loss often perform better on closed-set tests where choices are provided rather than in an open-set format.

Teachers can provide the resource room teacher or the speech-language pathologist with special vocabulary or topics that will be covered in class. These individuals can reinforce classroom instruction or work ahead on certain subjects, providing these students the edge they often require. In addition, it is helpful if the resource room teacher or speech-language pathologist can go into the child's class during key times to assist with instruction. This will also provide insights into the child's group learning style.

Teachers need to encourage students with hearing impairments to participate in extracurricular activities. Such involvement fosters acceptance and truly makes them a part of the school. Activities such as scouts, school sports, and school clubs are critical to a successful school experience. Music is an area often thought inappropriate for children with hearing impairments. After all, how could someone with impaired or distorted hearing succeed in such an auditory area? Most children with a hearing impairment enjoy music-related activities and gain significantly from them. Music improves listening skills and rhythm. Children should not be deprived of this school experience (Maxon & Brackett, 1992).

Teachers of younger children often speak negatively of comic books. These books can be excellent learning tools, particularly for the child with a hearing impairment (Ross et al, 1991). They use short, simple sentences, always paired with pictures. This assists the child in language development and reading acquisition. Comic books can assist the child in understanding idioms, one of the most difficult language structures they will encounter. During the language-learning process, children with hearing loss are very literal and concrete. The teacher must keep in mind that idiomatic expressions such as "Don't knock yourself out over this assignment" will be confusing; or "You're pulling my leg" will mean just that to children with hearing impairments. Comic books can help eliminate the confusion prompted by idioms through their use of pictures.

Teachers should be aware that school announcements over a public address system are difficult listening situations for the hearing impaired. Not only are they typically distorted and of poor quality, they provide no visual clues. Teachers should either repeat such announcements or have the buddy explain them to the child with a hearing impairment.

Teachers need to be aware of the safety in the classroom that may not be as obvious to the child who is hearing impaired. Precautions need to be taken against such hazards. School crossings and bus loading zones are hazardous areas for all children. Teachers need to be aware of areas of hazard where hearing acts as a signal or warning (fire alarm, cooking timer, traffic, etc.) (Maxon & Brackett, 1992).

Teachers need to recognize that the hearing of all children can fluctuate during the presence of colds or allergies and that children with documented hearing losses are not immune to the temporary acquisition of additional loss because of these illnesses (Johnson et al, 1997). Inattentiveness or decreased performance may not be due to conscious behavior on the part of the child, but rather temporary conductive involvement. Teachers should be alert to such problems and refer the child for needed evaluation.

To assist in making the child feel a part of the class and if the added attention would not cause discomfort, teachers can incorporate the child with a hearing impairment into an instructional activity. A unit on hearing loss or hearing aids can be taught during science. A speechreading lesson can be taught to the entire class. As pointed out in Case Study 18–2, a child with a hearing impairment could instruct the class about the use of hearing aids.

Teachers need to communicate frequently with parents. They are, after all, the "at home" teacher. Teachers need to be willing to discuss both the strengths and weaknesses of the child with a hearing impairment. They should be encouraged to keep a management diary for the child to take home daily. It could include vocabulary lists, a preview of subjects to come, or teaching strategies that work. Using parents to work on topics at home can only improve carryover. Parents can use certain vocabulary introduced at school in different contexts, which certainly facilitates comprehension of multiple meanings.

Special Adaptations

Although many of the teaching strategies previously described are applicable to all children exhibiting impaired hearing, regardless of type or degree, they are often associated only with those children with losses identified in the severe-to-profound range. Children "classified" as hearing impaired by most educational standards are those requiring special services, meaning those with academic deficits and more significant impairments.

However, there are many children attending school with hearing losses of varying types and degrees who may be functioning with no difficulty in academic or other school-related areas. They may not require the extent of intervention that the more severely impaired do, but they do require some amount of special classroom adaptation for their needs to be met.

Children exhibiting fluctuating, conductive hearing losses can cause a dilemma for the teacher. On many occasions, the child responds with no difficulty and without problems in comprehension. At other times, the child seems to be "in a dream world" and follows very little of what goes on in the class. These children may be exhibiting fluctuating degrees of hearing loss due to temporary episodes of upper respiratory involvement, middle ear disease, or some other interference.

At these times, they may perform and function just as the severely hearing impaired child does who reveals a permanent sensorineural loss. Teachers should be alert to changes in responsiveness and understanding. If a history of fluctuating hearing loss is documented in the child's records, then the teacher might assume such a loss is the cause of the changes and begin incorporating those necessary teaching practices already described. If this is the first indication of poor awareness, the teacher should refer the child for testing and consult with the district's specialists on hearing impairment.

For many years, the presence of a unilateral hearing loss was thought to have no effect on the educational achievement of children. As professionals, we now know that is certainly not the case. Unilateral losses (in the presence of one normal ear) have been found to play a significant role in the abilities of the child exhibiting such disorders (Ross et al, 1991).

The intent of this chapter is not to debate the controversies that surround the skills of the child with a unilateral hearing loss. Rather, it is only important that teachers be aware that if such a loss exists, they must program for it appropriately. After reading the child's records documenting a unilateral loss, teachers should not assume that the one normal ear would compensate for that disorder. Obviously, special consideration must be given to seating the child with the better ear directed toward the speaker. Also, as appropriate to the unilateral nature of the loss, modifications should be made to teaching styles, as previously described.

Children with high-frequency losses pose an even greater challenge for the classroom

Case Study 18–2   E.W., age 15, exhibits a bilaterally symmetrical, severe sensorineural hearing loss. She utilizes binaural ear-level hearing aids that provide her adequate benefit, improving her acuity to within the borderline mild-to-moderate hearing loss range. For the last 3 years, E.W. has become somewhat more self-conscious about her loss and hearing aids. E.W. often leaves her aids at home or fails to have spare batteries.

E.W. is currently enrolled in the tenth grade. Until this school year, she received the majority of her academic instruction in a resource room. E.W. was mainstreamed into regular classes for mathematics, physical education, and extracurricular activities only. School staff involved with E.W. had observed her motivation to be very high to return to regular classes for additional periods. Assessments had shown her abilities to be in the average range. Although E.W. was not on grade level for high-language-content courses such as civics, history, and English, staff agreed to attempt increased mainstreaming, with resource/tutoring services reduced to 1 hour a day.

Initial observation of E.W. in many of her classes revealed a high level of motivation to succeed. Teachers believed that she was capable of keeping up with the work as long as the resource teacher could review content with her on a one to one basis. Teachers were concerned, however, about E.W.'s reluctance to discuss her handicap with her peers and her inconsistent use of hearing aids. In addition, E.W.'s regular teachers had been relying on E.W. communicating to the resource teacher the class material with which she needed assistance. A 9-week conference revealed that E.W. was often confused about assignments and had a significant amount of missing information in her class notes.

In attempts to decrease E.W.'s self-conscious feelings about her handicap, her science and history teachers approached her with some ideas to introduce her classmates to hearing loss. Although reluctantly, E.W. did agree to the teachers' ideas. An entire unit in E.W.'s science class was devoted to anatomy of the ear and hearing disorders. Although E.W. initially was bothered by the increased attention drawn to her loss, she quickly was pleased to see her classmates were nothing but positive and supportive. The children's curiosity and frequent questions about her loss and her hearing aids seemed to improve E.W.'s self-concept and acceptance of her handicap. Following encouragement to bring her aids to school by her peers so that they could listen to them, E.W. exhibited more consistent use of amplification.

In addition to the science unit, E.W.'s history teacher prepared lectures on Alexander Graham Bell and his interest in deafness following his marriage to a deaf woman. This reinforced E.W.'s improved relationship and openness with her classmates. Once E.W.'s confidence was enhanced and she appeared more comfortable in her classes, her communication skills improved and her eagerness to participate in class discussion was obvious.

To ensure that E.W. was obtaining all material presented in her classes and comprehending all assignments, a buddy system was implemented. A good student in each class was assigned to make copies of all notes for E.W. and to repeat to her essential verbal instruction. Other strategies to assist E.W. with keeping up with new material presented in class included each teacher supplying the resource teacher a weekly preview of new topics and vocabulary.

Preteaching of material, the buddy system, improved self-concept, and consistent use of amplification all contributed to a successful year for E.W. She maintained a B or C average in all classes.

teacher. Similar to those children with fluctuating losses, these children exhibit inconsistent abilities in awareness and comprehension. Special consideration is necessary for children with high-frequency hearing loss, as well. These students will often respond normally and comprehend with little difficulty. However, the presence of such a loss will certainly prompt more evident problems when noise occurs, visual clues are absent, speech is complex, and so forth. These children will have greater difficulty processing plurals or other morphological elements that are high frequency in nature.

Resource Materials

Many discussions of resource materials useful with the hearing impaired might like readers to believe that there are not many materials available that are appropriate for use with this population (Leeper & Gotthoffer, 2001). Regular teachers, as well as special educators, then feel abandoned, at times. Their responsibility is to "teach" these children, yet there are no "tools of the trade" useful to them.

The theory that curriculum materials or resources appropriate to education of the hearing impaired are limited should be rejected. Instead, it is contended that there are published sources for this population, but most materials designed for all students are more than adequate for the hearing impaired, with some modification. Too often, professionals fall prey to the philosophy that teaching methods and materials must be "laboratory tested" on the designated population before their usefulness can be proven. With the implementation of the strategies previously described in this chapter, many of the traditional or established materials used in the classroom will teach all students, including the child with hearing impairment.

In surveying professionals involved with the education of the hearing impaired, many themes emerge in the description of their approaches for organizing activities and content. Emphasis is placed on a natural language/whole language approach and strategies that are based on normal developmental information. There should be reliance on teacher judgment and experience to organize content areas and individualized instruction that best meets the child's needs (Brackett, 1990b). There is little difference between these emphasized priorities for programming for the hearing impaired and those that would be beneficial to any student.

Although not a teacher by profession, this author's years of experience have provided exposure to many "tried and tested" curricula and programs. Each publisher or agency described in the Appendix has a variety of useful tools in the education of a child with a hearing loss. It must be emphasized, however, that these listings are not intended to represent all groups with materials beneficial to students who are hearing impaired. Although this listing only begins to identify some resources, readers might recognize a trend in publishers or distributors. This listing is only the beginning of what is available.

Summary

It is hoped that the information contained in this chapter eliminates the need for educators to live under the influence of the self-fulfilling prophecy. Students with hearing impairment deserve the chance to prove that they can be a successful member of any class. The inclusion of these children can have many positive effects on the teacher and all the children.

The teacher and class work together to make the student with a hearing impairment feel accepted. This cooperative effort results in a class enthusiastic and eager to learn (Sexton, 1991). Also, the experience of getting to know a child with a disability can emphasize the fact they are a child first, a child with similar needs, likes, and dislikes. Being hearing impaired certainly requires specific teaching strategies, but it also requires being allowed to be a child.

As detailed in this chapter, teachers need to be more precise and graphic in their teaching style for the child with a hearing loss to have a clear understanding of the information presented. Such precision and clarity can only benefit the entire class. Also, because the teacher serves as an example, the class will make an effort to be clear and specific in their communicative endeavors (Sexton, 1991).

Educating a child with a hearing impairment can certainly be both frightening and overwhelming, but it can also be exciting and rewarding. Is that not the case with educating any child?

Appendix

Academic Communications Associates
P.O. Box 4279
Oceanside, CA 92052

Academic Therapy Publications
20 Commercial Blvd.
Novato, CA 94949

Alexander Graham Bell Association for the Deaf and Hard of Hearing
3417 Volta Place NW
Washington, DC 20007

American Guidance Service, Inc.
P.O. Box 99
Circle Pines, MN 55014

Butte Publications, Inc.
P.O. Box 1328
Hillsboro, OR 97123

Captioned Films for the Deaf
5034 Wisconsin Avenue NW
Washington, DC 20016

Charles C. Thomas Publishers
301–327 East Lawrence Ave.
Springfield, IL

Communication Skill Builders
555 Academic Court
San Antonio, TX 78204

Council for Exceptional Children
1920 Association Dr.
Reston, VA 22091

Dawn Sign Press
6130 Nancy Ridge Dr.
San Diego, CA 92121

Edmark
P.O. Box 3218
Redmond, WA 98073

Educational Audiology Association
4319 Ehrlich Rd.
Tampa, FL 33624

Educators Publishing Service
75 Moulton St.
Cambridge, MA 02138

Foreworks
Box 9747
North Hollywood, CA 91609

Gallaudet University
800 Florida Blvd. NE
Washington, DC 2002

Great Ideas for Teaching
P.O. Box 444
Wrightsville Beach, NC 28480

Harris Communications
15155 Technology Dr.
Eden Prairie, MN 55344

Houston School for Deaf Children
726 Diamond Leaf
Houston, TX 77079

Interstate Printers and Publishers
19–27 North Jackson
Danville, IL 61832

Laureatte Learning Systems
110 E. Spring St.
Winooski, VT 05404

Lingui Systems
3100 4th Ave.
East Moline, IL 61244

Modern Signs Press
P.O. Box 1181
Los Alamitos, CA 90720

National Association for the Deaf
814 Thayer Ave.
Silver Springs, MD 20910

NTID
1 Lomb Memorial Dr.
Rochester, NY 14623–0887

Parrot Software
P.O. Box 1139
State College, PA 16804

PRO-ED
8700 Shoal Creek Blvd.
Austin, TX 78757

Psychological Corporation
555 Academic Court
San Antonio, TX 78204

See Sign Productions
116 Volusia Ave.
Dayton, OH 45409

St. John's School for the Deaf
3680 Kinnickinnic Ave.
Milwaukee, WI 53207

St.Joseph Institute for the Deaf
1483 82nd Blvd.
St.Louis, MO 63132

Scott Foresman and Company
1900 East Lake Ave.
Glenview, IL 60025

Super Duper Publications
P.O.Box 24997
Greenville, SC 29616

References

Berg, F.S. (1993). *Acoustic and Sound Systems in the Schools*. San Diego: Singular.

Brackett, D. (1990a). Communication management of the mainstreamed hearing impaired student . In: M. Ross (Ed.), *Hearing Impaired Children in the Mainstream* (pp. 119–130). Parkton, MD: York Press.

Brackett, D. (1990b). Developing an individual education program for the hearing impaired student. In: M. Ross (Ed.), *Hearing Impaired Children in the Mainstream* (pp. 81–94). Parkton, MD: York Press.

Conway, L. (1990). Issues relating to classroom management. In: M. Ross (Ed.), *Hearing Impaired Children in the Mainstream* (pp. 131–157). Parkton, MD: York Press.

English, K.M. (1995). *Educational Audiology Across the Lifespan*. Baltimore, MD: Paul Brookes and Company.

Flexer, C. (1994). *Facilitating Hearing and Listening in Young Children*. San Diego: Singular.

Hall, B.J., Oyer, H.G., & Hass, W.H. (2001). *Speech Language and Hearing Disorders: A Guide for Teachers* (3rd ed.). Boston: Allyn and Bacon.

Johnson, C.D., Bensen, P.U., & Seaton, J.B. (1997). *Educational Audiology Handbook*. San Diego: Singular.

Leeper, L.H., & Gotthoffer, D. (2001). *Communications Sciences and Disorders on the Net*. Boston: Allyn and Bacon.

Maxon, A.B., & Brackett, N. (1992). *The Hearing Impaired Child: Infancy through High School*. Boston: Andover Medical Publishers.

Northern, J.L., & Downs, M.P. (2002). *Hearing in Children* (5th ed.). Philadelphia: Lippincott Williams and Wilkins.

Ross, M. (1991). A future challenge: Educating the educators and public about hearing loss. *Seminars in Hearing, 12*, 402–403.

Ross, M., Brackett, D., & Maxon, A.B. (1991). *Assessment and Management of Mainstreamed Hearing Impaired Children: Principles and Practices*. Austin, TX: PRO-ED.

Schow, R.L., & Nerbonne, M.A. (2002). *Introduction to Audiologic Rehabilitation* (4th ed.). Boston: Allyn and Bacon.

Sexton, J.E. (1991). Team management of the child with hearing loss. *Seminars in Hearing, 12*, 329–339.

19

Counseling for Parents of Children with Auditory Disorders

DAVID M. LUTERMAN

I'm not a teacher: only a fellow-traveler of whom you asked the way. I pointed ahead of myself as well as you.

—George Bernard Shaw, 1856–1950

Education of individuals with deafness in the United States began essentially as a school-based program within a residential setting. Because deafness is a low-incidence disorder, prospective students were scattered throughout the countryside. Each state would set up one school supported with tax dollars, generally in a rural area. The prevailing belief was that children who were disabled should be educated in a setting that was structured for them and was not visible to the rest of society; consequently, parents often had to travel enormous distances to reach the school. Because travel was so difficult and communication between home and school so minimal, the school personnel assumed total responsibility for educating the child; in fact, it was common for parents to be required to sign release forms granting custody of their child to the school. Parents were seen as peripheral to the education of the child. There might be a year-end conference with the teacher and occasional visits but very little detailed involvement of the parents was expected in the educational program. When parents did try to be involved, it was often seen as a threat by the school personnel. The principal of the Ohio School for the Deaf in 1917 admonished parents "to accept the recommendations of the school

authorities. They know. It is their business to know." Thus the culture of excluding parents was established deeply within the structure of education of the deaf (Bodner-Johnson, 1986).

With the urbanization of the United States and the technological improvements in transportation and communication that occurred in the early to mid-twentieth century, schools for the deaf became more accessible to families, but attitudes did not change appreciably. School personnel (and parents themselves) still saw parents as peripheral to the educational process. However, now that the school was more accessible, parents were more available to the professionals; thus began the parent–teacher organization (PTO). In this model, parents were viewed as "resources" to the schools; often, they were enlisted as fundraisers and school volunteers to fill in for office personnel, and, occasionally, they were enlisted as classroom aides. Education of the parents consisted of lectures and hurried conferences with teachers in which parents were expected to be passive recipients of the professional expertise. There was no sense that educating the child who was deaf was in any way a collaborative effort between parents and educators. Parents were seen at best as helpers and at worst as potential adversaries. This attitude was reflected in the training of teachers in which there was no mention of parental involvement and no training facilities that would demonstrate to the neophyte teacher an attitude toward parents other than the restrictive, patronizing one that was then considered good, standard operating policy for the school.

It was not until 1940, with the establishment of the Tracy Clinic in Los Angeles, that parent education and active participation in the educational process were demonstrated. With this pioneering effort, which was confined to preschool children, the Tracy Clinic established the notion that parents can and should be participants in the education of their children. It has taken us quite a while to make that cultural shift, and now almost all training programs in the United States and almost all schools for the deaf pay at least lip service to the notion of a parent–school partnership. This attitude also reflects the greater cultural shift that has taken place in the United States in which "consumers" are afforded a great deal of influence on the final "product." It remains to be seen, however, whether active parental participation has truly filtered up from the preschool program to invade all aspects of academics. Most schools seem to involve parents heavily in the preschool years and then revert to the PTO model in the school years.

A computer search of the literature reveals almost no articles and very few chapters about parents of school-age children with auditory disorders. Although there is material on the parents of preschool children; it is as though parents of school-age children have fallen off the face of the educational map. This chapter, then, was written mainly from an experiential and anecdotal framework. To aid in preparation of this chapter, information was solicited from parents of children with hearing impairments who were associated with Emerson College's family-centered program when their children were young (0 to 3 years old). This program has been described elsewhere (Luterman, 1999). Parents were asked to comment

in an open-ended way on three questions: (1) What are or were your specific needs as the parents of a school-age hearing-impaired child? (2) What programs do (or did) you wish the school had or did provide for you? (3) Aside from the academic considerations, what were your child's needs and were they met by the school? Thirty-four parents responded out of 121 solicited with children ranging in age from 5 to 30 years. Many of the parents wrote lengthy responses going much beyond the scope of the questions posed. This chapter then is written mainly from over 40 years of personal clinical experience of working with families of children who are hearing impaired and data gleaned from the questionnaires.

To understand parents' behavior, one must first understand parental feelings. In the early stages of the diagnostic process, when the child is very young, the feelings are usually apparent and felt acutely. For the parents of the school-age child, the emotions are present but may not be readily apparent. After the initial upheaval of feelings subsides, the parents begin to live a life of deafness that seems normal to them. When their adjustment is challenged by change or by trigger events that remind them of their initial pain, such as a shift in the educational plan or a diminution of the child's hearing, parents will often regress to an earlier stage of emotional adjustment. Parents of school-aged children frequently do not display their emotions because they have learned over the years to keep them under wraps. Consequently, professionals in school-based programs are often unaware of the parents' vulnerabilities. One father of a 17-year-old child commented: "When you first find out your child is deaf it hurts like hell; then it becomes a dull ache that doesn't go away."

Grief

Parents grieve the lost dream that they had of how their life was going to be and how their child would turn out. This dream or expectation is very real, and when it must be abandoned, it is experienced as a fundamental loss much akin to the death of a loved one. This loss is not to be minimized; it determines much of the subsequent behavior of the parent. As with the death of a loved one, it is the little incidents in subsequent years that remind parents again of their loss and throw them back into acute grief. One frequently hears professionals commenting in amazement on how a parent of an older deaf child broke down in tears when they put an FM system on the child "And I thought," commented the teacher, "she had accepted it so well." In actuality this mother was accepting the deafness quite well, but seeing her child so wired for sound brought the abnormality and loss to light again, and she needed some space and time to grieve anew. It often does not take much to remind the parents of their loss. Birthday parties and family gatherings are particularly hard because they force a comparison of the skills of the child with deafness with the skills of the child who hears normally. Invariably, the child with deafness is found to be deficient and the parents' tenuous adjustment is shattered: at least for the moment. For hearing parents of children who are deaf, the deafness is a wound that when assaulted by reality bleeds a bit. Acceptance is not without pain nor is it a straight-line progression; and hearing parents of a child with hearing impairment break down and grieve the loss from time to time. These breakdowns in subsequent years are usually short-lived and are part of the normal adjustment process.

Inadequacy

To understand parenting is to understand that parents are scared. Any parent who is the least bit introspective recognizes the awesome responsibility that being a parent entails. Somehow, parents have to find the resources and wisdom to raise their child to responsible adulthood. Usually these feelings of inadequacy are submerged under the everyday matters of raising a child.

The feelings emerge acutely whenever there is a crisis to be confronted. Deafness in a child is a matter of confronting a series of crises for parents, beginning with the diagnosis and, for many parents, never ending, as they remain involved in the adult life of their child. When life-changing decisions need to be made, parents often feel overwhelmed and scared because they do not want to make a bad decision that, in their eyes, might "ruin their child's life."

The feelings of inadequacy often lead to attempts to find someone else to make the decisions and at least share the responsibility, if not take it entirely. In short, the parents want to be rescued from their feelings of inadequacy. Often this felt inadequacy corresponds to the strong need of helping professionals to be needed, and thus an unholy alliance is formed in which the professional does a great deal of dysfunctional rescuing. Rescuing persons from their felt inadequacy reinforces their low self-esteem and lack of confidence in their own ability to cope. The more parents are rescued from taking responsibility for the welfare of their child, the more their feelings of inadequacy are reinforced. This phenomenon has been called "the Annie Sullivan effect," whereby the excessive helping of parents by professionals leads to the ceding of responsibility for their child to the professional (Luterman, 2002). The "Annie Sullivan relationship" leads to a disempowered, impotent parent—the obverse of what is needed for a successful outcome. Schlessinger's (1992) research shows that the best predictor of literacy in a deaf child is the quality of the parent–child interaction and the degree to which the mother is empowered.

Empowerment of parents is best accomplished not by rescuing but by assuming that the parents are capable of making good decisions for themselves and their family when they have all the facts. The professional's responsibility is *to* the parents not *for* the parents, and to provide the facts as needed and trust the parents to eventually make good decisions for themselves and their child. This is often a difficult thing for most professionals to do because they see foundering parents and children not being immediately helped. To rescue only leads to more rescuing and it becomes difficult, if not impossible, to break the dependency cycle once it is initiated. To be sure, professionals need to help, but the helping should be covert and not so obvious that it diminishes the self-confidence of the parents. At all stages, there needs to be empowerment of the parents; all clinical and educational interactions need to be examined in light of whether they lead to parental empowerment.

There are no more potent clinical interventions than those that enhance parental self-esteem.

Anger

At some fundamental level, all hearing parents of children with deafness are angry. Anger occurs whenever there is a violation of an expectation. Parents of school-age children fully expected to be the parents of a "normal" child: whenever the disability of hearing loss asserts itself, the parents become angry because it reminds them of their failed expectations. The parents who go to school and see their child wired for sound and socially isolated will get angry. Anger is usually one of the first emotions to emerge, and it often masks other emotions, frequently becoming a cover for the chronic grief and fear that the parents feel.

Anger also stems from a loss of control. A need that almost all people have is to feel as though there is an unlimited degrees of freedom to control their lives. When that is thwarted, anger usually ensues. One of the angriest men this author ever encountered was the father of a 10-year-old child with deafness. He had been working for a number of years in his business trying to be promoted to regional sales manager. When he finally got the position, he found out he was required to move to a small town in the Midwest that had no services for children who are deaf. His child would have to be sent to the regional school for the deaf on a residential basis, which was an anathema to both him and his wife. If he took the job, then he would injure his child, and if he failed to take the job, he would hurt his own chances for promotion. He was furious.

Another source of anger stems from the feelings of impotency. It is a fury stemming from the feelings of powerlessness that parents experience when they cannot "fix" their child's deafness. All parents are pledged to make things better for a hurting child and when they find they cannot make it better—that this child will always have to wear hearing aids and probably be subject to the taunts of children who are hearing—the parents become furious. It is the kind of anger that makes them want to put a fist through the door, and anyone or anything that gets in the way had better watch out. Unfortunately, an unsuspecting professional often gets in the way of the parents' displaced anger.

Anger also frequently masks fear. Boorstein (1996), a clinical psychologist, has commented: "It is my thesis that with few exceptions the root of all anger is fear and that psychotherapy is most effective when it focuses on the fear behind the anger rather than on the anger itself." The most common fears of parents of school-aged children are (1) Will my child be accepted by the peers? (2) Have I made the right decision to enroll in this program? (3) Am I doing an adequate job? When working with parents it behooves the professional to hang in with the angry parent. It is hard to do because anger is something most people have trouble dealing with given that it is equated with a loss of love. In actuality, there is a great deal of caring in anger; the opposite of love is not hate but indifference. It is difficult for parents to see this, and the anger is often suppressed or displaced. These are the most common means we have to deal with anger; unfortunately, neither is psychologically healthy. Suppressed anger often leads to depression, and displacing the anger onto professionals who are trying to help often leads to alienation of the parents and the child from the people who can best ameliorate the situation. The professional must help the parents to acknowledge the anger they feel toward their child's deafness by helping the parents to see that they are really upset by the situation. This often means confronting a furious parent, something most professionals find difficult to do. Anger is a useful energy that can be harnessed to work in the child's best interest, and it can be harnessed by mindful counseling.

Guilt

Almost all mothers of children with hearing impairments feel guilt. It seems women in this society are acculturated to take responsibility for everything bad that happens; one mother shared, "I even feel guilty when it rains." Guilt at a very fundamental level is really a power statement; it is saying that one has some control over that event (worry does the same thing). Often that power is an illusion but it serves to assuage the feeling of powerlessness that many women feel. In the long run, this is a psychologically expensive way to feel power because the flip side to guilt is always resentment. Guilt is such a corrosive, uncomfortable, and controlling feeling that we resent the person or the event that causes us to feel guilty. Relationships that are built on a foundation of guilt are often unstable because the resentment can bubble up to sabotage them.

The mother's role is usually to protect the health of the family members. When someone is sick, the mother feels she has failed in her responsibility. Mother guilt is particularly evident around the cause of the deafness. In most cases of congenital deafness, the cause is not known, at least by the professional. The mother then goes over her pregnancy, day by day, looking for something untoward that happened that she can blame for having caused the deafness, and thus is born the guilty secret. Often the mother "knows" that she did something to cause the child's deafness; this leads her to dedicate her life to attempts to "fix" it. In effect, she tries to make it up to the child by devoting all her energy and time to becoming a super-dedicated parent. This often has very serious long-term repercussions in the family. A super-dedicated mother has little

or no energy or time for the marriage or for the hearing siblings.

Father-guilt stems from his role in the family as protector; when people are hurting the father has failed in some way. Fathers tend to play the guilt out by denying it. They try to make other family members feel better and do not respond directly to their pain or may even refuse to acknowledge it. If they cannot "fix" it, they tend to withdraw. Occasionally, one does get to see a super-dedicated father, but more often than not, the father's solution to guilt is to become very involved with work. The pattern of the dysfunctional family begins to be established early in the educational process as the mother becomes overinvolved in her child's deafness, the father becomes overinvolved in work, and there is less and less time and energy devoted to maintaining the marriage. When this happens, the relationship spirals down into increasing levels of marital dissatisfaction. It seems that the most successful hearing impaired children are the products of a happy marriage, and children from the dysfunctional families are often limited severely in their abilities to have satisfactory interpersonal relationships.

In the preschool years, the super-dedicated parent looks very good to the professionals who are working with the family. These are the parents who are in two or three different programs and who never fail to attend a PTO meeting or a conference. The negative consequences of super-dedication begin to emerge later. For the school-age child the dedication is apt to become suffocating. The super-dedicated, guilt-driven parent finds it very difficult to let go—trust of professionals is usually minimal ("If I let something bad happen how can I trust these less invested professionals with my child?") and the child is overprotected ("I let something bad happen (to my child) once; I am not going to let it happen again"). Because so much energy has gone into the parenting of this one child, there is little left for the marriage or for the other siblings. When one examines families of the super-dedicated parent of a school-age child, one often finds a marriage that is not functional and siblings who are at risk. It is not a happy or supportive environment in which to raise a deaf child.

Ultimately, all parents must give up their children. This is a painful process, and the super-dedicated, guilt-driven parent finds this almost impossible to do. So much of the parents' time and energy has revolved around the child's deafness that to let go of the child leaves a huge void; parents are often horrified at the prospect of losing their child and therefore a large chunk of their lives. The tight bonding that is created by the guilt-driven parent often leads to a dependent child who has not been allowed to have sufficient life experiences to enable development of the skills necessary for becoming a responsible adult. Counseling parents around their guilt feelings is essential if we hope to create independent, responsible adults who happen to be hearing impaired.

Vulnerability

The existential truth of life is that it is hard and there is no way to encounter life without, at some point, suffering pain. At some fundamental psychological level, there is an awareness of this truth, and it causes anguish. In the desire to assuage this pain, there is a pretense of invulnerability; "bad things only happen to other people" becomes the mantra and life is lived as though one were indeed invulnerable. When a bad thing does happen, one realizes anew at some fundamental level what has always been most feared; that one is naked and alone in the face of what seems to be an indifferent universe. Childhood deafness is just such a defense-piercing event and often leads parents to overprotective behaviors.

By counseling parents and having them recognize that the overprotection stemming from these feelings of vulnerability is leading to destructive behavior, the parents can begin the process of transforming these feelings into self-enhancing acts. The recognition and acknowledgment of vulnerability can lead to a restructuring of life's priorities;

parents can now live more authentically because they know what is truly important in life. Knowing that loved ones are fragile (they are just on loan) can lead to more appreciation of them.

The parent of a 16-year-old said: "Deafness in my child has been the best thing that ever happened to me. My life now has a focus and meaning that it never had before. I was fated to become a suburban housewife whose main concern was whether the neighbor thought my house was clean. I now see how shallow that life was."

There is a potential for much good in deafness—the deafness can become a powerful teacher. David Wright (1969), an adult who is deaf, had this to say about his hearing loss:

> The handicapped are less at the mercy of vague unhappiness that afflicts so many, especially those without an aim in life, whose consequent boredom promotes what used to be called spleen. The disabled have been given a built-in ready-packed objective, which is always present: a definite impediment to get the better of. Like the prospect of hanging, it concentrates the faculties wonderfully. (p. 111)

Counseling can help unlock and unleash the potential good that is in deafness.

Unfortunately for most professionals working with parents of school-age children, they must often undo the mistakes and insensitivities of professionals who encountered the families in the preschool years. These parents are often locked into the unproductive behavior arising from their unacknowledged feelings of inadequacy, guilt, anger, and vulnerability leading them to dependency, over-dedication, overprotection, and the displaced anger that alienates them from professionals seeking to help. With proper assistance, the anger can become a positive energy to make things happen, the guilt becomes commitment, and the acknowledged vulnerability becomes an opportunity to restructure lives and values. The grief becomes a sadness that will always be there and serves to intensify all other feelings.

There is also much joy in deafness. Deafness can be reframed to the parents in such a way that this child has come bearing a gift; albeit the gift is buried under much pain and sheer hard work, but it is a gift nonetheless. Their task is to find this gift because with it there is much joy. It is the joy of having a purpose and direction in life; it is the joy, for example, of hearing that first word and knowing who made it possible.

Counseling

It is beyond the scope of this chapter to go into detailed descriptions about the counseling process in communication disorders. The interested reader can pursue this subject further in other volumes (Luterman, 2002).

The notions of the discipline of humanistic counseling have great implications for the field of communication disorders. According to Carl Rogers (1951), the founder of humanistic counseling, there are three prerequisites to fostering client growth: counselor congruence, unconditional regard, and reflective listening. It is the relationship that is established between the counselor and the client that promotes growth. In this relationship the counselor needs to provide unconditional regard that releases the client from feelings of being judged that might inhibit risk. With openness and acceptance in the relationship, growth can take place. There also needs to be an authenticity (congruence) in the counselor and all counselor communication that enables trust to be established in the relationship. The key to growth is the nonjudgmental reflective listening that the counselor does. This listening and valuing of the client within an atmosphere of acceptance allows clients to work through their own problems. Information is provided as needed, and the counselor trusts the clients ultimately to make good decisions for themselves. We diminish parents' self-esteem when we advise and try to "fix" things for them.

Here are some notions about working with parental feelings:

1. Listening is the single most powerful skill for a professional to have. Listening enables the parent to work things out within a supportive framework.
2. People can take care of themselves: the corollary of this notion is that people are not fragile. Sensitive and reflective listening elicits feelings that need only to be acknowledged and validated. When that happens, the feelings no longer control the person's behavior.
3. Feelings are neither good nor bad, they just are. Parents do not have to be responsible for how they feel; they must always be held responsible for how they behave. Behavior can be judged as to whether it is productive for both the parents and the child.
4. We all have a need to control events in our lives. After feelings have been elicited and validated, the professional and the parents need to embark on a journey examining what can be done now. Mental health lies in doing what is doable, and accepting what is not subject to change, and wisdom, as the old saying goes, is knowing the difference between the two. Counseling should encourage that wisdom.

Counseling is often approached fearfully, if at all, by professionals working with the families of children who have auditory disorders. In part this stems from a lack of coursework at the training program levels (Crandell, 1997) and a mistaken notion that parents are extremely fragile. The profession needs to address the lack of training and also needs to recognize that someone cannot be hurt by using the reflective listening, valuing model proposed here. How can someone be hurt if listened to and supported in their competency? It is destructive when they are talked at and overhelped and when the important role that feelings play in determining behavior is ignored. It must always be borne in mind that we are dealing with people who are normally upset, not emotionally disturbed. Listening in a nonjudgmental manner and valuing other people's competency in order to build self-esteem are not clinical skills that are exotic. These skills are within the scope of all caring professionals and need to be a part of every professional encounter with families who are hearing impaired.

Parental Issues

The major parental issue of the school-age child is the "success" of the child (and really the success of the parents) in accordance with the parental dream established in the preschool years. In examining the questionnaires that were sent to the parents, it became clear that many of the parents could not distinguish between their needs and their child's needs, even though the question was clearly worded as "What were your needs?" Here are some typical responses (it must be borne in mind that these are all rather sophisticated parents who have participated in a family-centered program):

> "That he didn't lose out on his scholastic social classes that fit him in with his peers."
> "We want our child to live as normal a life as possible."
> "We want him to always be challenged further in his development mentally and physically."
> "Teaching faculty willing and able to adapt classroom activities and learning environment to the needs of a hearing impaired child."
> "To receive a good education."
> "Teachers able to sign well."

When they did get around to talking about their needs, it became readily apparent that no school program offered anything to the parents other than the rather haphazard catch-as-catch-can programs of the traditional PTO model. Many of the parents were turned off and angered by the insensitivities of school personnel to their needs. For example, parents of a 19-year-old needed:

> To have educators who themselves were the parents of school-age hearing im-

paired children. We found that the educators, while with good intentions, seldom showed that they truly understood how it was to not only be involved with the education of these children but how it was to deal with the daily parent–child problems which all parents deal with when working with hearing children but which are multiplied over and over when dealing with hearing impaired children.

A single-parent mother of 5- and 7-year-old children who are deaf needed:

> A support group consisting of parents that have (had) their hearing-impaired children mainstreamed. I still have trouble separating which problems are connected to their hearing loss and normal "growing pains." Now that the kids are becoming aware of their difference they are having all kinds of emotions—anger, pain, why me? I need advice on how to deal with their feelings as well as my own.

A parent of a 24-year-old listed the following needs:

> 1. Knowledge of programs available and quality
> 2. Other parents with similar experiences
> 3. Relationships with parents of hearing peers so that my child had experience and relationships with other kids in her class
> 4. Knowledge of how to make the public school system work for her and skills for me to provide in-service for working with the classroom teacher

From the mother of a mainstreamed 16-year-old boy:

> "Program" has become a dirty word. The term has come to symbolize a complex, generalized set of obstacles organized within a rigid academic institution which guarantees that no one child's needs be evaluated correctly, acknowledged, or met. Having witnessed (and suffered along with) my son's program of the absurd, I can only be thankful there were none for me.

The parent of a 20-year-old mainstreamed student:

Would have liked to have been more involved in decision making as far as what the parents felt was in their child's best interests: So often the "professionals" made decisions about the child's placement in programs that were not the choices of the child or parents. When parents raised questions about the choice, there was always a "sterile" explanation by the educator which the less informed could not challenge or succeed in changing any minds. Over a period of time it would often show that the child would suffer the consequences of a bad decision and would lose years of his education as a result of the changes necessary to correct the errors. Listen to the child and the parents more often.

The school-age years are when the methodological decisions made in the preschool years come home to roost. Often the results leave the parents subject to profound feelings of disappointment. The school-age years are those times when parents begin to compare their dream of what their child with deafness was going to turn out to be with the actual emerging reality. A common strategy for a hearing parent in dealing with the initial pain of having a child with hearing impairments is to adopt the notion that the child will be a special case; that he or she will become a super-adult with deafness in which there is at worst a very minimal handicap associated with the deafness. The reality for almost all parents is that the deafness has loomed large in their child's life and, although they still love the child very much, they are also experiencing disappointment at the result of the educational choices made. For many parents, this is still a child who is not "normal" and they are disappointed and must somehow come to grips with the child who is *there* as opposed to the child they wished they had. This is a painful, delicate time for all parents and professionals need to be sensitive to the parents' renewed pain. It seems that parents who opted for an oral–aural, mainstreaming route for their child were generally happy with their child's academic skills and communication abilities, but very concerned about the social isolation that a mainstreamed situation en-

tailed. Parents who chose a school for the deaf were generally happy about their child's social abilities but not pleased with the child's academic accomplishments.

One parent of a 13-year-old currently mainstreamed child summed it well when she wrote:

> A socially/culturally enriched deaf curriculum with high academics. ... He is grade appropriate in his hearing school—has been on the honor role [*sic*] every semester. My dream would be for 2 or 3 deaf 13-year-olds to move to our town and mainstream with Todd. I am now in favor of mainstreaming only because of my disappointment in deaf education: the low expectations—the limited offerings—the narrow curriculum. I wish it could all come together and we have tried by trying to split Todd (½ day hearing/½ day deaf).

The concern about the social isolation of their children and of themselves worries all parents of mainstreamed children. Although many of these children (and parents) would be considered successful by most educators, it is apparent that many problems are not being addressed by the school systems. Confining the definition of success mainly to speech, language, and academic competency is too narrow. Somehow the social and emotional consequences of the educational methodologies must be looked at as well. The message of the deaf community must be heeded; we all hunger for community. Many children who are hearing impaired and are oral successes are severely lacking in community, and although they seem to be educationally successful, they are lonely, isolated, and not very happy. The schools for the deaf, on the other hand, must look at their academic standards and low expectations for youngsters with hearing impairments, which severely limit the children's ability to compete vocationally in a very complex world.

The route through this educational morass is, in part, an educated, empowered parent who can keep the educators aware of the broader picture that education of students with hearing impairments should entail. A recent study examining factors leading to the successful integration of hearing-impaired children found that family support was a key ingredient of success (Luckner & Muir, 2001). Educators should look at the consequences of the methodological choices; it is the parent who must live with them. It is only through a true parent/educator partnership that the child benefits. Empowered parents seem to work out their own solutions, often quite creatively. The following letter was received from the mother of a 5-year-old child who is empowered and is fashioning her own program (note how she is not afraid to move her child in and out of programs as needed):

> Tyler was enrolled in a School for the Deaf for 2 years after he left Emerson. The first year he was in a total communication program. In January of his first year, he received a cochlear implant at the MEEI in Boston. He began to hear sounds and speech all around him and began to develop some oral skills. His second year at the School for the Deaf he was enrolled in an oral program that was just developed that year.
>
> Tyler did good both years, but I felt there was a lack of communication between the school, teachers, and parents. I think the parents need to be more informed and have an open line of communications with all of the teachers, speech therapist, and others that are all working with your child. I think everyone working together and keeping in communication on a regular basis would be very beneficial to everyone involved and you would see faster and more productive progress with your child.
>
> Tyler at age 5, has now had the cochlear implant for almost 2 years. He is now mainstreamed into a special needs pre-kindergarten program with his peers, but they have normal hearing. He is doing fine! I find the teachers to be open and cooperative with me and we all work as a team. We have a common journal that we all write in to keep everyone informed of Tyler's areas of need and progress. The team consists of a head teacher, asst. teacher, speech therapist, and a special aide. He also still sees an outside speech therapist once a week. I think I am fortunate to work with a team of professionals that don't feel intimidated by other professionals' opinions and most of all I get to share my opinions!
>
> Tyler's program is a language-based program, which is wonderful. Academically, Tyler needs to work hard in all areas, but math seems to be his best subject. Socially, he is so happy. He is making friends and talks about them all the time. They tell me he loves to sing and recite poems. I have not had the pleasure to see that yet!

There need to be more programs that offer an aggressive language-based program, teacher–parent teamwork with open lines of communication and a challenging environment that would give the child maximum opportunity to succeed. With the advent of newborn screening, sophisticated digital hearing aids, and cochlear implants the technological thrust clearly favors mainstreaming hearing-impaired children over placement in a school for the deaf. Which means that public school–based personnel need to be prepared to educate many more hearing-impaired children, wearing sophisticated amplification, than they currently are. There is little evidence that school personnel are prepared for these children and it is not certain that mainstreaming per se will turn out to be beneficial for hearing-impaired children.

For anyone who takes a dispassionate view of the learning/education process, it is obvious that parents do play a key, and perhaps primary, role in their child's education. At one level, it is a matter of sheer arithmetic that the mainstreamed child will spend many more hours with the parent than with the teacher. It seems logical, then, that a more efficient use of school personnel time would be to work with the families to ensure that the home environment is conducive to ameliorating the effects of childhood hearing impairment than with providing direct service to the child. In short, if we can make the home educationally responsive to the child's needs, we should be able to succeed mightily. To give a single example, deaf children are taught the pragmatics of language skills through conversation. It is obvious that the child would have the most opportunity to converse with the family and, in particular, the parents. Would it not be better to teach the parents how to converse with their child? This means that we must direct our energy at the parents and give them a much more central role in professional thinking than they currently seem to have.

Occasionally, one hears criticism of parental involvement with the statement that "parents should not be teachers." This begs the question because all parents, by virtue of their central role in their child's life, are teachers. The goal of parental education should be to enhance the natural teaching that all parents do so as to create a home environment in which the child who is hearing impaired can learn best. To accomplish this goal, we will need parents who are educated and empowered. The cogent studies of Schlessinger (1992) demonstrate the value of an empowered parent; she studied 40 families over a 20-year span and found that literacy in the child was most related to empowerment of the mother. An empowered mother was more important to the child learning to read than socioeconomic status, methodology, or hearing loss. This is an incredible finding, and it substantiates what most educators know intuitively: that they need to direct energy and time to incorporating the parents into their educational planning although this seldom seems to happen at the school-age level. Parental education and involvement pay huge dividends. An empowered parent is the greatest asset a child or the school has; it is clear that this asset must be fully cultivated if educating children with hearing impairments is to be successful. Beyond the preschool years, there is no evidence that schools are doing anything actively to educate and involve parents in the educational process so that there is truly a parent–school partnership. There is never any need for an adversarial relationship between the parents and the school because both want the same thing—

good things for the child. Yet it seems so difficult to achieve a true working partnership.

The following are some suggestions for school personnel to consider in thinking about parents and perhaps going beyond the limited PTO model that seems to be currently in vogue:

1. Before the school year begins, all parents should be visited at home by the teacher. The purpose of this visit is in part to draw up a contract of parent participation in their child's education for the year. The purpose of this meeting, on the parent's turf, is to discuss the nature of the parent's participation in the child's schooling. This can be minimal if it is arrived at by parent–teacher decision. These contracts need to be flexible in nature and renegotiated over the school year. There always needs to be some element of parental involvement in every contract.

2. Schools should try to establish support groups for parents. These groups need to deal with feeling issues as well as content discussions; the content should emerge from the needs of the group. For parents of mainstreamed children, the groups will probably have to be established on a regional basis and may take the format of an intensive day-long workshop whereby the parents receive information and also have an opportunity to network. School personnel need to look at the learning vacation model sponsored so enthusiastically by Gallaudet University, where parents and children are enrolled in a camplike environment to actively learn together and recreate together.

3. Attitudes of school personnel need to change. Parents must be seen as central to the educational process. Educators will need increased skills in dealing with parental needs, which they probably did not receive in their training programs. Schools, therefore, will have to provide ongoing in-service experience

for their personnel. All educators must understand fully the notion that if you take good care of the parents, the children will turn out well.

Summary

The emotions of fear, anger, guilt, and vulnerability, which are part of the grief reaction, are still present in the parents of the school-age child. The feelings generally manifest themselves at trigger events such as changes in the child's hearing ability or educational status, and school-based personnel need to be prepared to deal with the emotional aspects of the diagnosis. A listening/valuing model of counseling parents seems to have the most cogency. It seems evident from a survey of parents of school-aged children that most programs are not sufficiently addressing the parents' needs. In order to achieve better outcomes more professional energy needs to be directed toward the parents. In particular, parental self-esteem needs to be enhanced.

References

Bodner-Johnson B. (1986). The family in perspective. In: D. Luterman (Ed.), *Deafness in Perspective* (pp. 225–240). San Diego: College Hill Press.

Boorstein, S. (1996). *Transpersonal Psychotherapy*. Albany: State University of New York Press.

Crandell, C. (1997). An update on counseling instruction within audiology programs. *J Acad Rehab Audiol, 30,* 1–10.

Luckner, J., & Muir, S. (2001). Successful students who are deaf in general educational settings. *Am Ann Deaf, 146,* 435–446.

Luterman, D. (1999). *The Young Deaf Child*. Albion, MD: York Press.

Luterman, D. (2002). *Counseling Persons with Communication Disorders and Their Families* (4th ed.). Austin: PRO-ED.

Rogers, C. (1951). *Client Centered Therapy*. Boston: Houghton Mifflin.

Schlessinger, H. (1992). The elusive X factor: Parental contributions to literacy. In: M. Walworth, D. Modres, & T. O'Rourke (Eds.), *A Free Hand* (pp. 44–59). Silver Springs, MD: TS Publishers.

Wright, D. (1969). *Deafness*. New York: Stein & Day.

20

Enhancing the Self-Image of the Mainstream Child with Auditory Disorders

SUSAN P. RUSSELL

The greatest magnifying glasses in the world are a man's own eyes when they look upon his own person.

—Alexander Pope, 1688–1744

Self-image is most often defined as the manner in which people describe the way they perceive themselves. There are different domains of self-image. For children, some of the most important domains include the academic, where children define themselves as a student and perceive their own achievement in a classroom setting; the social/emotional or personal, which includes relationships within the family, as well as other interpersonal exchanges; and the physical, how children perceive their own outward physical appearance and related physical or athletic abilities. Each domain develops and changes as a child grows and matures and is impacted by the experiences encountered throughout the years. Within these domains, a child's self-image is going to be influenced by the people and experiences in two important environments: home and school.

Parents have the earliest and perhaps the major role in influencing the development of a positive self-image in their children. Parents have the opportunity, right from the start, to establish an atmosphere of acceptance, and to plant the seeds of confidence and competence in their children. As the child grows older, teachers join parents in this endeavor and play an important supporting role. There are many books and articles for parents and professionals on en-

hancing children's self-concept (Berne, 1985 and Table 20–1). These guidelines help the adults create an environment at home and at school conducive to and supportive of building a strong and positive self-image. Marshall (1989) addresses more skills on which to focus when a good self-concept is the goal (Table 20–2). Both the climate that is created for the child and the direct teaching of skills significantly impact the development of self-image.

Development of self-image for children who are deaf or hard of hearing will also be influenced by all of these factors and strategies, and each one can have a positive difference. However, there is much more to the picture. Each of the three domains mentioned, academic, social/emotional, and physical, is likely to be impacted by hearing loss.

There is no dispute that having a hearing loss has consequences within the parameters of a hearing world. Maxon and van den Berg (1991) delineates the potential separateness that a student who is deaf may experience in a mainstream setting: communication difficulties in both academic and social situations, the visibility of necessary amplification, difficulty in listening situations, and the need to leave the classroom for support services. Additionally, the following factors also impact on the self-concept of a student

Table 20–1. Seven Secrets for Building Kids' Self-Esteem*

Build in success	Success builds self-esteem, especially when the chain of successes remains continuous and unbroken
State the positive	Acknowledging the positive in a nonevaluative but validating way nurtures success
Capitalize on successes	Children will feel success is possible if you can help them build a history of similar successes
Watch for growth sparks	Children with low self-esteem tend to believe they cannot grow, learn, or successfully relate to other people. Often they do not until a spark of interest is ignited.
Value and acknowledge	Evidence of success that is visible and tangible has a strong positive effect on a child's self-esteem
Keep expectations realistic	Clearly stating reasonable expectations will help children with low self-esteem feel less anxious about pleasing others
Do not be boring	Boredom depresses self-esteem; interest and excitement increase a sense of self. Active involvement in life nourishes self-esteem

*From Berne (1985).

who is deaf: the global impact of language and communication skill development, the role of these skills in developing age-appropriate social interactions, and the often resulting isolation, exclusion, or rejection (Oblowitz, Green, & Heyns, 1991); the different settings or programs in which a student's self-image might be high or low (i.e., mainstream versus residential); the role that degree of hearing loss, age of onset, or gender plays; the significance of having deaf or hearing parents (Meadow, 1969; Yachnik, 1986).

The measures used for evaluating self-concept in students who are deaf have proved problematical in their own right. Oblowitz et al (1991) has examined the linguistic-related issues and problems for students who are deaf, using a variety of standard measures of evaluating self-concept. Suggestions that have come out of these studies include controlling the linguistic content of the test items and modifying the presentation to be more pictorial/conceptual. New items need to be added to current

Table 20–2. Ways to Influence Self-Concept*

Help children feel they are of value	Listen attentively to what they say; ask for their suggestions Help them identify their own positive and prosocial behavior
Help children feel they are competent	Provide experiences for children where they can succeed Provide new challenges and comment on positive attempts Teach strategies to accomplish tasks Allow them to carry out and complete tasks themselves
Help children feel they have some control	Provide opportunities for choice, initiative, and autonomy Avoid comparison between children; avoid competition Help children learn to evaluate their own accomplishments
Help children learn interpersonal skills	Help children learn skills to enter interactions with others
Become aware of your own expectations for children	Be open to perceiving new information about children and looking at them in new ways. Be aware of whether your expectations differ for boys and girls

*From Marshall (1989).

evaluation tools, including items related to communication, acceptance of disability, feelings of being different and excluded, perceptions of positive regard, and perceptions of academic competence in a context beyond the world of individuals who are hearing impaired. It will be beneficial to have further research in these areas because they are all issues that are important to examine when looking at the self-image of a student who is deaf.

When a child who is deaf has deaf parents, the overall process of development is more parallel to that of hearing children of hearing parents. Language growth goes through comparable stages of development, and the children are likely to see themselves as being like their parents. However, deaf children of hearing parents, as is the case in 90% of the families, may have a more difficult time sorting out how they see and define themselves and how they fit in as a member of their family. This often results in significant issues of acceptance that can adversely affect the development of self-image.

That same dynamic can occur with children who are deaf in a mainstream setting. The mainstream program in a public school system mirrors the scenario of a child who is deaf in a hearing family, and brings with it the same potential for feelings of isolation and rejection. Just as family dynamics differ, so do mainstream programs; like families, some are more successful at meeting these challenges.

When examining the concept of mainstreaming for students who are hard of hearing or deaf, and the qualities and destinies that these students may possess, the literature often begins with a look back at the period since the passage of Public Law 94–142 in 1975, and the successes and failures of the almost 30 years since that law was enacted. The field of education of children who are deaf or hard of hearing has been greatly affected by this legislation. However, this field of education has never been free of controversy and debate, and the law did not change this fact.

Today, as we learn and experience more about deaf culture, the concept of "least re-strictive environment" and, indeed, mainstream programs themselves, are under greater scrutiny. Regardless, today, mainstreaming is a reality. So is the likelihood that the parents of children who are deaf or hard of hearing will be hearing people. These are facts that are not going to disappear in the very near future. In light of these realities, the purpose of this discussion is not to look at what is good or bad about the law, and not to debate the merits of a residential school versus a mainstream experience. Rather, this discussion seeks to identify specific ways to enhance a deaf student's self-image in a mainstream setting. This is really the crux of the matter: maximizing a student's potential by making the mainstream setting as productive as possible within the parameters that exist.

Unfortunately, there has not been much written specifically for students with deafness in the mainstream for enhancing self-image. Skill-streaming techniques (McGinnis, Goldstein, Sprafkin, & Gershaw, 1984), although not specifically developed for deaf students, deal with special education students in general, and the increasing need for teaching prosocial skills. This is a tremendously important area for students in a mainstream setting, where social skills may lag behind other skills. In this "skill-streaming" book there are a total of 60 skills covered in five basic areas: classroom survival skills, friendship-making skills, skills for dealing with feelings, skill alternatives to aggression, and skills for dealing with stress. It is well laid out for parents and professionals and is an excellent resource for building students' confidence in social and mainstream settings.

Schwartz (1990) delineates four critical areas that impact on the psychosocial development of children who are in a mainstream setting: clear communication, parental support, extracurricular activities, and social skills. These issues are key in the development of children who are deaf, and are interwoven in many of the strategies related to strengthening self-image. Grimes and Prickett (1988) give an overview of the issues involved in self-concept of children who are deaf, and provide ideas for enhancing its positive development, although not specifically from a mainstream perspective. They describe a positive self-concept as being composed of many wonderful components including pride, acceptance, responsibility, and independence. These are indeed the positive qualities for which to strive.

The ideas presented in this chapter reflect personal experiences working with the staff, families, and students in the Montgomery County Public Schools, Programs for Students Who Are Deaf and Hard of Hearing (formerly the Auditory Program). This is a day program for children who are deaf and hard of hearing within the public school system in Montgomery County, Maryland, a suburb of Washington, D.C. This program has a total population of approximately 320 students, from birth through age 21 years. The students have a range of degree of hearing loss, receive a broad continuum of services, and use different communication approaches (sign language, cued speech, oral–aural). Reflecting the accepted statistics, hearing parents outnumber deaf parents. Although the focus here is on the mainstream environment, many of the following ideas are appropriate for public school programs where there are special classes for children who are deaf. Regardless of the placement, the more focused the attitudes are of the families and staff working with the students, and the more effectively home and school can work together, the stronger the self-image will be for these students who are deaf.

The mainstream life of a student with deafness and the strategies to achieve success will be divided into two environments: at home and at school. These two environments are both important when developing and enhancing self-image. Each of these environments will be examined from two perspectives: strategies that impact on the overall climate, making it more accepting and positive for the students with deafness; and those skills that students need to develop to strengthen and enhance their self-image.

At Home

Climate

Parents are the first and most important people who affect the development of a child's self-image. The single best predictor of self-concept among children with deafness is related to parental child-rearing attitudes (Warren & Hasenstab, 1986). The attitude that a parent projects acceptance of deafness, commitment to clear and consistent communication at home, and involvement in school with the related guidance and support all play an important role for building a positive self-image. Home should be a place of unconditional love and unconditional acceptance.

ACCEPTANCE OF DEAFNESS

When hearing parents have a child who is deaf, there is often a sense that the child is different from the parents. There is an emotional process of understanding and acceptance parents go through, each at their own rate. Professionals need to work with parents to help them arrive at the conclusion that their child, while unique in his or her deafness, is also special simply as their child. This relates to the social/emotional domain of self-image. What parents then do for their relationship with their child with deafness affects this child's self-concept as a member of the family, and as a potential member of both a hearing society and a deaf culture.

SUPPORT FOR PARENTS

Parents need support, in different ways, at every level of their child's development. Parents who feel confident and secure are more likely to be successful at developing a good self-concept in their child. A parent group can provide a venue for gaining information, validating practices, and sharing concerns. At the parent–infant or preschool level, this group addresses the parents' more basic and immediate needs about deafness, interacting and communicating with their young children, issues of amplification, and support from other parents.

For a parent with an older child, there is an additional need of being able to support and cope with a child who may be experiencing feelings of isolation or rejection. Although evidence shows that attendance at parent groups declines as the child progresses through school, the need for information and support continues. Talking with other parents continues to help put feelings and anxieties in perspective, to enable a parent to deal more effectively with the child.

In conjunction with, or as an alternative to, parent groups, a trained parent educator or counselor for parents of children who are deaf can be a tremendous resource for parents. This professional can help parents deal with all aspects of child-rearing, as well as with issues specifically related to deafness. Such a person should be available to parents in groups or individually to link up parents who may have similar needs or suggest a "veteran" parent for one facing a new experience. Knowing what is part of "normal" development (which many tend to lose sight of) is often helpful, as is having someone with whom to share thoughts, who can offer ideas and solutions. In our program there is a teacher who recruits the parent counselor for monthly discussion groups, where parents can come together and share ideas and concerns in conjunction with a planned topic presentation. Being able to deal with a child as an individual with deafness, and being able to say that deafness is fine, has an incredible effect on the child's self-perception and how the self-image develops. This is one of the basic tenets of self-concept.

ACCESS TO DEAF INDIVIDUALS

Having access to individuals with deafness can be beneficial for hearing parents to get a different perspective on what it is like to be deaf and perhaps to understand life from their child's viewpoint. One approach is to present a "panel" of teens who are deaf, or adults from different backgrounds and experiences, perhaps as part of a parent-meeting series, or the previously mentioned parent group. This kind of presentation provides an opportunity for sharing valuable information and feelings that books cannot adequately communicate. The Washington, D.C., area is fortunate to have a large population of individuals with deafness, and the opportunities that go along with this community. There are social events, dramatic performances, and sporting events through Gallaudet University and local organizations that are available for families. All of these can provide parents with an inside view of deaf culture.

A school program or parent organization can call on their resources to sponsor informational meetings and workshops. One well-received workshop is a Deaf Awareness Day for parents and the community. A variety of presentations on cultural topics, opportunities for questions and answers, as well as time for more informal social interactions can be scheduled. It can be a positive experience for the parents and can lead to a greater overall understanding of deaf culture.

In a different type of outreach, the Deaf and Hard of Hearing Program has developed an educational videotape series, through the Montgomery County Public Schools educational cable television channel. The series *Stop, Look and Listen*, is designed to inform and educate parents of young children with deafness. Each show, as part of the format, spotlights teens and adults from the community who are deaf. These segments, which have received positive feedback from parents, help present a view of what their child can grow up to be, supporting a positive sense of potential and possibility. This "can do" attitude is showcased on "About Me," which examines ways to build self-esteem in children who are deaf. The series is open-captioned, which in itself alerts parents to the technology available to serve individuals with deafness. Having a technological resource like television, and the ability to reach out to parents in their own homes through cable and videocassette, has proved to be very valuable.

COMMUNICATION

Part of accepting a child's deafness is understanding the kind of communication challenges that deafness can bring, and the commitment that parents and the family must make to be part of that communication system. It is widely accepted that one of the most powerful factors influencing a student's development and achievement is appropriate, clear, and consistent communication at home. For a deaf child with deaf parents, this communication happens automatically and naturally, from birth. No time is lost; the diagnosis of the child's hearing loss is secondary.

In contrast, with hearing parents, effective communication does not happen from the start. The hearing loss may not even be diagnosed for 2 or 3 valuable language-learning years. This starts the deaf child of hearing parents off at a disadvantage. If parents do not make the commitment for effective communication, the child can be more vulnerable to developing a negative self-image. A child who feels included as part of the family dynamic will feel positively about himself and his role in the family. Parents need to take the responsibility to develop their child's communication skills, while building their own, as well.

As a child goes through the normal stages of development, during childhood and adolescence, parents will have to deal with the range of feelings that will inevitably occur. Being a child who is deaf in a mainstream setting can magnify feelings of isolation and rejection, real or perceived; these same feelings should not have to be experienced at home, or, for that matter, away from home, at a store or restaurant. For example, the child needs to know that this commitment to communication is full-time, and neither child nor parent should feel any embarrassment about using their hands in public to communicate. Parents need to develop the communication skills and competence to discuss any thoughts, ideas, and issues on a level appropriate for their child. Parents and adolescents with deafness also need to be able to discuss honestly the differences between the deaf and hearing worlds, an openness that ultimately leads to a feeling of parental acceptance (Leigh, 1987). Communication at home addresses the social/emotional domain of self-image, the necessary ability to have meaningful relationships among family members. Parents who make that clear and consistent communication commitment have a greater ability to give the kind of support, and show the kind of acceptance, that a child needs to feel part of the family.

INSTRUCTIONAL CLASSES AND MATERIALS

Parents often need encouragement and assistance in finding appropriate instructional classes and materials to help them meet the communication needs of their child with deafness. Contacting a local college or the adult education office in their area about classes is a good place to start. Organizations for individuals who are deaf and their families have resources and materials available for parents.

Instructional classes for parents and family members may be offered through the local parent organization or the school program. Instructional classes such as these are welcomed by parents, and not only do the parents who attend feel good about themselves and their efforts, but teachers also report a positive impact on the children, which is ultimately the goal.

Building on the known accessibility of videotape technology, there are instructional videotape series for both sign language and cued speech, which the staff may provide to parents. Montgomery County Department of Public Libraries has a Special Needs Library devoted to materials and resources for people with disabilities. There is a wide range of videotape and print materials not only on developing communication skills, but on deafness in general. When a parent takes advantage of these classes and resources, it sends positive messages of support and value to the child, translating to a positive feeling of self-worth.

SCHOOL INVOLVEMENT

Parent involvement at school is important for all children, and this may be even more true for deaf children in a mainstream setting, where the school attended may not be their neighborhood school. Sometimes, as a result of not living in proximity to the school and not being part of that community, parents may have the feeling of needing to prove that they, and their child, "belong" to the school. Some parents view themselves in a "public relations" role in the school, feeling that a constructive level of visibility and contribution is necessary. Being involved in school activities and projects provides a way for parents to positively impact not only their child but also the whole school program with regard to having students with deafness as part of that program. In Montgomery County, schools have a "special needs chairperson" for the parent–teacher association (PTA). This role may be filled by a parent of a child with deafness, and can help ensure that programs and extracurricular events take into account the needs of deaf children (e.g., interpreting services for school programs).

SUPPORTING THE SCHOOL TEAM

Children need to feel that all the adults in their environment are working together for their benefit and that all fronts are united. Krupp (1991) supports the concept that parents and teachers who are willing to work together have the best chance of helping students develop a sense of higher self-esteem. Parents who openly work against the school team can cause confusion and doubts in their child regarding not only the child's support system but also his or her place in it.

This does not mean that parents should be spectators, simply sitting back and agreeing with the professionals. There should be an appropriate process in place for disagreement, discussion, and resolution. When a child sees that there is open communication between school and home, that everyone knows the same information, the child's confusion is lessened. Establishing appropriate channels of communication helps give parents feelings of comfort and control. For a child to feel comfortable and secure in a classroom setting, it is necessary to have teamwork among all the adults.

Student Skills

Parents have a critical role in the development of skills that will enable their children to feel positive and successful in life, and to develop a strong self-image. For a child with deafness in a mainstream setting, parental involvement is just as important, if not more so. Parents of children who are deaf have expressed that, although they practice their own child-rearing philosophies, nothing magical or different, they do so more consciously and purposefully for their child. A resource such as MegaSkills (Rich, 1988) can provide parents with useful and practical information on the kinds of skills that all students, including students who are deaf, need to develop to be confident and successful students. It may take more effort for students who are deaf, but the payoff is well worth it. The two major areas in which parents can play a direct role are language skills and social skills, addressing both the academic and social/emotional domains of self-image.

Language Skills

The most pervasive problem that a student with deafness can experience is one of a language delay. As discussed previously, when a child who is deaf is born to hearing parents, the hearing loss may not be detected for several years. In the meantime, valuable language-learning time is lost. If children are to be successful in school and in life and reach their potential, they need a strong language base on which to build. Therefore, language learning must take place at all times, not just at school. Home is a place for language input as well, and parents must be prepared to take on this task.

The parent first and foremost needs to develop the communication skills discussed previously. There is much communication and language that happens (or should happen) on a day to day basis. Experiences at the supermarket, at the dinner table, or at the gas station all contribute to a child's comprehension of the world at large. Clear communication impacts on overall language development, which correlates to how the student who is deaf is going to function in a mainstream class.

ACADEMIC SUPPORT

For a child in a mainstream setting, supporting academic goals at home is an area where parents can and should play an important role. Having the communication skills and understanding enables the parent to go over a spelling list, drill and practice mathematical facts, and review for a social studies or science test. These kinds of activities are important and contribute to increased confidence in the classroom. A child who is well-prepared for school each day, ready with homework, and familiar with the vocabulary used and the concepts being taught, will have more self-esteem, and be more willing to participate in the teacher's questions and classroom discussions. That feeling of success will build on itself.

There are other areas of language that a parent can and should continue to support, which may not seem at first glance directly related to school but are relevant to supporting a stronger self-image in a mainstream setting. An understanding of the language of the world around them is critical. This effortlessly "happens" for hearing students, but needs to be consciously presented to students with deafness. Knowledge of current local and world events can put a student who is deaf in a better position to participate in class discussions and understand references and comparisons presented in various subject areas. Just as important if not more

so is the awareness of the current pop culture. When children are concerned about "fitting in," there are few things that have the potential to impact them like the social concerns of television, movies, radio, fashion, and, of course, the latest social slang. These are media to which a child with deafness may not have access. Decoders are helpful, as are other printed materials, such as books, newspapers, and magazines. However parents can play a major role in presenting and discussing these concepts and supporting this aspect of language development.

Students may get academic support from school personnel, but the home support provided from parents can make a critical contribution to the child's self-perception as a student in a competitive classroom (see Case Study 20–1).

SOCIAL SKILLS

A child with deafness needs to have appropriate social behaviors and manners, as does any child. Children with appropriate manners and positive interpersonal skills are more attractive to other children, and for a child in a mainstream setting, these behaviors and skills help increase the likelihood of acceptance.

RESPONSIBILITY AND INDEPENDENCE

Building qualities such as responsibility and independence can contribute to school success and a positive sense of self for a child in a mainstream setting. There are many ways to build these qualities at home that carry over to school. It can be as simple as learning how to get dressed for school, doing household chores and duties, preparing books and materials to take to school, or getting out and completing homework exercises. All of these things can develop pride in a job well done independently. This pride in accomplishment and independence makes for a more confident student. Parents may be too overprotective, trying to compensate for a perceived deficiency they think comes with deafness. However, fostering independence

Case Study 20–1 D.G. is in the fourth grade and has been in mainstream classes since kindergarten. His parents demonstrate the kind of commitment to consistent communication that results in a child who feels part of his family and part of his class.

Starting with an oral education, investigating cued speech, and currently using sign language primarily, these parents saw the value in assessing what would work best for their son, and then how they worked to support it. Between them, they have taken many instructional classes to develop and refine their skills. To make communication as clear as possible for D.G., they use a combination of these communication approaches as appropriate.

Always thinking about ways to expand D.G.'s language and cognitive development, these parents make the effort to include him fully in all communication that takes place at home. For them, this ranges from explaining the humor of a popular television show to discussing the latest United States involvement overseas.

At home, D.G. knows that his parents are a dependable source of information, support, and guidance, and he takes this knowledge and support to school with him. Although the specific topics may not directly relate to the curriculum units, he is developing an understanding of the world around him. This knowledge is powerful. D.G. feels more confident in classroom discussions and peer interactions.

gives children a chance to do for themselves, perhaps to try and fail, but to learn from mistakes and then try again. These skills, when supported by parents, help develop confidence along with the risk-taking skills so critical for success.

SOCIAL OPPORTUNITIES

Having the opportunity to be in a variety of social situations helps to develop the familiarity and confidence that will be important for working in a mainstream setting as well as in society later in life. Parents should try to seek out a variety of playmates for their child, both deaf and hearing, to give the child the chance to learn how to deal with different people and personalities, experiment with different social strategies, and practice the interpersonal skills being learned in school or at home. Also helpful is providing opportunities out in the community, perhaps at a restaurant, where the child has the chance to build appropriate manners and etiquette and parents can be there as a support. These are opportunities and strategies built and supported by parents that will positively affect the child's behavior and comfort level in the mainstream and enhance self-image.

At School

Climate

The school environment encompasses a large number of people who can have an impact on the self-image of the student with deafness. The climate of a school sends a message to the child: one of acceptance or rejection. School climate encompasses all three of the domains of self-image: academic, social/emotional, and physical. One goal here is to examine strategies that help support a more positive and accepting environment, where deafness is respected and celebrated.

There are successful practices that positively influence a school's climate, which in turn affects the student's self-perception as a member of that school. History, or how long students have been part of the overall school population, influences this climate. The longer the history, the more there is a sense among staff and students of ownership and permanence, rather than a situation that is temporary. In the Montgomery County Program for Deaf and Hard of Hearing Students, schools are not dispersed throughout the county, as is often the case in public school programs. Instead, schools were selected that were in the same "cluster," so that the school population, deaf and hearing, stays constant as the students move through the grades from preschool through twelfth grade. The goal is for familiarity with deafness to foster understanding, sensitivity, and acceptance among students, staff, and principals who are hearing.

Deaf Awareness

In developing a positive climate in a school it is important to educate the staff, students, and community about deafness and the population of students with deafness. There are many practical and effective ways of providing this kind of information to the school community on an ongoing basis.

Staff and Student In-Service Programs

Providing information and ideas to the staff and hearing students in the school is one effective way of demystifying deafness. Included in a presentation would be the "physical" attributes of deafness: anatomical and audiological information, and explanations of equipment and assistive technology used [decoders, teletypwriters (TTYs), hearing aids, frequency modulation (FM) trainers]. Also important is the discussion of the communication systems used by people who are deaf (and by the students in that school, if different) and effective communication strategies that can be utilized.

Individuals who are deaf (students, staff, and community) can and should play an integral role in an in-service program. Consulting ahead of time with the student with deafness who may be in the mainstream class, explaining the presentation, and soliciting feedback, are all important steps to take before going into a classroom. Feedback shows that when done respectfully, the student who is deaf feels proud to be able to share something very unique to him- or herself.

BULLETIN BOARDS AND CLASSROOM DISPLAYS

Displays of information in and around the school can provide ongoing reinforcement of a variety of topics, from use of the national relay system and TTY etiquette, to audiological equipment, to people in history who were deaf. Bookcovers or clippings from recent newspaper articles can also be posted. Included should be whatever is most relevant not only to the population of students who are deaf in that particular school, but also items of interest and relevance to deaf culture and the larger circle of people with deafness.

Schoolwide Assemblies and Programs

Schoolwide functions can provide a way to present people who are deaf in a variety of roles. In our program, a visiting production by a deaf/hearing drama troupe from the National Technical Institute for the Deaf performed at several schools where students with deafness attend. The performances provided insight into the deaf perspective. In addition to theatrical presentations of fairy tales and stories, there were skits dealing with deaf culture as well.

A local performing arts academy has also incorporated students who are deaf into its productions, forming a deaf access company that performs publicly, including performances at school functions, for school staff and students during the school day, and in evening school programs for parents and the community.

Participation of students with deafness in school productions also sends a positive message to the students who are deaf and to the school as a whole. Students with deafness in Montgomery County schools have had leading and backstage roles in several productions at both the elementary and secondary levels. Some of the schools have taken a slightly different direction and have put on all-deaf student productions. These have been presented to the entire student body with voice interpretation, and in some cases to other school programs where there are students who are deaf. These types of productions put students who are deaf in a positive spotlight for the whole school to see, and it is an inspiring sight to see the hearing student audience wave their hands in applause.

One school program currently has a music teacher who cultivated an interest in sign language, developed her skills through classes, and then made sign language an integral part of her music program (Burdette, personal communication, 1993). She formed a unique choral group, "The Fabulous Flying Fingers," made up of fifth graders who are hearing and deaf, which performs all of their numbers in song and sign. It has developed a special reputation for all students in the school. The group travels and performs around the Washington, D.C., area, and showcases the recognition and respect in the school for students with deafness and sign language.

Presence of Interpreters

Working with interpreters for students with deafness and staff is new for many school staff members, but it should be an important part of the school program. Educating the school staff that interpreter coverage needs to be arranged not only for classroom instruction but also for assemblies and programs; lunchtime; "special subjects" like art, music, and physical education; as well as visits to the school nurse or principal, is important. The high visibility of interpreters can become a good source of public relations. Having staff who are deaf in the school provides an ongoing awareness of the need for including interpreters, for they will be seen at faculty meetings and conferences. Understanding this need for interpreters, and the role they play in and out of the classroom, contributes to the climate for students with deafness in the school.

Role of Deaf Students, Teens, and Adults

Recruiting a variety of persons who are deaf in different roles in a school is very important. Role models are invaluable in developing a greater understanding about deafness,

as well as creating a positive school climate. Adults who are deaf not only provide a perspective of "what it's like to be deaf," they also show that children with deafness grow up and can aspire to the same goals as other children. This can be accomplished by hiring staff who are deaf at the school, by inviting adults with deafness from the community as guest speakers or mentors, welcoming parents who are deaf as volunteers in the classroom, or inviting teens with deafness from the secondary program to the preschool or elementary level as interns or aides.

Staff with deafness at school give the rest of the school staff an ongoing learning opportunity, while providing them with a unique view of the needs of students with deafness as well. Such staff will require interpreters (as mentioned) or note takers at staff and team meetings and can share firsthand experiences with other staff members.

Montgomery County currently runs a program, "Montgomery Exceptional Leaders (MEL)," which was developed by the Superintendent's Advisory Committee on the Rights of Disabled Individuals. This group consists of teams of high school students with disabilities who travel across the county to different elementary schools, presenting firsthand accounts of their own disabilities, and more importantly, their own abilities. These presentations give young children not only the exposure to deafness but also the opportunity to ask questions and get to know a person who is deaf as an individual.

This program also plays an important role in the development of self-image for the high school students with deafness who participate. Students with deafness get a positive sense of contributing to a better acceptance and understanding of deafness. This leads not only to the development of poise and confidence in public presentations but also to a different understanding about being a deaf person and more positive feelings about themselves as shown in Case Study 20–2.

Having people with deafness in the environment is positive for the hearing students,

Case Study 20–2 M.H. is a 22-year-old college senior and a graduate of our program. In mainstream classes from the upper elementary years through high school, he was academically successful. During his high school years, he was a member of the Montgomery Exceptional Leaders (MEL) program. Looking back at the experience, M.H. was able to see how much his involvement in this program affected the way he saw himself as an individual, and as a deaf person.

As a child, M.H. was very shy and reserved. When he got to high school and joined the MEL program, he saw he had the chance to influence how young children develop an understanding and acceptance of deaf people. In preparing for this endeavor, he had to look closely at himself, at his strengths and at his limitations.

The actual presentations gave M.H. the confidence and poise that would carry over to his mainstream classes and his interpersonal relationships, both in high school and in college. He was able to compile a definition of himself that he liked and felt comfortable with. It helped him feel good not only as a person but as a deaf person.

numbers for a student TTY directory can be collected and distributed to students who are deaf and their families, to put them in touch with other students at different schools within the county. Pen pal letters or electronic bulletin boards can supplement these opportunities. Newspapers done by students at the elementary and secondary levels can be shared among deaf students at other schools. A newspaper of this sort is particularly beneficial for the itinerant population, where a student may indeed be the only student who is deaf or hard of hearing in the school. The *Montgomery Messenger* brings stories and experiences to the hundred or so students who are deaf and hard of hearing across the county who contribute to this newspaper. The students report positive feelings of knowing there are other students out there like themselves. Teachers and parents can use these connections to develop relationships further between students, who may be in different schools but share common experiences.

Young students always look up to the older students in their school or program. Older students with deafness can fill a variety of roles for the younger ones. Within a school, pairings of older and younger students who are deaf, perhaps for a story time, can give both parties a sense of connection and belonging. Teens who are deaf and doing their community service requirement or child development practicum in the preschool or elementary program, or volunteering in the summer school program, contribute to positive feelings among the younger students. Older students are uniquely able to support and advise younger students in a mainstream setting, as those who have "been there." Sharing feelings between those who have a special bond is invaluable for helping students feel comfortable with who they are.

Communication Skill Development

The nature of deafness means unique communication needs. How these needs are met is often the center of controversy. One main

but students who are deaf need appropriate role models who are deaf. This is particularly significant for those students in a mainstream setting. While getting an academically challenging program, these students also need opportunities to connect with other individuals with deafness. In Montgomery County, the program is fortunate to be large in comparison to other public school systems. There may be more than one student in a mainstream class; if not for the full day, for at least part of the day. This allows for some creative role modeling within the program.

There are effective strategies for widening the circle of peers who are deaf. Telephone concern is how to ensure that a mainstream setting will effectively meet the communication needs of students with deafness so that isolation can be minimized as much as possible. Obviously, a mainstream program has to be creative in its approach to achieving the goal of complete communication access for students who are deaf. Working successfully with interpreters, as already mentioned, certainly plays a critical role in the communication between both populations. However, there is value in developing the communication skills of the hearing staff and students, trying to build a bridge of acceptance for all.

Instructional Classes

Achieving a level of effective communication for both staff and students is critical to any successful school climate. It is made more challenging when students with deafness are part of that environment. Offering instructional classes and opportunities for learning sign language or cued speech, perhaps as a lunchtime or after-school activity, is one way to encourage direct interaction and communication between students and staff who are deaf and hearing. Where sign language and cued speech classes or clubs are offered, students who are hearing often develop excellent communication skills, which fosters positive relationships with students who are deaf. Staff members, from teachers to secretaries to cafeteria workers, should have the opportunity to develop these skills as well.

In-School Opportunities

Developing creative in-school activities for students who are hearing to build communication skills addresses students who may not be able to participate in after-school classes. By offering specific activities during the school day, an attitude of acceptance is reinforced.

One creative and effective approach involves the music teacher previously mentioned. In this case, sign language is integrated into the students' music program from kindergarten through grade 5. This is done regardless of whether there is a student with deafness in that class. This provides a uniquely comfortable atmosphere for the students with deafness, particularly considering that music is not often thought of as a positive activity for them. For the students who hear, the result is not only a greater familiarity, but often fluency in sign language. Students who are deaf are likely to feel more included in classroom activities if those around them have some comfort level with their communication method.

To encourage communication between classmates who are deaf and hearing outside of school, a TTY loaner program has been developed. Hearing students have a training session on using a TTY and then borrow one to take home to call deaf classmates. This gives students who are deaf a chance to develop relationships with classmates outside of school and provides a social link important to the development of a strong self-image (see Case Study 20–3).

Extracurricular Activities

Extracurricular activities are of great value and must be available to all students, including the students in the school who are deaf. Transportation may be an impeding factor, but it is well worth the effort on the part of parents to try to make necessary arrangements. In extracurricular activities students are often put on a more equal plane, quite different from the competition in the academic arena. Students have the opportunity to show different sides of their personalities, skills, and talents that may not be recognized in the classroom.

Athletic activities are an example of this. A student who has physical and athletic talents becomes a sought out classmate, as the respect and admiration from the playing field carries over to the classroom. A recognized schoolwide honor, like patrols, also relates directly to a student's self-concept. This special position, like participation in student government, is one that is highly regarded throughout the school. These activities provide the student who is deaf with a chance

Case Study 20–3 B.H. is in the seventh grade in mainstream classes, but the work does not come easily to him and he has to put forth a lot of effort. "Fitting in" and having friends are important to him, as they are to any child.

When in elementary school, B.H.'s class was involved in a TTY loaner program. The communication specialist in the school implemented the TTY loaner program, which was successful in his class. Many students were anxious to participate.

The result? B.H. was able to call his classmates. He was able to initiate communication comfortably. This provided the vehicle for sharing homework assignments and sports statistics. He had the opportunity to feel special in his experience and expertise, and the TTY activity helped him to see himself more as a member of the class. In fact, the program was so successful that Brian and other members of the school's student council raised money for a TTY for the school.

Case Study 20–4 A.L. is in the fifth grade and is fully mainstreamed. She had been struggling with her identity and self-esteem as a deaf person. The factors she perceived that made her feel "different," including hearing aids and an interpreter, are magnified in a mainstream setting.

A.L.'s school has started a Deaf Awareness Club. As part of this program, a graduate of our program, a young man who is now a professional athlete, was invited to be a guest speaker for the entire student body. Everyone was excited and enthusiastic.

A.L. was positively impressed by the presentation on several accounts. She saw a popular and successful adult with deafness wearing hearing aids, using his audition and speechreading skills to the maximum, without hesitation. She saw him use an interpreter in front of this large audience without embarrassment, and she saw that all of these "differences" had not made a difference in his aspirations and achievements. For A.L., having this experience helped her look at herself in a more positive light.

to develop not only a sense of responsibility and teamwork, but also confidence and a positive self-concept.

Deaf culture clubs, deaf awareness activities, "Deaf and Hearing Power," and the Junior National Association of the Deaf (NAD) are extracurricular types of activities that can be implemented at both the elementary and secondary levels. These groups may be made up of only students who are deaf, or mixed deaf and hearing. Planned events can include guest speakers and field trips in addition to the use of videotaped materials. These activities provide ongoing opportunities for all to learn more about Deaf Culture and American Sign Language through drama, literature, and informal interactions with other people who are deaf, as shown in Case Study 20–4. Exposure and acceptance from this perspective cannot come too early.

Teacher Attitudes

Attitude can be one of the most subtle, yet one of the most critical factors in how students perceive their place and success in the classroom. Difficult to measure objectively, the presence or absence of the "right" attitude can definitely be felt by students and staff alike. Does the teacher view the student with deafness as an individual? or are all of the students with deafness lumped together, as one mass composite? Teachers and other staff have the tendency to have one particular student in mind, and then define all students with deafness that way. Or, when there is more than one student who is deaf in the mainstream class at a given grade level, those students are often so closely identified together that it is easy for their individual identities to be lost. Teacher recognition of individual characteristics, preferences, skills, and needs is important to each student. And the teacher's attitude influences the other students' attitudes as well. Students with deafness want to be valued for who they are.

How the classroom teacher uses the interpreter in the classroom also sends a message. Teachers should talk to and face the student who is deaf, and not face the interpreter or say to the interpreter, "Tell him . . . " Even if the teacher does not know sign language or cued speech (whichever the student uses), communication should still be face to face. Direct communication reflects an attitude of respect.

Consistent Expectations and Equitable Treatment

It is important that accepted school rules and behavior exist. Students who are deaf need to know that they are responsible for their own actions, and the consequences are the same for them as for other students in the school. This not only influences the deaf student's self-concept as part of the school but also how the hearing students perceive the situation: what exceptions are necessary because a student is deaf, by nature of the deafness, and what exceptions are not made, in terms of academic and social behavior.

There are, of course, accepted classroom accommodations that a student who is deaf will require. It is important for teachers to understand what these accommodations are and their importance. Teachers then need to transmit this understanding to the other students. Interpreters and note takers are but two examples of these accommodations; they are services that may be vital to the student who is deaf in the mainstream and should be used appropriately.

For example, the interpreter should not be used as a disciplinarian for the student who is deaf alone or for the class as a whole. When the interpreter disciplines the student with deafness, the student feels judged by the person who should be there to facilitate communication objectively. No one should

feel they have their own personal "watch-dog." When the interpreter is put in the position of responsibility for the whole class and disciplinary action results, the entire class resents the student who is deaf for needing to have that person in the class. The interpreter as a professional understands the role, but the teacher must understand it too, for inappropriate use of the interpreter can greatly affect the way the student with deafness perceives his or her place in that classroom.

It is equally important not to be overly accommodating. Special treatment, which at some level may seem enticing, in fact works against what deaf students are looking for in the classroom, which is acceptance and appreciation. When a student who is deaf gets undue preferential treatment it can build resentment among hearing students in the classroom. For example, students with deafness should not be exempt from staying after school as punishment because they may live a great distance from school and need to catch the bus to get home. Academic and behavioral standards should be the same for the entire class, and students who are deaf need to know that they must follow the same rules.

It is also helpful for students who are deaf to know that they are not alone in being "pulled out" of class to work with a resource teacher or other specialist. It is often a revelation for a student who is deaf to realize that hearing students may also be pulled out of class for a different kind of resource or speech support. It may be psychologically beneficial in the design of a school to have these support personnel, for both students who are deaf and those who are hearing, located in proximity to one another. These attitudes of respect and equality contribute to a student's feelings of acceptance and belonging.

Student Skills

There are strategies and activities that may be used directly through teaching techniques or indirectly through attitudes that can make a difference not only in academic performance in the classroom but also in a deaf student's self-perception in a mainstream setting. The focus here is on the instructional program, and the roles of the speech or communication specialist and the resource (or itinerant) teacher. We often see what Reich, Hambleton, and Houldin (1977) found: the more available and the better the quality of the support services, the better the self-concept of the student. Through this instructional support, the academic, social/emotional, and physical components of a student's self-image are addressed.

Speech and Communication Skills

The words and the body language (including the facial expression) that teachers choose are often a reflection of their attitude toward the student who is deaf with whom they work. This may be especially true for the person responsible for speech teaching, because how this person deals with the child who is deaf, and the messages, direct or indirect, sent to the child are delicate yet very significant. In fact, in Montgomery County, the term "communication specialist" is preferred, with a departure from "speech teacher," putting more emphasis on overall communication skill development and not only on speech.

Development of oral and auditory skills presents potentially the most difficult skill area for a child with deafness. Although not a criterion for placement in a regular education classroom (in Montgomery County), it is often the one by which a child is judged by those unfamiliar with deaf people. The balance between communicating encouragement, praise, and realistic feedback can impact on the willingness of the child to continue to develop these skills, as well as the child's self-perception. The idea of "making mistakes" or "not achieving a goal" puts the student's work in a negative light, one that may build a barrier to further work and successes. Honesty and realism are critical in this area, but they need to be put in a constructive light: you are deaf, and this may mean limits, but it does not mean you make mistakes or fail. One communication specialist puts it very simply: "'Limit' is a place to go, not a place to stop" (Flecker, personal communication, 1993).

The communication specialist may focus on reviewing current vocabulary and content with respect to pronunciation (or speech approximation), speechreading, or audition, whichever skills are appropriate for the particular student. Related to less academic activities, the communication specialist may review the rhythm, lyrics, or signs for a musical performance, or go over the Boy Scout oath or the Pledge of Allegiance. This kind of reinforcement gives the student more comfort and confidence with the material, and a sense of "owning" the terminology.

Another area of focus is the oral presentations that are required in some classes. The communication specialist works closely with the student, the teacher, and the interpreter to make this a positive and successful activity. It is also relevant to the issue of respect because the student is not "required" to use his or her voice or speech. Not all students who are deaf feel comfortable using their voice in everyday classroom situations or formal presentations. The staff works with students to learn how to use visual aids effectively, and how to use the interpreter appropriately and effectively. Of course, for students who do want to speak for themselves, the communication specialist will review the presentation and give feedback regarding the rate, rhythm, and so forth, that will help that student be more intelligible and successful in this classroom endeavor.

Students who are deaf need to realize their own areas of strength and areas of need and learn how to accommodate for themselves. The goal is to maximize all of the students' communication skills, enabling them to feel more comfortable and confident with their communication in the mainstream classroom.

Audiology

The need for and the use of amplification relate to the physical domain of self-image. Deafness itself is not a visible disability, but hearing aids and the FM auditory trainer make it visible. This is an area that becomes a more sensitive issue as the student who is deaf gets older. With advances in technology, this kind of equipment has become smaller in size, and the hearing aids and auditory trainers of today are much smaller and more "acceptable" than in years past. But that still does not make it easy for a child or adolescent to accept wearing them.

At the elementary level, having an in-service program, as mentioned previously, can be effective for educating the hearing students in the mainstream about audiological equipment, while helping the student who is deaf try to have a more positive and accepting outlook. The in-service teaching should be done with respect for and in coop-

eration with the deaf student, in the effort to recruit the student and build self-esteem in this area. Suggested resources for a student in-service program are listed in Appendix A. Reviewing the equipment is basic, but it is in the explanation of what the equipment can and cannot do that there is an opportunity for the student who is deaf to see a positive response from classmates, as occurred for T.F. in Case Study 20–5. It is one experience that can bring this equipment into a positive light for the student with deafness.

Using the analogy of the hearing aid and a radio is an effective strategy. A radio can be tuned to a station, and different volumes can make it too hard to hear (too soft) or too distorted (too loud). Then if the tuner is moved between stations, it is too fuzzy, and turning up the volume does not make it better. It can be very meaningful for a student who is deaf to see looks of frustration and confusion on the faces of his classmates, as they begin to comprehend and empathize. These are feelings that may not have been previously attributed to students who are hearing. It makes a strong connection on a very human level.

As a student who is deaf enters adolescence, "looking like everyone else" becomes much more important, which is true in the development of self-concept for all children. One thing that has had a somewhat positive effect at the upper elementary and middle school grades is the newer, "behind the ear" FM system. The less visible and noticeable the apparatus is, the more likely a student is to use it and to admit that it is beneficial. This can also be enhanced by having opportunities to meet older students and adults who are deaf and who may have similarly rejected audiological equipment as a younger student, but perhaps returned to an FM system in college. The goal is to put it in a perspective of usefulness and benefit, with students being their own advocate for optimum amplification.

Academic Skills

Just as supporting academic skills is important at home, it is even more the business of

---

Case Study 20–5 T.F. is in the second grade and has been in the mainstream for the past year. He has a difficult time accepting his auditory trainer and often refuses to wear it. To start off this school year, his communication specialist went into his classroom to explain hearing loss and the audiological equipment that the students wear. She worked with T.F. ahead of time, to let him know what she would discuss and to see if he had any questions or concerns.

Initially, T.F. was not very enthusiastic about this activity. However, as the communication specialist explained that the FM trainer is wireless and can transmit as far as the length of a football field, through walls (even when the teacher is out in the hall, or in the bathroom), T.F. was surprised to hear the other students exclaim, "That's cool!" and "Can I listen?"

T.F.'s feelings changed from embarrassment to pride. He enjoyed "showing off" his equipment and giving other students a chance to listen through his hearing aids. This activity helped him feel more accepting of his need for amplification. He was more willing to wear his equipment and even willing to admit that it helps him.

school. The resource teacher works directly with deaf students with the goal of helping them develop the skills to become stronger students in the mainstream. The stronger and more confident these students feel, the more they will perform to their potential and feel good about themselves. This may include development or refinement of the following areas that may be challenging for a student with deafness: concept and vocabulary skills, written English skills, higher-order thinking skills, organizational and study skills, communication skills, and interpersonal and social skills. These skills impact on learning in all of the content and related areas.

The focus is on building a level of comfort with the information, language, and vocabulary being presented in class. The student needs to feel confident with the work and expectations of the teacher in order to be willing to participate appropriately in class. In addition to the internal feelings of success, there will more likely be recognition from classmates of achievement and "sameness," ideally leading to more acceptance of the deaf student.

Social Opportunities

In a mainstream setting, social acceptance can be a challenge to a student with deafness. Providing a variety of social opportunities within the parameters of the school day can be valuable and should include opportunities for interaction with both hearing and deaf classmates.

Within the mainstream class, the way the teacher arranges the seating or the class groupings can impact the student with deafness. For example, sometimes students are allowed to choose their own seats, but a deaf student may not, and is instead always assigned to the same seat in the front of the room. Although the front of the room is certainly preferable for a student who is deaf, there are choices even within that parameter, and perhaps giving the student some say as to seating choice gives some control over the student's environment and social arrangements. For small group work or pairings (as

in cooperative learning strategies), not always having the students with deafness together (if there is more than one in a class) can expand the social opportunities within a very structured situation.

Resource teachers or communication specialists may even allow the student who is deaf to choose a classmate who is hearing to join an occasional session. These opportunities provide the student who is deaf a chance to work with other students, to get to know them as peers.

Conversely, it is also important for a student with deafness in a mainstream setting to have opportunities to interact with friends who are deaf, whether in the classroom, in the resource room, or during the social times of the day, such as lunch and recess. A student who is deaf expends a lot of energy and effort attending and communicating in the regular education classroom, often through an interpreter. There is an ease of communication that exists between friends who are deaf, and that time and experience allows the student to relax and recharge.

Pragmatic Skills

Students need to develop the necessary and appropriate interpersonal and social skills. These skills can be developed with assistance from either the communication specialist or the resource teacher. One program, "POWER to Communicate (Practicing Oral and Written Expression Regularly)" (Nordfiord & Amann, 1991) is an integrated curriculum developed for the regular education program in Montgomery County and has been used effectively with students with deafness. It provides a vehicle for working on effective conflict resolution strategies while developing written expressive skills, a unique blend of strengthening both the academic and the interpersonal skills. Another resource, a pragmatics checklist, developed by the county's communication specialists specifically for students who are deaf is outlined in Appendix B (Fernandez et al, 1992). This compilation is designed to take a student from preschool through high school and develop the relevant and necessary pragmatic skills at each level. Much attention was given to the skills necessary for working in a mainstream classroom, as well as those for functioning successfully in society. In conjunction with this checklist, at the secondary level, students go out into the community to practice and refine these important skills. The goal is to maximize all of the student's skills, enabling him or her to feel more comfortable and confident in the classroom and more prepared to become a positive and productive member of society with an enhanced self-image.

Summary

The self-image of a student with deafness in a mainstream setting can be positively developed and enhanced by the people and experiences in two important environments: home and school.

At home, parents can positively influence the self-image of their child with deafness by understanding and accepting deafness, by continually developing their own communication skills, and by being a partner in the school team. Parents also play a major role in helping their child develop confidence and competence by building and reinforcing language and social skills.

At school, the overall awareness and understanding by the school administration and personnel, staff, and students will greatly affect the student's self-perception. A mainstream program that values students who are deaf in the school as individuals promotes greater understanding of deafness, fosters the development of appropriate communication skills, and works to develop constructive and positive teacher attitudes. Students with deafness will develop healthy, positive self-concepts when they have confidence in their own skills and feel acceptance from others through a variety of social opportunities; through effective training in the areas of academics, communication, and pragmatics; and through meaningful interaction with a variety of individuals who are deaf.

Although there is no one answer to the complex issue of enhancing the self-image of students with deafness in a mainstream setting, the ideas presented and discussed here represent an overview of strategies that have proved effective in the Programs for Students Who Are Deaf and Hard of Hearing in Montgomery County, Maryland. The underlying message found in all of the strategies is one of understanding, acceptance, and respect; this is what any program, mainstream or residential, should embrace.

Appendix A

In-Service Materials and Resources

Ear Gear: A Student Workbook on Hearing Aids
Carole Bugosh Simko
Gallaudet University Press
Washington, DC

Wired for Sound
Carole Bugosh Simko
Gallaudet University Press
Washington, DC

Hearing Aids for You and the Zoo
Richard Stoker and Janine Gaydos
Alexander Graham Bell Association for the Deaf and Hard of Hearing
Washington, DC

What Is an Audiogram?
Venita Gragg
Gallaudet University Press
Washington, DC

Let's Learn about Deafness
Rachel Stone
Gallaudet University Pre-College Programs
Washington, DC

How They Hear
RCA Victor
Gordon Stoke Associates
Custon Records Department
Northbrook, IL

Hearing Aid Demonstration
AV Resources
Minneapolis, MN

Using Your TTY/TDD
An Educational Videotape
Telecommunications for Deaf and Sign
  Media
Burtonsville, MD

Appendix B

Pragmatics Checklist*

I. Deaf culture
  A. Define culture
  B. Compare and contrast to other cultures
  C. American Sign Language and its history
  D. Who is a member of the deaf culture
  E. Values and beliefs; experiences and customs
  F. Civil rights and political organizations
  G. Social organizations for the deaf; clubs
  H. Gallaudet University
  I. Montgomery County Public School Deaf Culture Club

II. Deaf awareness
  A. Exposure to other deaf children
  B. Have pictures of children with hearing aids
  C. Exposure to variety of older children and adults
  D. Discuss audiology, assistive devices, and interpreting; communication approaches and skills
  E. Mainstream in-service: include communication strategies and interpersonal protocols

III. Historical perspectives of deafness
  A. History of deaf in ancient civilizations
  B. History of the education of the deaf
  C. History of the education of the deaf in the United States, including communication controversies

  D. Deaf president NOW organization—1988 student protest

IV. Sound and hearing
  A. Hearing: anatomy, audiology
  B. Hearing aids: types, parts, care, potentials/limitations

V. Social/interpersonal communication
  A. Nonverbal communication: body and facial expression
  B. Listening/attending skills
  C. Spoken communication
  D. Verbal communication
  E. Conversational skills
  F. Social communication

VI. Communication devices and support services
  A. Telephone
  B. Conversational skills and etiquette
  C. Related skills: operator, information, emergencies
  D. TTY/Telecommunication Device for the Deaf (TDD) calls/assistive devices/services
  E. Assistive services, including Telecommunication Relay Service (TRS)
  F. Assistive devices: decoders, flashing lights, alarms

VII. Situational topics
  A. Safety
  B. Community helpers
  C. On the bus
  D. Health room
  E. Restaurants
  F. Medical
  G. Mainstream classes
  H. Stores/shopping
  I. Family meals
  J. Celebrations
  K. Summertime
  L. Law/police
  M. Job applications
  N. College applications
  O. Job interviewing
  P. Banking
  Q. Transportation
  R. Renting apartments/rooms
  S. Budgeting

*Adapted from Pragmatics Checklist's (Fernandez et al, 1992)

References

Berne, P. (1985). Seven secrets for building kids' self-esteem. *Instructor, 14,* 63–65.

Fernandez, J., Smith, J., Flecker, P., Broe, M., Kittleman, R., Munshower, C., Michael, M., Smith, R., & Hunt, F. (1992). *Pragmatics Checklist.* Rockville, MD: Programs for Students Who Are Deaf and Hard of Hearing.

Grimes, V., & Prickett, H.T. (1988). Developing and enhancing a positive self-concept in deaf children. *Am Ann Deaf, 133,* 255–257.

Krupp, J. (1991). Self-esteem: How do you feel about yourself? *Teaching PreK–8, 21,* 63–64.

Leigh, I. (1987). Parenting and the hearing impaired: Attachment and coping. *Volta Rev, 89,* 11–21.

Marshall, H. (1989). The development of self-concept. *Young Children, 44,* 44–51.

Maxon, A.B., & van den Berg, D.S. (1991). Self-perception of socialization: the effects of hearing staus, age, and gender. *Volta Rev, 93,* 7–18.

McGinnis, E., Goldstein, A.P., Sprafkin, R., & Gershaw, N.J. (1984). *Skillstreaming the Elementary School Child: A Guide for Teaching Prosocial Skills.* Champaign, IL: Research Press.

Meadow, K. (1969). *Deafness and Child Development.* Berkeley, CA: University Press.

Nordfiord, G., & Amann, R. (1991). *POWER to Communicate.* Rockville, MD: Montgomery County Public Schools.

Oblowitz, N., Green, L., & Heyns, I. (1991). A self-concept scale for the hearing-impaired. *Volta Rev, 93,* 19–29.

Reich, C., Hambleton, D., & Houldin, B.K. (1977). The integration of hearing-impaired children in regular classrooms. *Am Ann Deaf, 122,* 534–543.

Rich, D. (1988). *MegaSkills: How Families Can Help Children Succeed in School and Beyond.* Boston: Houghton-Mifflin.

Schwartz, S. (1990). Psycho-social aspects of mainstreaming. *Hearing-Impaired Children in the Mainstream.* Parkton, MD: York Press.

Warren, C., & Hasenstab, S. (1986). Self-concept of severely to profoundly hearing-impaired children. *Volta Rev, 88,* 289–295.

Yachnik, M. (1986). Self-esteem in adolescents. *Am Ann Deaf, 131,* 305–310.

Index

Page numbers in italics indicate that the entry on that page is in a figure or a table.